CLINICAL PRACTICE AND SURGERY OF THE COLON, RECTUM AND ANUS

CLINICAL PRACTICE AND SURGERY OF THE COLON, RECTUM AND ANUS

Sisir Kumar Saha BSc MBBS FRCS
Consultant in General Surgery
with a special interest in Colorectal Surgery
United Kingdom

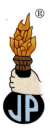

JAYPEE BROTHERS MEDICAL PUBLISHERS (P) LTD
New Delhi • St Louis • Panama City • London

Published by
Jaypee Brothers Medical Publishers (P) Ltd

Corporate Office
4838/24 Ansari Road, Daryaganj, **New Delhi** - 110002, India
Phone: +91-11-43574357, Fax: +91-11-43574314

Offices in India
- **Ahmedabad**, e-mail: ahmedabad@jaypeebrothers.com
- **Bengaluru**, e-mail: bangalore@jaypeebrothers.com
- **Chennai**, e-mail: chennai@jaypeebrothers.com
- **Delhi**, e-mail: jaypee@jaypeebrothers.com
- **Hyderabad**, e-mail: hyderabad@jaypeebrothers.com
- **Kochi**, e-mail: kochi@jaypeebrothers.com
- **Kolkata**, e-mail: kolkata@jaypeebrothers.com
- **Lucknow**, e-mail: lucknow@jaypeebrothers.com
- **Mumbai**, e-mail: mumbai@jaypeebrothers.com
- **Nagpur**, e-mail: nagpur@jaypeebrothers.com

Overseas Offices
- **North America Office, USA,** Ph: 001-636-6279734
  e-mail: jaypee@jaypeebrothers.com   anjulav@jaypeebrothers.com
- **Central America Office, Panama City, Panama,** Ph: 001-507-317-0160,
  e-mail: cservice@jphmedical.com, Website: www.jphmedical.com
- **Europe Office, UK,** Ph: +44 (0) 2031708910, e-mail: info@jpmedpub.com

Clinical Practice and Surgery of the Colon, Rectum and Anus

© 2011, Jaypee Brothers Medical Publishers

All rights reserved. No part of this publication should be reproduced, stored in a retrieval system, or transmitted in any form or by any means: electronic, mechanical, photocopying, recording, or otherwise, without the prior written permission of the author and the publisher.

This book has been published in good faith that the material provided by author is original. Every effort is made to ensure accuracy of material, but the publisher, printer and author will not be held responsible for any inadvertent error(s). In case of any dispute, all legal matters are to be settled under Delhi jurisdiction only.

First Edition: **2011**
ISBN 978-81-8448-992-7
Typeset at JPBMP typesetting unit
Printed at Ajanta Offset & Packagings Ltd., New Delhi

Dedicated to

Elder brother – Amulya
Wife – Dipika
Daughter – Mowe
Son – Shironjit
Daughter-in-law – Sue
Granddaughter – Sophie

Preface

Specialization in every modality has become a new breed in the medical practice. To be an expert, requires thorough knowledge in other fields of medicine, outside the choice of specialty. I believe one needs to be a good physician to be a good surgeon. Because of these reasons, a comprehensive training, practical experience and understanding of the disease are important. It is imperative for every surgeon to know the entire surgical physiology and surgical anatomy in dealing with a particular or multiple surgical problems developed in the same patient. It would be totally wrong to assume that one organ specialist does not need to know other fields of medicine.

Although I had gone through most of the surgical fields of training, my knowledge and experience will be focused on the particular specialty, where I have developed a particular interest and where I can provide a better care to my patients.

During my residency, I recognized the deficiency in understanding the basic principle in the management of diseases. And at times, I needed to ask my senior or to consult other books in order to understand the particular issue. With that experience in my mind, this book has been comprehensively compiled with all aspects of surgical anatomy, surgical physiology, and dealing with all sorts of clinical and operative skills in the field of colorectal surgery.

In ageing populations, carcinoma of the colon and rectum seems to be a major concern to the families and to the medical profession, in particular when the surgical science has been changing faster than one can grasp it. To meet this challenge, this new book has been written, covering all aspects of new revelations and ideas with a particular interest in colorectal surgery.

In this book, I have described the symptoms, clinical examination, investigations and merits of different treatments reported in the literature. I have highlighted the recent trend in surgical treatment for the rectal carcinoma. I hope this book will assist the trainee surgeons to understand the difference between the two schools of thought, difference between two surgical approaches and technical benefits between the conventional and new operative procedures for the same surgical pathology.

I have highlighted the conflicting surgical anatomy between the textbook of clinical surgery and the textbook of anatomy. At the same time, I have focused the consistency between two arguments along with my own views, based upon my own anatomical dissection, clinical and operative experience.

Although one can learn a skill and gain a practical experience by working in the field of colorectal surgery, it is not possible for everyone to be fully aware of the recent changes, published in the literature. It has been well established that colonoscopy provides additional diagnostic evidences, but it is not without problems. To improve the clinical management, colonography has been a new diagnostic tool in clinical medicine. Its clinical importance and its pitfalls have been highlighted in this book. Apart from these technologies, many radiological evidences, such as modern role of CT scan, MRI scan and PET scan have been compiled in this book. This would provide immense clinical value in the management of diseases. This book will provide the necessary diet to meet individual quest without searching for further information in other literature.

Since 1973, I had started working in the specialty of colorectal surgery and developed interest in both surgical techniques and improving the postoperative stay in the hospital. I am pleased to highlight that I am pioneer of many new innovative surgical techniques. Among many of my original contributions reported to the surgical and medical literature, primary perineal wound healing that provides a great comfort to the patients after total excision of the rectum, is a great achievement. During my prospective study, I have noticed a great deal of difference in the management of the carcinoma of the rectum, wound infection, postoperative pain relief and fecal peritonitis. With the background of my research and practical experiences, this book has been written entirely by me. I hope this book would provide valuable facts to the surgical students, in particular to those who intend to practice in colorectal surgery and to those who have been working in this specialty.

Since colonoscopic tools are widely available, radiological investigations are less frequently used in the investigation of the colonic diseases. As a result, academic input to the postgraduate students has become a problem in the absence of true radiological features of certain colonic diseases such as ischemic colitis, ulcerative colitis and Crohn's colitis or familial polyposis coli. I have, therefore, retrieved a few rare radiological images from other literatures for the benefit of the postgraduate students. And I would like to express my appreciation and gratitude to Dr AK Dutta Munshi, Dr Cornah and Dr S Sinha for providing me several radiological illustrations from their collections. I am grateful to Prof Subir Kumar Chatterjee, Professor of Anatomy, for assisting me in the dissection of the rectum in his department, NRS Medical College and Hospital.

Sisir Kumar Saha

Other Publications

- Foundation in Operative Surgery 2009.
- A list of my innovative contributions in the leading journals since 1976.
- Carcinoma of the rectum.
  1. A Study of Perineal Wound Healing after Abdominoperineal Resection. *British Journal of Surgery* 1976;555-58.
  2. Synopsis on the Primary Closure of the Perineal Wound after Abdominoperineal Resection of the Rectum and Primary Wound Healing. *Review of Surgery* USA 1977;345.
  3. Care of Perineal Wound in Abdominoperineal Resection. *Journal of the Royal College of Surgeons* Edinburgh 1983;324-27.
  4. A Critical Evaluation of Dissection of the Perineum in Synchronous Combined Abdominoperineal Excision of the Rectum. *Surgery, Gynecology and Obstetrics Journal*, 1984 (It is now known as American College of Surgeons Journal) USA; 33-38.
  5. Primary Suture of the Perineal Wound using Constant and Irrigation, following Rectal Excision for Inflammatory Bowel Disease: A Letter to the Editor. *Annals of the Royal College of Surgeons of England* 1985;268.
  6. Merits of perineal dissection of AP Resection of the Rectum for Rectal Carcinoma, *Synopsis at the Amscon*, (Ima-Kolkata) March 2003.
- A New Operative Technique for Undescended Testis.
  7. Cordopexy: A New Approach to Undescended Testis. *British Journal of Urology* 1978;39-42.
  8. Cordopexy: A New Approach to the Treatment of Undescended Testis. *Journal of the Royal College of Surgeons of Edinburgh* 1984;105-106.
  9. Cordopexy: A New Approach to the Undescended testis; A Review of 2-5 Year Follow-up. *The Journal of Urology* USA, 1983;561-64.
  10. Cordopexy: A New Approach to the Treatment of Undescended Testis. A Letter to the Editor. *The Journal of the Royal College of Surgeons, Edinburgh* 1985;139.
  11. Orchidopexy: Planned 2 Stage Technique; A Letter to the Editor. *Journal of Urology,* USA 1986;479.
  12. Cordopexy: A new Operative technique for undescended testis, synopsis published in a book by the *Royal College of Surgeons of Edinburgh* 1988.
- New Operative Technique for Enlarged Prostate Gland.
  13. Transcervical Prostatectomy Urology—*Journal*, USA 1980;481-84.
  14. Saha Bladder Neck Spreader: A New Surgical Instrument. *Urology Journal,* USA 1985;180.
  15. The Evaluation of Transcervical Prostatectomy, Journal of International Urology and Nephrology, 1985; 61-69.
  16. Synopsis of the Evaluation of Transcervical Prostatectomy. *Urology Digest,* USA 1986;13-14.
  17. Bladder Irrigation with Chlorhexidine for the Prevention of Urinary Infection after Transurethral Operation: A Prospective controlled study. *A letter to the Editor Journal of Urology*, USA 1989;142:829-30.
  18. Transcervical Prostatectomy in Perspective. *Scandinavian Journal of Urology and Nephrology,* 1992;339-43.
  19. How Complete is Transurethral Resection of the Prostate? *A letter to the Editor British Journal of Urology* 1996;662.
  20. Transcervical Prostatectomy: A new Rational Technique. *Published in the Bulletin RG Kar Medical College* 1996; 4-5.
  21. Surgical Efficiency and Cost in Transurethral Resection of the Prostate Versus Transcervical Prostatectomy: A Perspective View. *Published in Surgical Efficiency and Economy, Proceedings of the third World Conference, University of Kiel, Thieme Medical Publishers Inc.* 1997;178.
  22. Quality and Cost between Transcervical and Transurethral prostatectomy, Synopsis: A Key Advances in Clinical Management Benign Prostatic Disease. *Royal Society of Medicine* 2000;30 Nov.
  23. Quality and Cost between Transcervical and transurethral Prostatectomy. *International Urology and Nephrology* 2002;34:515-18.

- Research on the Carcinoma of the Stomach and Peptic Ulcer Disease, Gallbladder and Pancreas.
  24. A Cyst in the Stomach. *Journal of the Royal College of Surgeons of Edinburgh* 1980;125-28.
  25. Smoking Habits in Carcinoma of the Stomach: A Prospective Study. *Journal of Clinical Gastroenterology*, USA 1990; 475-78.
  26. Smoking Habits in Carcinoma of the Stomach: A Case Control Study. *Japanese Journal of Cancer Research* 1990;82:497-502.
  27. Concept of Mucosal Plug in the Etiology of Duodenal Ulcer: A Prospective study in Perspective. *Indian Journal of Gastroenterology*, 2002;39-40.
  28. Mucosal Plug in the Etiology of Peptic Ulcer. *Disease, Digestive Diseases and Sciences*, USA, http://dx.doi. org/10.1007/s10620-006-9659-2 (Published on 31/3/07 Online first) and in the hard copy of the Journal in August 2007.
  29. Clinical Significance of Pyloric Aperture in the Etiology of Peptic Ulcer Disease: A Prospective Study. *Jl of Indian Medical Association*, 2009;107 (4):226.
  30. Calcium Disturbances in Acute Pancreatitis. *British Journal of Clinical Practice*, 1982;146-51.
  31. Ligating the Cystic Duct in Laparoscopic Cholecystectomy. *The American Journal of Surgery* 2000;179:494-96.
- A List of Other Specialties
  32. Bradycardia in Acute Mesenteric Vascular Occlusion. *British Journal of Clinical Practice*, 1978;227-28.
  33. Retroperitoneal Liposarcoma. *British Journal of Urology*, 1977;92.
  34. Continuous Intravenous Infusion of Papaveretum for relief of postoperative pain. *Postgraduate Medical Journal*, 1981;686-89.
  35. Peritoneal Lavage with Metronidazole. *Surgery, Gynecology and Obstetrics Journal*, USA, 1985;335-38.
  36. Efficacy of Metronidazole Lavage in the treatment of Intraperitoneal Sepsis: A Prospective Study. *Digestive Diseases and Sciences*, 1996;1313-18.
  37. A New Concept and New Treatment for the Relief of Postoperative Pain. *Amscon*, (IMA-Kolkata) March 2003.
  38. Hernioplasty: A new approach against the recurrences. *Journal Hernia*, 2005;134-39.
- Lecture Delivered on the Following Subjects
  1. Royal College of Surgeons of Edinburgh, 1988 on Cordopexy
  2. Royal College of Surgeons of England with collaboration of Association of surgeons of India, New Delhi, 1991
  3. The Royal Society of Medicine of London, the Quality and Cost Between Transcervical Prostatectomy and *TURP*, 2000 and many other learned societies on many subjects:

My works have been cited in many TextBooks:
1. My name appeared in the Textbook of Operative Surgery, by FARQUHARSON, for Carcinoma of the rectum, 1978.
2. Member of the Commission set up by the Royal College of Surgeons of England and Royal College of Anaesthesia, for the management of the postoperative pain, published in 1990.
3. In the Textbook of Anesthesia, by Prof. Nimmo and Prof. Smith, my study on the treatment of postoperative pain has been described.
4. In the Textbook of Pediatric Urology, 1996, by Prof. O'Donnell and Dr. Koff, my technique on Cordopexy for undescended testis has been described in the book.

Contents

1. **Applied Anatomy of the Colon and the Rectum and Disease of the Colon 1**
   - A Brief Description of Surgical Anatomy and Physiology of the Colon and the Rectum   1
   - The Rectum and Anus   1
   - Function of the Colon   3
   - Applied Anatomy and Physiology in the Mechanism for defecation   4
   - Diseases of the Colon   6
   - Pathological Lesions of the Colon   6
   - Clinical Importance of Benign Colonic Lesions   6
   - Characteristic Features of a Polyp   6
   - Epidemiological and Pathological Features   7
   - Broad Outline of Treatment   7
   - Polypectomy through the Colonoscope   7
   - Complications of the Procedure   8
   - Clinical Features and Treatment of Villous Papilloma   8
   - Criteria for Considering Malignancy in the Benign Adenoma or Villous Papilloma   9
   - Difference between the Adenoma and Villous Papilloma   10
   - Familial Polyposis   10
   - Clinical Presentation   10
   - Choices of Treatment Modalities   10
   - Difference Between Adenoma, Peutz-Jeghers Syndrome and Familial Polyposis   10
   - Other Benign Polyp in the Colon, Rectum and Anus   11
   - Papilloma of the Anus   11

2. **Malignant Tumors of the Colon and Spread of the Colonic Tumor 13**
   - Malignant Tumors of the Colon, Rectum and Anus   13
   - Description of the Macroscopical Features of the Malignant Tumors   13
   - Macroscopical Appearance of the Tumors   13
   - Macroscopical Changes in the Colon, Presented with Malignant Tumor   14
   - Pathological Changes in the Gut Wall   14
   - Sites for the Colonic Carcinoma   15
   - Spread of the Colonic and Rectal Carcinoma   15
   - Prognostic Factors of the Colorectal Carcinoma   19
   - Dukes Stage of the Colorectal Tumor   19
   - Histological Staging   19

3. **Presentation of Symptoms 21**
   - Striking Symptoms of Colonic Carcinoma   21
   - Loss of Appetite, Loss of Body Weight and not Feeling Well   22
   - Symptoms of Abdominal Pain   22
   - Burping and Funny Noise in the Abdomen   23
   - Discharge of slime, Mucus and Blood per Rectum   23
   - Symptoms Associated with the Growth in the Right Side of the Colon   23
   - Symptoms Associated with the Growth in the Left Side of the Colon   23
   - Symptoms Associated with the Growth in the Distal Part of the Sigmoid Colon, the Rectum or Anal Canal   24
   - Malignant Growth in the Anal Canal   24

4. **Clinical Examination 25**
   - Clinical Examination and Investigations   25
   - Examination of the Abdomen   26
   - Techniques for Palpation   26
   - Superficial Palpation   26
   - Deep Palpation   27
   - Technique for Percussion   28
   - Technique for the test of Fluid Thrill   29
   - Rectal Digital Examination, Proctoscopy and Rigid Sigmoidoscopy   29
   - Important Features of the Rectal Carcinoma, recorded on Rectal Digital Palpation   31
   - Features of Advanced and Poor Prognosis   31
   - Method of Instrumentations through the Anal Canal and the Rectum   31
   - Method of Proctoscopy   33
   - Technique for Sigmoidoscopy   34
   - Position of the Patient   34
   - Sigmoidoscopy   34
   - Indication for Sigmoidoscopy   35

5. Investigations 37

- Radiological Investigations 38
- Important Radiological Features of Abdomen 40
- Specific Line of Radiological Investigations 41
- Clinical Significance of Barium Enema Study 41
- Principle of Bowel Preparations 42
- Advice to the Patient on Diets and Oral Fluid 42
- Complications with Bowel Preparation 42
- Contraindication of Oral Purgatives 42
- A Brief Review of Barium Enema Study 42
- Important Radiological Features of the Carcinoma of the Colon and the Rectum 43
- Radiological Features of Nonmalignant Disease 43
- Method of Small Bowel Enema 46
- Intravenous Pyelogram 47
- For Intravenous Pyelogram (IVP) 47
- Clinical Value of Colonography 48
- Normal Mucosal Features of the Sigmoid Colon 49
- PET Scan 51
- Colonoscopy 53

6. Preoperative Preparation 67

- For Elective Surgery 67
- Policy for Parenteral Fluid Infusion 67
- Crystalloids used in Hypovolemic Shock 68
- Sites of Parenteral Infusion 68
- Total Body Fluid and Management of Fluid Therapy 68
- How much Fluid is necessary for a Normal Healthy Person? 68
- Daily Fluid Requirement 69
- How to Evaluate the Daily Requirement for Electrolyte? 69
- Treatment of Hypokalemia 70
- Treatment of Hyperkalemia 71
- How to Deal with Daily Fluid Balance? 71
- How to Work Out the Rate of Infusion to be given per hour? 71
- How to Set up the Central Venous Pressure (CVP)? 72
- How to Decide how much Fluid is to be given per day? 72
- Interpretation of Unusual and Conflicting Results of Serum Electrolytes 72
- Serum Creatinine (Normal Value 75–150 mmol/l) 72
- Evidences of Dehydration 72
- Evidences of Rehydration 73
- Evidences of Overhydration 73
- A Broad Guideline for Blood Transfusion 73
- Indication and Preparation for Blood Transfusion 73
- Adverse Effects of Blood Stored in the Bag 74
- Instruction to the Nurses 74

7. A Broad Outline for the Surgical Treatment 75

- Principle of Operative Preparations 75
- Technique for holding the Knife 76
- Basic Principle and Technique for the Wound Closure 76
- Precaution in Suturing the Skin Wound 78
- Closure of Burst Abdomen 79
- Operative Technique for the Closure of the Burst Abdomen 79
- Postoperative Care 80
- Broad outline for Suture Materials 80
- Principle of Anastomosis 81
- Stapling Gun 82
- Anastomotic Clamps 82

8. Principle and Policy for Postoperative Care 83

- Metabolic Response to Stress and Shock 83
- Postoperative Stress to Injury 83
- Policy for Postoperative Parenteral Infusion 84
- Surgical physiology of the Gut 84
- Physiological changes of the postoperative Gut 84
- Clinical Application of Nasogastric Tube (Ryle's Tube) 85
- Physiological Value for Gastric Aspiration 86
- Policy for Oral Feeding to Postoperative Patients 86
- Policy for Antibiotic Therapy 87
- Certain Pharmacological Restrictions 87
- Indications for Antibiotic Therapy 88
- A New Therapeutic Approach to Primary Wound Healing 89
- Indications for stopping the Antibiotic Therapy 90
- Clinical Value of Maintaining the Temperature Chart 90
- Postoperative Pain Relief 92
- Complications of Postoperative Pain Relief 93
- Treatment for Postoperative Complications 93

- Postoperative Chest Complications 94
- Management of Wound Drain 95
- Daily Wound Discharge 95
- Closed Drainage System 96
- Merits and Morbidity 96
- Management of Constipation 96
- Etiology for Constipation 96
- Clinical Responsibility of the Doctors 96
- Management of Deep Vein Thrombosis 97
- Treatment for Deep Vein Thrombosis 98

9. The Colon 99

- Techniques for Anastomosis 99
- Types of Anastomosis 100
- Technique for End-to-end Anastomosis (Single Layer) 100
- Technique for End-to-end Anastomosis in Two Layers 101
- Indication for Side-to-side Anastomosis 101
- Technique for Side-to-side Anastomosis 101
- Alternative to Side-to-side Anastomosis 102
- Right Hemicolectomy 102
- Preoperative Preparation 103
- Operative Procedure 104
- Proceeding with the Same Operative Technique for the Right Hemicolectomy 105
- Technique for the Resection of the Growth 105
- Dealing with the Problems 107
- Resection of the Transverse Colon 107
- Operative Procedure 108
- Resection of the Tumor in the Splenic Flexure 109
- Left Hemicolectomy 109
- Preoperative Preparation 110
- Operative Procedure for Left Hemicolectomy 110
- How to Resolve the Problems 111
- Resection of the Sigmoid Colon 112
- Etiology of Anastomotic Leakage 114

10. The Rectum 115

- Preview of the Operative Techniques 115
- Criteria for the Anterior Resection 116
- Preoperative Assessment and Consultation 117
- Technique for the Anterior Resection 117
- Anastomosis by Autosuture 119
- Dealing with the Problems 120
- Technique for the Hartmann's Procedure 120
- Preoperative Consultation for the Terminal Colostomy 121
- Operative Procedure for the Construction of Colostomy 121
- Postoperative Care and Complications 122
- Construction of the Transverse Loop Colostomy 122
- Construction of the Pelvic Loop Colostomy 124
- Telescopic Pelvic Loop or Terminal Colostomy 125
- Construction of Telescopic Colostomy 125
- Complication of the Pelvic Loop Colostomy 125
- Complication of the Telescopic Colostomy 125
- Sphincter-saving Low Anterior Resection of the Rectum 126
- Preoperative Adjuvant Treatment 126
- Preoperative Preparation 127
- Preoperative Consultation 128
- Technique for the Sphincter-Saving Low Anterior Resection 128
- Anastomosis by Stapling Gun 128
- Alternative Approach to Deal with the Resection 129
- Construction of Loop Ileostomy 131
- Construction of Terminal Ileostomy 132
- Postoperative Care for the Low Anterior Resection and the Ileostomy 133
- Postoperative Complication 134
- Postoperative Care and Morbidity with Ileostomy 134
- Clinical presentation of Anastomotic Leakage and Management 135
- Etiology of Anastomotic Leakage 135
- Anal Sphincteric Dysfunction 137
- Review of Local Recurrence 138
- A Summary of the Potential Risk Factors for the Local Recurrence of the Tumor 138
- What is the Safe Level of Resection? 140

11. Abdominoperineal Resection of the Rectum 142

- Preoperative Consultation 143
- Preoperative Preparation for the APR 144
- Technique for Abdominoperineal Resection (APR) of the Rectum 144
- A Preliminary Rectal Digital Examination 145
- Skin Preparation 145
- Procedure for the Synchronous Combined APR 145

- Methods of Perineal Dissection of the Rectum 147
- The landmark for the Perineal Incisions 147
- SAHA Retrograde Dissection of the Rectum 148
- Postoperative Care 152
- Care of Urethral Catheter 152
- Care of Colostomy 152
- Care of Perineal Wound 153
- Merits of Different Techniques used for the Perineal Dissection of the Rectum 153
- Postoperative Bladder Dysfunction and Management 154
- A study of Postoperative Sexual Function among the men 156
- Merits of the Perineal Wound Closure 156
- Review of the Primary Perineal Wound Healing 156
- Continuous Perineal Wound Irrigation 157
- Merits of the Pelvic floor Reconstruction 157
- Merits between the Sphincter-saving Low Anterior resection and Abdominoperineal Resection of the Rectum for the Rectal Carcinoma 157
- Criteria for Curative and Palliative Resection 158
- Merits of Abdominoperineal Resection 159
- Evaluation of Survival Rate after Abdominoperineal Resection of the Rectum 159
- Merits of Abdominoperineal Resection 161
- Factors Affecting the Survival Rate after the Resection of the Rectal Carcinoma 162

12. Prolapse of the Rectum 164

- Partial Prolapse 164
- Epidemiology of the Prolapse Rectum 164
- Etiology 164
- Symptoms 164
- Examination 164
- Treatment 165
- Surgical Treatment for the Complete Prolapse 165
- Operative Technique for Thiersch Operation 166
- Preoperative Preparation 166
- Operative Technique 166
- Postoperative Care 167
- Complications 167
- Delorme Operation 167
- Postoperative Care 168
- Operative Technique for Devadhar Operation 168
- Operative Technique for Abdominal Rectopexy 168
- Operative Technique for Well's Operation 169

13. Emergency Admissions 170

- Clinical Presentations in Emergency Admissions 170
- A Broad Outline of Management for Acute Surgical Patients 170
- Care of Septic Abdomen 171
- A Prospective Study of Septic Abdomen 173
- Emergency Operative Procedure 173
- Outcome of the Operative Treatment 173
- Postoperative Morbidity and Mortality 174
- Surgical Physiology in Emergency Surgery 175
- Epidemiological Study of the Colonic Obstruction 178
- Presentation of Acute Colonic Obstruction 179
- Palpation of the Abdomen 180
- Plain X-ray of Chest and Abdomen 180
- Interpretation of the Radiological Investigations 180
- Plain X-ray of the Abdomen 181
- Interpretation of the Colonic Gas in the Plain X-ray 181
- Preoperative Assessment and Treatment for Dehydration and Correction of Electrolyte Imbalance 182
- Procedure for Emergency Laparotomy 183

14. Ulcerative Colitis 185

- Pathogenesis of Ulcerative Colitis 185
- Epidemiological Study 187
- Pathological Features of the Colon 187
- Power of Healing 188
- Clinical Presentation 188
- Chronic Ulcerative Colitis 189
- Proctoscopy 189
- Sigmoidoscopy 189
- Hematological Investigations 190
- Plain X-ray 190
- Colonoscopy 190
- Management of Ulcerative Colitis 190
- Complications with Drug Therapy 191
- Complications with Long-standing Ulcerative Colitis 191
- Surgical Intervention 192
- Preoperative Preparation for the Elective Surgery 192
- Types of the Operative Procedure 192
- Management of Acute Dilation of the Colon 192

- Appropriate Time for Emergency Laparotomy   193
- Choice of Operative Procedure for Emergency Operation for the Toxic Dilatation of the Colon   194

15. Management of Ulcerative Colitis 198

- Operative Treatment for Ulcerative Colitis   198
- Preoperative Treatment   199
- Preoperative Consultation and Preparation   199
- Operative Procedure for Total Panproctocolectomy   199
- Postoperative Care   200
- Operative Procedures for Subtotal Colectomy and Ileostomy   200
- Operative Procedure   200
- Postoperative Care   201
- Fluid Balance and Correction of Fluid and Electrolytes Deficit   201
- Description of Specific Complications   202
- Delayed Complication of Ileostomy   202
- Problems of Prolapse of the Ileostomy   202
- Various Methods of Correction   203
- Amputation of the Ileostomy Spout   203
- Refashioning of the Terminal Ileostomy   203
- Dysfunction of Ileostomy   204
- Management of the Obstruction   204
- Technique for Surgical Correction of Stenosis of the Stoma   204
- Operative Treatment for Parastomal Hernia   204
- Long-term Follow-Up   206
- Indications for Surgery   206
- Ischemic Colitis   206
- Amebic Colitis   207
- Proctitis   207

16. Diverticula of the Colon 209

- Surgical Anatomy and Physiology   209
- Pathogenesis of the Diverticulosis   210
- Pathology   210
- Description of the Clinical Presentation   211
- Problems with the Diverticulosis   212
- Management of Diverticulosis   213
- Elective Operative Treatment   214
- Preoperative Assessment of the Patient   214
- Resection of the Stricture   215

- Surgical Treatment for Internal Fistula   216
- Colovesical Fistula   216
- Ileocolic Fistula   216
- Management for Emergency Admission   217
- Colonic Hemorrhage   218
- Management for the Perforated Diverticulitis   218
- Care of Septic Abdomen and Perforated Diverticulitis   218
- Angiodysplasia   220
- Pathology   221
- Pharmacological Action of the Drug   221
- A New Therapeutic Approach   221
- Results   222
- Background of the Disease   222

17. The Vermiform Appendix 225

- Surgical Anatomy and Clinical Pathology   225
- Diseases of the Appendix   225
- Epidemiology of the Appendicitis   226
- Etiology   226
- Obstructive Appendicitis   226
- Pathological Changes   226
- Composition of Fecolith   226
- Appendicitis due to Parasites   226
- Nonobstructive Appendicitis   227
- Symptoms of Acute Appendicitis   227
- General Inspection and Examination   228
- Abdominal Examination   229
- Surgical Physiology of Pain and Vomiting in Acute Appendicitis   230
- Clinical Features Associated with Unusual Type of Appendicitis   231
- Differential Diagnosis with Other Abdominal Condition   232
- Important Differential Diagnostic Features   232
- Right Renal and Ureteric Stone   233
- Clinical Features of Pyelonephritis   233
- Crohn's Ileitis   233
- Bilateral Acute Salpingitis   233
- Twisted Ovarian Mass   233
- Rupture of the Right Corpus Luteal Cyst   234
- Ruptured Ectopic Pregnancy   234
- Nonspecific Acute Mesenteric Adenitis   234
- Tuberculosis of the Mesenteric Lymph Nodes   234

- Pathology of the Appendicular Mass or Abscess 235
- Composition of the Appendicular Mass 235
- Surgical Procedure for Acute Appendicitis 235
- The Criteria for Deferring the Operation 236
- Evidences of Responding to Conservative Treatment 236
- Initial Therapeutic Measure 236
- Preoperative Preparation 236
- Technique for Appendicectomy 236
- Dealing with the Problems 238
- Postoperative Care 239
- Postoperative Complications 239
- Tumors of the Appendix 239
- Pathology 239
- Biochemical Effect of the Tumor 239

18. Reversal of Transverse Loop Colostomy 241

- Preoperative Assessment 241
- Technique for Intraperitoneal Closure 241
- Technique for Extraperitoneal Closure 243
- Postoperative Care 243
- Postoperative Complications 243
- Reversal of the Hartmann's Procedure 243
- Postoperative Care and Complications 244

19. The Anus 245

- Hemorrhoids 245
- Etiology 245
- Pathology 245
- Indication for Hemorrhoidectomy 247
- Treatment of Piles with Injection of Phenol in Oil 247
- Treatment of Piles with Rubber Band Ligation 247
- Operative Treatment for Larger Piles 247
- Technique for Hemorrhoidectomy 247
- Postoperative Care 248
- Postoperative Complications 248
- Treatment for Thrombosed Piles 250
- Expected Outcome of the Acute Thrombosed Piles 250
- Strangulated Prolapsed Piles 250

20. Anorectal Abscess 251

- Perianal Abscess 254
- Operative Procedure for Drainage of Abscess 255
- Perianal Fistula 257
- High Anal Fistula 258

21 Fissure-in-Ano 262

- Pathology 262
- The Anatomy of the Anal Canal 264
- Background of the Etiology of Anal Fissure 267
- Pathogenesis of Anal Fissure 268
- Preoperative Preparation 271
- Pruritus Ani 271
- Malignant Tumors of the Anus 272
- Treatment of the Carcinoma of the Anus 273

22. Volvulus of the Colon and Intussusception of the Intestine 278

- Volvulus of the Colon 278
- Volvulus of the Sigmoid Colon 279
- Operative Procedure 280
- Intussusception of the Intestine 281

23. A Bird's Eye View of the Surgical Practice 284

- Potential risk of Problems at Induction 284
- Problems developed in the Operating Room 284
- Problems in the Recovery Room 285
- Problems in the Recovery Ward 286
- Postoperative Chest Problems 286
- Distention of the Abdomen 287
- Attention to the acute abdomen 288
- Wound Hematoma and Infection 288
- Deep Vein Thrombosis and Pulmonary Embolism 288
- Pulmonary Embolism 289
- Other Chronic Debility Conditions 289
- Delayed Complications 289

Index 291

1

Applied Anatomy of the Colon and the Rectum and Disease of the Colon

A BRIEF DESCRIPTION OF SURGICAL ANATOMY AND PHYSIOLOGY OF THE COLON AND THE RECTUM

■ Anatomical Review of the Colon and its Surgical Importance

The large intestine begins from the cecum and ends at the anal orifice (Fig. 1.1).

The medial wall of the cecum is connected to the terminal ileum and its bottom to the appendix. The large intestine has three distinct anatomical names. They are known as colon, rectum and anus. Unlike the small intestine, the longitudinal fibers that appear to be like a thin ribbon are present on the external wall of the colon and are located at three sites of its circumference. They are known as taeniae coli. They begin from the base of the appendix and are shorter in length than the true length of the colon, thus forming sacculations or outpouching between the taeniae coli. Apart from the taeniae coli, the colonic wall is constructed by the circular smooth muscles that keep protruding outwards between the taeniae coli.

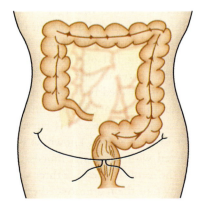

Fig. 1.1: The anatomical features of the large intestine

Its significance is to make a large mucosal surface area of the colonic wall that would provide a greater absorbing power of fluid that is discharged through the ileocecal valve.

As a result, the loose motion tends to be semisolid, as they are pushed further down the colon and these feces are held in these sacculations a bit longer in contact with the colonic mucosa. The main purpose is to delay in transit, thus enhancing the absorption of water from the feces.

The taeniae coli are absent in the appendix, rectum and anus, but the longitudinal fibers cover all around the circumference of the appendix, rectum and anus. Its physiological function will be touched in brief in the respective section.

The ileocecal junction has a valve that regulates the discharge of the liquid motion from the terminal ileum to the cecum. It remains closed as a rule that allows the small intestine to absorb the bile salts, vitamins, and all other nutritional materials. The ileocecal valve opens up briefly at the force of the peristaltic waves— thus permitting the liquid materials from the terminal ileum into the lumen of the cecum. Both ascending and descending colon remains in the retroperitoneal space, but the transverse and sigmoid colon has a mesentery. They are mobile.

The physiological importance of the sigmoid colon is to accommodate the excess lumps of feces that could not be pushed down through the rectum. Because of this reason, the sigmoid colon and its mesentery get elongated along its long axis as well as circumferentially. In certain cases, the sigmoid colon along with its long mesentery becomes folded, forming various shapes of loops in the lower abdomen.

THE RECTUM AND ANUS

The meaning of the word 'Rectus' in Latin is straight. This means the rectus abdominis muscle is consistent with the above meaning, but the true meaning of the rectum is not clear in

Latin. This could be interpreted in the same way that it is also a straight tube, constructed with circular and longitudinal muscles. The rectum is the continuation of the sigmoid colon and it begins anatomically at the level of third sacrum. It is around 15 cm in length.

Unlike the sigmoid colon, it has no mesocolon, nor does it have appendices epiploicae, but three taeniae coli merge together in order to invest around the outer wall of the rectum. The longitudinal muscle fibers are inserted into four main sites. One set of the fibers is attached to the dentate line below the internal anal sphincter, another set that passes down between the internal and external sphincters descends further to be inserted into three directions; some of the fibers pass through the space between the superficial external sphincter and subcutaneous external anal sphincters, and other fibers pass over the subcutaneous external anal sphincter to be attached to the skin and a few strands pass down vertically to be attached directly to the skin of the anal verge.

The purpose of the longitudinal muscles of the rectum is to provide continuous support to the circular muscle uniformly all around and to sustain the intra-luminal pressure uniformly all around the rectal wall, when needed for discharging flatus or feces through the anus. These fibers play a major role in the operation of opening of the anal orifice during defecation.

However, the entire rectum remains in the retroperitoneal space and lies loosely attached to the fascia of Waldeyer by the areolar tissue. In the resection of the rectum, mobilization from this fascia becomes easier, and the posterior wall of the rectum comes off from the fascia of Waldeyer by just blind finger mobilization. The middle rectal artery that lies behind the rectum may cause some degree of bleeding, but the surgeon needs not to be alarmed, if there appears to be bleeding from the torn vessels. A detailed account about the resection of the rectum is available in the section of the rectal surgery.

The upper one-third of the rectum is covered by the peritoneum anteriorly and laterally but the middle-third is covered by the peritoneum only anteriorly. The lower-third of the rectum is devoid of peritoneal covering. The infraperitoneal part of the rectum, known as ampulla, which can distend all around rests upon the pelvic floor, formed by the levator ani muscle and the anococcygeal raphe. This could be the reason as to why the sacrum has been gradually tapered down towards the bottom thus making a large space available outside the rigid bony wall for the distention of the ampulla.

The pelvic peritoneum that covers the anterior wall of the middle-third of the rectum is reflected anteriorly to cover the back and dome of the bladder, forming rectovesical pouch in male and to cover the back of the upper vagina and uterus, forming rectouterine pouch, known as pouch of Douglas in female subject.

In some literature, contrary to the textbook of anatomy and surgery, mesorectum has been referred in the operation of sphincter-saving low anterior resection. But this literature has not produced any cadaveric specimen of the mesorectum to support the description.[1] There is no conclusive evidence in the Human Anatomy to suggest that the rectum has mesorectum like mesocolon. Such evidence has been recorded over 100 years in the Gray's Anatomy[2] and all other textbooks of anatomy.[3] Here is the conclusive evidence in the whole specimen of the rectum, removed during the operation of abdominoperineal resection of the rectum which has no mesorectum (Fig. 1.2).[4]

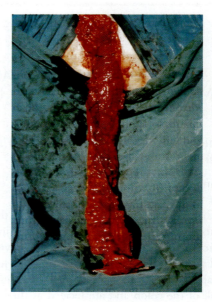

Fig. 1.2: Operative specimen of the rectum with no evidence of mesorectum

However, both upper and the lower end of the rectum lie in the same midline despite the fact that it is resting on the sacral curvature. In sagittal plane, the rectum has two curvatures, the proximal one is directed towards the left, and the lower one directed towards the right. In coronal plane, the rectum has three curvatures, but the proximal convexity is directed towards the left, the middle one to the right and the lower one towards the left of the midsacral line before it passes through the center of the pelvic floor.

These curvatures are formed because of disparity between the length of the sacrum and that of the rectum which is greater than that of the sacral curvature. This curvature has been designed in order to form valves, known as Houston valve. It is not constructed with the rectal mucosa; but with the circular muscle of the rectum. There are three valves altogether in the rectal wall; two of them are situated on the left lateral wall and the third one on the right side of the rectum (Fig. 1.3).

Nevertheless, the physiological role of the rectum being placed under the peritoneum is to enhance the propagative

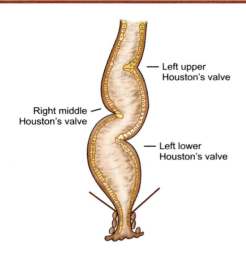

Fig. 1.3: The rectum in sagittal section, displaying the Houston valves

In the past, the rectum used to be the usual site and route for infusion of saline and dextrose. Surprisingly, it does not induce transmission of bacteria into the circulatory system. Although it is much less traumatic and commonly used in the children, it is no longer in practice for various reasons. But this route is still used in the clinical practice for the absorption of drugs. These are antibiotics, narcotics, steroids and bronchodilators and it is often used in the treatment of ulcerative colitis and proctitis with other drugs, used as enema.

Nevertheless, the functional state of the colon plays an important part in maintaining the body fluid and nutrition that depends upon the total transport time from the pylorus to the sigmoid colon. According to literature, the transport time from the pylorus to the ileocecal valve is 6 hours, and it is 12 hours between the ileocecal valve and the sigmoid colon. This function could be affected adversely by other diseases. They are food poison, cholera, salmonella typhoid, ulcerative colitis, Crohn's ileitis and colitis or intraperitoneal abscess. Inflammation of mucosa, or inflammation surrounding the intestine may delay the absorption of the fluid or it may cause increased secretion of fluid from the inflamed or ulcerated mucosal wall that leads to rapid transit of motion, often referred to as bouts of intestinal hurry.

Loose motion may occur, if the functional state of the colon is interfered with, by shortening of the transit time for the feces. This may result from the partial resection of the colon or bypass procedure—thus shortening its transit length and time, or it could be interfered with, by the advanced diseases causing communication between the colon and small intestine or between the colon and the stomach. These conditions are referred to as fistula.

Colon has no somatic nerves supply. Hence, it does not elicit pain when its wall is cut with cutting diathermy needle, but it has a parasympathetic and sympathetic nerve supply, known as Auerbach's myenteric plexus that maintains the peristaltic movement. Apart from these neural plexus, the movement of the gut, known as peristalsis is also initiated by the tone of the muscles. The peristalsis has two components of movements. One is segmentation, that helps needing and mixing up the intestinal contents; and other one is propagative movement that assists in moving the contents forwards.

Evidence of bowel sounds on auscultation through the abdominal wall suggests turbulence of gas and water. This is due to the effect of two peristaltic movements of the gut, but passage of flatus through the anus is mainly the result of propagative peristalsis. It implies that the continuity of the lumen or passage of the gut and functional state of the neural plexus has recovered. Absence of flatus suggests that there is either mechanical obstruction or paralytic ileus. The latter could be associated with peritonitis, or with the hypokalemia.

Again, the peritonitis may result from inflammation, infection or injury to the peritoneum. Hence, bowel sounds

movement of the feces in one direction, but the physiological function of the Houston valves has not been fully defined in the literature.

It seems it acts as a shelf, upon which the lumps of solid feces are stuck up, one after another, thus protecting the lower rectum from being overloaded and distended. At the same time, the anal sphincters are spared from being subjected to a constant gravitational pressure that could have imposed downwards by the solid feces.

It also permits the flatus, passing through the space that is maintained between the rectal wall and contralateral Houston valves. If these valves were not existing in the rectal wall, the lower rectum and the anal canal would have been packed with the solid feces that would not permit the flatus to get through the anal orifice. Its physiological function in the defecation of the feces will be described later.

FUNCTION OF THE COLON

The average volume of the liquid, known as chimes, passing through the large gut would be around 300 – 500 ml. And they are isotonic. This volume eventually transforms into solid feces, by the time it arrives into the rectum. It is related to the duration of the transit time and related to total length of the gut.

The main function of the colon is to absorb water, electrolytes, and certain vitamins and possibly amino acids, but it does not absorb carbohydrates, fats, proteins and calcium. Most of the absorption of water and nutritional elements takes place along the right half of the colon, and left half of the colon acts as reservoir for the feces to be shifted down to the rectum at a suitable duration. Because of this functional difference, the blood supply to the right colon is also different and greater than that in the left colon.

and flatus remain silent in all these conditions. In all postoperative cases, bowel sounds return sooner than the passage of flatus. The reasons for the delay in the passage of flatus are associated with the edema and inflammation around the site of the anastomosis. It takes four to five days to settle the edema around the site of anastomosis, to restore the continuity through the gut anastomosis and to return the functional state of the neural plexus. Oral feeding should not be commenced until the patient has admitted that flatus has passed per rectum.

The functional movement of the gut, known as gut motility is judged by the frequency of defecation per day. Mass movement of the semisolid feces is initiated by the combination of intrinsic neural innervations and tone of the colonic muscles. Hence, volume is one of the important factors, causing local distention of both circular and longitudinal fibers of the colon. Overdistention may cause atony of the muscles. Constipation is the result of either lack of local stimulation of the tone of the gut wall or due to atony of the gut wall.

In dehydration, colon tends to absorb fluid from the feces, thus reducing its volume into round dry balls, often referred to as pellets. As a result, lots of dry hard feces are necessary to induce the tone of the colon, but pellets of feces delay the initiation of the local tonicity of the circular muscles of the colon. Hence, bulky feces is the main factor for maintaining the tone of the muscles and transit time, from the cecum to the rectum. Average time for the test meal is around 6 hours from the stomach to the cecum and another 6-12 hours are required for the motion to pass from the cecum to the rectum, but the transport time is much slower in the rectum.

APPLIED ANATOMY AND PHYSIOLOGY IN THE MECHANISM FOR DEFECATION

The ampulla of the rectum is a storing house for both wind and feces. It has Houston's valves incorporated with the rectal wall. These valves keep holding the lumps of feces on its shelf, thus delaying its descent and at the same time protecting the anal orifice from being subjected to overloading with the feces. This delay may allow the small round feces like pellet to be held up in the ampulla of the rectum, until they build up the pressure, causing distention of the rectal wall.

The circular muscles of the rectum such as Houston's valves keep on squeezing and pushing the feces downwards, concurrently and sequentially. This peristaltic action is carried out by contraction of the circular muscles and the Houston's valves of the rectum.

As a result, the puborectalis muscles and the distal rectum are forced to be stretched up by those lumps of feces. Its purpose is to accommodate more lumps of feces, forming a continuous sausage-shaped or pipe stem type of feces in most cases.

When the distention of the rectal wall and the puborectalis muscles exceeds its limit, the stretch receptors present in the rectal wall and the puborectalis muscles are triggered off in order to induce reflex action that conveys the inhibitory effect on the tone of the sphincteric muscles. This inhibitory reflex that is mediated through the spinal cord, produces relaxation of muscle, thus allowing the anal canal to be distended by those feces and air. In sequence, the propagating peristalsis sets in propelling, the lumps of feces further downwards through the anal canal— thus exerting pressure upon the anal sphincters and the anal orifice. The consequent effect would be a gentle awareness for defecation. All these actions lead to progressive discomfort around the perineum.

In some cases, defecation could be held back by squeezing the anal sphincters for some time, until a suitable time and/ or place is available, but eventually the desire for defecation is triggered off, once the puborectalis muscles exceeds their limit of stretch. The consequent effect would be squeezing the rectal wall forcing the feces further down. It would act like squeezing the toothpaste tube. At that moment of time, a constant discomfort around the perineum is experienced because of the fact that feces are trapped within the anal canal, by the contraction of the puborectalis muscles at the upper end and closure of the anal orifice at the distal end of the feces.

The circular sphincteric muscles surrounding the impacted anal canal are subjected to rhythmic contraction. This may generate discomfort through the perineal muscles. And eventually, it would not be possible any longer in holding the defecation back.

While sitting on the commode, the longitudinal muscles of the rectum play an important part in opening the anal orifice. In normal condition, anal canal and anal orifice remain closed at rest by the tone of the sphincteric muscles. It opens up passively by a combination of descent of the feces and by inhibitory reflex action, resulting from the distention of the rectal wall and the puborectalis muscles. The loss of muscle tone of the anal sphincters allows opening of the anal orifice, thus propelling the bulk of the feces down through the anal orifice. It is assisted by raising the intraabdominal pressure, which is maintained by the contraction of the abdominal muscles and by holding the inspiration. During this process of defecation, the longitudinal muscle of the anal canal keeps pulling the anal sphincters upwards or holding them *in situ*, while the feces continue moving slowly down, out of the anal orifice concurrently.

As a result, the descent of the feces is accelerated by the combined contraction of the abdominal muscles, circular muscles of the rectum and the puborectalis muscles; all of which exert together, squeezing the feces concurrently, until the bolus of the feces pushes down through the anal orifice, where the circular muscles of the subcutaneous external anal sphincters are stretched passively in pari passu with the delivery of the feces, like delivery of a baby through the cervix uteri. All the anal skin covering the anal verge is stretched and rolled out when the bulky motion is coming out slowly.

The final act of defecation is completed by the contraction of the subcutaneous external anal sphincter; but the latter will only work after the feces being expelled out of the anal orifice. This contraction is the result of return of the muscle tone of the external anal sphincters, and it acts like a wiper of the bottom; but its action is repeated at the end of each spell, until the defecation is completed, while sitting on the commode.

However, the defecation is a complex physiological action regulated by the spinal reflex action, and operated by the combination of the rectum, puborectalis muscles, and anal sphincters. Puborectalis muscle is a U-shaped sling that remains attached across the lateral and posterior wall of the rectum and its fibers pass across the longitudinal fibers of the rectum and keep holding the rectum angulated forwards at the level of anorectal ring (Figs 1.2 and 1.4). It is striated muscle and a part of the levator ani muscle. Therefore, the position of the rectum that is held angulated forward at the level of anorectal ring is regarded to be another break to the descent and defecation of the feces.

This muscle that lies above the upper border of the deep external anal sphincter is stretched by the distention of the rectal wall. Hence, the Levator ani muscles are also affected by such distention. The puborectalis muscle holds the key for the urge defecation and keeps holding the feces back, thus protecting the anal sphincters from its continuous sphincteric action.

Previous study suggested that the pressure of the anal canal was found reduced, when the rectal wall was distended by inserting a balloon into the rectum. And the authors claimed in their study that this loss of pressure was evident despite paralyzing the external anal sphincters.[5,6] Their inference was that this change in pressure of the anal canal was attributable to relaxation of the internal anal sphincter. Such conclusion was not consistent with the function of the anal sphincters.

In all instances, the anal canal remains closed not by voluntary action of the anal sphincters, but by the muscles tone of the external anal sphincters. These muscles are striated muscles and ten times thicker than that of internal sphincter. Hence, these muscles keep the anal canal closed by the muscle tone. Of course, paralysis of these striated muscles would obviously lose its muscles tone and would lose the intraluminal pressure of the anal canal. In contrast, the internal anal sphincter is composed of smooth muscles, similar to that of the rectum. Hence the above inference, derived from their studies was not consistent with the facts.

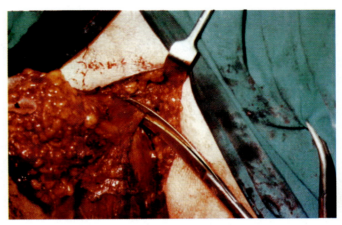

Fig. 1.4: The one of the U-shaped sling of the puborectalis muscles to be divided by the scissors

Nevertheless, further study confirmed that dilatation of the rectum by the balloon showed inhibition of the electrical response in the external anal sphincters and the levator ani muscles.[7] In another study, incontinence was reported in the results of sphincter saving low anterior resection of the rectum, where most of the rectum was removed at the operation.[8]

Despite all these conflicting reports, the fact has to be recognized that volume of the stool mass seems to be the primary factor for rectal dilatation. This induces urge defecation that is mediated via the spinal reflex neural action. The latter is triggered off through the stretch receptors present in the rectal wall, and puborectalis muscle. Therefore, the urge to defecate will not be initiated until the rectal wall and the puborectalis muscles exceed their limit of distention that depends upon the volume of the feces present in the rectum or anal canal.

In the literature, it has been postulated that this reflex action is initiated by the distention of the ampulla of the rectum, it is debatable whether the defecation is initiated by the distention of the rectal wall or by the puborectalis muscles or by a combination of both muscles. It is more likely that the urge to defecate is induced by the effect of stretch receptors present in the rectal wall and puborectalis muscles. Obviously, these receptors are stimulated by the distention of the rectum and puborectalis muscles.

Furthermore, this will also affect the levator ani muscles that continue resisting the intraabdominal pressure during defecation. At the same time, it will keep holding the sphincters steadily in places against the downwards forces of the feces. Furthermore, puborectalis muscles, levator ani muscles and external anal sphincters are innervated by the same pudendal nerves (S_2, S_3 and S_4). It seems more likely that the reflex action for urge defecation is mediated through these neural flexus, supplying to those muscles.

The circular muscles of the external anal sphincters are striated muscles; they keep the anal canal closed by its muscle tone alone and have no power to keep the anal canal open, unless these muscles are relaxed by voluntary action. The same mechanism plays in the subcutaneous external anal sphincter, which also has no physiological power to open the anal orifice voluntarily; but they have a power to defer the defecation that is carried out by just squeezing the anal orifice voluntarily. This voluntary action keeps the orifice closed further tight. This is due to the fact that they are not attached to the levator ani or anococcygeal raphe.

When the subcutaneous anal sphincter squeezes voluntarily, the anal orifice is closed and drawn inwards and upwards. As a result, the longitudinal muscle of the rectum, being a smooth muscle goes into spontaneous retraction. Ano-coccygeal raphe that lies between the coccyx and the external anal sphincters does not participate in defecation but it supports the pelvic floor and keeps holding the anus in place during defecation.

DISEASES OF THE COLON

Colonic diseases remain silent for many months, until it interferes with its physiological functions. These are loss of appetite, dehydration, malnutrition, weakness or feeling of discomfort in the belly or having abnormal bowel movements. For the ordinary people, it is not easy to recognize the abnormal symptoms that may develop slowly. Patients may anticipate that something in their belly is not right but they do not know exactly the reasons for being unwell or whether something serious has been growing in their belly. The symptoms that persist over many weeks are usually referred to as chronic and in other cases; the symptoms that appear abruptly without prior warning are referred to as acute condition that needs urgent attention of medical care.

Before discussing the individual medical problems, trainee surgeons need to understand the function of the gut. The whole length of the intestine has been anatomically divided into small and large intestine. Again the latter is subdivided into colon, rectum and anus.

PATHOLOGICAL LESIONS OF THE COLON

Colonic diseases could be classified in the following groups:
1. Benign tumor.
2. Malignant tumor.
3. Inflammatory disease.
4. Other benign lesions.

1. **Benign Tumors**
   a. Benign epithelial tumor – Adenoma
   Villous papilloma
   Familial polyposis.
   b. Other varieties – Lipoma
   Leiomyoma
   Neurofibroma
   Hemangioma.
   c. Hamartomas – Juvenile polyp
   Polyps of Peutz-Jeghers syndrome.
2. **Malignant Tumor** – Mainly adenocarcinoma
   Carcinoid syndrome.
3. **Inflammatory Diseases** – Ulcerative colitis
   Crohn's colitis
   Diverticulitis
   Amebic colitis
   Benign lymphoma.
4. **Other Benign Lesions** – Hyperplastic or metaplastic mucosal polyps
   Pneumatosis cystoids intestinalis
   Hypertrophied anal polyp or papillae.

CLINICAL IMPORTANCE OF BENIGN COLONIC LESIONS

■ A Broad Presentation of Polyps or Papilloma

Although this pathological lesion is simple to understand, it is often misunderstood and is neglected, because of rare clinical presentation. First of all, it arises from the epithelium of the colonic mucosa and remains initially as a tiny and localized growth in any part of the colon or rectum. It grows slowly and becomes either sessile without a stalk or large with a stalk. It has various names. These are polyp, adenoma, familial polyp, adenomatous polyp, and villous adenoma or villous polyps. One needs to understand the difference between the polyp and the adenoma. The latter, contrary to polyp contains the glands arising from the mucosa. Although it is a benign lesion, it may change to malignant condition later in life.

CHARACTERISTIC FEATURES OF A POLYP

The normal color of the colonic mucosa is pale, but the adenomatous polyp would appear to be pink or red color, because of increased vascularity.

In most instances, adenoma or papilloma remains symptoms-free. Nevertheless, they may present with bleeding, discharge of mucus, diarrhea and tenesmus. It may prolapse through the anus; if it is located in the lower rectum and has a long pedicle. It may present as anemia or as intussusception or recurrent spasm in the abdomen. The etiology of anemia could be attributable to chronic blood loss from its surface. In most instances, they are identified during investigations for other conditions.

Applied Anatomy of the Colon and the Rectum and Disease of the Colon

These investigations are rectal digital examination, rigid or flexible sigmoidoscopy and colonoscopy or double-contrast barium enema. These investigations are carried out for routine cancer screening program, constipation, and change in bowel habit or bleeding per rectum or anemia.

These lesions are also suspected in routine radiological investigation such as double-contrast barium enema, which may suggest a localized filling defect, whether or not it was a lump of feces or colonic lesion. This suspicious looking lesion needs to be confirmed by colonoscopy or by flexible sigmoidoscopy that depends upon the site of the lesion, shown on the barium enema films. In most cases, the report turns out to be no pathological lesion in the colon, provided the colonoscopy has been carried out with a good bowel preparation.

EPIDEMIOLOGICAL AND PATHOLOGICAL FEATURES

The adenoma is used to be regarded as premalignant lesion. It is often present, concomitant with the malignant growth and the commonest site for adenoma is in the sigmoid colon and the rectum. Its incidence varies between 2 to 8 percent. It may present with various shapes and sizes, ranging from a split pea to a small cherry or plum. It could be sessile or pedunculated. The pedunculated lesion moves around within the lumen of the colon and could be of mushroom like appearance. The length of the pedicle varies between half an inch and one and a half inch.

Most adenoma has a smooth or mildly lobulated mucosal covering and its color is similar to the surrounding colonic or rectal mucosa, but it could be pink or red. All lesions must be removed for tissue diagnosis and to exclude malignancy. Further review should be done in every six months with a view to checking whether it has recurred. It is also possible that a separate lesion may be identified in the same anatomical region.

BROAD OUTLINE OF TREATMENT

If the lesion is pedunculated or sessile and located within the reach of the rigid sigmoidoscope, it could be removed by a long biopsy forceps through the rigid sigmoidoscope. The procedure is more often done while having the rectal examination in the outpatient clinic. No bowel preparation or sedation is necessary, but patient must be explained about the merits of the treatment and the procedure involved.

If the lesion is located beyond the reach of the rigid sigmoidoscope, then patient should be brought back for flexible or colonoscopy or is referred to the colleague for such procedure being carried out. It is also possible to carry out the same procedure at the end of the clinic, if there is such facility available for performing the flexible sigmoidoscopy to be carried out in the outpatient clinic.

POLYPECTOMY THROUGH THE COLONOSCOPE

Before considering for colonoscopy, it is important to document other medical conditions which could prevent the procedure for colonoscopy. These are:

Recent myocardial infarction in less than 6 weeks—This procedure may cause cardiac arrhythmias. Other contraindications are acute or chronic ulcerative colitis and Crohn's colitis, diverticulitis, ischemic colitis, postradiation proctitis. These cases remain at greater risk of perforation of the gut due to inflammation of the bowel.

Polypectomy must not be done, if the patient is on anticoagulant therapy, or on aspirin.

Patient must be explained again about the complication and procedure, before a written consent is obtained. Rectal wash-out is normally given a few minutes before procedure being undertaken in the colonoscopic theater, the treatment is by snaring of the polyp either through the colonoscope or flexible sigmoidoscopy (70-110 cm). Two types of colonoscopes are available. One is longer ranging from 165 to 180 cm. This is suitable for the examination of the cecum. Durability of this type of colonoscope is short due to the fact that its wires may breakdown due to manipulation. The shorter one is between 130 cm and 140 cm.

Performance of the colonoscopy depends upon the cooperation of the patient and experience of the colonoscopist. It is advisable to carry out this procedure under short-acting intravenous sedation. The popular choice is midazolam. The recommended dose is between 2.5 mg and 5 mg. In addition, injection of pethidine 50 mg may be given either at the outset or later, if necessary. These drugs are given slowly. In some cases, injection of Buscopan 20-40 mg could be used, during the procedure.

In this procedure, the patient must have intravenous cannula onto the dorsal vein of the hand. Patient lies on the left lateral position with both knees onto brought towards the pelvis. First rectal digital examination should be carried out with right index finger, using a generous KY jelly. The end view of the colonoscope is first examined for sharpness of the focus, brightness of the light, air flow and suction apparatus, before it is gently inserted into the rectum by the right hand.

Generous lubrication is used all around the scope, every time it is pushed inside, under direct vision. It should not be pushed until the lumen of the gut is well-visualized with minimum air insufflations used. Overdistention of the gut may cause pain and discomfort and it may also cause angulation of the colon. To avoid this problem, air is again sucked out, after the scope has moved further forward.

The procedure is repeated and the tip of the scope is manipulated around the bends or around the mucosal folds, until the lesion is recognized. At times, saline wash-out needs to be given through the side channel in order to clean the lens and to push the solid feces out of the field of vision. If the patient is in distress, it could be due to overdistention of the belly, short-acting sedation and buscopan could be given through the cannula. Alternatively, all air could be sucked out by a combination of manipulation of instrument over the lower abdomen along with the suction of air and feces. Both procedures could be done concurrently.

Patient must have electrode pad attached to the thigh or on the buttock, in case the polyp needs to be snared by electrocoagulation. The power setting should be around 35-50W. If the size of the stalk of the polyp is greater than 1cm, power setting should be increased in order to coagulate the vessels running through the thick-walled part of the stalk.

Having identified the polyp, a long flexible snare loop connected to diathermy electrode is passed through the side channel of the instrument, until the snare loop is seen protruding out of the plastic tube. Once the lesion is recognized, the loop of the snare is manipulated to be pushed around the pedicle and the snare is slowly withdrawn towards the end of the plastic tube, until the pedicle is snugly caught within the loop.

The plastic tube is pushed down and away from the scope and under vision, while the diathermy-peddle is touched by the foot. This allows cauterization and severance of the polyp.

In case the snaring has failed despite using the higher power setting, then following items need to be checked, whether the complete circuit has been maintained and whether the electropad has been placed under the buttock or across the thigh, whether the snare has been placed properly around the stalk and connected to the electrocoagulation circuit.

When the polyp has been snared successfully, the snare is pulled out and biopsy forceps is next passed through the same side channel in order to grasp the said detached polyp. If it has been picked up by the forceps, the scope is slowly withdrawn along the biopsy forceps that keep holding the polyp.

If the polyp appears to be sessile, it could be removed with a long flexible biopsy forceps passed through the side channel of the telescope. Any remnant, left *in situ*, is cauterized with coagulation diathermy. The tissue is sent for histology. It does not cause great deal of complication for this procedure.

COMPLICATIONS OF THE PROCEDURE

First, there could be a false passage of the colon due to a faulty technique, poor visibility and poor bowel preparation. Mucosal trauma may be possible due to lack of experience in handling the instrument, or by reversing the tip of the colonoscope, forming an inverted U loop, within the lumen of the rectum.

The immediate complication is perforation, and bleeding from the site of operation. The lesion may be lost in the lumen. In this case, colonoscopy is withdrawn slowly, while looking for the tumor. Alternative procedure is to give a rectal wash-out on the same table and the patient is asked to open the bowel in a bedpan, where the resected specimen is discharged with the motion. It is then retrieved from the pan. Alternatively, patient is admitted in the ward for a bedpan in which the specimen may drop.

If the patient complains of pain in lower abdomen and appears to be in a state of shock, patient needs to be admitted straightaway for urgent resuscitation. In a state of hemorrhagic shock, patient will appear pale looking, sweating and there would be low blood pressure and rapid pulse rate. The first medical care is to start resuscitation with intravenous infusion of colloids and blood, sedation and antibiotics. Blood transfusion should be considered, if the hemoglobin is less than 10 gm/dl.

Once the patient has recovered from the shock, examination of the abdomen is carried out, whether or not there is any evidence of peritonitis and paralytic ileus. Both rectal digital and sigmoidoscopy are carried out, if possible. In most cases, bleeding stops but for persisting bleeding, the bleeding points may require to be controlled by a gentle touch with electrocoagulation under general anesthesia and on the operating table.

Later, a plain X-ray of abdomen in both erect and supine position is taken. This may reveal any gas under the diaphragm or around the colon. If the diagnosis is in doubt, water-soluble contrast known as gastrograffin enema should be carried out. Once the diagnosis has been confirmed, emergency laparotomy should be carried out for the repair of perforation and for the construction of a transverse-loop colostomy.

In other cases, secondary hemorrhage may occur after two weeks. It occurs when the necrotic tissue tends to be dislodged from the site of electrocoagulation. Patient may collapse in the bathroom at home. For a mild type of bleeding that may be noticed along with the defecation, no more special care is necessary, but blood hemoglobin should be checked, before prescribing iron tablets to the patient.

CLINICAL FEATURES AND TREATMENT OF VILLOUS PAPILLOMA

A villous papilloma is another variety of adenoma, usually develops in the rectum. It has shaggy surface with characteristic frond-like appearances and ill-defined edges. It has a wider base, covering a large area, but it is mobile. In most instances, they are located in the posterior wall of the rectum. It discharges jelly-like mucoid material and thick watery motion that contains high-rich potassium.

Patient may be dehydrated with electrolyte abnormality in which hypokalemia would be the major concern to the surgeon. Histologically, it is regarded to be benign but malignant change may occur unless dysplastic changes are noticed on histological examination.

All those patients, usually above the age of 30, are investigated in order to exclude any other pathological lesion present in the colon. These include, sigmoidoscopy, ultrasound scan of the liver, kidneys and abdomen, contrast barium enema, and blood tests for electrolytes and full blood count, blood sugar. After reviewing all these results, colonoscopy should be arranged in order to complete the investigation.

Patient needs to be admitted for correction of dehydration and electrolytes imbalance with the supplementation of potassium, either in the infusion or orally. Preoperative bowel preparation is carried out with oral laxative and rectal phosphate enema followed by rectal saline wash-out; before the patient is operated upon. A full discussion should be held with the patient, for obtaining consent for the operation. Patient must be informed that the tumor needs to be resected locally. And there remains further possibility for developing a local recurrence. It is also important to draw his attention that malignant change may be noticed in the resected tumor or it may develop later that depends upon the local treatment and the report of the histology.

The treatment entails a fulguration of the tumor with a ball pointed electrode or a wide submucosal resection of the tumor under direct vision. This depends upon the size and location of the tumor.

Operative Procedure

Under general anesthesia, patient is put on the lithotomy position. Sterile drapes are put around the perineum and legs. Rectal digital examination is done in order to palpate the tumor about its size and mobility. Rigid sigmoidoscopy is also carried out in order to see the rectum and a part of the sigmoid colon, whether there is any other additional growth located higher up.

Anal orifice is dilated with 2-3 fingers. A self-retaining retractor with two blades is inserted through the anus. And it is held in position by retracting the two blades *in situ*.

The proximal edge of the tumor is grabbed with a Babcock forceps. It is gently brought down in order to define the edge of the attachment of the tumor with the rectal mucosa. Assessment is made whether the defect of the submucosal space could be covered technically with the mobilization of the surrounding rectal mucosa after resection of the tumor is carried out with a cutting diathermy needle. This assessment is done by pulling the tumor down, measuring its size and by evaluating the mobility of healthy mucosa, around the base of the tumor; before the resection is contemplated.

After this assessment, a stay suture is inserted a little above the upper edge of the tumor. A few more Babcock forceps are applied to the edge of the tumor in order to act as traction, during the process of cutting the tumor edge, using an angled diathermy needle. Submucosal resection of the tumor is continued from the proximal side, and at the same time the surrounding cut edge of the mucosa is mobilized to be stitched together. This bridging across the defect is made by a continuous suture. The procedure is continued downwards until the whole tumor is resected out. During resection, bleeding points are stopped with diathermy forceps. At the conclusion, the retractors are removed. The wound is covered with jelly net. The specimen is sent for histology.

Postoperative Care

Patient should be kept nil by mouth for a few days, until flatus has passed. Once bowel has moved, patient is allowed home, but is reviewed six weeks later.

Alternative to submucosal resection is the resection of the tumor with a special form of resectoscope, through an operating sigmoidoscope, like TURP. Other approach is to destroy the surface of the papilloma by diathermy; but total ablation of the tumor is not possible in this procedure. There are many disadvantages in undertaking this procedure. However, patient may experience with wet bottom and foul smell due to discharge of mucous, soiling the under-pants or dress.

Every six weeks, the patient is reviewed at the outpatient clinic and further surgical intervention may be necessary within 3-6 months time. The condition is not curable but it requires regular surveillance.

If the villous tumor is located in the sigmoid colon or in the rectum, laparotomy is necessary for resection of the gut that depends upon the location and histological grade of the tumor.

CRITERIA FOR CONSIDERING MALIGNANCY IN THE BENIGN ADENOMA OR VILLOUS PAPILLOMA

a. Age: If the polyp develops in a young child, it is known as juvenile polyp, and is regarded to be benign but if it occurs in the older age group, the lesion could be either of the pathology.
b. A family history should be obtained in order to exclude familial polyposis coli. They are treated like malignancy.
c. Histology report is not 100 percent reliable. Negative report does not exclude malignance. It is more likely to happen that biopsy was taken from the non-malignant site of the adenoma.

d. Characteristic appearance of the growth—Malignancy should be suspected, if the surface is ulcerated or the growth appears to be large in size and indurated.

DIFFERENCE BETWEEN THE ADENOMA AND VILLOUS PAPILLOMA

The incidence of adenoma is reported to be 84.6 percent and that of villous papilloma 11.6 percent. And the average size of the former is between 2 and 7 cm and that of the latter ranges from a few mm to 9 cm. Majority of the adenoma is pedunculated but villous papilloma is sessile in almost 90 percent of the cases, or finger like projection and rarely pedunculated. And they are almost solitary compared to the adenomatous lesions. The commonest anatomical sites for the adenoma remain in the sigmoid colon but the villous papilloma develops by contrast in the rectum more frequently than in the sigmoid colon.

FAMILIAL POLYPOSIS

Familial polyposis is an autosomal dominant condition. The name familial polyposis implies that it is hereditary and genetic disease, transmitted by the father to the offspring in both sexes, but only half of the children are likely to inherit the disease and the affected member will pass the gene to the next generation. The average age for the development of symptoms is 20 and it takes 10-15 years to develop cancer in these polyps. It is diffusely present in the large bowel, right down to the anal canal. It is more in numbers in the left side, but they are generally uniformly distributed between the cecum and anal canal. They are adenoma and are of various sizes. Eventually, malignancy develops in these adenomas.

CLINICAL PRESENTATION

In early life, they remain silent, but with the age, the symptoms are presented initially with a slight soft motion, that may progress to increased number of frequency. In most cases, either the parent or the child may not pay much attention to the unusual symptoms, until it becomes evident that bowel movements are getting worse and associated with frank diarrhea, discharge of mucus and blood in the motion.

These cases are often presented with multiple sebaceous cysts, dermoid cysts, bony exostoses. If the patient is presented with multiple soft and hard tissue tumors, while attending the clinics, suspicion should arise and further investigation should be contemplated to exclude familial polyposis of colon. Suspicion should also arise in the investigation of ulcerative colitis among the younger patients.

In the routine examination, rectal digital examination would reveal the features of adenomatous polyps. Sigmoidoscopy will show multiple polyps and normal looking mucosa in the intervening space. In contrast, the findings would be quite different in the case of proctocolitis, in which, there would be no classical vascular pattern in the rectal mucosa, and there would be contact bleeding associated with pus and blood in the lumen.

Other investigations include colonoscopy and double-contrast barium enema. It is also important to remember how to differentiate the distinct features between the ulcerative colitis and the familial intestinal polyposis in barium enema. In the former case, the barium enema will show contraction, and lack of haustration.

CHOICES OF TREATMENT MODALITIES

It is a difficult situation in which surgeons could not predict the prognosis for any conservative surgical procedures used in dealing with this case. If total colectomy followed by ileorectal anastomosis is carried out, patient needs to be followed up every three months that includes check sigmoidoscopy. This would be expensive and would render psychological trauma. As a result, patient would be tied down to a particular medical team or a hospital.

Again, there remains a further risk of multiple operative procedures. In these cases, tissue diagnosis is first done by biopsy and then fulguration of the recurrent polyps is done, if the histology report suggests benign lesion. And eventually abdominoperineal resection of the rectum is undertaken for the recurrence of malignant tumor in the rectal stump or anal canal. Again, this procedure would be much more difficult because of previous operative adhesions developed in the pelvis or in the abdomen.

Therefore, considering the morbidity and financial implication, it is safer to do total panproctocolectomy and terminal ileostomy, before the age of 30 or when the disease has reached to a period of 10 years, and when the symptoms have developed. The only problem remains with the young patients whether they are prepared to accept the burden of permanent ileostomy and to sacrifice the enjoyments of family or married life. Regrettably there is no satisfactory alternative choice in the safe treatment for this inherited disease.

Postoperative complication following total colectomy or panproctocolectomy or AP resection has been described in the respective chapter. It is especially important to add one import complication associated with this disease. There remains a risk of developing desmoids tumor in the abdominal scar.

DIFFERENCE BETWEEN ADENOMA, PEUTZ-JEGHERS SYNDROME AND FAMILIAL POLYPOSIS

Polyps also develop in other parts of the alimentary tract, but it is associated with pigmentation in the skin and buccal mucosa. It is a benign clinical condition and a hereditary condition.

The commonest site for developing polyp is in the jejunum but it can occur in other parts of the small intestine. The pigmentation usually appears to be irregular flakes over the lips and commonly in the mucocutaneous junction of the lower lip, buccal mucosa and over the plates, but not on the tongue, fingers and toes.

Polyp could be of various sizes and similar in appearance to other adenomas or familial polyposis, but not associated with buccal or lips pigmentation. Nevertheless, it presents confusion when these polyps develop intussusception or bleeding or recurrent episodes of pain in upper abdomen. Investigation is necessary to establish the differential diagnosis and to establish the causes of symptoms. Surgical intervention is only indicated if they pose persistent problems not resolving spontaneously.

OTHER BENIGN POLYP IN THE COLON, RECTUM AND ANUS

Lymphoma

This benign tumor remains silent in most cases and is diagnosed incidentally during routine rectal examination. It appears like any other polyp. Although a polyp found on proctoscopy or sigmoidoscopy in the rectum, may be innocent or benign pathology, thorough clinical history and investigation is necessary. It should be removed for tissue diagnosis. If the histology report suggests that the tissue removed from the rectum is lymphoma, no further treatment is necessary and complete excision is not important, because of the fact that it does not change into lymphosarcoma.

Lipoma

Lipoma is a lobulated and capsulated fatty benign tumor. It can develop in any part of the body, but it is rarely found in the alimentary tract. If it is present in the gut, commonest site would be in the cecum, but it can develop in other sites of the colon and rectum. In most cases, it remains symptoms-free, but it may cause intussusception in the cecum and it may cause some discomfort. It lies in the submucosal layer and unlikely in the subserous layer. This fatty lump may be palpable on abdominal examination.

Differential diagnosis may be difficult, if barium enema shows a filling defect in the wall of the cecum or colon. Because of the radiological finding, further investigation should be arranged. These are ultrasound scan, CT scan, MRI scan and colonoscopy. Conservative line of approach may be recommended, if the colonoscopy confirms no evidence of mucosal growth, but laparotomy should be considered because of symptoms of pain, and obstructive features. Although lipoma is a benign tumor, it cannot be certain of its pathology without histological examination. In this scenario, one should not ignore the radiological or CT scan report.

Leiomyoma

Leiomyoma is also a rare variety and a benign tumor, but it may change to malignancy, presenting as leiomyosarcoma. It develops usually in the smooth muscle layer of the gut.

It can affect both sexes and at any age. Its size and consistency varies. When it is small in size, it would appear to be rubbery and firm but when it is large, it could be lobulated. It may project through the overlying mucosa into the lumen, causing discomfort and partial obstruction. It may also project through the serosal wall into the peritoneal cavity. Those tumors develop in the intramural part of the colon, are not capsulated, but others in the rectum may have a capsule. It may ulcerate through the mucosa, causing bleeding.

This rare tumor is diagnosed at the laparotomy or through the sigmoidoscopy. Total excision will protect the patient from any risk of malignant change. Hence, histology report will guide the surgeon whether or not it has been excised completely.

Other rare variety of pathological lesions present in the colon or rectum is Hemangioma. If they are encountered in any clinical examination, conservative line of approach should be observed. In any condition of acute hemorrhage, the lesion needs to be excised along with a segment of bowel. Coagulation diathermy or sclerosing injection into the vessels would be ineffective in most instances.

PAPILLOMA OF THE ANUS

Papilloma may develop around the anus. It may be associated with penile or vaginal warts. Its etiology is not known, but viral in origin has been referred to the literature. Poor local hygiene and anal sexual intercourse are the alternative cause for these benign conditions. It could be transmitted to sexual partner.

They are multiple and may develop into the lower part of the anal canal. It causes discomfort and produces foul odor. Differential diagnosis has to be made between the condyloma latum due to syphilis and squamous cell carcinoma. In the latter case, induration is a distinct feature around the lesions and tissue diagnosis is done while dealing with this lesion.

Treatment is the recurrent fulguration or a partial excision like hemorrhoidectomy. Specimen must be sent for histology following each surgical treatment.

REFERENCES

1. Heald RJ, Husband EM, Ryall RD. The mesorectum in rectal cancer surgery: The clue to pelvic recurrence? Br J Surg 1982;69:613-16.
2. Textbook of Gray's Anatomy, 37th Edition, 1989.
3. Last RJ. Anatomy Regional and Applied, 4th Edition, J and A Churchill Ltd: London, 1966.
4. Saha SK. Critical evaluation of dissection of the perineum in synchronous combined abdominoperineal excision of the rectum. Surgery Gynecology and Obstetrics. 1984;158:33-38.
5. Denny-Brown D, Robertson EG. An investigation of the nervous control of defecation. Brain 1935;58:256.
6. Duthie HL, Watts JM. Contribution of the external anal sphincter to the pressure zone in the anal canal. Gut 1965;6:64.
7. Porter NH. Megacolon: A physiological study. Proc Roy Soc Med 1961;54:1043.
8. Parks AG, Porter NH, Melzak J. Experimental study of the reflex mechanism controlling the muscles of the pelvic floor. Dis Colon and Rectum 1962;5:407.

2 Malignant Tumors of the Colon and Spread of the Colonic Tumor

MALIGNANT TUMORS OF THE COLON, RECTUM AND ANUS

Distribution of Sex and Age

By and large, both sexes are equally affected by the colonic carcinoma, found in clinical studies,[1,2] but the incidence of the rectal carcinoma was found greater in men than in women and the sex ratio was 5:3. In other studies, the difference was 3:1.[3-5] Difference in statistical data may often be affected by the different interpretation of the growth located in the rectosigmoid region, where it could be classified as sigmoid tumor included in one study and as rectal tumor in another study.

Similarly, the younger age group below the age of 40 is less frequently affected by the carcinoma of the rectum. Its incidence was found to be 3.85 percent under the age of 30, but it was over 50 percent found above the age of 60, in a series of 1171 cases included in the study.[6] It has also been found in another series that women are affected more frequently at younger age than that in men.[7]

DESCRIPTION OF THE MACROSCOPICAL FEATURES OF THE MALIGNANT TUMORS

Large bowel carcinoma may develop into various shapes and sizes. There are five varieties of the tumor mass, identified in clinical surgery. They are:
- Polypoidal type
- Ulcerative type
- Infiltrating
- Colloidal type
- Annular type.

MACROSCOPICAL APPEARANCE OF THE TUMORS

The macroscopic feature of polypoidal growth would look like a cauliflower. Its surface tends to be ulcerated and projected into the lumen of the colon or rectum. In some instances, it may change into fungating appearance in extreme circumstance. The commonest site for polypoidal type of growth is in the cecum but annular type of growth is more prevalent in the left colon, particularly in the lower descending or sigmoid colon.

The ulcerative carcinoma is another macroscopical variety, in which the edges are irregular and everted, its middle part undergoes sloughing and it appears to be firmer in consistency. They tend to grow transversely, covering nearly 75 percent of the lumen of the colon or the rectum. It invades the colonic wall causing indentation or deformity.

The infiltrating carcinoma presents as a diffuse type, like linitis plastica—thus producing a diffuse thickening of the gut wall. Although its intraluminal surface remains covered with intact mucosa in major surface, certain part may breakdown into ulceration. It is associated with ulcerative colitis.

The colloidal carcinoma is generally bulky, and may present with gelatinous appearance.

According to the literature, the commonest sites for the annular type of the cancer are in the sigmoid colon and in the rectum, compared to other sites of the colon, but the sigmoid colon seems to be more frequently affected than the rectum. It is hard in consistency. It begins with a small tumor that grows slowly around the wall of the gut, causing stricture, encircling the whole girth of the gut. Furthermore, feces in the pelvic colon is relatively solid in consistency. Because of this reason, patients present with a large bowel obstruction much sooner. By contrast, the cauliflower type of growth developed in the ascending colon behaves differently, where the feces by contrast remains liquid. Hence the incidence of obstruction of the right colon has been found much less.

In most instances, malignant tumor develops in a single site, but about 3 percent of the cases had more than one primary site.[8] The photograph of the rectum removed after abdominoperineal resection shows multiple tumors of different sizes at different places in the mucosal wall of the rectum, and whether each one was a primary tumor or seedling, derived from the primary tumor would be difficult to draw a definitive conclusion.[4]

In the past, metastasis of the tumor by implantation was disputed, but such doubt has been overcome by the *in vitro* study, in which implantation of malignant cells in the healthy tissue has been established. These issues would be highlighted in appropriate section on metastasis.

Colonic carcinoma has been found concurrently in the cecum as well as in the sigmoid colon. Both tumors were regarded to be two primary tumors. In one case, the sigmoid colon has been found stuck to the cecal carcinoma, thus producing a fistula, but it was difficult to confirm whether the tumors in both sites were two primary growths or one invaded the other site; because of abnormal position of the loop of the sigmoid colon over the cecum. But they should be regarded to be the two primary growths.

MACROSCOPICAL CHANGES IN THE COLON, PRESENTED WITH MALIGNANT TUMOR

Due to chronic process of partial obstruction, the large bowel proximal to the tumor tends to be working hard in order to push the liquid or semisolid feces through the narrow lumen of the colon. Due to incomplete passage of feces, the colon tends to get dilated in order to accommodate the excess contents. Reverse peristalsis is not possible sometimes due to competent ileocecal valve.

As a result, colonic wall continues to work hard against the resistance that leads to increased intraluminal pressure. These peristaltic waves enhance the thickening of the wall known as hypertrophy of the colonic muscles. Eventually, the intraluminal pressure, proximal to the tumor is held back by the iliocecal valve like a closed loop for some time, but it gives away eventually, releasing the pressure into the terminal ileum. In this process, reverse peristalsis starts working—thus refluxing the colonic contents into the terminal ileum.

PATHOLOGICAL CHANGES IN THE GUT WALL

In some extreme circumstance, in which the obstruction is not dealt with, the taeniae coli may show a partial split up known as serosal tear. This would permit to accommodate more luminal pressure. Apart from thickening of the colonic wall, and serosal tear, the mucosa may be ulcerated which may look like 'stercoral' ulcers or a moth-eaten appearance.

In acute obstruction, gangrene of the colonic wall or perforation through this tear or through the stercoral ulcer may occur. The commonest site is the cecum. This may cause localized peritonitis and retroperitoneal or paracecal abscess. Acute appendicitis in elderly patient should be suspicious. In the past, abscess due to cecal perforation had been found at the operation of acute appendicitis.[9–11] The remaining part of the colon, distal to the tumor, remains collapsed and it contains lots of solid round feces.

If the obstruction continues, the terminal ileum gets dilated if the small intestine cannot empty its contents into the cecum. And this dilatation continues progressively and the gut gets elongated, thus making the small intestine into many loops, forming like step-ladder pattern. In a thin belly, these features could be visible from outside the abdomen. To accommodate these distended guts, the stomach is distended, the gallbladder may be congested or dilated and the diaphragm is elevated, causing the compression to the bases of the lungs. This back pressure to the chest may delay as well as reduce the venous return to the heart.

Furthermore, there would be accumulation of air and increased collection of fluid into the dilated intestine due to lack of absorption and due to back-pressure from colonic obstruction. Because of dilatation, venous channels are compressed and it occurs along the circumference of the gut wall and along the mesenteric border of the colon. This compression is due to a thin wall of the vein that is affected by the dilatation of the gut wall.

As a result, there would be mucosal congestion and exudation. And absorption of the fluid or nutrients from the intestinal contents will be reduced or ceased. On the contrary, exudation would add to the existing intestinal contents, causing further distention.

In addition, the arterial blood flow would eventually be reduced, affecting the antimesenteric border of the gut, thus developing ischemic changes in this area. Through these devitalized tissues, bacterial toxins may transmigrate into the peritoneal cavity along with the exudation of the tissue fluid from the gut wall. In this process, migration of bacteria from the peritoneal cavity and through the gut wall takes place that may set into septicemia and peritonitis. There would be exudation of fluid both inside the gut as well as outside the gut wall, thus reducing the total blood volume. In colonic obstruction, perforation of the small intestine is very rare.

Apart from the perforation of the large bowel, perforation may also occur through the center of the tumor bed. It is not unusual in the pelvic colon or in the rectum. The clinical presentation in both cases would be localized peritonitis and localized abscess, behind the bowel. Patients will present a tense distended abdomen, associated with dehydration and shock.

SITES FOR THE COLONIC CARCINOMA

The frequency of the carcinoma in the colon and rectum varies from one study to another. By and large, carcinoma develops more frequently in the distal colon and the rectum (Fig. 2.1). In 1963, the Registrar-General's death registry in England and Wales showed that the incidence of the rectal carcinoma was 38 percent, but in another study, it was 57.4 percent.[1] Distribution of the carcinoma in different anatomical sites of the colon and the rectum has been compiled in Table 2.1 from the literature.[1]

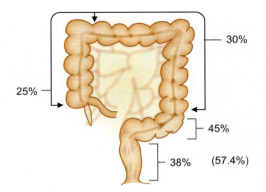

Fig. 2.1: The incidence of the tumor in different areas of the colon and the rectum

Table 2.1: Distribution of the carcinoma in different anatomical sites of the colon, and the rectum		
Sites	Sexes Male (Females)	No.
Cecum	48(53)	101
Ascending colon	24(24)	48
Hepatic flexure	20(9)	29
Transverse colon	37(40)	77
Splenic flexure	25(25)	50
Descending colon	18(27)	45
Sigmoid colon	176(174)	350
Rectum	559(385)	944
Total	907(737)	1644

Goligher recognizes the significant differences and has highlighted the reason for this difference that depends upon whether the tumor located in the rectosigmoid region was regarded to be colonic or rectal tumor. The literature suggests that the incidence of the carcinoma of the colon would be nearly 45 percent in the sigmoid colon, around 25 percent in the cecum and ascending colon. The remaining may occur in the transverse colon, splenic flexure, descending colon and the hepatic flexure, in that order of frequency (Fig. 2.1).

The frequency of the rectal carcinoma would be 30.8 percent in the upper-third, 32.6 percent in the middle-third and 36.6 percent in the lower-third that includes the anal canal.[4] This distribution was based upon those specimens removed at the operation. According to Goligher, the frequency was determined on the findings of the sigmoidoscope from the anal verge.[6] He excluded those tumors located above 15 cm. They were regarded to be in the sigmoid colon. The incidence of those tumors, below the level of 15 cm were reported to be 36 percent, found in the upper-third at a level of greater than 11 cm, 28.7 percent in the middle-third at a level greater than 6cm and 35.3 percent in the lower-third, located below the level of 6cm from the anal verge.

He also found that the incidence of annular growth was 31.7 percent and that of non-annular tumor was 68.3 percent. It was also reported that the tumor developed in the posterior wall of the rectum was found to be 24.9 percent, 22.2 percent in the anterior wall, and 21.2 percent in each lateral wall.

SPREAD OF THE COLONIC AND RECTAL CARCINOMA

Malignant tumors traverse macroscopically and microscopically. The common routes of spread are:
a. Direct spread
b. Lymphatic spread
c. Venous spread
d. Transplantation spread
e. Transcelomic spread.

■ Direct Spread

Cancer initially develops in the mucosa of the gut. It increases in size in both direction and progresses across the bowel wall through the submucosal, and muscle layers until it reaches the peritoneal surface. The tumor reaches the pericolic fat or perirectal fat or to the surface of peritoneum. This sort of spread depends upon the location of the tumor.

The tumor located in the posterior wall of the rectum eventually reaches the fascia of Waldeyer. In advanced cases; sacral plexus, sacrum and coccyx may be invaded by those tumor cells. In other areas, the tumor developed in the anterior wall and below the peritoneal reflection invades the prostate gland, seminal vesicle, or bladder in male and posterior vaginal wall or cervix uteri in the female. These infiltrations occur by a direct invasion.

If the tumor remains very close to any other gut or organ, it would invade that wall of the organ. It may communicate with other hollow viscus, forming a fistula, such as gastrocolic fistula, colovesical fistula and rectovaginal or recto-uterine fistula.

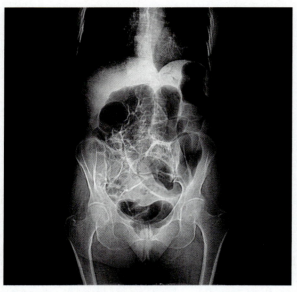

Fig. 2.2: Plain X-ray abdomen shows the dilation of the colon and small intestine. This was due to obstruction by the tumor in the sigmoid colon

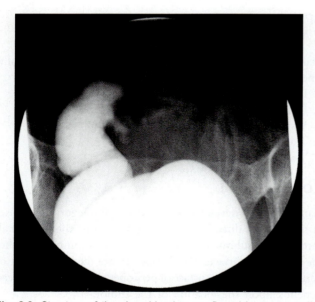

Fig. 2.3: Structure of the sigmoid colon, confirmed by gastrograffin enema

It may invade the ureter, duodenum, renal pelvis or psoas muscle and iliac vessel that depend upon the location of the tumor.

Although a small site of the gut is initially inflicted by the malignant cells, they traverse transversely more rapidly as a malignant ulcer. Its edges begin to advance transversely in both directions, until they meet at the opposite wall. This leads to constriction of the lumen of the gut, and it is known as annular ulcerating growth. There are evidences that the tumor also continues advancing along its long axis; but it spreads slowly and its longitudinal axis would be around 2-3 inches and it is much less in longitudinal axis of the colon. Annular tumor is a unique example of the transverse spread and the sigmoid colon seems to be affected more frequently than other colonic sites (Figs 2.2 and 2.3). Annular tumor presents as colonic obstruction. Plain X-ray abdomen provides the evidence of gaseous distention of the gut.

At laparotomy, the sigmoid colon would appear to be constricted as if it has been tied around by a string and by external palpation; it would appear to be stony hard and irregular. Furthermore, the lumen surrounded by the tumor would appear to be narrowed or no lumen could be felt through the tumor, when the tips of the index finger and the thumb are attempted to push through concurrently from sides of the lumen of the colon, held up by other hand in the air.

Study showed that the average duration required for developing this type of growth would be around two years. The biological behavior also suggests that the spread of the cancer in the rectum required six months to cover only one quadrant of the rectal wall.[12] In my past experiences, it became evident that recollection of patients' memory was consistent between the duration of symptoms and the circumferential spread of the tumor, when the specimen of the colon was opened longitudinally. Apart from the local advancement of the tumor, transcelomic spread does occur and it produces ascites, omental cake and parietal peritoneal seedling. These are evidences of poor prognosis.

■ Lymphatic Spread

Microscopic spread takes the route of both lymphatic and vascular channels. Prognosis of the survival rate depends upon the local and distant spread. Dukes classified the rectal and colonic tumors into three groups, and each one has been defined by the local and lymphatic spread. They are known as Dukes A, Dukes B and Dukes C.[7]

Dukes A are those tumors that remain confined within the wall of the rectum and the colon without involvement of the extrarectal or colonic tissue and without any evidence of metastasis into the lymph nodes; Dukes B are those tumors that have extended further beyond the wall but without invading the lymphatic channels or lymph nodes and Dukes C are those tumors which had invaded the lymph nodes (Fig. 2.4).

Invasion or spread of the tumor to other organs or other segment of the gut would not alter the tumor staging from Dukes B to C, if the lymph glands were not invaded by the tumor.

Since then, further classification has been made in order to define the further stage of the spread. Those tumors which have invaded the lymph nodes close to serosal surface known as epicolic glands are regarded to be Dukes C1, and those tumors which have invaded the lymph nodes further away

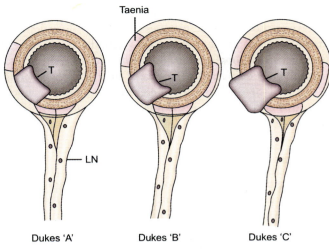

Fig. 2.4: Dukes Tumor Stage

A = The tumor confined within the wall of the rectum
B = The tumor has extended further beyond the wall. But not invading the lymph nodes
C = The tumor has advanced further and invaded the lymph nodes

from the epicolic glands and lie along the main arterial vessels, are referred to as Dukes C2.

The prevalence of the Dukes A, Dukes B and Dukes C was found to be 15 percent, 35 percent and 50 percent respectively in his study.[7] The long established classification has been well recognized among the surgeons, but further classification has been made in those cases in which the tumors where found in the liver. They are regarded to be Dukes D but this additional classification now referred to as Dukes D stage was not included in his original classification.

However, the mode of spread is by embolization. The lymphatic channels, known as lymphatic plexus begin at the submucosal layers, and they are also present in the intermural and subfascial planes. In this spread, the striking feature is that microscopical spread does not extend distally beyond a few millimeters from the macroscopical edge of the tumor.[13,14] Further studies claimed that it did not extend beyond 20 mm distal to the lower edge of the tumor.[15,16] Because of this evidence, distal resection of the rectum at 2.5 cm from the tumor margin has been regarded to be a safe level of resection. Therefore, sphincter-saving low anterior resection of the rectum has become a popular choice.[17]

Although the resection of the rectum, at 2 cm below the macroscopical margin of the rectal tumor has become a standard operative procedure, in sphincter-saving low anterior resection, the recurrence of tumor at the anastomotic site or in the pelvis suggests contrary to the histological report.[18] Recent follow-up study showed a correlation of local recurrence with the anastomotic leakage, despite the fact that histology did not reveal any evidence of the tumor in the doughnut specimen retrieved from the autosuture gun.[18] It could be postulated that those recurrences developed later could be attributed to the dislodgement of the malignant cells that had dropped into the distal rectum. These cells are expelled in the pelvis later through the anastomotic leakage.

Hence, the question remains to be highlighted in perspective, how safe it would be in the resection of the rectum at 2.5 cm clear margin from the lower margin of the tumor? And how could the safe level be identified by palpation from outside the bowel before resection being carried out seems to be unfathomable?

In this restrictive and a limited access, one could infer from the evidences of local recurrences that the risk of dislodgement of the tumor cells from the parent tumor is much greater during mobilization of the rectum and it would be technically difficult to apply the clamps across the so-called holy plane of the rectum at 2 cm below the tumor margin.

Radical or curative resection of the colonic tumor is guided by the local or distal lymphatic spread. Evidence of enlarged lymph nodes does not indicate that they are invaded by the tumor cells. Apart from the invasion of the malignant cells, paracolic glands could be enlarged in some cases by the spread of infection from the ulcerated bed of the tumor. And in some cases, glands may not be palpable despite the fact that they have been invaded by the cancer cells at the very early stage.

Hence, these findings do not influence upon the surgeon whether or not radical or curative resection should be undertaken. Prognosis depends upon the histology report on those enlarged glands removed along with the specimen. The decision to carry out the curative resection is influenced by a number of criteria. These are mobility of the growth, local invasion to other structures and evidence of distal metastasis and ascites.

All these studies suggest that paracolic glands that lie close to the colonic wall near the growth are first invaded by the tumor cells. The malignant cells then continue to traverse further through the chains of the lymph glands along the superior hemorrhoidal arteries and or along the inferior mesenteric arteries. In due course, the tumor cells invade the paraaortic lymph glands. This implies that the lymphatic drainage follows the corresponding arteries supplying to the primary tumor in the sigmoid colon and the rectum.

Miles, in his study, had outlined the lymphatic pathways in three directions. These are upward pathways, lateral pathways and downward pathways.[12]

The upwards pathways comprise of lymphatic spread from the primary growth. They follow through the lymphatic chains along the superior or inferior mesenteric arteries and finally to the abdominal aortic glands.

The lateral pathways involve the lymphatic drainage from the primary rectal growth into the lymph glands in the lateral ligaments, between the pelvic peritoneum and the levator ani muscles and finally into those glands lying along the internal iliac artery.

The downwards pathways are those spread that follow the lymphatic channels through the sphincteric muscle, the perianal skin and the ischeorectal fat and finally drain into the glands located in the groins.

Despite these extensive studies, subsequent studies had disputed those claims, apart from the upward spread.

Technical difficulty may be encountered in establishing the lateral spread. This is due to the fact that internal iliac lymph glands are often not included in the rectal specimen removed by a combined abdominoperineal resection. The prognosis could not be fully documented unless the internal iliac glands are removed separately with a view to confirming, whether or not these were invaded by the tumor.

Later in the follow up patients, enlargement of the internal iliac glands would provide further evidences, whether those glands were invaded by the rectal tumor. If histology confirms such evidence, then it would be regarded that those glands have been invaded by the rectal tumor, which was present in the posterior wall of the rectum and below the peritoneal reflection.[19-21]

Furthermore, the study confirmed that no lateral lymphatic spread did occur in those patients, whose rectal tumors were located above the peritoneal reflection.[21] From these clinical evidences, it was evident that lateral spread from the tumor below the level of peritoneal reflection does occur.

The lymphatic spread from the tumors in the anal canal or around the anal orifice drains into the lymph glands present in the inguinal region.

The lymphatic spread from the tumors present in the cecum, ascending colon and transverse colon follows the same principle, in that paracolic glands are invaded first. It continues to traverse the lymphatic plexuses along the tributaries and arterial branches of the right colic, or middle colic arteries, until they reach those glands present around the roots of the superior mesenteric vessels. Evidence of enlarged lymph glands at the root of the superior mesenteric vessels is a poor prognosis and curative resection of the tumor would be impossible.

■ Venous Spread

Like lymphatic channels, venous invasion by microscopical malignant cells does occur, but it occurs after the lymphatic spread has commenced and its invasion begins after the tumor has invaded the serosal layer.[22] This may lead to distant metastasis in the liver, and lung (Figs 2.5A and B).

The incidence varies from one study to another study and it depends upon the position of the tumor. Venous thrombosis may supervene in those cases, in which, venous invasion has occurred. A correlation with lymphatic spread has been reported. It seems to be more common among the cases with lymphatic spreads and its incidence was 21.6 percent. By contrast it was 13.7 percent found among other cases not invaded by the lymphatic channels.[7]

Furthermore, the incidence of venous invasion is associated with the tumor grades in that it was 5 percent found with grade I growth, 11.8 percent with grade II, 25 percent with grade III and 31 percent with grade IV tumors.[7]

Despite all these evidence, the prognosis does not always correlate with the evidence of venous invasion. Dukes reported that patient died of liver metastasis without venous invasion, on the other hand, patients had survived over 5 years despite the evidence of venous invasion being present.[22,23]

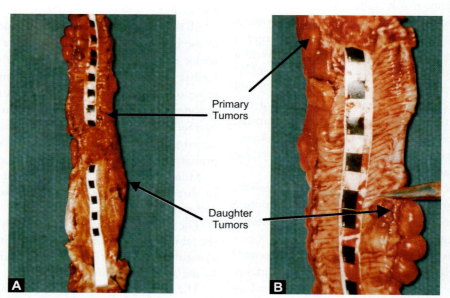

Figs 2.5A and B: Showing primary tumors; daughter tumors shown a little below the primary tumors

Spread of the Cancer by Transplantation

There are now conclusive evidences found in ex-foliated cytology that metastasis does occur by transplantation in the *in vitro* study and in clinical practice.[24,25]

Local implantation of the malignant cells into the mucosa, distal to the tumor may not occur by the lymphatic or vascular spread; but by spillage from the tumor. Such evidence has been found in the rectum, where multiple daughter tumors had been grown distal to the primary growth (Fig. 2.5A).

And dislodgement of the tumor may occur during mobilization of the rectum. In *in vitro* study, viable cancer cells were found to have shed into the lumen of the colon.[24,25]

Recurrence of cancer at the site of anastomosis could be the result of local implantation of the malignant cells. Furthermore, it has been claimed that a high incidence of local recurrence was found associated with the anastomotic leakage following a curative resection being carried out.

The incidence was 25.5 percent, compared with 10 percent found among the nonleaked cases in five years follow-up.[18]

Transcelomic Spread

This is another form of transplantation of the malignant cells, but its method of spread is quite different from the former category. It begins after the malignant cells have invaded the serosal surface, where they produce an inflammatory reaction leading to a secretion of exudates. It contains a lot of fibrin that enhances adhesions of the tumor to the adjacent viscera. And malignant cells are embedded into the fibrinous exudates that may induce local collection in which these fibrinous exudates may be floating and detached, or proliferated, leading to seedlings. In this process, the exudates with malignant cells may drop into the peritoneal cavity producing peritoneal ascites. Omental cake is the end result of transcelomic spread. It is commonly seen in carcinoma of the stomach and the tumor of the colon.

PROGNOSTIC FACTORS OF THE COLORECTAL CARCINOMA

Prognosis of the treatment is evaluated by macroscopical analysis of the tumor spread and by the histological analysis of the tumor cells.

Macroscopical features are apparent observation at the operation, but the tumor has already progressed beyond the apparent finding. Nevertheless, it provides a basic guideline to the surgeon on how the operative procedures need to be planned. To set up a common understanding of the tumor prognosis among the clinicians, and surgeon, a consensus policy has been established, on the tumor spread, and histological grade. The tumor spread takes place by various routes. These are direct spread, lymphatic spread, venous spread and transcelomic spread.

The direct spread extends beyond the palpation of the tumor. Because of these reasons, a wider field of resection is included in the curative excision of the primary tumor. This is an arbitrary decision of the surgeon on how far the level of resection is to be considered to be a curative operation. After the operative procedure being completed, the extent of the direct and other indirect spread is evaluated by the histology.

In addition to macroscopical spread of the tumor, the behavior of the malignant cells has been studied by the mitotic division and its character of the cell's nuclei. The histological studies have been compiled in four grades. They are Grade I, Grade II, Grade III and Grade IV.

DUKES STAGE OF THE COLORECTAL TUMOR

Stage I is the Dukes A – In this category, the malignant cells remain confined within the muscular wall of the colon or rectum. Its incidence is reported to be 15 percent in his study, but it could be variable that depends upon, how soon the diagnosis is made.

Stage II is the Dukes B – in this category, the tumor has invaded in continuity the extrarectal tissues, without invading the lymphatic channels and lymph glands. Its incidence is reported to be 35 percent.

Stage III is the Dukes C – In this category, the perirectal and distal lymph glands are invaded by the tumor cells. They migrate as emboli. Its incidence would be 50 percent.[26,7] This group has been again subdivided into Dukes C_1 and Dukes C_2. Dukes C_1 are those cases in which the perirectal glands have been invaded by the tumor and Dukes C_2 is referred in those cases in which the distal lymph glands are infiltrated by the malignant cells.

Stage IV is the Dukes D and are those cases in which the liver has been metastasized by the colorectal cancer cells.

HISTOLOGICAL STAGING

Although histological staging is also important in order to assess the prognostic factors histologically, readers are encouraged to seek further knowledge through the histology book. Only important aspects of histological features are outlined here in order to grasp the subject. The histological features have been classified into four grades. They are as follows:

Grade I – The tumor cells would appear like adenoma, but the difference from the adenoma is the evidence of increased epithelial proliferation and invasion. Its incidence was found to be 6.7 percent.

Grade II – In this section, the nuclei of the cancer cells will show deeply stained and they would appear to be irregular mitotic figures. Its incidence was 56.7 percent.

Grade III – In this section, the cells would appear to be less differentiated and mitotic figures would be more in numbers compared to the Grade II, and its incidence was 2.7 percent.

Grade IV – In this section, the tumor cells would be more anaplastic. Its incidence was 1.4 percent.

Colloid tumors – It is referred to as mucoid carcinoma. They are all grouped together, instead of classifying them into separate grades. Its incidence was 12.4 percent.[7]

In 1946, Dukes had revised his earlier classifications and changed to 4 categories. These are low grade, equivalent to Grade I, average grade to Grade II, and high grade are Grade III and Grade IV; and colloid carcinoma.[27]

Further conclusion could be made on the correlation between the macroscopical grading such as Dukes A,B, and C and the histological staging such as Grade I, II, III, and IV. Dukes concluded that Dukes A would have correspondence to Grade I and Dukes C to Grade IV.[7,28,29]

Although, Dukes tumor staging is an established map to the surgeons in certain countries, further consensus has been developed throughout the whole world by another form of tumor classifications. They are known as TNM classification and they are internationally used.

T_1, T_2, T_3, T_4 are related to the size of the tumors, but it is not possible to define the size of the colorectal tumor by any measurement.

N_0 is related to no involvement of the lymph nodes.

N_1, N_2, N_3, N_4 refer to the involvement of the regional lymph nodes by numerical number.

M_0 and M_2 would suggest presence or absence of distal metastasis.

The value of these types of prognostic factors is to correlate internationally how a particular modality has responded to a particular circumstance of the tumor behaviors.

REFERENCES

1. Smiddy FG, Goligher JC. Results of surgery in treatment of cancer of the large intestine. Br Med J 1957;1:793.
2. Frazer Sir John. Malignant disease of the large intestine. Br J Surg 1938;25-647.
3. Saha SK, Robinson AF. A study of perineal wound healing after abdominoperineal resection. Br J Surg 1976;63:555.
4. Saha SK Care of perineal wound in abdominoperineal resection. J Royal College of Surgeons, 1983;28:324.
5. Saha SK. A critical evaluation of dissection of the perineum in synchronous combined abdominoperineal excision of the rectum. Surg Gynec Obstet 1984;158:33.
6. Goligher JC. The operability of carcinoma of the rectum. Br Med J 1941;2:393.
7. Dukes CE. Cancer of the rectum: An analysis of 1000 cases. J Path Bact 1940;50:527.
8. Goligher JC, Dukes CE. Bussey HJR. Local recurrence after sphincter-saving excision for carcinoma of the rectum and rectosigmoid. Br J Surg 1951;39-199.
9. Ewing MR. Inflammatory complications of cancer of the cecum and ascending colon. Postgraduate Med J 1951;27-515.
10. Goligher JC, Smiddy FG. The treatment of acute obstruction or perforation with carcinoma of the colon and rectum. Br J Surg 1957;45-270.
11. Saha SK. Carcinoma of the cecum in elder lady presented with acute appendicitis 1981 (Unpublished report).
12. Miles WE. Cancer of the rectum. London: Harrison 1926.
13. Cole PP. The intramural spread of rectal carcinoma. Br Med J 1913;1:431.
14. Leitch A. Quoted by Miles WE 1926.
15. Westhues H. Die pathologisch-anatomischen Grundlagen der Chirurgie des Rektumkarzinoms. Leipzig: Thieme 1934.
16. Black WA, Waugh JM. The intramural extension of carcinoma of the descending colon, sigmoid and rectosigmoid. Surg Gynec Obstet 1948;87:457.
17. Quer EA, Dahlin DC, Mayo CW. Retrograde intramural spread of carcinoma of the rectum and rectosigmoid. Surg Gyne Obstet 1953;96:24.
18. Bell SW, Walker KG, Richard MJFX, et al. Anastomotic leakage after curative anterior resection results in a higher prevalence of local recurrence. Br J Surg 2003;90:1261.
19. Gilchrist RK. Fundamental factors governing lateral spread of rectal carcinoma. Ann Surg 1940;111:630.
20. Gilchrist RK, David VC. A consideration of pathological factors influencing five-year survival in radical resection of the large bowel and rectum for carcinoma. 1947;126:421.
21. Sauer FD, Bacon HE. A new approach for excision of carcinoma of the lower portion of the rectum and anal canal. Surg Gynec Obstet 1952;95:229.
22. Dukes CE, Bussey HJR. The spread of rectal cancer and its effect on prognosis. Br J Cancer 1958;12:309.
23. Sunderland DA. The significance of vein invasion by cancer of the rectum and sigmoid: A microscopic study of 210 cases. Cancer 1949;2:429.
24. Skipper D, Cooper AJ, Marston JE, et al. Exfoliated cells and in vitro growth in colorectal cancer. Br J Surg 1987;74:1049-52.
25. Umpleby HC, Fermor B, et al. Viability of exfoliated colorectal carcinoma cells. Br J Surg 1984;71:659-63.
26. Dukes CE. The spread of cancer of the rectum. Subsection in paper by C Gordon-Watson, Dukes CE. Brit J Surg 1930;17:643.
27. Dukes CE. The Dukes Classification of the rectum (or colon). Proce Roy Soc Med 1936.
28. Dukes CE. Histological grading of rectal cancer. Proc Roy Soc Med 1936;30:371.
29. Dukes CE. Personal communication 1946.

3 Presentation of Symptoms

In most instances, public remains ignorant about the symptoms arising from the cancer of the intestine. It would be difficult for them to recognize the seriousness of the symptoms attributable to colonic cancer from other nonmalignant bowel diseases. And they are sometimes misguided by the neighbors, relatives, and local practitioners. Patients from the developing or underdeveloped countries seek medical advice at the terminal stage, when the malignant tumor turns out to be inoperable.

In many instances, the symptoms attributable to malignant tumor may not be straightforward, and may mask with other disease such as amebic colitis. In these cases, they are often treated blindly, in line with the amebic colitis. And chronic anemia is often overlooked, because of ignorance. This condition is more often believed to be associated with poor nutritional diet, peptic ulcer disease and amebiasis.

Furthermore, screening program would be regarded to be luxury and expensive to the developing countries. To set up such a clinic requires public education and awareness, but it is a debatable issue whether it would be cost-effective, where the provision of free comprehensive health services is bare minimum to the needs of ordinary indigenous people.

Despite all these practical problems, symptoms of colonic carcinoma, in particular to those tumors developed in the cecum or ascending colon remain silent for several months. Constipation is very rare due to the fact that the cecum has a spacious capacity. This delays the symptoms to develop late and when it develops, the tumor has caused obstruction to the ileocecal valve or it has invaded to the parietal wall. In these cases, symptoms could be of various forms. These are loose motion, tiredness and anemia. In some cases, patient is presented with a loose motion and in other cases, anemia is recognized in routine blood test. These are often overlooked.

In this case, the investigation must include both upper and lower gastrointestinal tract in order to exclude malignancy in the stomach, pancreas, enlarged spleen and colorectal cancer.

Patients, in most instances, cannot remember their previous pattern of bowel habits, and when the change in habit has started. They are often vague about the duration of the symptoms. In all instances, leading questions should be put forward to the patient, asking specific question. This may assist in retrieving the near accurate symptoms, instead of relying upon their own description of their versions.

STRIKING SYMPTOMS OF COLONIC CARCINOMA

- Initially weakness or not feeling well
- May look pale or suffering from jaundice (in advanced condition)
- Loss of appetite
- Loss of body weight
- Abdominal pain or pain in the back or lumbosacral region
- Constipation – Requiring laxative
- Change in bowel habit
- Burping, funny noise in the belly
- Fullness either in lower or upper abdomen
- Discharge of mucus mixed with blood per rectum.

All these symptoms are nonspecific, until a detailed account of each symptom has been documented with duration of onset and associated changes in the well-being of the patients.

In routine blood test, low hemoglobin (<10 gm) is not uncommon without any evidence of blood loss. But it is very common among the laborers in the developing countries and is more often associated with amebic colitis and hook-worm sufferers. Nevertheless, a full investigation must be carried out to exclude malignancy.

It has been frequently found that carcinoma of the cecum remains symptoms-free or presented with an acute appendicitis or loose motions. Let me highlight a sad experience with one lady patient, aged 70. She was admitted with an acute appendicitis and her daughter was a theater sister in the District Hospital in Wales.

Clinically, there was a tender localized palpable mass in the right iliac fossa (RIF), but emergency operation was deferred because of her low hemoglobin. She had no bowel symptom and no other symptoms related to cecal carcinoma known to her, despite the fact that she was fully aware of the colonic tumor. Her hemoglobin on admission was around 8 gm/dl. This is very rare among the European people.

Initially, she was treated with conservative line of approach because of misleading diagnosis. The tender palpable mass in the right iliac fossa was considered to be appendicular mass. She responded to the conservative treatment, despite the fact that it was cecal carcinoma. Since she recovered well with conservative treatment, she had barium enema done a few weeks later, but the finding was inconclusive. Surprisingly, her hemoglobin dropped again. This prompted for undertaking an elective laparotomy. This turned out to be advanced cecal carcinoma with metastasis in the mesenteric lymph glands. Of course, it was regrettable that prognosis would have been better, if emergency operation were carried out on admission.

LOSS OF APPETITE, LOSS OF BODY WEIGHT AND NOT FEELING WELL

Many patients do not recognize the significance of these nonspecific symptoms, until they are questioned. They are correlated with the duration of the tumor and metastasis. In most instances, they do not know their body weight. In these situations, the loss of body weight could be established by asking them whether the present clothes are loose to their body or have noticed some changes in their fittings over the last few weeks.

Since this question has been referred to them, they started wondering in order to recollect their old memory and to find out the difference between what used to be six months ago and what has been the present fittings. From these differences, they would reply with a definitive answer without referring to the actual body weight. The loss of body weight may be associated with diabetes and hyperthyroidism. And in malignant disease, it denotes that this loss of body weight could be attributable to a poor appetite and it could be due to secondaries in the liver. Hence, it reflects a bad prognosis.

SYMPTOMS OF ABDOMINAL PAIN

It is regarded to be a late presentation and it would suggest obstructive feature of the large bowel, resulting from a partial obstruction by the tumor, advance growth, invading the parietal peritoneum, psoas muscle or other structures such as sacral plexus, posterior vagina, prostate gland, bladder or anal canal. In most cases, other symptoms such as poor appetite, loss of body weight and change in bowel habits would appear concurrently.

A change in bowel habit may be of various types. It could be either progressive constipation or a change in consistency of the feces. The usual presentation is constipation that requires laxative which may not be effective with regular usual dose. In some cases, patient may demand a larger dose. Constipation means less frequency of bowel action, and it also implies to hard feces. Period of constipation that is followed by loose motion at irregular pattern is the important clinical bowel symptom related to tumor in the distal colon or in the rectum. Persistent increasing constipation that requires laxatives is also regarded to be serious clinical feature of distal colonic tumor that requires an immediate investigation.

Other type is a change in bowel habit. It is one of the important classical symptoms associated with the colonic carcinoma, but it is frequently associated with the tumor in the distal colon and the rectum. It refers to abnormal habit, pattern or frequency of going to the toilet that would be quite different from his or her regular habit in everyday or week.

In other words, it denotes something different from his or her usual habit and it may refer to a frequency of bowel movement everyday, or every week over a month. Furthermore, this change in bowel habit is also measured by frequency per day or per week, and consistency of the feces. Any evidence of discharge of mucus mixed with or without blood is very important. Soft feces, loose motion, motion mixed with slime, associated with or without blood are also pathognomonic.

All these bowel symptoms may be missed, if the clinicians rely upon the patient's own description of symptoms. This may lead to a wrong diagnosis or the latter may be delayed and when the correct diagnosis has been made, it would be too late for the patient to be treated with a good prognosis. A curable disease would turn out to be incurable state of affairs at the end.

In this respect, the patient should be reassured and explained the merits of such questions prior to put specific question to the patient on those points.

These questions are:
a. When did you notice that you tend to open bowel less frequently and how long this problem has been going on?
b. Do you take laxative, for bowel action?
c. Have you noticed that the motion has become softer than usual over many weeks?
d. Have you noticed a lot of mucus or slime in the motion or when the bottom is wiped out with tissue paper or with water, as the case may be?
e. Have you noticed any blood mixed with motion or with slime?

In this way, it is better to extract the correct answer from the patients than relying upon the description of symptoms which may not be relevant to the lesion in the colon.

When a particular type of question is referred to the patients, they would try to recollect the symptoms which could be a difference between the old forgotten habit and the present symptoms.

BURPING AND FUNNY NOISE IN THE ABDOMEN

Burping denotes belching which is more often referred to as dyspepsia after a meal is taken. Physician tries to reassure the patient by referring to indigestion, duodenal ulcer, biliary dyspepsia due to gallstones, but in fact it may be associated with a serious and hidden pathological condition that may interfere with propagative peristalsis at the distal gut. It results from reverse peristalsis, initiated by the partial obstruction in the ileocecal region or thereafter.

It has been a unique experience, in dealing with a man of 70 referred to the clinic, because of complaining of dyspepsia. But surprisingly, simple history and rectal digital examination revealed the true pathology located in the other end of the abdomen. The diagnosis was carcinoma of the rectum and later gastroscopy did not show evidence of peptic ulcer disease.[1]

Therefore, burping may be an innocent symptom, but the primary pathology could be located anywhere between the cecum and the rectum. Advanced carcinoma, or annular growth may interfere with the passage of feces and flatus. This triggers exaggerated bowel sounds, due to increased or turbulent peristalsis, thus causing loud sound or excessive borborygmi. This may put the patient in an embarrassing position in the public place. Passage of flatus may relieve the symptoms and may reduce the fullness of the abdomen.

Apart from burping, patient may notice that the lower abdomen tends to be full or distended and may complain that their fitting around the waist seems to be tight. One has to bear in mind that many men and women tend to develop a pot belly in lower abdomen after the age of 40.

In sharp contrast, the upper abdomen tends to be full or blown up more than that in the lower abdomen, in those instances in which the colonic obstruction is in the sigmoid colon. In these cases, the transverse colon tends to be dilated and patient may have developed other bowel symptoms, as described before. These distinct clinical findings could be apparent on both inspections of the abdominal wall and by palpation.

DISCHARGE OF SLIME, MUCUS AND BLOOD PER RECTUM

In the developed countries, patient becomes alerted by the apparent painless discharge of fresh blood noticed in the commode, or in the toilet tissue paper. More often, it is associated with internal piles and constipation. This condition could also be attributed to an acute fissure-in-ano, if the fresh bleeding is associated with acute sharp pain in the anal orifice. Nevertheless, it should not be ignored unless proved otherwise.

But motion mixed with blood is regarded to be a serious clinical pathology. It could be due to a polyp, adenoma, rectal or colonic carcinoma, ulcerative colitis, proctitis, Crohn's colitis or amebic colitis. Many a times, patient recognizes the abnormal consistency in the feces and discharge of mucus or slime. The latter is usually associated with the growth in the rectum or anal canal. It is very unlikely to be attributed to the growth in the cecum or right colon. Discharge of slime or mucus is also associated with a foul odor. In amebic colitis or proctitis, feces are usually soft, mixed with yellowish jelly-like mucus, mixed with streaks of blood.

Despite all these symptoms being accurately recorded, exact location of the tumor could not be tentatively diagnosed without clinical examination and investigations. Nevertheless, statistically there are distinct differences in the symptoms that could refer to the possible site of the tumor, but these statistics are not reliable in clinical practice. In this section, all these differences have been compiled for the purpose of better clinical understanding and to avoid any pitfalls in clinical diagnosis.

SYMPTOMS ASSOCIATED WITH THE GROWTH IN THE RIGHT SIDE OF THE COLON

1. Patients remain symptoms-free for the early stage, but anemia may be early indication for cecal carcinoma, if pernicious anemia, piles or peptic ulcer disease could be excluded. Nevertheless, concomitant carcinoma in the colon must be excluded by all investigation.
2. Fullness in lower abdomen, with or without palpable lump in the right side of the abdomen would suggest cecal carcinoma, and Crohn's ileitis. Renal carcinoma or right hydronephrosis, volvulus of the cecum or sigmoid colon remains an alternative diagnosis. In female patient, ovarian cyst or ovarian tumor or fibroid of the uterus may be found concomitantly on clinical examination. In some cases, cecal carcinoma is diagnosed during emergency appendicectomy.
3. Discharge of slime per rectum or diarrhea is rare in this case.

SYMPTOMS ASSOCIATED WITH THE GROWTH IN THE LEFT SIDE OF THE COLON

1. Constipation could be a predominant presentation. In this situation, ignorant patients start treating themselves, without seeking any medical advice. They may take laxatives, add high roughage diet. If the constipation is a striking feature, patients tend to seek early medical advice. Or they could be admitted with an acute large bowel

obstruction. In this acute admission, the tumor is usually annular type of growth in the descending or sigmoid colon. Because of this early presentation, prognosis seems to be brighter. Around 25 percent of cases are admitted with acute large bowel obstruction.
2. A change in bowel habit, such as persisting constipation followed by diarrhea is also more prominent in clinical presentation among these cases. Mucus or slime in the soft motion are more often recognized by the patient, while wiping the bottom with a toilet tissue or with water that depends upon the hygiene habits of a particular country.
3. Fullness of upper abdomen, exaggerated bowel sounds or borborygmi could be an embarrassing situation in the public place. In chronic obstruction, the cecum takes the brunt of back pressure first, before the transverse colon is distended. It behaves like blowing up a balloon, where the distal end is first seen to be expanded.

SYMPTOMS ASSOCIATED WITH THE GROWTH IN THE DISTAL PART OF THE SIGMOID COLON, THE RECTUM OR ANAL CANAL

Clinical presentation for the growth developed in the sigmoid colon, rectum or anal canal depends upon the exact location and macroscopical features of the tumor. All symptoms may not correlate to the anatomical site of the tumor, but they may provide a broad clue for possible sites of the growth.
1. Annular type of the tumor is frequently located in the lower sigmoid colon and less frequently in the rectum. The symptoms develop much earlier and they are of colicky type of discomfort, associated with increasing period of constipation. In this situation, patient starts seeking medical advice and taking laxative, without realizing the true cause for progressive tendency for not going to the toilet.
2. In all other cases, the early symptom, if any, is the painless bleeding per rectum. More often, it is treated like piles or a fissure-in-ano. But on closer questioning, it would reveal that bleeding occurs at the end of the defecation or it comes mixed with feces. In some cases, patient notices blood in the underpant, although he did not go to the toilet. Pain is usually absent in the cancer of the rectum, but pain or discomfort seems to be a part of other symptoms, then it has to be considered that the tumor has invaded to the parietal wall, sacral plexus, prostate gland or vagina.
3. Constipation is the next striking feature. It tends to be increasing despite taking laxative. It may be associated with alternate episodes of diarrhea, followed by a period of constipation. This is often due to a change in bowel habit or alteration of bowel habit. In some patients, episodes of diarrhea become more frequent than constipation.

Many a times, patient develops urge defecation that forces him to get up early morning. This is not the usual habit of getting up out of bed and collection of mucus or slime and blood derived from the rectal tumor gives rise to urge defecation, but in the toilet, patient experiences discharging mucus and blood along with a little soft pipe stem type feces. This is referred to as a spurious diarrhea, bloody slime. These symptoms are frequently present in those cases in which the tumor is in the lower rectum.
4. Patient also experiences incomplete emptying of the bowel, after being to the toilet. This is another classical presentation in the cancer of the lower rectum.

Patient tends to strain in order to empty the rectum. This feature is known as tenesmus and patient uses toilet several times in the morning and throughout the day, because of an urge defecation and feeling of incomplete emptiness of the rectum at each attempt.

Various terminologies for these sorts of bowel actions have been referred to in the literature. They are morning diarrhea, bloody diarrhea, mucus diarrhea or spurious diarrhea. Early morning diarrhea and incomplete emptying of the rectum are frequently associated with the cauliflower type of tumor in the ampulla of the rectum.
5. Apart from the bowel symptoms, patient may experience pain in the lumbosacral region, believing of sciatica pain. In fact, the tumor has advanced and found fixed to the parietal wall, invading the sacral plexus. In other cases, patient may complain of pain around the anus, like fissure-in-ano, but in fact the tumor has invaded the lower anal canal, covered by the skin.

Bleeding per vagina may be associated with the invasion of the rectal cancer into the posterior fornix, thus forming a rectovaginal fistula. In male patient, passing of bubbles and feces per urethra may be reported because of rectovesical fistula.

MALIGNANT GROWTH IN THE ANAL CANAL

In most instances, the lesion in the anus is squamous cell carcinoma. It may occur in the chronic anal fissure. In this case, patient complains of pain in the anus. Rectal digital examination may reveal the hidden bomb as squamous cell carcinoma. Confusion may also arise for other carcinoma. Although, it may seem to be squamous cell carcinoma, but histology report may turn out to be adenocarcinoma in the anal canal. It is concluded that the tumor originally developed in the mucosa of the upper part of the anal canal but it has protruded further down to be palpable in the anal orifice. Other rare variety is the basal cell carcinoma, which develops at the area near to dentate line. Commonly it occurs at the anal verge and is a low grade tumor.

REFERENCE

1. Saha SK. Carcinoma of the rectum diagnosed as diverticulitis and later presented with dyspepsia. 1991 (personal experience).

4. Clinical Examination

CLINICAL EXAMINATION AND INVESTIGATIONS

General Examination

Although many clinicians start examining the particular part associated with the symptoms, assuming that the particular symptom has developed from the particular anatomical site. This practice is misleading. For instance, patient may complain of tiredness, loss of appetite and breathlessness on exertion. These symptoms may often be associated with chronic iron deficiency anemia, but these symptoms may be attributable to malignant disease. Patients are often ignorant in defining the accurate description of the symptoms. Therefore, methodical process must be adopted in all systematic examinations. It would take five more minutes, to complete the examination of all the systems. And the patient will have confidence that the surgeon has taken due care in the investigation of his or her illness.

It has been a recent trend in developed countries that one organ specialist seems to have been emerging from the training program, but the diseases are not confined to one organ. It affects the whole body. For instance, laparoscopic cholecystectomy is more often carried out by a specially trained laparoscopic surgeon who may not need to be trained for other specialties, but he needs to know everything on the way to enter into the peritoneal cavity. In this case, skin, muscle, blood vessels, peritoneum and all those organs inside the abdomen are each regarded to be one organ. But the surgeon should have full knowledge and training in handling with the operative injury to any one of those organs, before he reaches the gallbladder. Hence, a limited training program is detrimental to the patients.

The purpose of general physical examination of the patient is to establish the positive clinical findings and to assess the general state of the health. General clinical findings would be used to assess whether the patient would be reasonably fit for surgery; if that question arises in due course, once a definitive diagnosis has been made.

In the clinical examination, patient's cooperation is necessary. He should be asked to empty the bladder before all clothes, apart from the area of private parts are taken off. Patient is first asked to sit on a stool facing the clinician. In this position, inspection around the head, face, neck and chest is carried out.

First initial examination is the inspection. It begins from face and ends to toes. In the face, the lower eyelids are gently drawn down by the tip of the index finger. The purpose is to see the color of the lower conjunctiva. This may reveal whether the patient is anemic. Pale color reflects anemia, (Hb < 10 gm/dl). Yellow pigmentation in, the sclera of the eyes suggests jaundice which could be due to obstruction of the bile ducts, or hepatitis or cirrhosis of the liver. Suspicion for the latter should creep in, if there are evidence of spider naevi on the cheek.

Next examination is to see the mouth and tongue. Crack on the angles of the mouth and painless glossitis are the signs of iron deficiency anemia. In this case, the shape of the finger nails should be looked for. It may appear to be spoon-shaped in some cases of iron deficiency anemia. Coated tongue suggests irregular bowel movements and constipation. Malignant lesion should be excluded from the oral cavity or around the fauces. Evidence of fissure in the tongue or leukoplakia should be recorded and its significance must be evaluated with other investigation.

In the inspection of neck and supraclavicular fossa, dilated jugular veins suggest congestive cardiac failure or constrictive pericarditis or metastasis in the mediastinum causing pressure upon the superior vena cava. Any change in voice, evidence of goiter and enlarged lymph glands are recorded. Palpation around the neck should be carried out simultaneously. Evidence of enlarged lymph glands in both supraclavicular fossa, particularly on the left side of the neck requires further investigation in order to exclude malignancy in the guts or in the lung or thyroid glands.

For the assessment of nutrition and dehydration, both forearms are inspected, and nails of the fingers are examined. Clubbing of the finger nail and pale color of the palm are suggestive of heart-lung disease. Elasticity of the skin is tested by gently lifting a skin fold from the forearm, between the thumb and index finger. Lack of elasticity suggests poor nutritional state, loss of body weight and possibly dehydration. Whitish powder like skin flakes also suggests dehydration and poor nutritional state.

Before proceeding further down, permission of the patient is sought for the palpation of the breasts in order to exclude any discharge from the nipple or suspicious lump present in the breasts. This examination must be done in the presence of a female nurse and this is followed by the examination of both axillas. The right axilla is examined by the left and *vice versa* for the left axilla. During examination, patient's right forearm should rest upon across the surgeon's left forearm and *vice versa*.

If lymph nodes are palpable, their mobility and consistency must be recorded simultaneously. In addition, it is necessary to evaluate the axillary glands, whether or not they are tethered together and fixed to the overlying skin. During examination of the breast, distortion or retraction of nipple is examined by asking the patient to raise both forearms above the shoulder. This may reveal that one nipple is elevated to a higher level, compared to the contralateral one. This could be related to malignant tumor arising from the ducts. There could be appearance of any dimpling or puckering of the skin over the breast lump or peau d'orange present in the overlying skin around the breast lump. These are suggestive of malignant lump developed in the breast. These are broad clinical matters that may require further examination, methodically, if there is evidence of palpable breast lump.

EXAMINATION OF THE ABDOMEN

▪ Inspection

For the inspection and examination of the abdomen, patient is asked to lie flat on the back with knees straight on the examination table. Patient must lay in a comfortable position and in a relaxed state of mind. For this reason, the head must rest upon the pillows. Blanket or sheets should cover across the chest and also across the mid thigh. Surgeon should stand on the right side of the abdomen and should keep on chatting with the patient for a few minutes before proceeding with the examination. This gives a reassurance and provides a relaxation to the patient.

In the inspection, it is important to look for evidence of dehydration, nutritional state, and anemia.

Before examining the abdomen, inspection is also carried out in order to notice the size of the abdomen, shape of the umbilicus, visible peristalsis, known as step-ladder pattern of the small intestine, pulsatile mass, skin discoloration, any localized lump and dilated veins on either side of the umbilicus. And a conclusion could be made whether the abdomen is distended centrally, and umbilicus is protuberant. The next inspection is to see any evidence of distention along the flank, or upper or lower abdomen.

Patient is next asked kindly to take a deep breath in and then out through the mouth. After a pause, patient is next asked to give a cough. This will reveal free movement of abdominal wall and may show any evidence of bulging through the umbilicus or through the inguinal rings, in pari passu with the coughing. A painless free movement of the anterior abdominal wall on coughing excludes peritonitis.

At last, the lower limbs and both forearms are inspected for evidence of tissue dehydration or retention of tissue fluid.

TECHNIQUES FOR PALPATION

Before proceeding with palpation, patient's permission must be obtained whether he or she could be examined. It is also important to be sure that the palm of the hand must be warm, before touching the patient. Palpation begins from the face and is continued systematically downwards, one after another.

Abdominal palpation requires some degree of sensitivity in the palms and fingers. It also requires skill on how to palpate the mass under the abdominal wall. You can miss it, despite palpating the area, unless you know the difference between a normal abdominal wall and the abnormal one. There are a few types of palpation. They are superficial palpation, deep palpation and bimanual palpation. Deep palpation requires learning the skill on how to use the hand and fingers in the palpation.

Some patients particularly, female ones do not feel relaxed with their bare abdomen. In this situation, initial palpation should be done over her clothes or a thin sheet is left spread across her abdomen, and superficial palpation could be carried out through this sheet. Once she seems to be relaxed, the procedure could be repeated without this sheet.

SUPERFICIAL PALPATION

First the superficial palpation is just to palpate and feel the abdominal wall gently with the flat palm and straight fingers. It would reveal whether, the abdominal wall is soft, rigid, and flat or distended, associated with or without tenderness all around or around the localized area.

The palpation begins from epigastric region and it is continued right down to suprapubic regions and then all around the abdomen. This will give a general impression whether there is any palpable mass in any particular site of the abdomen and whether the patient experiences some discomfort or pain while moving around his abdomen.

DEEP PALPATION

After initial examination is completed, deep palpation is carried out but it requires technique on how to proceed with the fingers.

In this procedure, clinician should sit close to the couch and the level of abdomen should be near the level of forearm of the clinician. Once this position has been arranged, the thenar part of the palm is rested firmly on a particular site to be examined and then four fingers are placed together in straight position and gently over the surface of the abdomen. These fingers are pushed together, slowly and deep down through the abdominal wall.

The movement of those fingers is regulated by the flexor tendons at the metacarpophalangeal joints, where the gentle flexor movements will be like hinge movement. Tip of the fingers should be avoided in this palpation, but pulp of the fingers will try to feel something while pushing down. If there is a lump present under the fingers, it will resist the fingers for pushing further and the clinician will recognize resistance encountered with the lump.

All four fingers are slowly moved back in the same way, while the abdominal wall returns concurrently to its normal position. By this maneuver or technique, lump or mass could be palpated because of some gentle resistance encountered while pushing the fingers down through the abdominal wall.

In this method of palpation, firm or soft lump under the abdominal wall could be recognized. Once this finding becomes apparent in the deep palpation, the next procedure is to define its size, consistency and mobility.

Therefore, to complete the deep palpation, the clinician should decide how the palpation of the entire abdomen is completed. It is recommended that this palpation should begin from the left iliac fossa. While palpating in this area, it is important to palpate the groin. In this area, a few things could be palpated. These are lymph glands, lump in the inguinal region and pulsation of the femoral artery. Poor arterial pulsation could be attributed to atherosclerosis in the abdominal aorta and / or common iliac artery or a pulsatile lump would suggest aneurysm of the femoral artery.

After this quick palpation, the examination is continued along the left flank of the abdomen, using the right flat hand. In certain cases, deep palpation could be performed by both palms together, in that the right hand is first placed over the particular site of the abdomen and the left hand is placed over the dorsum of the right hand. Then the right hand is pushed down passively by the left hand. All other techniques of palpation remain the same.

During palpation along the left side of the abdomen, abdominal aorta must be palpated, whether it is pulsatile and tender to touch. In my clinic, an 80 years old man was referred, because of symptom of painless bleeding per rectum without any other bowel symptoms, but abdominal aortic aneurysm was diagnosed by a routine palpation and the rectal carcinoma was found on rectal digital examination. It was then confirmed by a rigid sigmoidoscopic examination at the same clinical examination. This was not my first experience and neither my last.

Therefore, it became apparent that the primary symptom did not have any correlation with the two major pathological lesions, found at the clinical examination in the outpatient clinic. It is a lesson to every clinician that thorough and systematic examination must be carried out, irrespective of the presentation of symptoms.

At the completion of the deep palpation, bimanual examination is carried out, between the left and right hands. In this case, the left hand is placed behind the left flank and right hand across the front of the left flank.

The purpose of the left hand being placed behind the left flank is to push the kidney or the colon forwards and keep holding them in position. This would push the organ or colonic mass forwards, closer to anterior abdominal wall and it would be easier to be palpated by the right hand palpated concurrently through the anterior abdominal wall. In some cases, both hands are pressed concurrently, one against the other, one from behind and other one from the front.

This maneuver is to push the anterior wall down against the posterior wall of the lumbar region, and it would assist to identify whether there is any abnormal mass, palpable between the two hands. If so, enlarged kidney, dilated renal pelvis, fatty lumps or palpable lump in the colon should be considered for differential diagnosis.

Apart from the colonic carcinoma, renal clear cell carcinoma, hydronephrosis, or retroperitoneal lipoma or liposarcoma remain the alternative diagnosis in some cases. Negative finding does not exclude malignancy.

If the left colon is palpable and appeared to have contained mass along the left colon, it is more likely to impact soft and lobulated hard feces, lying inside the descending or sigmoid colon. In most cases, this impaction of feces is attributable to the annular tumor or large colonic tumor mass, obliterating the lumen of the colon.

Multiple diverticula may contribute a narrow segment of the colon. This pathological condition may also lead to constipation.

Nevertheless, this finding could be clinically significant and consistent with the symptom of progressive constipation. A diverticular mass could not be ruled out in some cases. If tenderness is elicited on palpation, then diverticulitis or paracolic abscess remain a strong possibility.

The next examination is concentrated along the left subcostal margin, by the same bimanual examination. Patient is asked to breathe in deeply and slowly while palpating the spleen and the splenic flexure of the colon and then to relax after breathing is out. This is repeated a few times before proceeding to the right side of the abdomen.

Difficulty may be experienced in those cases in which the left kidney has enlarged, pushing the spleen and colon forward. In this case, diagnosis is made by other investigations. Enlarged spleen moves downwards and towards the midline or umbilicus. And it would have a smooth surface. In some cases, a notch in the anterior edge may be recognized by palpation.

After examination of the left flank, the right side of the abdomen is next examined. Deep palpation is commenced from the right groin. Like in left groin, inguinal canal, lymph glands and femoral artery pulsation are examined. Palpation is next continued along the right flank towards the right hypochondrium, where the gallbladder, liver and stomach are palpated in that order.

In chronic distal obstruction, the cecum seems to the first to be blown up slowly. Therefore, deep palpation may reveal whether the cecum is palpable, whether it is blown up or solid in consistency. In this examination, the flat surface of the right hand is gently moved around in clockwise and anticlockwise direction and side-to-side over the surface of the palpable lump. This maneuver may give some impression on the size, mobility and contour of the cecum or cecal mass.

For better assessment, bimanual palpation is also carried out; but it is done by placing hands in two directions. In first approach, the left palm is placed behind the right flank, with the fingers directed towards the loin and right hand is also placed in the same way over the anterior abdominal wall.

As stated before, the main purpose of placing the left hand behind the right flank is to push the colon forward, so that it comes to closure to the anterior abdominal wall and the cecum becomes easily palpable by the right hand. In addition, both hands are pressed one against the other concurrently. This will assist in defining the size and consistency of the mass in the cecum or in the ascending colon.

Apart from this palpation, deep palpation in the same area could also be carried out by changing the direction of both hands. In this case, the fingers of the left hand are directed towards the midline, and right hand towards the liver first and then towards the umbilicus. In this maneuver, the mobility and consistency of the tumor mass, if palpable between the two hands, are evaluated.

At the end, the right kidney is also examined like the left one. Liver and gallbladder are next palpated, whether the liver edge and boundary of the gallbladder could be mapped out beyond the costal margin.

During this examination, patient is asked to inspire deeply and slowly. This will allow the liver to move down with the descent of the diaphragm. In this position, the edge and surface of the liver could be palpated. During expiration, the liver will return to its original position with the elevation of the diaphragm. Furthermore, bimanual deep palpation should be undertaken in the palpation of the hepatic flexure of the colon, while examining the liver.

Finding of sharp liver edge is suggestive of cirrhosis of the liver and palpation of nodular surface of the liver is also suggestive of metastatic tumors, but it is not easily palpable, unless the liver has extended down, covering upper quadrant of the abdomen. Nevertheless, such finding reflects a poor prognosis.

TECHNIQUE FOR PERCUSSION

After palpation, percussion is done in order to determine any evidence of ascites, or solid tumor mass in any quadrant of the abdomen. This should be done methodically and systematically.

First, the percussion is performed by placing the three straight fingers on the patient's abdominal wall. The three fingers are index finger, middle finger and ring finger. They are placed apart from each other. The dorsal side of the middle finger is tapped or percussed by the tip of the right index finger in semiflexed position. It would be like hammering on the wooden board.

Each tapping will elicit either resonance or dullness in the note. To be sure, tapping is done on the side fingers alternatively with the middle finger. This may be necessary to be certain about the difference between the sound of resonance and that of dullness. And this question may arise if there is doubt or the site of percussion seems to be the site between the level of fluid and the loops of gut.

The procedure is carried out along the midline of the abdomen, from the epigastrium right down to the suprapubic region, then from the subcostal border along the flank, right down to the iliac fossa.

Then the procedure is repeated transversely across the abdominal wall, preferably at the level of umbilicus. If there is evidence of dullness along the flank, then it is necessary to confirm whether this is due to collection of intraperitoneal fluid or solid mass. Shifting dullness is the conclusive evidence of intraperitoneal fluid. It is associated with any one of these conditions. They are cirrhosis of the liver, carcinomatosis peritonei, tuberculosis peritonitis, congestive cardiac failure.

Shifting dullness could be demonstrated by two methods. If there is suspicion of a small amount of peritoneal fluid, the patient is asked to turn the abdomen to one side, for instance, he lies upon the right lateral flank. This will permit all fluid to be collected in the dependent side of the abdomen, occupying along the right flank or it may occupy one half of the belly.

After a few minutes, percussion is repeated, commencing from the contralateral flank or from the left side of the abdomen and it is continued transversely across the abdomen towards the other flank. The percussion in the area of left flank will be tympanitic or resonance note but it will begin to change to dullness on percussion in the area of right flank upon which the patient is resting or *vice versa* by changing the position, turning the patient to the opposite flank.

Alternative method is to carry out the percussion in supine position of the abdomen. It is commenced from the center of the abdomen and continued towards the one flank, where a difference note is elicited due to collection of fluid or solid mass. This is confirmed by repeating the percussion backward and forward on the same area, until the level of dullness is determined. And it is marked with skin pencil, if available.

The surgeon keeps his fingers over the site of dullness, while the patient is next asked to turn the body and belly to the other side with a view to lying on the other flank. Percussion is repeated. If resonance is elicited on percussion, then the conclusion would be that the dullness has shifted concurrently with the movement of fluid, thus confirming shifting of dullness, which is attributable to the transfer of fluid to the other side of the abdomen.

To confirm this finding further, the percussion is continued backwards towards the other side of the abdomen, where the intraperitoneal fluid has moved. The site which was in resonance on percussion before, will turn out to be in dullness on percussion.

By this maneuver the outline of appendicular mass, ovarian mass and full bladder could be mapped out. In female patient, cystic lump of the ovary could be confirmed by both palpation and by percussion.

Apart from the technique of percussion, intraperitoneal fluid could be demonstrated by the clinical method known as fluid thrill, peritoneal aspiration and by ultrasound scan.

TECHNIQUE FOR THE TEST OF FLUID THRILL

For the test of a fluid thrill, assistant is asked to put the ulna border of his or her hand along the linea alba of the midline. In this case, the fingers are directed either towards the epigastrium or towards the bladder that depends upon which hand is being used. This ulna border of the hand is kept pressing down through the linea alba of the patient's abdomen, thus obliterating the dead space.

The surgeon keeps his left palm in close contact over the flank, while he starts tapping over the contralateral flank. As a result, the fluid thrill is transmitted across to the other side of the abdomen, thus hitting to the abdominal wall where the surgeon could feel the fluid thrill in his left hand.

The evidences of peritoneal fluid are:
a. Centrally bulging abdomen.
b. Protuberance of the umbilicus.
c. Dilated veins running on either side of the umbilicus from groins towards the upper abdomen.
d. Shifting dullness.
e. Fluid thrill.

Apart from those examinations, difficulty may arise whether the localized mass or lump has been arising from the intraperitoneal organ or it remains all along outside the peritoneal cavity.

This doubt could be resolved by asking the patient to elevate in straight position of both lower limbs in the air above the couch. The intraperitoneal lump will not be palpable but extraperitoneal lump would be palpable.

At the end, both groins are examined for any evidence of inguinal or femoral hernia and any evidence of palpable lymph glands in the groin. Furthermore, in male patient, testes are palpated whether they are atrophic or one of them would appear to be large in size, heavy and hard in consistency. The clinical diagnosis would be testicular tumor. This finding would be significant, if there are enlarged para-aortic lymph nodes and cannonball type opacities noticed in the chest X-ray.

After the examination of the abdomen and groins is completed, a quick look around the ankles and feet should be done in order to demonstrate pitting edema over the medial malleolus, and dorsum of the feet. Both posterior tibial pulsation and pulsation of the dorsalis pedis should be recorded.

RECTAL DIGITAL EXAMINATION, PROCTOSCOPY AND RIGID SIGMOIDOSCOPY

Rectal Digital Examination

In this procedure, patient must be explained about the purpose of this local investigation. Permission must be obtained for internal examination that includes examination of vagina. In female patient, pressury or tamponade is removed by the patient or by the nurse, before rectal or vaginal examination is commenced.

No special preparation is necessary. The examination is normally carried out on the ordinary bed. A good illumination light that could be moved around for visual inspection of the lesion present around the anus is necessary.

Patient is asked to turn and lie on the left lateral position with both knees held up towards the groins. The pelvis is covered with sheet but underpant needs to be taken down. All necessary equipments must be assembled in a tray. The fiberoptic light source and its fittings must be checked before instrument is inserted into the rectum. Long biopsy forceps, suction machine and long swab holding forceps must be available and is kept nearby for ready use if necessary.

The perineum and anal orifice are inspected and palpated under direct illumination in order to see any evidence of acute or chronic fissure-in-ano. It is normally located in the posterior wall of the anal orifice. In rare cases, and in female patient, it may be present in the anterior wall of the anal orifice. There may be anal skin tags hanging from the anal verge or from the posterior edge of the chronic posterior fissure-in-ano. Multiple anal warts could be present around the anus. In addition, a few may be found inside or around the posterior vaginal wall.

After this initial inspection and examination, the right index finger, soaked with KY jelly is gently inserted into the anal canal. If the patient experiences pain or discomfort, no further procedure should be done. Rarely, anal-stenosis may be encountered, in which case, insertion of index finger may be difficult. This condition is the result of chronic fissure-in-ano.

Therefore, the anal orifice needs to be examined under spinal or general anesthesia in the theater. A separate arrangement has to be organized for the patient and a provision for a surgical treatment for this condition should be made with the consent of the patient. Otherwise, patient may need a second anesthesia for a definitive surgery to be done later on.

During this digital examination, the palmar surface of the index finger is moved around keeping in close contact with the wall of the anal canal and the rectum. It moves sideways in clockwise and anticlockwise directions, and follows the posterior concave curvature of the sacrum. This movement first takes place in clockwise direction, commencing from the 6 O'clock position and then the finger continues sideways along its wall towards the right lateral direction, until it reaches at around 11 or 12 O'clock position. The finger is brought back to 6 O'clock position and it is moved other ways in anticlockwise direction along the left lateral wall of the anal canal and rectum, until it reaches to around 1 O'clock or 12 O'clock position.

During this palpation, concentration is kept on about the smooth or irregular mucosal surface, mobility of the mucosa and any irregularity felt or any induration of the mucosa felt, while moving and palpating the anal canal and rectum. And finally the hand is turned around, in order to bring the palmar surface of the index finger across the anterior wall of the anal canal and rectum.

In performing this maneuver, the surgeon needs to turn his body and face in a half-circle and in an anticlockwise direction, thus facing backwards. This would allow the rotating half circle of his right forearm and arm in similar anti-clock wise direction, in straight position. The palmar surface of the index finger will face the anterior wall of the anal canal and the rectum.

Without this maneuver, the anterior wall of the rectum and anal canal cannot be palpated. And by this maneuver, the surgeon will be able to palpate the cervix uteri through the anterior wall of the rectum. By this method, any invasion of the tumor into the vaginal canal could be identified.

In male patient, the surface of the prostate gland is examined in the same position, by the palmar surface of the index finger. It requires side-to-side movement of the fingers like the movement of a pendulum, in order to palpate its anatomical features. In this assessment, the following features are examined: These are the size and consistency of the prostate glands, mobility of the rectal mucosa over the posterior surface of the prostate gland, and any evidence of irregularity of the posterior surface of the gland, palpation of its midline sulcus and that of the lateral gutter that lies around the outer edge of the glands with the parietal rectal wall.

During palpation over the convex surface of the gland, a firm nodularity could be felt by the palmar surface of the index finger. These findings could be suggestive of carcinoma or it could be attributable to prostatic stones imbedded in the prostate glands. Straight X-ray of the pelvis or transrectal ultrasound scan could assist the differential diagnosis.

In addition, attempt is made to reach to the upper limit of the prostate gland. This would assist the approximate weight of the gland, although such evaluation requires experience over many years. It assumed that the weight of the gland could be in excess of 50gm, if the upper limit of the gland cannot be reached.

All these findings would be invaluable later, if the patient develops acute retention, or difficulty in voiding urine or chronic retention and if the patient requires abdominoperineal resection of the rectum.

Among all these features, obliteration of the midline sulcus or the lateral gutter is suggestive of carcinoma of the prostate glands. Furthermore, invasion of the gland by the rectal carcinoma sitting just behind the prostate gland would indicate a poor prognosis and it would alarm the surgeon in advance whether the tumor would be resectable or how to take necessary measure in mobilizing the rectum from the prostate gland.

During the examination, concentration is also focused on whether the tip of the index finger could feel something hard higher up or outside the rectum. There are two possibilities in this finding. One of the possibilities is the growth located a little above the reach of the finger and the second possibility is the annular tumor, although developed in the sigmoid colon, has been lying in the rectovesical or rectouterine pouch. Sometimes, hard feces in the sigmoid colon may give a misleading impression.

At the completion of the rectal examination, the finger stall is examined for any evidence of blood and slime. Presence of slime may give rise to foul smell; the source of the blood is more likely to be from the friable or ulcerated tumor. If it is dark in color, it should be venous blood. In the absence of any evidence of tumor, one could assume that tumor could be located further up, beyond the reach of the tip of the finger. In other cases, it may arise by contact with the inflamed rectal mucosa. This is known as contact bleeding and the blood is more likely to be of arterial origin. And it could be associated with postradiation proctitis, ulcerative colitis or from the hemangioma.

After rectal digital examination, vagina is next examined by the index finger. Glove is changed and patient's permission is obtained. This examination is carried out in the left lateral position, but the position may require to be changed, from lateral to supine position with both knees in flexed and partial abducted position, if necessary.

The purpose of vaginal examination is to confirm the evidence of invasion of the rectal tumor into the posterior fornix and to confirm whether the rectal tumor has invaded the entire posterior vaginal wall. The cervix uteri are also palpated in order to exclude the evidence of ulcer in the osteum of the cervix, unrelated to the rectal carcinoma. Bimanual examination should be done whether uterus is free from the rectal growth. At the completion of digital palpation, the vaginal canal needs to be inspected by direct vision with a speculum inserted into the canal, but biopsy should not be taken without giving general anesthesia.

IMPORTANT FEATURES OF THE RECTAL CARCINOMA, RECORDED ON RECTAL DIGITAL PALPATION

a. Edge of the ulcerated tumor elevated, everted, and hard in consistency.
b. Evidence of deep ulcer crater in the base or center of the growth.
c. Evidence of annular growth through which the finger could be negotiated without causing pain or discomfort—an indication of poor prognosis. It implies that the duration of the tumor is more likely to be greater than 2 years of age.
d. Palpation of induration around the base of the growth.

FEATURES OF ADVANCED AND POOR PROGNOSIS

a. Dislodgement of necrotic and friable tumors.
b. Evidence of fixity of the base of the tumor either over the sacral wall, or in regard to anterior wall of the rectum.
c. Evidence of rectovaginal invasion or rectovesical fistula.
d. Annular carcinoma.

During this procedure, any abnormal tissue, lump or ulcer or growth is kept in memory until the examination is completed and recorded in the case notes. This is a blind procedure, but certain characteristic features appreciated by the direct palpation will give the diagnostic clue and lead to further invasive examination.

An over-all impression could be drawn up from this palpation on the basis of certain characteristic macroscopical features. These are induration, elevation of edges, ulceration, cauliflower type or annular type of the growth.

If the tumor appears to be encircling all around the circumference of the rectal wall, gentle attempt is made to negotiate the index finger through the narrow stricture in order to palpate the size and fixity of the growth.

If no tumor is palpable in the rectum, but the symptoms are suggestive of cancer in the bowel, then it is wise to pursue the rectal examination further, whether something could be felt higher up.

In this case, the finger can slowly be advanced like a cork-screw and it could be pushed further up, upto the knuckle of the finger through the anal orifice. If successful, the position of the tip of the index finger will reach near the upper third of the rectum, which could be around 10 cm from the anal verge. When the finger is withdrawn, the finger stall is examined for blood, or slime.

If the growth is palpable by the tip of the finger, its edge, its consistency, mobility and shape are documented. In this instance, it is important to assess simultaneously during rectal digital examination about other macroscopical features of the tumor, whether or not it is nodular, ulcerative, and annular or cauliflower type of the growth and whether it has a broad base or a pedunculated stalk.

The evidence of circumferential spread around the wall, its mobility, and induration are very important. These findings would indicate the age of the tumor and prognosis of the surgical treatment. The anatomical position of the tumor, whether it is located in posterior wall, anterior wall, lateral wall and covering all around or a particular quadrant of the rectal wall, must be documented. This would guide the perineal surgeon on how the growth could carefully be mobilized from the surrounding wall, without breaking the specimen of the rectum through the tumor bed. All these findings are important and carry a prognostic prediction.

Apart from the malignant growth, benign adenoma, pedunculated polyp, villous adenoma could be palpated by this simple examination.

METHOD OF INSTRUMENTATIONS THROUGH THE ANAL CANAL AND THE RECTUM

Description of Proctoscope

The common instruments used are; proctoscope, sigmoidoscope, biopsy forceps, fiberoptic light source, suction apparatus, swab holding forceps, and a flexible standing lamp for the perineal illumination. No rectal washout or any special preparation is necessary.

In the past, metal proctoscope was the only instrument that used to be employed for the inspection of the anal canal. Now, disposable plastic type proctoscope is available. The proctoscope, whether made with steel or plastic has different sizes, both in length and diameter. It has an obturator, and a handle for holding the instrument. Its main purpose is to establish the cause for painless fresh bleeding, identification of fistula-in-ano, anal polyps or villous adenomatous lesion. Its therapeutic purpose is to inject the phenol in almond oil to the internal piles or to the partial mucosal prolapse. It is also used for taking tissue from the growth in the anal canal.

Milligan-Morgan proctoscope is commonly used in most instances. Its length is 2¾ inches, and diameter is 7/8inch at the terminal end and 1¼ inch at the other end or base. The reason for making the base wider is to make easier for withdrawing the obturator and probably it helps the surgeon to visualize the structure inside the anal canal through the wider opening.

The end of the proctoscope could be an oblique or a transverse cut. The oblique cut facilitates to isolate the particular pile that needs to be injected with injection of phenol in almond oil. This isolation is done by pressing the oblique tip against the wall of the anal canal. But for the purpose of diagnosis, the transverse cut is suitable and all three piles could be seen through the one field of vision that is only possible through the transverse cut end.

The handle through which a tunnel has been created for the insertion of fiberoptic light bulb has been mounted on the side wall at the broader end of the proctoscope and it is fixed obliquely to the shaft of the tube, so that instrument could be pushed into the anal canal slightly obliquely that would not obscure the anal orifice while inserting the instrument.

For the children and for the cases with acute anal fissure, a narrower tube is available, but it should not be used in the presence of acute pain in the anus.

The new disposable variety of the plastic proctoscope is slightly longer and narrower.

■ Description of Sigmoidoscope

Sigmoidoscope is another instrument, used for the examination of the rectum and sigmoid colon. No bowel preparation is necessary in most cases. It is a diagnostic tool for various types of lesions. These are tumors, diverticulosis, ulcerative colitis, and proctitis. It is used for the location and identification for the various macroscopical features and types of the rectal and colonic tumors. It is used for removal of foreign body, biopsy and for polypectomy.

It is a straight, long, metallic and rigid tube. It has different sizes in length and diameters. Its length varies between 25 and 30 cm, its diameter is between ½ and ¾ inch. There is a detachable eyepiece to be fitted at the proximal end and its distal end is open through which the terminal end of the obturator is passed. The eyepiece has glass window and other fittings. One of them is the setting of the fiberoptic light bulb that is attached with a long flexible fiberoptic cable. The latter is connected to the main fiberoptic light source.

In addition, the eyepiece has a nozzle to be attached with bellows and rubber tube. The latter is used for air insufflations, in order to inflate the rectum and the sigmoid colon. In some cases, the detachable eyepiece fitted with magnifying lens could be used for better visualization of the mucosa and growth, but it has no other operating value.

Nowadays the metallic sigmoidoscope is less used, instead a disposable sigmoidoscope is commonly used. It is made up with transparent plastic rigid tube of same design. Although it is around 25 cm in length, only 22 cm in length could be inserted into the rectum and sigmoid colon.

All variety of sigmoidoscope has been marked with numerical number by each cm on the surface of the tube. This will indicate to the clinician on how far the rectum or the sigmoid colon has been examined by this instrument from the anal verge. And by this measurement, the lower margin of the tumor from the level of anal verge could be identified. Such measurement will guide the surgeon about selection of a particular operative technique to be used in his patient.

The clinician will also recognize, by reading the marking on the surface of the sigmoidoscope, whether the tip of the sigmoidoscope has reached the rectum or sigmoid colon or at what level the examination has been carried out. Such reference is very important in subsequent examination. If the polyp has been snared from a particular site, and its anatomical level is recorded by measurement of the sigmoidoscope, then in future follow-up, repeat sigmoidoscopic examination will reveal whether the tumor has recurred in the same place from the anal verge.

This is only possible if the tip of the sigmoidoscope has reached around the site, by looking at the measurement on the wall of the instrument at the level of anal verge and it would be easier to be ascertained whether the tumor has recurred in the previous site, that is only possible by placing the tip of the sigmoidoscope at the corresponding level. This is a broad assessment and it is not a foolproof clinical practice.

In this new design, the eyepiece is made by contrast with a metal and it has a lid, fitted with a glass window. This glass window lid, fitted with the metallic eyepiece tube is operated by a hinge joint attached to one side. The whole eyepiece, unlike that of the old design, is fitted by clockwise rotation over the proximal end of the tube. Its purpose is to prevent from blow-out if a high intraluminal rectal pressure is built up. It is reuseable after sterilization.

All other fittings with the eyepiece are the same like the old one, but the fiberoptic light is incorporated at the distal end and is illuminated when the fiberoptic light source is switched on. All the fittings should be completed before it is pushed through the anus.

Furthermore, its outer wall has a thin layer of dry lubricating material, coated all around, at the source of manufacture. Therefore, no further lubricating jelly would be necessary. But the sigmoidoscope needs to be run through warm water, before it is used.

Nevertheless, the obturator that is inserted through the proximal window of the eyepiece, needs to be soaked with lubricating jelly. Many surgeons assemble the fittings after the sigmoidoscope along with its obturator, has been inserted into the rectum. This procedure may cause injury to the rectal mucosa; while the eyepiece is fitted by clockwise rotation. Therefore, it is safe to assemble all the fittings first with the sigmoidoscope, before it is pushed into the anal canal.

The length of the biopsy forceps and suction tube must be longer than the length of the sigmoidoscope.

Apart from the rigid sigmoidoscope, flexible fiberoptic sigmoidoscope up to 100 cm in length is used very frequently. Its operation and function are no different from the colonoscope, apart from its length. It has many clinical and operative advantages in the management of colorectal diseases, but bowel preparation is necessary in most instances and patient may need short-acting sedation and anti-spasmodic agent or analgesia in certain cases.

METHOD OF PROCTOSCOPY

Many patients do have apprehensions regarding any kind of instrumentation to be used for internal examination. They need to be explained about the purpose and benefit for such examination and they need to be reassured in every stage before, during and after the procedure being completed. Furthermore, the patient should be asked whether the procedure is hurting or is it uncomfortable. Procedure should be discontinued straightaway, if there is any sign of discomfort or resistance experienced.

■ Procedure

Position of the Examination Table in the Outpatient Clinic

In most hospitals, the height of the table could be adjusted by the paddle fitted to the table and it should be according to the choice of the surgeon. He does not need to bend too much forward and he should be in comfortable position. Therefore, he should adjust the height of the table according to his choice.

Position of the Patient

Attending nurse should assist the patient how and in what position the patient should lie on the table. Patient should take off the underpant before lying on the left lateral position and the bottom of the body and legs are covered with long cotton sheet. It is preferable to keep the buttock resting on the edge of the table near the surgeon and to lay the patient's body obliquely across the table and away from the surgeon. Both knees are forward towards the belly in flexed position, but both feet should be away from the surgeon's side or near the other edge of the table. Adjustable light source should be standing at the bottom of the table.

■ Procedure for Proctoscopy

It is important to exclude any evidence of acute anal fissure, before the proctoscope is inserted through the anal orifice and for establishing this acute condition, index and middle fingers of both hands are placed on either side of the anal verge. It is preferable to lay the swabs over each side of the anal verge, upon which the fingers are placed. The swabs, held by the fingers assist in retracting the perianal skin of the anal verge, away from the anal orifice.

If there is no acute fissure-in-ano, internal examination is done by the right index finger, using generous KY jelly. Before proceeding with this approach, patient should be notified in advance about each step of procedure, reassuring him that there is no need to be frightened. The purpose of gentle digital examination prior to proctoscopic examination is to assess whether there is anal stenosis and whether there is any growth in the anal canal. Furthermore, it gives a reassurance to the patient.

Proctoscope fitted with the obturator is soaked with KY jelly. It is held firmly around its flange, between right index finger at one side and middle finger on the other side of the flange and handle of the proctoscope is firmly grabbed by other fingers. In addition, end of the obturator handle is held down firmly by the thumb, so that the obturator butt does not slip out from the proctoscope, when the instrument is pushed through the anal orifice.

During the negotiation through the anal orifice, the patient is again asked to be relaxed and breathe in and out gently. This will assist to relax the sphincteric muscles. The upper buttock and the perineum are both retracted gently up by the left thumb or fingers, thus revealing the anal orifice in sight. The butt of the obturator is gently pushed through the anal orifice and it is directed towards the sacral curvature. Gentle and steady pressure onto the obturator is maintained, while it is progressing through, until it enters into the anal canal. Simultaneously, surgeon should ask the patient by saying: "Are you all right? Am I hurting you?"

Once the proctoscope has passed the anal orifice, it is gently pushed further until the flange has reached the anal verge. The flange is next grabbed by the left index and middle fingers.

This is necessary to keep the proctoscope steady in position, when the obturator is gently withdrawn from the proctoscope. Any evidence of blood or necrotic tissue gives an advance indication for pathological lesions. This could be proctocolitis, postradiation proctitis or it could result from mechanical trauma to the mucosa.

The proctoscope is next held in position by holding its handle with the left hand. For convenience and for a better visualization, the position of the handle could be moved around, but it should be at 9 O'clock position of the anal orifice. The surgeon's right hand is now free. For a better illumination, the fiberoptic light bulb is inserted through the tunnel, incorporated in the body of the handle.

Surgeon needs to see inside the anal canal and end of the proctoscope may require to change its position and direction in various ways, until, a good view is obtained. The loose motion may need to be cleaned up and wiped out with a small swab, held in the forceps.

The lumen of the rectum may be obscured either by the lumps of feces or the distal opening end is touching against the wall of the anal canal. In this situation, the proctoscope could be moved around in different directions or it could be pulled out for a short distance, until the view of the anal canal is in sight.

Once the position of the proctoscope has been set up, the color and macroscopical abnormal mucosal features are noted. In normal state of the anal canal, submucosal veins could be seen clearly, but they would be obscured if there are features of granular proctitis, ulcerative proctocolitis or tumor or contact bleeding.

After withdrawing the proctoscope for a few millimeters, internal pile will appear protruding through, showing congested and dilated veins in the lump of the anal mucosa that may occupy a part of the distal opening of the proctoscope. By changing the position or angle of the proctoscope, each quadrant could be examined separately, whether there is a pile in each anatomical site. Their anatomical positions are located at 4 O'clock, 7 O'clock and 11 O'clock position.

At the completion of the inspection, decision has to be taken whether any one of these piles needs to be treated, either by injection of 5 percent phenol in almond oil, or with rubberband ligation or by operation. This depends upon the frequency of episodes of bleeding and size of the pile, provided there is no malignant growth higher up in the rectum.

Apart from the findings of piles, other abnormal condition needs to be looked for, whether there is any evidence of fistula-in-ano, anal polyps, papilloma, or carcinoma. For the diagnosis of perianal fistula, the internal opening could be seen either anteriorly or posteriorly. It is not easy to locate the osteum, unless, a streak of watery or pus discharge is seen leaking through the opening. A gentle massage on the perineal skin may assist the diagnosis.

The treatment of piles has been described in another chapter.

TECHNIQUE FOR SIGMOIDOSCOPY

Like proctoscopy, bowel preparation is not necessary, but it may be necessary, if the rectum contains impacted feces. In this case, procedure should be abandoned with a view to bringing him back in another day. In the mean time, he should be prescribed to take laxative for a few days prior to the procedure being re-booked. Alternatively, he should be given glycerine or Dulcolax suppository in the rectum two hours before putting him on the table.

Alternative to suppository is the phosphate enema that could be given a few hours before the procedure is carried out. Soap and water enema or rectal wash-out would make worse due to the fact that there would be lot of watery motion retained inside the lumen of the sigmoid colon and the rectum. If such preparation is indicated, then this has to be done a day before.

POSITION OF THE PATIENT

Position of the patient is similar to the one described for proctoscopy. It is advisable to put pillow underneath the buttock, and the latter should be brought further towards the surgeon's side of the table, i.e. over the edge of the table, so that sigmoidoscopy could be manipulated easily in many direction. If this simple maneuver is not carried out, movements of the surgeon's head will be restricted due to a limited space below the level of the anus.

Furthermore, elevation of the anal orifice may enhance a better manipulation of the sigmoidoscope inside the rectum, in which, the round feces tend to drop down in the bottom of the rectal wall, because of gravity, when the rectum is inflated by the air that occupies above the lumps of feces. As a result, the end of the sigmoidoscope could easily be advanced under direct vision through this air-space—thus, by-passing the lumps of feces.

Again the perineum and anal orifice are examined, as described before, before the instrument is inserted through the anus. Rectal digital examination is also carried out, as described before. This gives reassurance and confidence to the patient. All these preliminary procedures, as described before with proctoscope, are repeated in this procedure.

The instruments are assembled, as described in the previous pages. Nowadays, disposable plastic sigmoidoscope is commonly used.

SIGMOIDOSCOPY

Sigmoidoscopy requires technical skill and understanding of the anatomy of the sigmoid colon and the rectum. The difficult area is the rectosigmoid bend where gentleness and skill of manipulation of the instrument is necessary. This will be highlighted later.

INDICATION FOR SIGMOIDOSCOPY

It is an investigation. It confirms clinical and tissue diagnosis. It can provide a limited operative treatment in certain cases.

■ Procedure

Surgeon keeps holding the proximal end of the sigmoidoscope along with the handle of the obturator firmly in his right hand and keeps his left elbow gently resting on the patient's right buttock. Due care is taken that the butt of the obturator is not slipped back into the lumen of the distal opening, while the sigmoidoscope is pushing through the anus. To stop this happening, the other end of the obturator is held firmly down with the proximal end of the sigmoidoscope by the right hand.

Next job is to display the anal orifice. This is done by retracting the over-hanging right buttock and perineal skin away from the anal orifice by his left thumb or by index and middle fingers, as described with the procedure of proctoscope.

Under direct vision, the distal end of the obturator along with the distal end of the sigmoidoscope is slowly negotiated through the anal orifice. At the same time, patient is asked to breathe in and out gently, while pushing the end of the sigmoidoscope through the anal orifice.

The direction of the obturator is directed towards the sacral curvature at horizontal level. Once it has passed beyond the anal canal for a distance of about 5 cm, the obturator is withdrawn slowly. Sometimes, resistance may be encountered in removing the obturator. It may be found jammed at the distal end, if old type instrument is used, but it is unknown in the new disposal sigmoidoscope. The eyepiece is next fitted and light source is switched on.

The surgeon now needs to look through the window of the eyepiece, in a good illumination, whether the end of the sigmoidoscope has reached the anal canal or rectum or is it still in the anal orifice? If so, the instrument is withdrawn and the procedure is repeated. At this time, it is important to be sure that the instrument has at least entered into the anal canal.

The obturator should not be withdrawn from the lumen, until 5 cm in length of the sigmoidoscope has entered into the rectum. Further internal inspection is done through the window of the eyepiece, in order to be sure that it is in the rectum and to see whether there is a lot of loose motion entering into the distal end of the instrument; if so, the eyelid is removed, and a long suction tube is passed through the proximal end in order to suck out all liquid feces.

If the loose motion is running into the lumen of the instrument and the problem could not be overcome by repeated suction, the procedure should be abandoned.

If there are soft feces at the entrance of the tube, this could be wiped out by passing a long swab stick. The eyelid is put back and further examination is repeated, by pushing some air by squeezing the bellows. This air will open up the lumen of the rectum.

If on the other hand, the distal opening of the sigmoidoscope appears to be partially obscured due to sticky lumps of feces, in this situation, air is pushed by squeezing the bellows. It has two benefits; in that air pressure would by-pass those lumps of feces, and the lumps of feces may drop down by gravity and by intraluminal air-pressure, concurrently with the distention of the rectal wall. A clear air space becomes evident along the upper half of the lumen of the rectum.

The sigmoidoscope is now advanced slowly through the air-space under direct vision, seen through the window of the eyelid, until the lumen of the rectum becomes obscured once again. In some cases of partial obscurity inside the rectum, the distal end of the instrument could be negotiated, by pushing the feces sideways.

In some cases, the vision within the lumen of the sigmoidoscope turns out to be obscured, this could be attributable to poor light, fault in the bellows or loose motion or soft feces, sticking around the terminal edge of the instrument. In this case, further air could be pushed at the same time, while looking around inside by moving the scope in different directions by the left hand. If no better, then the tube is pulled back for a centimeter until the lumen is in sight again.

Too much distention of the rectal wall may cause distention of the lower abdomen and patient may experience colicky pain. Furthermore, there could be acute bend by the distended gut. Hence it is advisable not to push too much air. It may cause further angulation, obscuring the vision within the passage.

In most cases, sigmoidoscopy is not a difficult task up to the level at 10 cm from the anal verge. In fact, many surgeons or clinicians are contended with this limited examination. They rely upon other investigation, such as colonoscopy, barium enema and CT scan.

But, surgeon needs to know the accurate level of the tumor, any other primary smaller tumor present nearby. And tissue diagnosis is very important for a definitive mode of treatment. Therefore, further examination above the level of 10 cm should be attempted, if possible.

The upper end of the rectum takes a different course at the rectosigmoid junction, where, it bends forward and then turns towards the right and finally towards the left to be continued as descending colon. At this level, the rectum would appear like a blind end, popularly known as cul-de-sac in the western people. Overdistention may cause further bend in this area.

To overcome this bend, the direction of the distal opening of the instrument may need to be moved forwards first through the lumen of the rectum and then towards the right under direct vision, seen through the window of the eyelid. To follow this bend, the eyepiece of the instrument is moved by the left hand concurrently, while keeping busy in seeing through the window of the eyelid. No maneuver must be attempted blindly.

The instrument must not be manipulated through the course of the bend blindly and without displaying the clear view of the lumen, which could be of semilunar shape because of rectal valve or acute bend. Sometimes, this partial view could be overcome by just gently elevating the bend with the terminal edge of the instrument.

Every attempt should be made to display the lumen of the rectum, before proceeding further. In this maneuver the instrument may need to be swung in different directions under direct vision through the eyelid. Once the lumen is evident, the instrument is safe to advance again until it has reached at the rectosigmoid region which is around 12-15 cm from the anal verge. This position is identified by looking at the measurement, printed on the surface of the instrument.

Despite a careful procedure being undertaken, the instrument may not reach the sigmoid colon and once this difficult bend has been overcome, further advancement of the instrument would no more be difficult.

The instrument could reach to its full length easily up to 22 cm, if disposal instrument is used. A sigmoidoscopist should be aware of the macroscopical features of diverticulum present in the wall of the sigmoid colon. It may simulate like a true lumen of the rectum or colon. Therefore, there remains a potential risk of perforation through this diverticulum, if the instrument is forced through as if, believing of a true lumen of the gut. This may lead to bleeding, and fecal peritonitis and eventually septic shock.

Therefore, the clinician must be aware of the danger, once the instrument has exceeded above the level of 15 cm. These are the general principles to be followed, while understanding this examination in the passage of the rectum and sigmoid colon.

The following important findings must not be overlooked or ignored:

Loose motion, mixed with mucus and blood is more likely to be associated with ulcerative or proctocolitis. Finding of undigested food has a clinical importance that would be reevaluated with other investigation.

Anatomical feature of the colonic and rectal mucosa should be recorded. In normal condition, the mucosa would appear to be shining and pale-pink in color. And submucosal veins are seen clearly, but they may be obscured due to inflamed mucosa. The commonest conditions are proctocolitis, postradiation colitis, and amebic colitis.

Evidence of stricture, diverticula in the sigmoid colon, narrow lumen due to multiple diverticula, and discharge of altered or fresh blood are all important findings. Evidence of fresh blood could be associated with diverticulitis, ischemic colitis, angiodysplasia, intussusception, and that of altered blood may be attributable to bleeding peptic ulcer disease.

Evidence of slight oozing of blood in the mucosa may be due to direct mucosal contact with the instrument. This is known as contact bleeding associated with proctocolitis.

Abnormal color and loss of mucosal shining are pathological. Granular appearance in the mucosa could be recognized. These are features of chronic inflammation, and are attributable to proctitis, proctocolitis or postradiation proctitis. Mucosal biopsy must be taken for tissue diagnosis.

Other macroscopical features could be, pedunculated adenoma, flat polyp, and villus adenoma, associated with fronds-like appearances. Mucus and thick watery discharge is quite common in this lesion.

Ulcerated growth associated with firm raised and everted irregular edge is a classical feature of malignant growth in the rectum. A narrow lumen, surrounded by the growth, encircling all around the wall of the sigmoid colon or the rectum is a classical feature of annular growth. Among other macroscopical features of the rectal tumor is the cauliflower type, in which case, the tissue would be friable and necrotic in nature. These sorts of tumors are commonly developed in the ampulla of the rectum.

Evidence of broad-based ulcerated tumor invading circumferentially provides a clue for the duration of the growth and prognosis. In all instances, tissue is removed by the biopsy forceps for histology.

5 Investigations

There are two sets of investigation; one of them is the routine investigation for blood profiles irrespective of the pathological conditions. And other investigation should be specific, related to the provisional diagnosis. There is no need to arrange expensive type of investigations which would be of little value in the initial treatment of the disease. But the special type of investigation may be needed, if the surgeon is seeking further information on the etiology of unknown clinical problems. Every clinician should bear in mind that no investigation is fool proof in the diagnosis of the surgical condition.

First line of investigations:
- Hematological investigations.
- Plain X-ray of the chest and abdomen.
- Ultrasound scan of the abdomen or pelvis.

Second line of investigations:
- Barium enema, small bowel enema.
- Endoscopy.

Third line of investigations:
- Computerized Tomography Scan (CT Scan).
- Colonography.
- PET Scan.
- Magnetic Resonance Image Scan (MRI Scan).
- Magnetic Resonance Cholangiopancreatic Scan (MRCP).
- Laparotomy.

Hematological profile:
- Full Blood Count (FBC), Hemoglobin, (Hb/dl), PCV, ESR, C reactive protein.
- Liver Function Test (LFT).
- Serum Electrolytes, Urea, Creatinine, Serum Calcium, Serum Phosphate, Albumin and Globulin.

Specific investigations:
- **Radiological investigations:**
  - Plain X-ray of the chest, X-ray of the abdomen, barium enema, and Ultrasound scan (USS).
  - Computerized Tomography Scan (CT scan) and Magnetic Resonance Image Scan (MRI scan) are reserved for particular clinical conditions.
- **Hematological profile:**
  - FBC: It may reveal polycythemia by the increased number of RBC, greater than 7 million/c. mm and Hb./dl, greater than 16 gm/dl. Such incidental finding is very rare and it is probably related to:
    - Living in a high altitude.
    - Chronic pulmonary disease.
    - Cardiac disease.
    - Renal tumor.

Resident surgeon must be concerned with the incidental hematological report. In this case, there remains a high risk of perioperative bleeding and risk of postoperative thrombosis. Patient may be confused, and may present with a raised serum urea, creatinine and high potassium. Preoperative venesection for a liter of blood should be considered. And blood collected from this sort of patients must not be used in blood transfusion to any other patients.
- Hb < 10 Hb < 10 gm/dl may be associated with cecal carcinoma, ulcerative colitis, Crohn's ileitis, piles or peptic ulcer disease, pernicious anemia, bone marrow depression, multiple myeloma, iron deficiency, and hemolytic anemia. Patient may need preoperative blood transfusion before major operative procedure is undertaken. In this case, packed cell blood is preferable and transfused in elderly patient, because of preexisting cardiac problems.

- **Serum electrolytes:** Low serum potassium could be associated with medical condition, diuretics, vomiting, and villus adenoma. Elevation of high potassium may be associated with renal failure, or postrenal condition. Low serum sodium with normal serum potassium and urea could be the result of hemodilution, but it could be due to secretion of inappropriate antidiuretic hormone (ADH) from the tumor of the lung.
- **Serum urea:** High level of serum urea could be attributable to dehydration, and other urological and medical conditions. Its clinical value has to be evaluated with the blood result on serum sodium, serum potassium and other clinical conditions.
- **Serum creatinine:** It may be due to prerenal, renal or postrenal condition. The prerenal condition is dehydration, or cardiac failure. Again, its elevation without the elevation of potassium may be related to gross dehydration. But its elevation associated with high potassium may be attributed to intrinsic renal disease or prerenal condition.
- **Serum calcium:** Hypercalcemia is associated with hyperparathyroidism, but bone metastasis may produce high serum calcium.
- **Plasma protein:** Normal range is between 35 gm and 45 gm/l (average 40 gm/l). It remains below 30 gm/l in postoperative period or in cancer patient.
- If it is less than 25 gm/l, it could be associated with many medical and surgical conditions. Preoperative supplementation with infusion of human albumin (100 ml per day) should be considered. Patient may develop into cardiac failure due to reabsorption of fluid from the tissue and transferring to the heart, and it may also lead to retention of fluid in the tissue, in some clinical conditions.

It is a debatable issue that whether supplementation with human albumin is effective therapy in order to treat the gross tissue edema; but postoperative risk would be much greater, if its level remains less than 20 gm/l. In my experience, it is advisable to bring the serum albumin up to the level of 30 gm/l at least with the infusion of human albumin. During this therapy, diuretic should be prescribed everyday in order to combat against the potential risk of developing acute left ventricular failure. This therapeutic measure provides a better hemodynamic support, during and after operation being carried out. In some cases, whole blood transfusion should be considered, if the level of hemoglobin is less than 10 gm/dl.

All these results are discussed in brief but resident doctors and medical students are advised to read the reference book on specific reports.

RADIOLOGICAL INVESTIGATIONS

Important Radiological Features of the Chest

Chest X-ray is frequently requested in emergency condition, but it would be of no benefit to the patient, if the film could not be interpreted straightaway. Consultant radiologist is not always available when needed. Hence, it is equally important for the clinician to interpret the normal and abnormal radiological features present in the chest X-ray.

Among the important features are size of the heart, lung fields, costophrenic angles, pleural effusion, pneumothorax and consolidation or collapsed lung. At emergency medical care, it would not be possible for the resident doctors to read many other rare pathological features present in the same X-ray, which may be attributable to other primary lesions.

In this chapter, only important radiological features would be highlighted. In normal chest X-ray, the lung fields are clear right up to the costophrenic angle, which remains in acute angle, but it would be obliterated by pleural effusion, hemothorax, basal consolidation or collapsed lung.

Although the chest X-ray in Figure 5.1A suggests that the size of the heart, costophrenic angles and lung fields are normal in appearance, nevertheless it has multiple metastasis as nodules in the lung fields.

In sharp contrast, the next X-ray of the chest (Fig. 5.1B) shows pleural effusion in both sides but it is worse in left side with obliteration of the costophrenic angle and enlarged heart.

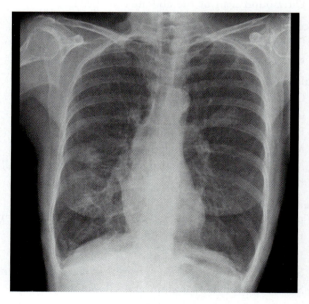

Fig. 5.1A: Chest X-ray showing normal sized heart, normal costophrenic angles, but there are evidences of metastasis in both lungs (by courtesy of Dr S Sinha)

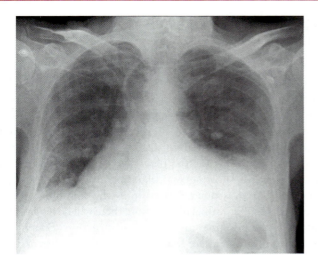

Fig. 5.1B: X-ray of chest in erect position showing enlarged heart, pleural effusion in both sides of the chest, but it is worse in the left side of the chest. Metastasis is present in both the lung fields (By courtesy of Dr S Sinha)

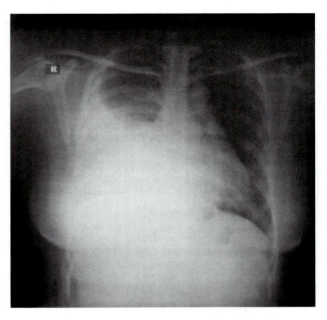

Fig. 5.1C: X-ray of chest with right-sided pleural effusion due to TB lung (by courtesy of Dr AK Dutta-Munshi)

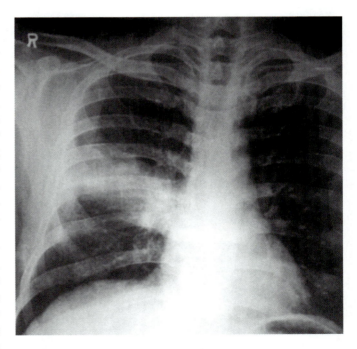

Fig. 5.1D: Chest X-ray showing consolidation of the right middle lobe of the lung

In most benign conditions, the pleural effusion occurs in both sides of the chest and its etiology is associated with congestive cardiac failure, pulmonary tuberculosis or subphrenic abscess. If there is evidence of pleural effusion in the X-ray of the chest in erect position, its minimum volume would be over 500 ml that is required to show the obliteration of the costophrenic angle. Aspiration of this fluid will provide for the diagnosis of the disease. And it would improve a better capacity of breathing, increase the vital capacity of the lung and enhance the oxygen saturation of the blood. All these benefits are due to the expansion of lungs. Patients will feel much comfortable, energetic and will be relieved from shortness of breath. Blood gas analysis will reveal better oxygen saturation.

Unilateral pleural effusion may be associated with tumor in the lung and tuberculous lesions (Fig. 5.1C). If round opacities are present in the lungs, they are often known as cannon ball appearance and regarded to be the classical features of secondary tumors, arising from the renal carcinoma or testicular tumor. CT scan should be done for better assessment of the lung metastasis. Such evidences are available in CT scan (Figs 5.1E and F).

This is another chest X-ray which shows the right-sided pleural effusion. This was due to pulmonary tuberculosis.

The consolidation shown in right middle lobe of the chest was due to chest infection.

In reviewing the progress of chest infection, repeat X-ray would be necessary, but it should not be repeated everyday. The average dose for each exposure to the chest is around 0.2mSV and it would be 8mSV if CT scan for chest is done. These doses are very small but cumulative doses could be much higher, if the chest X-ray or CT scan for chest is repeated several times in a week.

There are many other abnormal lesions that could be identified from the X-ray of chest. They are osteolytic lesions in the ribs with or without pathological fracture, pneumothorax, collapsed lung or consolidation. The commonest site for consolidation is the base of the lung but this particular chest X-ray showed the features of consolidation in the right middle lobe of the lung (Fig. 5.1D). This resulted from chest infection. These findings will assist the clinician whether the patient is fit for general anesthesia.

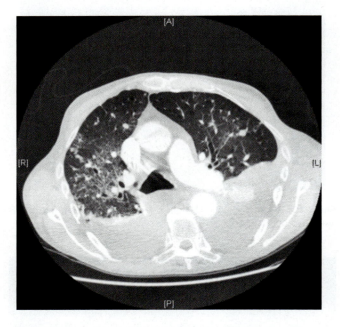

Fig.5.1E: CT scan of chest showing bilateral pleural effusion, collapsed both lungs and metastasis in the lungs

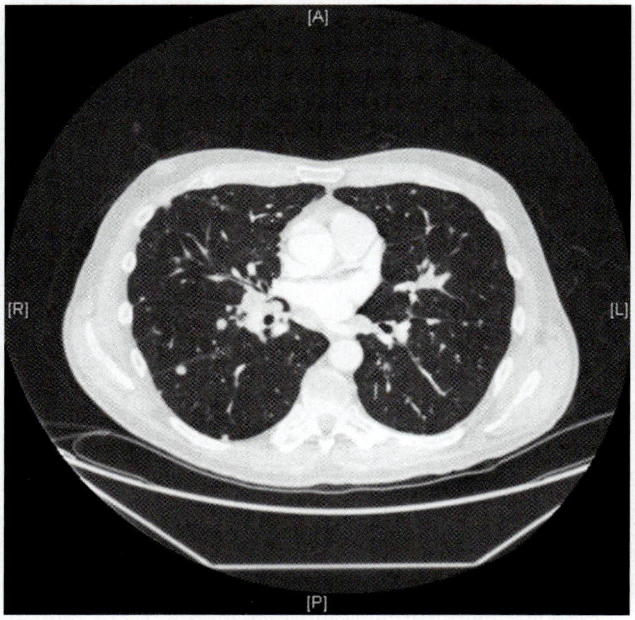

IMPORTANT RADIOLOGICAL FEATURES OF ABDOMEN

Plain X-ray of the abdomen (Fig. 5.2): In the past, abdominal X-ray used to be taken in two views; one for supine and the other one for erect or decubitus position. This is rarely recommended nowadays. A plain X-ray of abdomen in supine position is necessary. In this film, colonic obstruction could be identified by the distention of the colon, proximal to the obstruction. In this case, the plain X-ray of the abdomen in supine position shows gross dilatation of small and large intestine. This was due to stricture in the sigmoid colon.

In all cases of intestinal obstruction, there will be no gaseous pattern in the intestine, distal to the obstruction. Distention of small intestine is a late feature of the colonic obstruction. But it would appear earlier if the cecal tumor has caused obstruction to the ileocecal valve.

If the X-ray film shows gaseous distention in all parts of the colon and in the rectum, the possible diagnosis would be paralytic ileus. It is associated with generalized peritonitis that may cause distention of the abdomen. In plain X-ray of the abdomen, psoas shadows are well-defined, but its obliteration is due to intraperitoneal sepsis or collection of inflammatory fluid and it would appear like a ground glass appearance in the plain X-ray of the abdomen.

Straight plain X-ray of the abdomen may reveal abnormal radiopaque opacities. These could be calcified lymph glands, gallstones, renal or ureteric stone, aneurysmal sac or atherosclerosis in the walls of aorta, or iliac arteries.

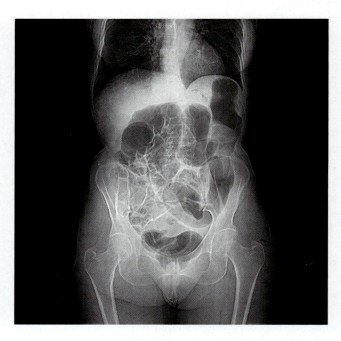

Fig. 5.1F: CT scan of chest showing multiple secondaries in the lungs due to primary colonic carcinoma

Fig. 5.2: Plain X-ray of abdomen showing gaseous distention of the gut right up to the rectum

If the opacity is suggestive of gallstones, renal or ureteric stone, this could be differentiated by further plain X-rays. In this case, one X-ray is taken at inspiration and another one taken at expiration. These two films may assist to distinguish the renal stone from the calcified lymph nodes or gall stone.

The position of the opacity in the renal parenchyma will remain constant with relation to the cortical border of the kidney, despite the fact that the kidney has moved up or down with the inspiration or with expiration of the chest respectively. This change in positions of the kidney is due to movement of the diaphragm, but the position of the opacity in the renal parenchyma remains unchanged. Hence, it is regarded to be renal stone. In other cases, stag-horn calculus will show a characteristic feature occupying the whole or a part of the renal pelvis or calyces.

Gallstones could be diagnosed in a plain X-ray by thier classical shapes with various facets and they could be differentiated from the renal stone, by taking a lateral exposure of the abdomen. In case of gallstones, they could be either multiple faceted or solitary and round opacity in the area of right hypochondrium and these opacities will appear to be located anterior to the lumbar spine, compared to those renal stones, if such doubt is raised in the clinical diagnosis.

The plain X-ray will also reveal the shape and size of the soft tissue shadow of the kidneys, liver and spleen. The classical soft tissue shadow of the renal carcinoma will reveal that the lower or the upper pole of the kidney will appear to be broader, compared to the lower pole or compared to the contralateral kidney. In contrast, the enlargement of the upper pole in children may be due to Wilms' tumor.

A soft tissue shadow showing a smaller sized kidney in one side would suggest atrophic kidney and it could be of congenital in origin or it could be attributable to chronic infection or renal artery stenosis.

In the plain X-ray of a healthy patient, the hilum of each kidney will show parallel to the outer border of the psoas muscle but this relationship may be lost in abnormal conditions. These are horse-shoe shaped kidney, polycystic kidney and renal tumor.

Enlargement of the spleen may show the indentation on the splenic flexure of the colon. In rare occasion, any evidence of calcification in the region of left hypochondrium in elderly patient could be related to aneurysm or stenosis of the splenic artery.

In the same way, enlarged liver or enlarged gallbladder could be visualized by their soft tissue shadow in the plain X-ray.

The plain X-ray of the abdomen may reveal localized opacity over the anatomical site of the psoas muscle, which could be psoas abscess or perinephric abscess. In this case, the psoas shadow of one side would be missing or obliterated by the large soft tissue shadow around the kidney or in the paravertebral region. Abdominal aortic aneurysm may be diagnosed by the evidences of abnormal pattern of calcification, representing the aortic aneurysmal wall.

All these radiological features may lead to tentative diagnosis, but further investigation may be recommended by the radiologists, if there is any doubt. Resident surgeons and medical students must keep on examining the plain X-ray that contains many hidden abnormal features.

SPECIFIC LINE OF RADIOLOGICAL INVESTIGATIONS

Many opportunities have opened up to establish the diagnosis of the tumor in the colon and to establish the tumor staging. These are barium enema, gastrograffin enema, colonoscopy, CT scan, CT colonography, ultrasound scan of the abdomen and MRI scan.

CLINICAL SIGNIFICANCE OF BARIUM ENEMA STUDY

The initial line of investigation should be barium enema or colonoscopy that depends upon the facilities available to the surgeon.

For the abnormal bowel actions, barium enema is arranged first, but the growth in the anal canal and the rectum must be excluded first by the proctoscopic and by the sigmoidoscopic examination.

Barium enema will only reveal the anatomical pattern, above the level of the rectum. This is due to the fact that the barium is inserted into the rectum by a rectal tube that may go up to the upper part of the rectum. As a result, the tumor in the rectum and the anal canal could not be diagnosed by barium enema. And many times, this investigation had failed to diagnose the rectal tumor because of the sigmoidoscopy not being done, before a request form was sent to the X-ray department. It is a routine procedure that request form will be returned to the signatory, if the form does not state about the finding of the sigmoidoscopy.

This investigation should not be recommended if there are evidences of acute colonic obstruction, peritonitis and volvulus or gross dilatation of the colon shown on plain X-ray of the abdomen. It is also contraindicated in acute ulcerative colitis or acute dilatation of the colon due to known diagnosis of ulcerative colitis.

Barium enema technique has been improved over the last 50 years. The major study reported that the incidence of false-positive was 0.8 percent and false-negative was 6.9 percent.[1]

These negative results in barium enema are less concerned to the surgeons, since the surgeons and gastroenterologist have started using colonoscope and CT scan in establishing the colonic lesions routinely in colorectal clinics. Nevertheless, no technique is infallible but one is complementary to others.

Nevertheless, double contrast barium enema should be the first line of diagnostic tool. It requires a good bowel preparation. The detailed description of technique used for the contrast barium enema is not important to surgical students. Nevertheless, a broad outline is highlighted in this section and they should develop interest in understanding the method used in contrast barium enema, how to read the X-ray films independently and must learn how to recognize the abnormal mucosal features shown in the X-ray films.

PRINCIPLE OF BOWEL PREPARATIONS

In most cases, bowel preparation is done at home without medical supervision, but elderly patient should be admitted for this preparation. They may go into severe hypovolemic shock due to gross dehydration that may result from repeated watery motion. In these cases, patient needs encouragement in drinking isotonic fluids containing some amount of salt. Alternatively, intravenous infusion with dextrose-saline should be commenced to overcome the acute hypovolemic shock. This prophylactic measure should be taken if the patient is above 60 years of age or lives alone at home.

Types of Bowel Preparations

- Oral laxatives
- Oral lavage regimens
- Rectal enema.

Oral Preparations

There are many commercial products available for oral laxatives, but the common products used are:
- Senna
- Picolax
- Mannitol
- Klean-preparation.

Rectal Enemas

- Soap and water enema
- Phosphate enema.

Rectal Suppositories

- Glycerine suppositories
- Bisacodyl suppositories.

ADVICE TO THE PATIENT ON DIETS AND ORAL FLUID

Patient is advised to stay on a low residue diet for a few days and to stop taking iron tablets. This tablet tends to cause constipation. Patient is advised to take either senna or picolax orally, a day before the barium enema is scheduled. And patient is advised to continue drinking clear fluid. A better bowel clearance is achieved with double dose than with a single dose of picolax. In this case, the second dose is taken 6-8 hours later. No rectal wash-out or enema is necessary in this case.

The main objective is to have watery motion and if it contains undigested foods, a good bowel clearance is most likely to be expected. In most cases, oral laxative starts working within 2 hours, but in some cases, it may take over 6 hours.

Alternative to those oral preparations, a good purgation could be achieved, if the patient could drink around 3-4 liters of isotonic saline mixed with orange juice, a day before the X-ray is taken, but patient may experience nausea or vomiting, and it should not be prescribed to those patients suffering from high blood pressure and heart disease. If such problems are encountered, phosphate enema followed by soap and water enema could be supplemented two hours before the barium enema is due.

COMPLICATIONS WITH BOWEL PREPARATION

- Gross dehydration, hypotension and lack of concentration.
- Electrolytes imbalance, hyponatrium and hypokalemia.
- Nausea and vomiting.
- Colicky abdominal pain and perforation of the colon.
- Poor bowel preparation, recognized by the retention of residual lumps in the colon and rectum.
- There may be accumulation of hydrogen ion gas; if mannitol is used. Cauterization may cause explosion during polypectomy. Hence, this solution should be avoided, if colonoscopy is necessary.

CONTRAINDICATION OF ORAL PURGATIVES

- Evidence of colonic obstruction
- Peritonitis
- Paralytic ileus
- Postoperative patients
- Habitual constipation
- Megacolon
- Volvulus.

A BRIEF REVIEW OF BARIUM ENEMA STUDY

In the past, colon used to be radiologically examined by barium that was poured into the rectum through a rubber tube. Patient is screened in the darkroom and a series of X-rays used to be taken, when necessary, if there was evidence of abnormality in the mucosal wall, or in the colonic lumen. After evacuation of the barium stuff, further X-rays used to be taken, when the colon was empty apart from a thin layer of barium being retained in the lumen of the colon.

But this method of examination could not detect small sized growth, like polyp. In 1946, the technique included tannic acid in the barium. The purpose was to inhibit the secretion of mucus and induce increased peristaltic contraction, thus, assisting a quick empty of the barium from the colon. As a result, barium used to stay adherent to the colonic mucosa. A better radiological feature of the colonic mucosa was obtained.[2]

To overcome these pitfalls, a new technique has been devised by using both barium and air.[3] It is now known as double contrast enema. This technique provides an early diagnosis of early lesion presented with mucosal plaque, polyps, multiple familial polyposis coli, and multiple ulcerations. The classical radiological features in these cases would be a 'mosaic of negative shadows'. In other cases, pattern of large tumor will be evident by the barium coat inside the air-filled lumen of the gut.

IMPORTANT RADIOLOGICAL FEATURES OF THE CARCINOMA OF THE COLON AND THE RECTUM

The classical diagnostic radiological feature is the persistent filling defect in the wall of the gut in all sorts of views taken during screening. There are various names for these filling defects shown in the wall of the colon by the double contrasts. They are apple-core, napkin-ring, and string stricture. These features are attributable to polypoidal growth, projecting into the lumen of the gut, causing narrowing of the lumen. It all depends upon the circumferential involvement of the gut by the growth. The radiological feature with annular growth would be quite different from that with cauliflower or polypoidal growth developed from one quadrant of the gut wall.

The other diagnostic features are persistent filling defect and its mobility in the same site, during the process of screening being undertaken in the darkroom, despite changing the position of the patient on the examination table. A false-positive finding is not impossible due to incomplete bowel clearance and presence of residual solid lump found stuck to the wall.

RADIOLOGICAL FEATURES OF NONMALIGNANT DISEASE

Apart from the diagnosis of the tumor, this double-contrast barium enema will reveal the size of the tumor and patency of the lumen, evidence of diverticulum, stricture, and abnormal position of the colon such as redundant loop of the transverse colon, lying in the pelvis or sigmoid colon lying across into the right iliac fossa, high position of the cecum, evidence of indentation of the hepatic or splenic flexure by the liver or spleen.

It may show fistula track either between the colon and bladder, or vagina or the other parts of the intestine. They are referred to as colovesical, colovaginal and colocutaneous or ileocolic fistula. In some cases, barium may leak into the retroperitoneal space through the chronic perforation of the diverticulum or perforation of the ulcerated growth.

In early stage of the diverticular disease, barium enema may reveal sea-saw or saw-teeth appearance in the wall of the colon, it may show loss of haustration along the gut, and multiple round-shaped pouches, coated with thin layer of barium and it may also reveal the opening of these pouches, connected to the colon. These pouches are blind mucosal sacs, referred to as cul-de-sac to the lay person and are known as diverticular pouch in the medical literature.

In ulcerative colitis, barium enema will show a tubular pattern without any features of haustration and it may reveal smaller multiple feeling defects which are suggestive of pseudopolyposis. The loss of haustration and shortening in length of the colon are attributed to chronic inflammation affecting the circular muscles as well as taeniae coli of the colon. In fact, fibrosis develops in these muscles, resulting in reduction of girth and length of the colon.

In ischemic colitis, radiological features would be the thumb printing, or copper beaten appearance, lack of haustration, ragged saw-tooth pattern of the bowel, or it would appear like a tubular narrow segment between the healthy looking segments of the colon.[4,5]

Other Investigations

If the double contrast barium enema does not reveal any malignant growth, but the symptoms are strongly suggestive of carcinoma of the colon or the rectum; in this case, there are a few options available to the surgeon to arrange further investigation. These are:

a. Repeat the barium enema in 4 weeks time.
b. Small bowel enema.
c. Colonoscopy.
d. Contrast CT scan for the colon known as colonography.
e. CT scan for the abdomen for secondaries in liver and for the colonic tumor. PET scan has been a new tool for the purpose of investigation that could be done along with the CT scan or MRI scan.
f. MRI scan for the rectal tumor for establishing the tumor stage and for resectability of the tumor.
g. Occult blood test.
h. Exfoliative cytology.
i. Laparoscopy.
j. Laparotomy.

Experiences suggest that double-contrast barium enema may not reveal the ulcerated lesion in the cecum. If this investigation turns out to be inconclusive or inconsistent with the provisional diagnosis or clinical presentation, small bowel enema should be arranged, if the initial presentation was anemia or low hemoglobin. It may reveal the abnormal features in the cecum. It may show that the cecum would appear to be deformed or contracted or it may reveal obstruction at the ileocecal valve.

Alternative to radiological investigations is colonoscopy. It is another diagnostic tool but in certain cases, the tip of the colonoscope may not reach the cecum for many reasons. The reason for not being able to see the cecum could be a technical error, redundant sigmoid loop or transverse loop of the colon lying over the cecum, incomplete bowel preparation or lack of skill of the radiologist.

In double-contrast barium enema, the cross section of the colon that will appear to be round, hollow cavity will show two types of media. The inferior or lower half of the circumference of the colon that depends upon the position of the colon or position of the abdomen on the screening table, will be filled up with liquid medium such as barium that will not reveal the normal or abnormal mucosal wall of the colon, because of the fact that the liquid barium will rest on the colonic wall due to gravity and dependent part of the colon—thus obscuring the features of the colonic mucosa.

But the upper or superior half of the same circumference of the colon will be filled up with air medium that will show clear and distinct mucosal features, coated with a thin layer of barium, filling defect or abnormal size of the lumen. To demonstrate these images, patient needs to be screened in darkroom in different positions, which are in supine, prone, right lateral, left lateral or standing position. For each position, images of the colon, filled with air medium are recorded in the X-ray films. As a result, the liquid barium will rest at the dependent and the contrast air will float above the barium, thus, occupying the superior part of the colon, when the patient is placed in lateral or supine positions on the table.

In this way, a complete examination of the colon is carried out. These sequences will continue commencing from the upper third of the rectum until the terminal ileum is reached (Figs 5.3A to I).

The two lateral views, one taken on the right lateral position and other one taken on the left lateral position have outlined around the near full circumference of the colon from the cecum to the sigmoid colon up to the level of the sigmoid stricture. It is a broad principle that how a complete examination of the colon could be performed by a double contrast barium.

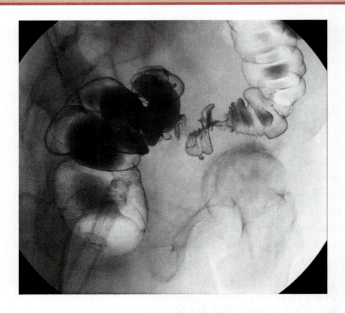

Fig. 5.3A: The stricture of the sigmoid colon. In this plate, a large amount of air contrast is held in the distal sigmoid colon and a small amount of air is above the stricture

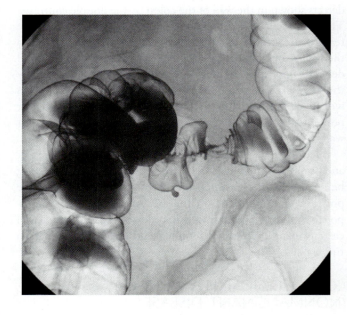

Fig. 5.3B: In the same patient, it shows the stricture in the sigmoid colon, and the rectal tube is seen in the lower part of the pelvis. It was taken in supine position. As a result, the proximal segment of the sigmoid colon contains a thin layer of liquid barium contrast showing the normal colonic wall, proximal to the stricture, and a larger amount of air contrast just distal to the stricture

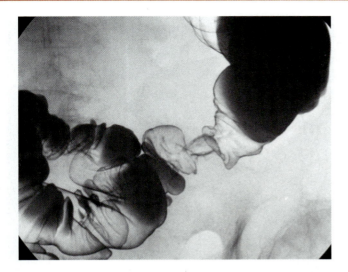

Fig. 5.3C: This image was taken when the patient was probably in erect oblique position. As a result, air contrast is in the descending and proximal sigmoid colon, but the stricture is clear due to a thin layer of barium. Some amount of air contrast is held in the sigmoid colon distal to the stricture

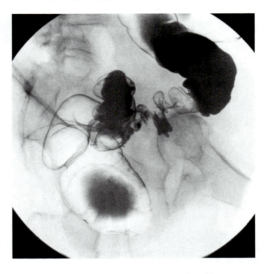

Fig. 5.3D: This is a left lateral view showing the sigmoid colon anteriorly and the lateral profile of the sacrum shown on the right side posteriorly. The radiological image of the stricture in the sigmoid colon remains persistently unchanged in this plate, like other previous views. This confirms that it was not a spasm due to peristalsis. It was an annular tumor developed in the sigmoid colon

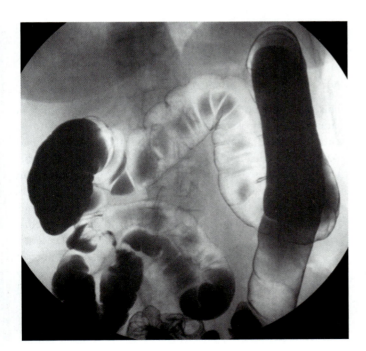

Fig. 5.3E: This X-ray shows the images of the descending colon, splenic flexure, transverse colon, ascending colon and a loop of the terminal ileum. On the left side, the cecum appears to be contracted showing a string, containing air contrast between the cecum and terminal ileum. Further views are necessary to establish the true evidence

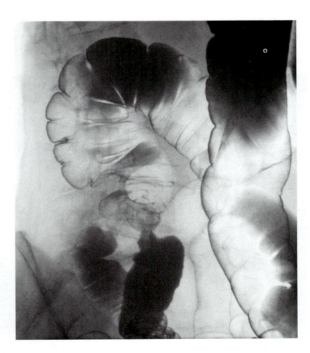

Fig. 5.3F: This film appears to have been taken in left lateral position, thus, showing the cecum closer to the descending colon. An apple-core filling defect appears to be present in the lateral wall of the cecum and a narrow lumen of the ileocecal junction

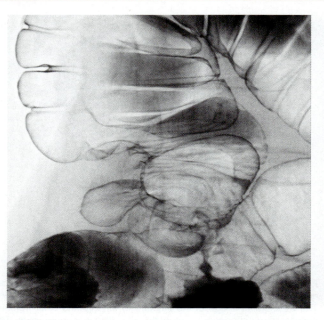

Fig. 5.3G: This plate shows a clear image of apple-core appearance on the lateral wall of the cecum and a string-like stricture between the cecum and the ileum. It suggests a second primary tumor of the cecum affecting the opening of the ileocecal valve. All these plates were taken from the same patient

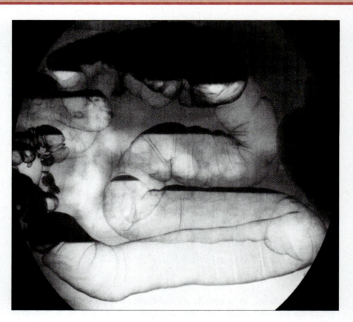

Fig. 5.3H: This X-ray shows multiple fluid level in horizontal lines, thus, suggesting the dark shadows lying above a thin liquid barium. This X-ray was taken in left lateral position, thus, displaying the loops of the descending colon, transverse colon and a part of the ascending colon. A few round opacities that appear to be well-defined and whiter in color because of thin barium coating are shown in the mid-transverse colon, but a narrow stricture is evident on the left side distal to the dark shadow. This could be a primary tumor. There was no other evidence of filling defect in any part of the descending colon and transverse colon, shown in this X-ray

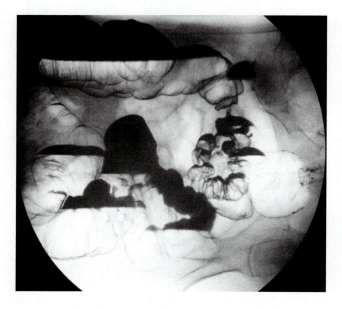

Fig. 5.3I: This X-ray was taken in right lateral position and the rectal tube is seen on the right side of the plate. It shows multiple fluid levels like intestinal obstruction. The parallel horizontal levels are between the liquid thin barium contrast and the air contrast that lies floating over the liquid contrast. Again a small stricture is seen on the upper left side of the rectum and proximal to the level of dark shadows. The evidence of an ill-defined filling defect in the cecum is not very clear in this plate

METHOD OF SMALL BOWEL ENEMA

This new technique was reported in 1943.[6] In this method of barium study, stomach is excluded. For this reason, barium mixed with 90 ml saline is introduced directly and rapidly into the second part of the duodenum, using a 50 ml syringe attached to a tube. The latter is inserted into the duodenum, before the liquid barium is pushed through rapidly. The flow of barium that continues running through the jejunum and then through the segments of ileum is followed constantly and important area of abnormal features are recorded in the X-ray films, as and when necessary.

This particular investigation is used to reveal any abnormal features in the terminal ileum and cecum, although any pathological lesions present in the proximal gut are recorded concurrently.

In Crohn's ileitis, the most striking feature is the long segment of stricture in the terminal ileum, referred to as string of Kantor. Other characteristic features are lack of peristalsis, multiple filling defects. These abnormal features develop because of ulceration in the wall of the terminal ileum. And they become apparent in the postevacuated barium films. This finding is known as cobblestone reticulation. And there may be evidence of linear fissures through the thick mucosal layer. They are often referred to as raspberry thorn, rose thorn, seen in the X-ray films.

Investigations

In tuberculous intestine, a similar radiological feature, like regional ileitis may be apparent. There could be a long stricture or filling defect in the terminal ileum, cecum and ascending colon.

It would be a difficult task to differentiate the TB intestine from Crohn's colitis, or carcinoma of the cecum. In this case, ultrasound scan, and CT scan guided mesenteric lymph node biopsy must be done to exclude the tuberculous lymphadenitis. In addition, other investigations should be done, these are:
- Sputum examination for TB bacilli
- Mantoux skin test
- X-ray of the chest.

X-ray of the chest may be normal in intestinal tuberculosis.

In my clinic,[7] one 25 years old male patient was referred to for a loss of appetite and body weight. He had colonoscopic examination done two years ago and a large area of granulomatous lesion in the ascending colon was found. He was treated on the line of Crohn's colitis, but no one had thought of possibility of tuberculous colitis. Although he was from an Asian country and cook in the UK for many years, suspicion arose on the abdominal examination. Eventually, TB colitis was diagnosed on mesenteric lymph glands biopsy that was carried out through the guidance of the CT scan.

Therefore, it is important to exclude other possibilities. In this study, delay in barium movement, and deformity of the cecum are pathognomonic. Alternative to those benign conditions is the cecal carcinoma.

Small bowel enema may reveal multiple congenital diverticulosis in the proximal small intestine, abnormal large curvature of the second part of the duodenum, papillary carcinoma of the pancreas, jejunal polyps, small stricture or carcinoma and Meckel's diverticulum.

INTRAVENOUS PYELOGRAM

This particular investigation is indicated only in those cases in which the carcinoma has been identified in the cecum, ascending colon, lower descending colon, sigmoid colon or rectosigmoid region. The main objective is to see whether there is obstructive uropathy. This may result from the infiltration of the adjacent tumor to the urinary tract. In addition, it confirms the renal function of both kidneys. If one of the ureter is invaded by the colonic tumor, then it would be safe to excise the affected kidney along with the colonic tumor.

Complete evacuation of barium from the intestine has to be carried out before Intravenous Pyelogram (IVP) being arranged. It is also important to find out about iodine allergy from the patient, before the contrast is infused. It is safer to do skin test, by injecting into the dorsum of the hand with a small drop of iodine preparation to be used in pyelogram, before undertaking the IVP.

FOR INTRAVENOUS PYELOGRAM (IVP)

Initially, a control X-ray film is taken. Its purpose is to assess the quality of the picture shown in the control film. If it turns out to be unsatisfactory, then the exposure dose of the X-ray may need to be adjusted.

Other purposes are to see whether there are evidences of residual barium particles, present in the wall of the gut, if so, procedure has to be deferred, until those barium particles are cleared off completely. Apart from these technical matters, the clinical purpose is to record whether there is any radiopaque opacity, present in the anatomical line of the kidneys, ureters and bladder. It also provides soft tissue shadow of the kidney parenchyma. A broad-sized lower pole of one kidney suggests malignant tumor. This finding should not be ignored.

The opacity in the renal parenchyma should be suspected to be renal stone, if its position with relation to the cortex of the kidney remains unchanged in the subsequent film, taken on deep inspiration and then on expiration. The kidney moves up and down with the movement of the diaphragm. Because the fibrous strands arising from the perinephric capsule pass through the perinephric fat to be attached with the undersurface of the diaphragm. The same relationship could not be relied upon, for the smaller stone present in the renal pelvis.

The plain X-ray may also show any radiopaque opacity in the renal parenchyma or along the line of ureter or in the pelvis. These findings have to be reviewed along with the IVP films, whether they are present within the renal parenchyma, ureter or within the boundary of the bladder.

After this initial review, IVP contrast is injected into the vein. The preferable site is on the dorsum of the hand, but any prominent vein present along the forearm or in the cubital fossa could be used. Extravasation of the contrast into the soft tissue may cause discomfort and swelling around the punctured vein. If this complication is encountered, a new site is chosen on the other hand.

If IVP is done soon after emergency admission for a sharp pain in the loin or in the lumbar region, the first film taken 5 minutes later will show delayed excretion of contrast in one kidney, suggesting acute urinary tract obstruction by the stone present in the renal tract. In addition, there could be extravasations of the contrast in the perinephric fat suggesting of acute impaction of stone in the renal tract. Sometimes, delayed excretion may occur after several hours.

In all normal circumstances, this particular investigation will demonstrate the function of the kidneys by the excretion of the contrast on 5 or 10 minutes films. It also reveals the soft tissue shadow of the kidneys, in relation to the size and shape of the kidney. Subsequent films taken at 15 or 30 minutes may display the filling defect or gross distention of the renal pelvis, and renal calyces. This finding indicates an outflow obstruction, which could be either at the pelvic ureteric junction (PUJ) or any site below the renal pelvis.

It may show duplex renal pelvis or double ureters. In most cases, double ureters join at the lower-third before entering into the bladder. There could be a lot of congenital variation, but its incidence is less than 4 percent. If double ureters open separately into the bladder, then the one draining the upper pole of the kidney opens below and medially and the other ureter, by contrast arising from the lower pole of the kidney opens above the opening of the upper ureter.

In the films, the contrast will show the outline, the anatomical position and any filling defect in the lumen of the ureter or abnormal size or position of the ureter. It would also display the filling defect in the full or empty bladder, with or without prostatic impression at the bladder neck.

Postmicturition film may show residual contrast in the renal pelvis, ureter or in the bladder. Bladder tumor or bladder diverticula could be seen in full bladder; but filling defect in the bladder wall or retention of the contrast in the diverticula of the bladder could be seen well on postmicturition film.

If the X-ray film taken at 1-hour seems to be inconclusive, further films should be taken on induced diuretic excretion; but a larger volume of contrast may need to be infused into the vein, or delayed films should be taken at 6 and 24 hours later. This may reveal dilated renal pelvis and hydroureter.

If both ureters are shown to be medially displaced from the sacroiliac joints and dilated to the level of displacement, it is more likely to be associated with retroperitoneal fibrosis that is more likely to be around the bifurcation of the aorta. More often, it is attributable to certain drugs; methyldopa is one of them.

IVP is contraindicated for pregnant patient and noniodine preparation should be used if any other patient is known to be allergic to iodine.

Other Types of Investigations:

- Ultrasound scan (USS).
- CT scan, colonography and PET scan.
- MRI scan.
- USS is done to reveal any abnormality in the liver, gallbladder, spleen, pancreas, mesenteric and paraaortic lymph glands, kidneys, prostate gland, and bladder.

It is an important diagnostic tool. It will confirm the following pathological lesions:
- Peritoneal collection.
- Localized abscess.
- Appendicular mass.
- Ovarian cyst.
- Fibroid of the uterus.
- Renal stones, renal cyst, renal tumor.
- Hydroureter, hydronephrosis, dilatation of calyces.
- Polycystic kidney.
- Size of the spleen.
- Cystic lesion in the spleen or liver.
- Dilated biliary ducts, gallstones, stone in the bile duct.
- Polyp in the gallbladder, carcinoma of the gallbladder.
- Pancreatic mass, pseudopancreatic cyst.

It is used for many clinical conditions and for diagnosis. The principal purpose is:
1. To differentiate between a solid and a cystic lesion.
2. To make the diagnosis of the diseases, and the tumor.
3. To assist biopsy from the liver, lymph gland and kidney.
4. To diagnose the aortic aneurysm; whether or not, it has extended beyond or encroached upon the renal arteries, whether or not the iliac arteries are affected. It could assist the diagnosis of any arterial disease.
5. To measure the size of the abdominal aortic aneurysm, blood flow, patency of the vessels, the size of the kidney, and spleen, prostate gland and post-micturition residue in the bladder.
6. To assist paracentesis of the peritoneal fluid for the purpose of diagnosis. The fluid collected could be used for cytology. The paracentesis could be used for a continuous drainage of ascitic fluid as a part of therapeutic procedure. The catheter inserted into the peritoneal cavity could also be used for peritoneal dialysis.
7. To perform suprapubic cystostomy in order to relieve the acute retention.

- CT Scan, like USS, serves the same purposes. It is used for tumor staging and diagnostic purposes. In cases of difficult circumstances, colonic cancer could be diagnosed with a contrast medium. The exact location and size of the tumor could be identified and it would confirm the findings of the barium enema. It could define the size and extent of the aortic aneurysm in detail, whether there is intramural thrombus, tear of the aneurysmal sac. It would reveal whether it has extended beyond the renal vessels or beyond the bifurcation of the abdominal aorta. It could reveal the luminal size of the aorta.

Metastasis in the liver, lung, brain, and bones can be diagnosed. It has a wider field of application in order to establish the diagnosis and to evaluate the prognosis of the surgical treatment.

CLINICAL VALUE OF COLONOGRAPHY

Colonography is a new approach and a part of CT scan, alternative to barium enema. It has a limited diagnostic value for the colonic carcinoma and liver metastasis, but there are some benefits from this investigation. Among the benefits, barium is not required and the question of evacuation of the barium from the colon does not arise and no further bowel preparation is necessary, if patient needs immediate colonic surgery. Patient feels much comfortable apart from discomfort if the colon is distended too much with a gas. But this new investigation would be unsuitable for the diagnosis of small mucosal lesion, Crohn's colitis or ulcerative colitis. Hence, it has a limited diagnostic benefit.

In undertaking this procedure, bowel preparation remains the same like barium enema, but instead of barium being used, either carbon dioxide or air alone is insufflated via a catheter inserted into the rectum. There is no such guideline on how much air or gas is to be pushed into the colon for this investigation, but it is stopped pushing, as soon as the patient experiences discomfort due to distention of the colon. This technique may not be suitable in those cases in which straight plain X-ray of the abdomen shows that the colon is dilated with full of gas. Further addition of air or gas for the purpose of colonography would be detrimental to the patient, because, the amount of air to be pushed through the stricture or narrow lumen of the colon would cause further dilatation of the colon or it may cause splitting of the taeniae coli or serosal tear.

At the conclusion of the investigation, it would not be possible for this gas or air to get out through the stricture. In other cases, patient would not be able to pass this gas through the back passage, like flatus. It does not affect to the blood biochemistry, if it is absorbed into the circulation.

NORMAL MUCOSAL FEATURES OF THE SIGMOID COLON

This is the normal internal feature of the sigmoid colon, performed through the CT scan. It seems, as if, this new approach will eventually replace the function of colonoscopy and barium enema, but it is very unlikely. In this technique, air or carbon dioxide is pushed via catheter into the rectum. CT scan starts working, displaying the normal internal features of the mucosal lining. It seems it would serve the purpose of colonoscope, but it has a limited diagnostic value at this stage.

In figure 5.4, the top figure on the upper left corner is the CT scan of the pelvis and that on the upper right corner is the colonography showing the normal mucosal feature of the lumen of the lower sigmoid colon. The figure on the lower left corner is the CT scan of the sigmoid colon and the figure on the lower right corner is the normal mucosal feature of the lumen of the upper sigmoid colon.

This is the normal feature of the sigmoid colon, performed through the CT scan. In this technique, a good bowel preparation is necessary and air is pushed into the rectum via a catheter inserted into the rectum. The technique for clearance of colon remains the same as used in barium enema, but no

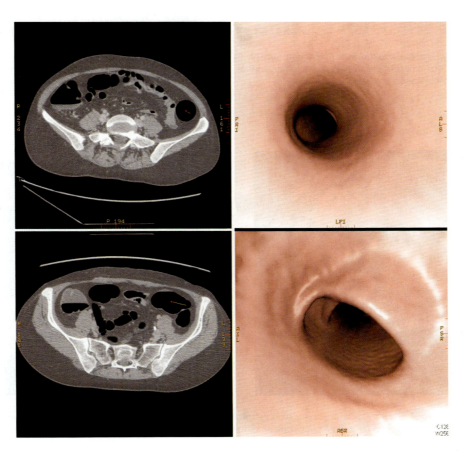

Fig. 5.4: Colonography via CT scan revealing the internal features of the colon (by courtesy of Dr S Sinha)

radiopaque liquid contrast is inserted per rectum or injected intravenously in this technique. Instead, air or carbon dioxide is pushed via catheter into the rectum. CT scan starts working, displaying the normal features of the colonic mucosa. It serves the purpose of colonoscope, but it has a limited diagnostic value at this stage. And this new approach has been advanced in the diagnosis of the malignant tumor or abnormal state of the colon, by just pushing air or carbon dioxide. It is a noninvasive procedure that provides a simple diagnosis of the diseases of the colon.

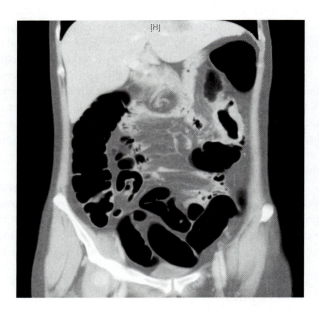

Fig. 5.5A: Colonography, first plate taken from the same patient. In this plate, stricture in the distal part of the transverse colon is evident. And a few small sized metastases are seen in the liver

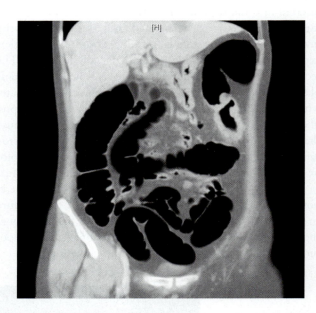

Fig. 5.5B: Colonography taken from the same patient shows dilatation of the proximal part of the transverse colon due to stricture in the distal part of the transverse colon. On the left upper flank of the patient, a small sausage-shaped black shadow is seen surrounded by a whitish soft tissue mass, which was the colonic carcinoma shown in this plate

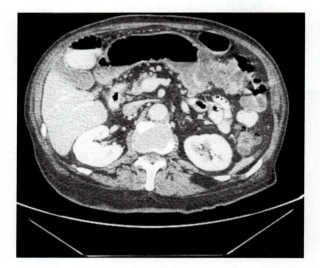

Fig. 5.5C: CT scan of abdomen of the same patient, whose colonography has been displayed in Figures 5.5A and B. This plate shows the stricture of the transverse colon and metastasis in the liver

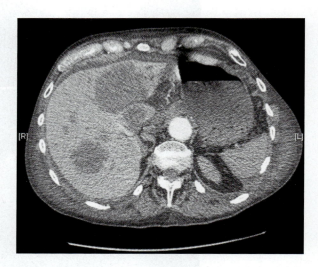

Fig. 5.5D: CT scan of abdomen shows multiple metastasis in the liver

In figure 5.4 of colonography, the proximal part of the transverse colon shows a feature of dilatation of colon compared to that of the distal part of the transverse colon, which would be attributable to obstruction between the two dilated segments of the transverse colon. This difference in diameter is the diagnostic feature for obstruction whether it is due to kinking of the colon or tumor. This differential diagnosis could be resolved by the CT scan. This plate of colonography showed stricture in the distal transverse colon and it showed secondaries in the liver (Fig. 5.5A). Detailed features of colonic obstruction has been shown in Figures 5.5B to D.

- MRI scan has a limited use in the investigation of the rectal carcinoma. It cannot be used if there is metal implant in the joints or in the limbs. It cannot be used against the bones. It is useful to establish the spread of the soft tissue mass and to establish the tumor staging of the rectum.

MRI scan of the rectal tumor showed that the tumor appeared to be invasive in one patient (Figs 5.6A and B) and it appeared to be localized within the rectum in another patient.

The advantage of this investigation would be that it can delineate the space around the rectal wall and between the fascia of Waldeyer and rectal wall in sagittal view. Such finding may indicate preoperatively, whether or not the tumor would be resectable. But, absence or reduced size of the space may be due to edema around the rectal wall or soft tissue layer. Hence, it would be misleading interpretation of the MRI scan.

In these two MRI plates, the rectal tumor has invaded the prostate gland.

In this sagittal view of MRI scan, the rectal tumor is located at the level between sacral 2 and 4. It enhances the accurate clinical diagnosis and assists the surgeon and radiotherapist to find out whether the patient would be benefited from preoperative adjuvant radiotherapy.

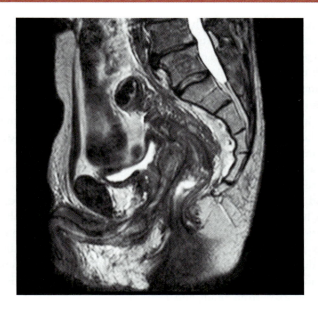

Fig. 5.6B: MRI scan of the rectum in sagittal view, showing the sacral curvature and the rectal tumor within the wall of the rectum. The tumor is at the level between sacral 2 and 4 (By courtesy of Dr S Sinha)

MRI scan has other disadvantage. For instance, peristaltic movement of the gut may interfere with the accurate feature of the tumor, present in the colon.

PET SCAN

Clinical Application

PET is known as positron emission tomography. PET scan is a new technique used in nuclear medicine imaging technology and is incorporated to the existing CT and MRI scans. It produces 3-dimensional images of a functional organ in the body. It enhances the information on biological function of many various tissues, in which the glucose metabolism is much higher. Among all tissues, malignant tissues consume a higher proportion of glucose than by any other healthy organ. Because of this abnormal glucose metabolism, the radionuclide is picked up by the cancer cells. Because of this metabolic affinity, the concentration of radioactive substance is much greater in areas of altered tissue metabolism, which is commonly present in the malignant tumors (Figs 5.6C and D).

Positron is a positively charged electron. It is a short half-life radioactive tracer isotope that undergoes decaying by emitting positron gamma rays. They are detected by special sensors. It is incorporated into a biologically active molecule or natural compounds, before it is injected into the blood.

PET scan is more often used to read the images along with the CT or MRI scan, and both scans could be done at the same time without changing the position of the patient between the two types of scans taken in the same session. They are

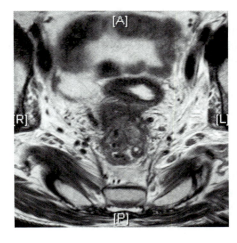

Fig. 5.6A: MRI scan of the rectum in axial view showing the rectal tumor (By courtesy of Dr S Sinha)

complementary to each other. The combined procedure provides lots of precise information in three dimensions about the site, size and shapes of the organ and these anatomic features are merged with the metabolic function of the organ, at the same session. This is the basis for a comprehensive diagnostic scan taken from the moving image.

In this technology, a cyclotron is required to produce the radioactive isotope that is then tagged with normal body compounds. It is known as Fleurodeoxy-glucose (FDG), which is a sugar-based molecule that undergoes positron emission decays. This sugar-based radioisotope is injected into the blood, and the dose is 200- 400 MBQ for an adult patient. It takes an hour before being deposited into the tissue. Hence the patient needs to wait for one hour before being placed into the scanner. This short half life isotope is picked up by the malignant cells due to the fact that the glucose metabolism is much higher in cancerous cells than that in any other healthy organ apart from brain and heart.

Hence, the PET scan can identify the malignant tumor much quicker than any other diagnostic tools available in clinical practice and it provides most accurate diagnosis (Fig. 5.6D).

The system then recognizes the pairs of gamma rays emitted indirectly by a positron-emitting radionuclide. The computer reconstructs a single image of tracer concentration, present in 3-dimensional space.

Clinical Value of the New Technology

This new technology assists in diagnosis, tumor staging and progress in treatment. As a result, it would provide information to the medical and surgical oncologist in review of the diseases, whether the metastatic or primary tumor such as Hodgkin, non-Hodgkin lymphoma are responding to the treatment, whether there is recurrence of tumor either in the same site or in other parts of the body, after excision of the tumor is carried out.

A short summary of clinical benefits:
- Diagnosis is much quicker and without other investigation.
- It can differentiate the malignant tumors from benign tumor, metastasis from the scar tissue or fibrosis.
- It can identify the metastasis in lymph nodes, liver and bone.
- It can assist in monitoring the response to treatment, aggressiveness of the tumor and spread of the tumor.
- This technology could be used in other specialties such as brain and heart, because of high consumption of glucose being used. It is frequently used in the diagnosis of dementia, epilepsies and Parkinson disease. It is also used for the evaluation of ischemic or viability of the cardiac muscles.
- This technology could be used in the treatment with radiotherapy where the target organ could be focused precisely to the pin-point on the proposed site of the tumor to be treated with gamma rays before the treatment is commenced by the linear accelerator. The radiation is given all around the tumor. As a result, tissue damage would be minimum because of the distribution of the total dose, uniformly all around the tumor. This new technology was available before.

Clinical Pharmacology

Nuclides are short half life isotope. These isotopes are added into the compounds or molecules. The compounds normally used in the body are glucose or glucose analogues, water and ammonia and the molecules bind the receptors or other sites of drug action.

These labelled compounds, known as radiotracers get distributed into the tissues by metabolic pathways of their natural analogues and other compounds. They bind with the specific tissue that contains particular receptor proteins.

The purpose of using the PET technology is to trace the biologic pathway of any compound that could be radio-leveled with a PET isotope. But there may be technical difficulty in producing the short half lives isotope locally, closer to the site of PET scan room.

Most of the isotope tracers must be manufactured using cyclotron in a radiochemistry or radiopharmaceutical laboratory near the PET imaging room, but such facility is not always available in many district hospitals. Instead, Fluorine-18 isotope, which has a long half life could be used, because of the fact that it has a half life of around 2 hours and could be transported to a distance away from the site of manufacture.

Relative Risk to the Patient

Although it is noninvasive, it has a small risk of ionizing radiation to the patient, but the dose of radiation is 7mSv, which is smaller than the dose required for CT scan. It does not cause radiation to other family members or to the attending nurses. Patient is encouraged to drink plenty of water that would eliminate the isotope through urine. Patient can resume his normal work after the investigation is finished.

This is an image of the PET scan taken in coronal plane, showing the images of the chest and abdominal organs (Fig. 5.6C). Among the abdominal organs, a radioisotope has been concentrated in the right colon, which appears to be much brighter and suspicious. This is confirmed by further PET scan taken through the cross-section of a particular anatomical organ of the abdomen and the sharp bright color in the right side of the colon was the cecal carcinoma, shown in a separate PET scan (Fig. 5.6D). The uptake of FDG isotope appears to be much greater in the cecal carcinoma due to the fact that glucose metabolism in the malignant cells of the cecum is much higher.

This is an image of carcinoma of the cecum shown on the PET scan, taken in cross-section, by the CT scan (Fig. 5.6D). Obviously, colonoscopy or contrast barium enema will confirm the diagnosis. This scan has been included in the book for the purpose of teaching to the postgraduate students and for a better understanding about the scope for advanced special investigation.

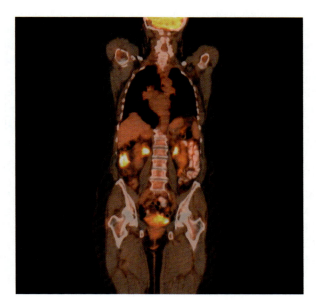

Fig. 5.6C: PET scan in coronal section showing a few bright illuminations, but one in the right colon could be colonic carcinoma (By courtesy of Dr S Sinha)

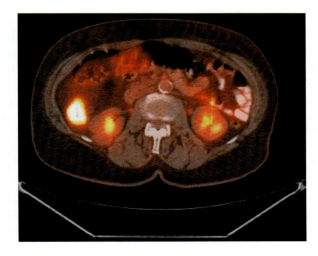

Fig. 5.6D: PET scan in transverse section is showing a bright color spot in the right side of the abdomen. It was suggestive of carcinoma of the cecum. (By courtesy of Dr S Sinha)

COLONOSCOPY

▪ Indication for Colonoscope

This investigation is supplementary to other radiological investigations. It is not without complication and it may not be possible to carry out the complete colonoscopy. It is an ideal tool for surveillance of polyps and to confirm whether ulcerative colitis or Crohn's disease has been responding to drug therapy or there is any malignant change in the ulcerated lesion.

Its main purpose is to confirm the abnormal condition, and evidence of tumor. It provides a route for tissue diagnose. It is also a diagnostic tool for confirming the diagnosis of diverticula, polyp, ulcerative colitis, ischemic colitis, and the source of colonic bleeding. Apart from collecting the tissue from the colon or snaring of the polyps with electrocoagulation, it could be used for the correction of volvulus. It is an expensive tool and its maintenance requires a trained personnel.

▪ Contraindications

- Recent heart attack.
- Acute ulcerative colitis and acute dilatation of the colon.
- Ischemic colitis.
- Peritonitis.
- Diverticulitis.
- Recent radiotherapy to the pelvis.
- Ascites.
- Hemorrhagic shock.
- Megacolon.
- Hirschsprung's disease.

Special measures against the following diseases:
- Tuberculous intestine.
- AIDS patients.
- Hepatitis.
- Patient is on immunosuppressive drugs.
- Known heart valve replacement.

▪ Prophylactic Measures in these Cases

For cases with AIDS and TB patients, a thorough cleaning of the colonoscope, along with all channels is carried out by immersing the instrument into the solution of 2 percent glutaraldehyde for 60 minutes and a particular care is taken to clean the channels with a special type of brush.

Prophylactic antibiotic therapy should be commenced prior to colonoscopy in the following cases:
- Known heart valve replacement.
- Immunosuppressive cases.

It has been reported to the literature that colonic bacteria may be transmitted into the circulation during the procedure of colonoscopy, because of mucosal abrasion being caused by the shaft of the colonoscope.

Bowel Preparation

Prior to colonoscopy, patient should be advised to stop taking the iron tablets for 3-5 days and should be discouraged against taking high fiber diet for a few days, before the day of oral bowel preparation is due. The color of the iron pigmentation in the stool and residual lumpy feces may obscure the true feature of colonic mucosa. The aim of cleaning the colonic mucosa is to visualize the abnormal mucosa. Therefore, a good preparation is essential and this could be achieved with water diarrhea. Patient must stay on oral clear fluid after the bowel preparation being completed.

These are the oral bowel preparations:
- Magnesium sulphate.
- Senna cot.
- Picolax.
- Mannitol 10 percent (1000ml).
- Castor oil (30-40 ml).

In other cases, where oral bowel preparation is contraindicated or the history and clinical examination indicates that the symptoms may be related to benign conditions or related to the pathology located in the left colon, flexible sigmoidoscopy could be undertaken to exclude the growth in the sigmoid colon or descending colon. In this case, rectal enema such as phosphate enema, soap and water enema or both in combination would suffice the purpose. And, phosphate enema could be given 30 minutes, prior to the procedure. It has a limited diagnostic and a therapeutic value.

Contraindications for Oral Bowel Preparations

- Intestinal obstruction.
- Peritonitis.
- Paralytic ileus.
- Immediate postoperative patients.
- Massive colonic hemorrhage.
- Septic shock.
- Abdominal pain.
- Megacolon.
- Hirschsprung's disease.
- Acute dilatation of colon.
- Acute ulcerative colitis.
- Acute diverticulitis.
- Ischemic colitis.
- Volvulus.

Policy for Oral Bowel Preparation

In most clinical practice, picolax in double dose or klean preparation is commonly used. Total duration of bowel clearance varies from person-to-person. In some cases, picolax starts working within 2 hours, but in other cases it takes around 6-8 hours. By and large, patient is advised to drink picolax preparation at 4 pm, if the colonoscopy has been planned to be done on the following morning. After the first dose, he should drink the second dose after 8 hours. During the period of repeated diarrhea, patient is encouraged to drink plain salty water to replace the fluid being lost with the loose motion.

Mannitol is prepared with sugar but it is not absorbed. If the solution of 10 percent in concentration is used in bowel preparation, it would lose a lot of body fluid, because of hypertonicity. In this case, it is not suitable for elderly patient. Apart from this, it should be avoided, in case polypectomy is necessary by using the electrocoagulations. This may cause explosion of methane gas inside the colon, because mannitol solution produces hydrogen ion or methane gas inside the colon, which is inflammable.

Bowel preparation depends upon the individual practice. Choice of oral preparation is not important, but a good guidance is necessary to obtain a good result in the oral purgative.

Complications with Oral Purgative

- Nausea, vomiting
- Dehydration
- Hypovolemic shock
- Confused
- Hyponatremia and hypokalemia.

Drugs used for Short-Acting Sedation

- Diazepam 5-10 mg
- Midazolam 2-5 mg
- Pethidine 25 – 50 mg
- Buscopan 20-40 mg.

Merit of Sedation

Colonoscopist requires acquiring a skill, a full knowledge of the patient's attitude and level of pain-threshold and the anatomical status of the colon. Hence, barium enema films should be available. If patient's apprehension could not be overcome, despite listening to a full reassuring talk, sedation should be given. In this case, patient remains at a greater risk of noncooperation that may cause damage to the bowel as well as to the instrument.

Pain is a safety factor that may remind the colonoscopist to be gentle, careful and to limit the procedure. It may be elicited, if the gut is overdistended, or if force is applied in the manipulation of the tip of the instrument to be negotiated through the acute bend, through the wall or through the diverticulum. Evidence of pain or discomfort becomes apparent by restlessness, facial expression, and by a rapid pulse rate.

Experiences tell us that without sedation, colonoscopy tends to be easier. This is due to the tonic state of the gut wall that keeps the gut shorter in length. For a limited colonoscopy, sedation may not be necessary in many cases. And some patient who accepts the procedure without sedation will respond to change in position of the body during colonoscopy. In this case, patient may feel embarrassed as if he or she wants to pass flatus. This is due to distention of the colon.

The success rate for total colonoscopy would be much less, if the procedure is undertaken under sedation. It all depends upon many factors. The situation has to be judged after a full consultation with the patient and after reviewing the barium X-ray. If the X-ray shows redundant transverse or sigmoid colon, sedation should be given, for colonoscopy.

Despite all this discussion, colonoscopy is not without complication. Therefore, merit of this particular investigation is to be judged and an appropriate decision should be taken on the merits, whether the patient would be benefited from colonoscopy.

Merits of the Drugs to be used for Colonoscopy

There are varieties of sedative drugs available for this procedure. Midazolam is a short-acting sedative and it relaxes the gut muscle, but it has no pharmacological effect on the relief of pain.

Buscopan should be administered if difficulty in negotiating the tip is encountered in the bend or the segment of diverticular diseases. It is effective for advancing the instrument through the narrow lumen, but it is not effective if the colon has redundant loop and is atonic. It cannot relieve the pain. Although its effect lasts for 10 minutes, the visual side effect of the patient lasts longer than 10 minutes. Patient should be discouraged against driving the car.

Preoperative Consultation and Preparation

During consultation, patient must be explained about the procedure involved. The possible risk of perforation of the colon, incomplete examination, or failure to reach to the cecum must be disclosed. In addition; pain, feeling of bloating of the abdomen, feeling of passing flatus, and poor bowel preparation should be discussed with the patient. Consent is taken on the prescribed form, if available. Patient should wear the theater gown.

Denture must be removed from the mouth. The blood pressure is recorded. Oxy-thermometer is put on in the finger. This will show the oxygen saturation of the peripheral blood in the tissue. A venous access is set up, preferably on the dorsal vein of the right hand, by inserting a fine venous cannula.

Position of the Patient

Patient is asked to lie on the left lateral position bringing both knees towards the pelvis. The buttock is brought towards the edge of the couch, on the surgeon's side. It is preferable and it would be comfortable if the buttock is rested on the pillow, covered with a plastic sheet. The feet should be along the other edge of the couch. The space between the legs and edge of the couch nearer to the surgeon is used to lay down the whole length of the colonoscope in U-shaped position, with the tip and the grip end directed towards the perineum.

In middle of the procedure, if difficulty is experienced in advancing the tip of the colonoscope through the redundant sigmoid loop, patient may need to be turned on the supine or right lateral position.

Procedure for Sedation

Before sedation is given, rectal digital examination should be carried out in order to assess about the status of the anus and the rectum and bowel preparation. If the bowel preparation seems to be inadequate, procedure should be postponed, otherwise, the sedation should be commenced with a choice of drug.

Surgeon should draw the drugs himself in the syringe, and each syringe must be labelled with the name of the drug. Initially, normal saline is injected into the cannula inserted into the vein. This will confirm whether the cannula is in the vein and is patent. It is followed by the injection midazolam 2.5 mg; and wait for a few seconds to see the level of sedation. It varies from person-to-person. Further dose should be considered later during the procedure.

Injection buscopan or pethidine could be given if necessary that depends upon the circumstances. If no difficulty is encountered with the advancement of the colonoscope, further sedation is unnecessary.

Procedure for Colonoscopy

Selection of Colonoscope

For a diagnostic purpose and for adjuvant diagnostic tool, colonoscope which is smaller in diameter will serve the purpose, but for a minor operating procedure such as polypectomy, a larger diameter of the colonoscope should be used. It has a wide-bore side channel, incorporated within the wall of the colonoscope. It is necessary for passing the biopsy forceps and other tool for snaring the polyp or adenoma. The length of the colonoscope is not important. Nevertheless, it would not cause any harm, if a longer one is used.

To avoid unnecessary waste of time, all instruments should be tested. The tip of the colonoscope is dipped into the bucket of water in order to see air-bubble in the water and to see the suction mechanism working perfectly. Next inspection is to see the brightness of the illumination and sharpness of the object seen through the eyepiece. The lens at the terminal end may need to be cleaned with a silicone stick. When the colonoscope appears to be in perfect operating condition, insertion of the distal end could be started.

General Description

It is a long flexible telescope that could be manipulated in various directions. It has a built-in lens, fitted at the distal end and viewing lens fitted at the proximal end. There are 4 channels built within the shaft of the telescope. They are fiber optic light channel, operating channel used for squirting water and for taking biopsy or snaring the polyp, a common channel used for inflating the colon and for suction of the loose motion.

At the proximal end, there are two rotating knobs, fitted on the side of the instrument, one used for changing the tip up or down and other one for changing the tip towards the right or left direction (Fig. 5.7). These knobs are operated by the left thumb alone, but at times, both left thumb and left middle finger may be required to be used in the operation of these knobs that depends upon the circumstances.

Some endoscopists prefer assistance for advancing the distal part of the instrument through the anus, while he or she keeps concentrating on viewing the lumen of the rectum or colon through the eye-window, held in by the left hand and at the same time, the other hand is kept busy in the operation of the two knobs, fitted to section of the eye-window. It all depends upon the individual preference and practice.

But the new type of colonoscope does not require viewing the pictures of the colon through the eye-window. The pictures of the colonic wall, lumen and bends of the rectum and colon are relayed on the television screen. This new technology allows every person and the patient to view those pictures displayed on the screen of the television.

Apart from the two knobs, fitted with the set of eye-window, there are two operating buttons fitted on the side wall of the proximal end. One is used for insufflation of air or carbon dioxide into the colon, and the other one for suction of the air or liquid feces from the colon. These buttons are operated by the left index and middle fingers. There is a large channel mounted on the shaft, but a little below the other two buttons.

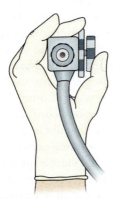

Fig. 5.7: The left hand, holding the colonoscope is displaying how the knobs are operated by the left middle finger and left thumb

It is usually covered with a stop-cork, when it is not used. Its main function is to permit either a biopsy forceps, snaring instrument or for squirting water with a view to cleaning the lens and loosening the residual soft feces. This is done by injecting 50 ml water in a 50 ml syringe, which can be fitted with an adopter, inserted into this operating channel at times when necessary. The loose motion is sucked out concurrently by the other channel. This channel is also used for taking biopsy and snaring the polyps.

The fiberoptic illuminating light channel is built in a thick cable, fitted opposite to those two buttons. This fiberoptic light cable rests upon the left thumb, particularly in the first web between the left thumb and left index finger, when the proximal part of the colonoscope is firmly held in the palm of the left hand between the left thumb at one side and middle ring and little fingers on the other side of the instrument (Fig. 5.7).

The left thumb is used to rotate the smaller knob and middle finger for the larger knob, if the colonoscopy is carried out by a single person. These knobs have been designed for manipulating the change in direction of the terminal end of the colonoscope.

The air insufflations or suction apparatus is operated by the tip of the left index and middle fingers. The right hand is left free to be used in negotiating the terminal end, through the anus and through the difficult bends (Figs 5.8A and B). The latter is more often overcome by a combination of twisting and torqueing and by changing the direction of the terminal end of the instrument. In that maneuver, the twisting of the shaft is done by the right hand and the change in direction of the tip is done by rotating the knobs with left thumb or middle finger.

The right hand is mainly used for advancing the instrument towards the proximal part of the colon by half twisting in clockwise and anticlockwise direction, and/or by pulling backwards and pushing forwards, as and when indicated (Fig. 5.9). It is also used for colonic wash out with 50 ml syringe or for taking biopsy with biopsy forceps, passed through the large operating channel or for snaring the polyp using electrocoagulation.

The distal end of the instrument is negotiated through the bends and through the redundant loop of the sigmoid or transverse colon by just applying half twisting of the shaft in clockwise and anticlockwise direction, by the right hand. In this maneuver, a small swab soaked with lubricating jelly should be used wrapped around the instrument, during the manipulation or advance movement of the colonoscope.

The acute bends of the colon are negotiated by manipulation of the terminal end under direct vision either seen through the window of the eyepiece or through the Television screen (Fig. 5.10A). The tip of the instrument must not be pushed forwards blindly. It must be advanced slowly when the tunnel is seen clearly through the screen or through the eyepiece

Investigations

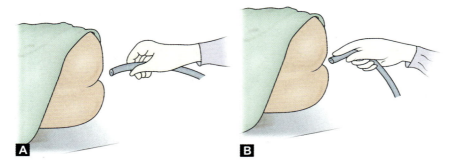

Figs 5.8A and B: (A) The tip of the colonoscope is focusing with light around the anal orifice. (B) The tip of the colonoscope is pushing into the anal orifice, under the direction of the right index finger

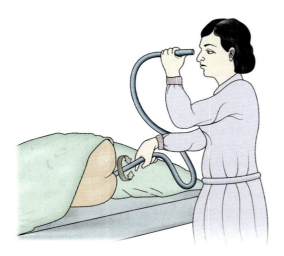

Fig. 5.9: This figure shows how the gastroenterologist looks at the lumen of the colon through the eyepiece, but it used to be regular practice 10 years ago. Now, this type of instrument is no longer used and internal visualization of the gut is carried out through the television screen. It relieves the endoscopist from undue strain in the eyes and around the neck. Furthermore, every person in the theater could see the normal and pathological features present inside the colon

(Fig. 5.9). It requires skill and anatomical knowledge of the internal features of the colon. This manipulation of the distal end of the colonoscope is regulated by the knobs operated by the left hand (Fig. 5.7).

If the clear view of the colonic lumen is not in sight, despite changing the direction of the terminal end, the tip of the colonoscope is withdrawn slowly until the lumen is in sight (Fig. 5.10B).

The procedure reduces the length of the bend of the colon and permits straightening of the sigmoid colon (Figs 5.10B and C). The procedure should be repeated until the difficulty is overcome, before the colonoscope is advanced through the redundant loop or bend of the colon. This is the basic principle in learning and handling the colonoscope that could be acquired through training. Every person then develops the individual technique and skill in performing the colonoscopy.

From time-to-time, a few things need to be followed. The colon must not be inflated with too much air or gas. If it appears to be overdilated, this needs to be deflated by sucking the air out, and liquid motions out of the gut. The patient must be assessed from time-to-time whether he/she is experiencing discomfort or restlessness. This is evaluated by palpating the lower abdomen (Fig. 5.21).

This is an outline of the mechanism involved and how to handle the colonoscope. Practical experience is acquired by handling the colonoscope in the colonoscopic theater and by learning the operating techniques while working with an experienced colonoscopist.

How to Proceed with the Colonoscopy

Despite checking the functional state of all the gadgets and operating function of the air channel, suction channel, biopsy channel and light source, it is equally important to take a decision on whether colon is to be inflated with air or CO_2 insufflation. The latter is absorbed from the gut much quicker than air and it is first absorbed into the blood and then is expelled through the expiration of the lung. By contrast, air remains in the colon longer and absorbed less quickly.

First, generous lubricating jelly is coated for several inches all around the distal segment of the colonoscope, using a small swab and the anus is also lubricated with jelly by the right index finger. The fiberoptic light source is switched on, while the tip of the colonoscope is gently pushed through the anus under the guidance of right index finger (Fig. 5.7).

The whole length of the instrument should be laid down on the sterile sheet that has been laid down over the couch and its tip is directed towards the anus. This layout would prevent the colonoscope from slipping out of the rectum and this position should be maintained that will stop dragging the shaft down from the anal canal. If the shaft of the colonoscope keeps hanging down by the side of the couch, the weight of

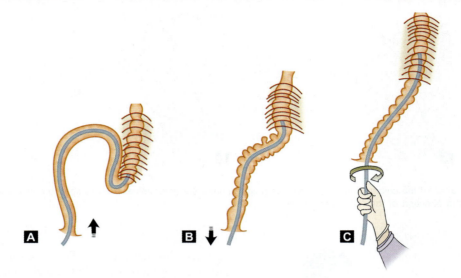

Figs 5.10A to C: (A) Showing the tip of the colonoscope in the junction of the sigmoid colon with the descending colon. (B) Displaying the technique on how the loop of the sigmoid colon is made straight. The colonoscope is pulled back, after its tip is hooked to the bend or to the side wall. Without anchoring its distal end, straightening of the coiled colonic loop is not possible. (C) Showing the technique on how the colon is advancing with clockwise half-twist and turn

the colonoscope may act as gravitational force that may slip down the tip of the colonoscope from the site of examination.

Once the tip of the colonoscope has passed for a few centimeters, the proximal end of the colonoscope is lifted up from the couch to be held in the left grip as described in the previous section. The anal canal is now identified through the eyepiece and a few air insufflations are pushed, in order to open up the lumen of the lower rectum.

In some cases, a pool of water may be seen resting on the left lateral wall of the rectum or a few lumps of feces could be hanging down from the right lateral wall of the rectum and they may obscure the field of vision or may be found stuck to the tip of the colonoscope. From time-to-time, those fluid or loose motion may need to be sucked out. In most cases, the lumen of the rectum becomes clearer, after the rectum is inflated with air. At the same time, lumps of feces may drop on the floor, concurrently, when the rectum is inflated with air.

The shaft of the instrument outside the anus is lubricated with jelly using a small swab and the shaft is advanced, if the lumen could be seen clearly. In some cases, it could be advanced in pari passu with the insufflations of air into the rectum, provided the lumen could be seen clearly.

Through the eyepiece, one could see a semilunar type of opening of the lumen by the rectal valve or haustration. This may guide the direction of the lumen. Some degree of intuition is necessary in the maneuver of colonoscope, but instrument should not be pushed further through the mucosal wall on blind intuition. In this situation, the tip could be manipulated through this semilunar opening, either by changing its position, as described before or by half twist in both directions under direct vision seen through the eyepiece or through the television screen.

Under any circumstance, the tip must not be pushed blindly and too much air must not be pushed with a view to displaying the better visualization of the lumen. Once the lumen is in sight, the tip is advanced by twisting in clockwise and anticlockwise direction (Figs 5.11 and 5.12).

Once it has been successfully advanced for a few centimeters, colon is decompressed. This would reduce its girth, its bend and patient would not experience any discomfort and would not desire to pass flatus.

If the bowel preparation is poor or it contains lumps of feces, or they are stuck to the lens, these need to be washed out by squirting water through the operating channel using 50 ml syringe, as described before. The pool of loose motion is sucked out. Once the vision is brighter and the passage of the lumen seems to be well-defined, the tip is advanced once again in the same way.

The ascending colon, descending colon and the rectum remain fixed to the posterior wall by the peritoneum (Fig. 5.13A). They are not mobile, but the transverse colon and the sigmoid colon have a mesentery (Fig. 5.13B), thus permitting these segments of the colon mobile. The transverse colon has a short and broad mesentery, known as mesocolon that lies between the transverse colon and the posterior wall along the pancreas, and between the colon and the greater curvature of the stomach.

This mesocolon may be stretched down and may be expanded by the weight of the colon, thus bringing it down to be rested in the pelvis. Volvulus of the transverse colon does

Investigations

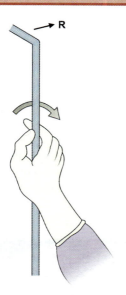
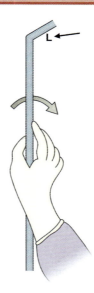

Fig. 5.11: Showing the technique for clockwise twist in two directions. If the tip is directed upwards, it would turn to the right in clockwise rotation

Fig. 5.12: Shown the change of direction of the tip of the instrument. If it remains directed downwards, it would turn to the left when the shaft is twisted in clockwise direction. Therefore, it is important to remember the direction of the tip during half-twist of the shaft

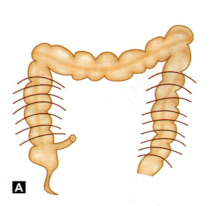
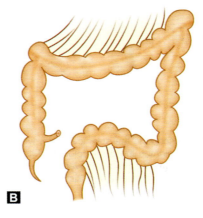

Figs 5.13A and B: (A) The figure shows the ascending and descending colon in the retroperitoneal space. They are fixed to the posterior wall by the peritoneum and are immobile. (B) The transverse colon has a broader mesentery and the sigmoid colon has a narrow mesentery

not occur because of broad mesocolon. On the contrary, the sigmoid colon has a narrow base of the sigmoid mesocolon like an inverted V.

It may form sigmoid volvulus if the sigmoid colon is elongated along with a long mesentery.

Because of these anatomical changes, difficulty may be experienced in advancing the tip of the colonoscope through these bends and through the angulations formed at the junction between the sigmoid colon and the descending colon, and at the splenic and the hepatic flexures in some cases (Fig. 5.14).

Identification of the Anatomical Site of the Colon

Unlike the rigid sigmoidoscope, the position of the splenic flexure is usually not recognized by the measurement in length of the colonoscope from the anal verge. Its location depends upon the length of the sigmoid loop and phrenicocolic ligament. The apparent position of the splenic flexure which appears to be 80 cm from the anal verge, may turn out to be 50- 60 cm. This change in difference is due to the

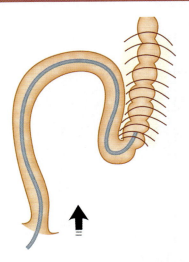

Fig. 5.14: The acute bend at the junction with the descending colon. It is referred to as 'hairpin' bend

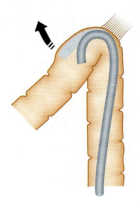

Fig. 5.15: The tip of the colonoscope in the splenic flexure, where it has been hooked in order to straighten the distal colon, and its tip is next deangulated like walking-stick. By this maneuver, the lumen of the distal transverse colon becomes clearer that assists in advancing the tip further

withdrawing of the shaft of the colonoscope for a short length from the colon, resulting in shortening of the sigmoid colon, while the tip of the instrument is held in position by hooking in the splenic flexure (Fig. 5.15). It is important to overcome the large sigmoid loop and the acute bend at the junction with the descending colon, before proceeding further and before straightening both sigmoid colon and descending colon.

Therefore, the correct position is usually determined by the internal anatomical feature and by the bluish color of the spleen seen through the wall of the colon and by the illuminating light seen through the posterior abdominal wall in the darkroom. In sharp contrast, no such illumination could be seen through the anterior abdominal wall for the left colon because of its location in the posterior paravertebral gutter.

The same rule is also applied for the hepatic flexure.

The internal anatomical feature of the transverse colon has a distinct shape. The cross-section of the colon would appear to be circular (Fig. 5.16A), but it would appear to be triangular in shape particularly in the transverse colon, seen through the colonoscope (Fig. 5.16B).

The position of the cecum is variable, but it has a thin-wall and large space. It is recognized by the longitudinal fold projecting inwards. These prominent inward projections are the longitudinal muscle of the taeniae coli. These bands are fused at the cecal pole where the osteum of the appendix could be evident, if the cecum does not contain scattered loose motion (Fig. 5.16C).

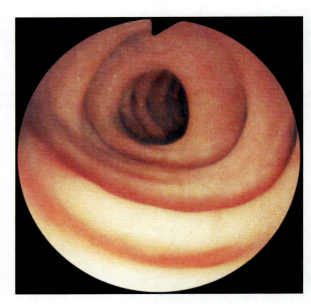

Fig. 5.16A: Colonoscopic view displaying the feature of the lumen of the descending colon

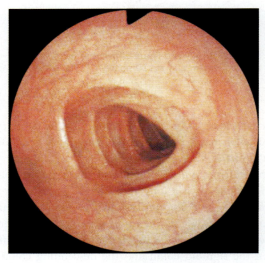

Fig. 5.16B: Colonoscopic view showing the triangular shape of the lumen of the transverse colon

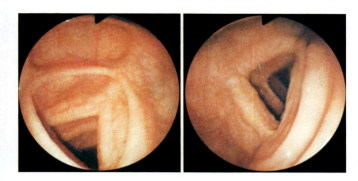

Fig. 5.16C: Triangular folds of the ascending colon are relatively thicker than the triangular folds in the transverse colon

The sigmoid colon has a mesentery and it makes an inverted U-shaped loop in most cases. The length of the sigmoid mesocolon may be increased in diverticular disease or habitual constipation. Overdistention of the sigmoid colon may be possible by the excessive insufflation of air during colonoscopy and this may form an alpha loop (Fig. 5.17A and B), thus causing distress of the mesentery and anterior abdominal wall.

As a result, patient may experience with sickly feeling, distention of the lower abdomen and distress or colicky pain. Sweating and restlessness are the clinical features of distention of the sigmoid loop.

If the appendix is very short in length, it may appear like a diverticulum. In cases with postappendicectomy, invaginated appendicular stump may appear to be looking like a polyp. Care should be taken before considering for polypectomy.

The cecal wall could also be recognized by the features of outpouchings or bulging outwards between these longitudinal folds and marked cecal haustra (Fig. 5.16D).

Other identification feature is the iliocecal valve present on the medial wall and 5 cm proximal to the opening of the appendix (Fig. 5.16E). It looks like a slit and remains closed more often. It is not easy to recognize it, unless some loose contents emerge through this slit.

Illumination seen through the abdominal wall in the right iliac fossa or in the right flank provides further confirmation. And it could also be recognized by the movement of the cecal wall in and out concurrently with the movement of the abdominal wall, when the latter is pushed up and down repeatedly.

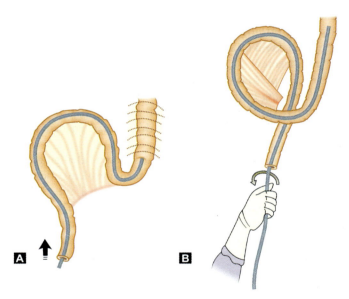

Figs 5.17A and B: (A) Over distention: It shows the long mesentery attached to the wide loop of the sigmoid colon. Because of acute bend at the upper end of the sigmoid colon, the tip of the colon could not be advanced, but instead, it has made the sigmoid colon much wider. (B) Alpha Loop: It shows how the large sigmoid loop could be twisted, transforming into a right alpha loop, while pushing the colonoscope

How to Overcome the Difficult Anatomical Sites

Difficult Anatomical Sites

a. The ampulla of the rectum.
b. Rectosigmoid junction.
c. Redundant large sigmoid loop.
d. Junction of the large sigmoid loop with the descending colon, simulating like an N loop or alpha loop.
e. Splenic flexure of the colon.
f. Junction of the redundant transverse loop and the hepatic flexure.
g. Identification of the iliocecal valve.

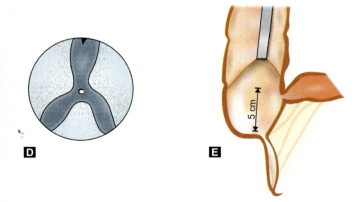

Figs 5.16D and E: (D) Base of the cecum and opening of the appendix in the center of the taeniae coli. (E) It shows the features of the cecum and the opening of the terminal ileum

Clinical Practice and Surgery of the Colon, Rectum and Anus

Colonoscope could be Advanced in Four Ways

1. Twisting of the colonoscope in straight position is one of the techniques used in advancing the instrument. It requires the shaft to be straight along with the terminal end. In this maneuver, the shaft is made half twisted in clockwise and then anticlockwise direction and *vice versa*, under direct vision seen through the eyepiece.

   The distal part of the shaft is held by the right hand, 5-10 centimeters away from the anus and twisting is carried out along the same axis of the shaft, when the lumen is seen open through the eyepiece. The change in direction of the tip may be necessary in pari passu, regulated by the knobs (Fig. 5.7). This operation is done by the left thumb or left middle finger or both in combination, if necessary. If single-handed operation turns out to be difficult, right hand could be used in turning the knob at times. In this situation, the right hand could be used in focusing the lumen alternate with the advancement of the tip.

   Or an experienced assistant could assist in the operation of half-twisting of the shaft and advancement, but he would respond to pushing the shaft at the command of the endoscopist. The difficult site for this delicate maneuver is at the bend of the colon.

   If the lumen appears to be obscured, despite changing the direction of the tip, or the tip is not seen advancing, despite the shaft has been pushed through the anal canal, then it has to be considered that the sigmoid loop is causing the problem, producing an acute bend with the descending colon. This is known as 'hairpin' bend (Fig. 5.18). In this position, the elastic sigmoid loop gets expanded by pushing the shaft of the colonoscope, while its tip being stuck at the acute bend of the sigmoid colon with the descending colon.

   To overcome these problems, the shaft of the colon is pulled back for a good length and the procedure is repeated again, as shown in Figures 5.19A to C.

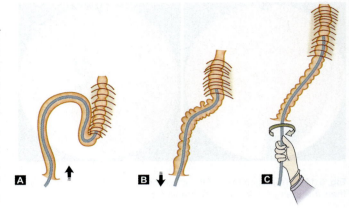

Figs 5.19A to C: (A) It shows the wide sigmoid loop and the tip of the colonoscope at the acute bend of the sigmoid colon with the descending colon. (B) It shows the withdrawal of the shaft of the colonoscope from the colon. This would assist in both straightening and shortening of the sigmoid loop, in line with the descending colon. (C) It shows how to advance the shaft of the colonoscope, by half twisting clockwise and anticlockwise, thus pushing it up in order to get into the descending colon

2. Twisting the shaft in straight position and the tip is directed upwards. In this procedure, the tip of the instrument that has been directed upwards, will turn towards the right, when the shaft is rotated in clockwise direction and it would turn to the left if the tip has been directed downwards.

3. Twisting the shaft in the position of the bend of the shaft (Fig. 5.19A). Here, one needs to understand the layout of the redundant sigmoid colon when viewing from the anal canal. The sigmoid colon remains anteriorly away from the sacral cavity and it turns left laterally and downwards before it meets the lower part of the descending colon, thus forming a clockwise loop. It would be worse if too much air insufflation is allowed, thus causing the sigmoid colon further dilatation and further bending.

   To overcome this preexisting loop, the shaft of the colonoscope is twisted clockwise while viewing the tip through the eyepiece (Fig. 5.19B). This will reduce the convex curvature of the sigmoid loop which may be pushed over the shaft towards the rectum (like sleeve of the shirt rolling up above the elbow). This would facilitate at the same time, pushing the tip slipping into the descending colon (Fig. 5.19C). Suction should be done and air insufflation should be restricted during this maneuver.

4. Torque is another maneuver which requires twisting the shaft of the instrument while the latter is withdrawing or pushing upwards concurrently (Figs 5.20A to C). In this procedure, twisting of the shaft in clockwise direction should be done if the sigmoid colon needs to be straightened. Clockwise twisting should also be carried out along the descending and transverse colon. This will reduce the tension upon the peritoneal attachment to the left paracolic gutter and upon the transverse mesocolon. This is rational from the anatomical point of view.

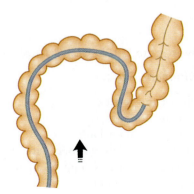

Fig. 5.18: Fixed 'hairpin' bend at the junction of the sigmoid and descending colon

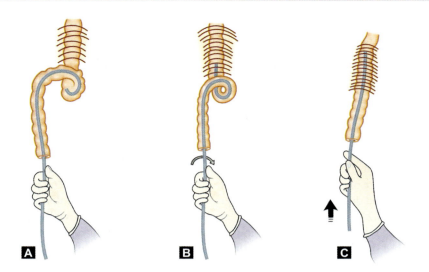

Figs 5.20A to C: (A) Sigmoid colon forms N loop with the tip of the colonoscope at the entrance of the descending colon. (B) The shaft of the colonoscope is kept on twisting clockwise until the lumen of the descending colon is in sight. (C) The tip of the colonoscope is advanced upwards while carrying out half twisting in clockwise and anticlockwise direction

▪ Problem in the Ampulla of the Rectum

The rectum has a spacious lumen. A beginner or an inexperienced endoscopist may find it difficult to follow the lumen of the rectum when the tip reaches the spacious space of the ampulla of the rectum. Beginner continues searching the proximal lumen by turning the tip of the instrument in various directions. As a result, the tip may turn back facing down towards the anus, thus forming an umbrella loop. Anatomical orientation is totally lost until the black color of the shaft is seen through the eyepiece.

It would be a similar position in the stomach where the shaft of the gastroscope could be seen coming out through the cardiac end of the stomach, when the end of the gastroscope is turned upwards in order to see the fundus, cardiac end of the stomach and the hiatus hernia, if it is present. This would be the similar position in the ampulla of the rectum where the tip of the colonoscope has turned back towards the anus, but here it occurs without recognizing the error. In this situation, the rectal wall may be split up, causing active bleeding, and patient may be restless or is experiencing pain.

To overcome this false turning, the end of the shaft needs to be straightened by rotating the two knobs methodically and slowly and decompression of the ampulla is done by the suction of the rectal fluid and gas.

The procedure is recommended with a view to advancing the tip in straight position, by half twisting in clockwise and anticlockwise direction under direct vision seen through the eyepiece or through the television screen. In every move, first decompression is followed by a minimum air insufflation. This is necessary just to open up the lumen.

▪ How to Overcome the Large Sigmoid Loop

This is the most difficult segment of the colon that may go wrong forming either N (Fig. 5.20A) or alpha loop while advancing the tip into the descending colon (Fig. 5.18B). This resulted from inexperience in handling the colonoscope. Overdistention of the sigmoid colon may contribute to further problem over the preexisting redundant sigmoid loop.

In reducing the length of the sigmoid loop, the following measures should be adopted:

a. Frequent decompression is followed by minimum air insufflation which should be the primary procedure in colonoscopy.
b. A frequent pulling and pushing the shaft in half-twisting clockwise rotation of the shaft should be attempted in conjunction with hooking of the tip of the colonoscope at the entry of the descending colon or in the mucosal fold of the sigmoid colon.

This maneuver will keep holding the junction steady by hooking the tip, while the shaft keeps on moving in and out in half-twisting clockwise direction, thus shortening the loop of the sigmoid colon and making the acute angulation of the sigmoid colon with the descending colon near straight.

This maneuver is conducted by an individual endoscopist, using the right hand for twisting, pulling and pushing the shaft, the left hand is used for holding the proximal operating tools, at the same time viewing the inner anatomical features either though the television screen or directly through the eyepiece of the proximal window.

It becomes difficult to recognize the acute bend of the sigmoid colon with the descending colon during colonoscopy.

Sometimes, this junction appears to be blind end, and it makes the anatomy worse due to overdistention of the sigmoid colon. It becomes impossible to wriggle the terminal end of the colonoscope through this acute bend.

In this situation, alternative approach is to follow the longitudinal fold seen in the mucosal wall of the sigmoid colon that provides direction of lumen of the descending colon. This longitudinal fold is the taeniae coli lying on the serosal wall of the colon.

If this approach seems to be ineffective, then the patient is next turned in order to lie flat on the back. The loop of the sigmoid colon is gently pushed down by pressing the lower anterior abdominal wall (Fig.5.21).

At times, it has been observed that the tip of the instrument has spontaneously entered in the descending colon. Nevertheless, the procedure is repeated for decompression of the sigmoid loop. This is done by sucking the air and loose motion.

This procedure is carried out in conjuction with the pulling down of the shaft by twisting halfway forwards and backwards, as described before. While undertaking the procedure, the tip of the instrument is kept on watching through the eyepiece or through the television screen, whether it remains in the same place, despite withdrawing a good length of the shaft of the instrument.

Once the tip starts moving down, then it would seem that the colonoscope is in straight position and the sigmoid loop has been corrected. After reviewing this achievement, the next approach is to push the shaft in a half-twisting clockwise direction, and see whether the tip is advancing simultaneously.

If no good result has been achieved, the patient is next turned on the right lateral position, thus sigmoid loop falls onto the right side. This may assist in reducing the mechanical compression from the descending colon. As a result, the descending colon will be lying in the superior position in the abdomen. This will permit the trapped air into the descending colon, thus visualization of the lower descending colon may be easier. The same procedure is repeated.

In the sigmoid colon, negotiation of the tip would be difficult if the sigmoid colon contains multiple diverticula. In this area, the lumen will appear to be rigid and narrow due to hypertrophy of the circular muscles and unusual multiple haustration around the chronic diverticula. Sometimes, the tip may enter into the diverticular pouch, believing to be in the true lumen of the colon (Fig. 5.22).

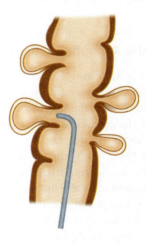

Fig. 5.22: It shows how the tip of the colonoscope may enter into the colonic diverticulum by mistake, believing to be in the true lumen of the colon

How to Overcome the Problem in the Splenic Flexure of the Colon

In left lateral position of the patient's body, the splenic flexure tends to be squashed by the drooping of the distal transverse colon down, over the descending colon. As a result, the splenic flexure becomes acutely angulated, as if the distal transverse colon is lying parallel to or resting upon by the side of the proximal descending colon. The problem may be more difficult, if there is a large sigmoid loop.

To overcome these problems, it is important to keep watching whether the tip is advancing further in pari passu with the half-twisting clockwise and anticlockwise movements

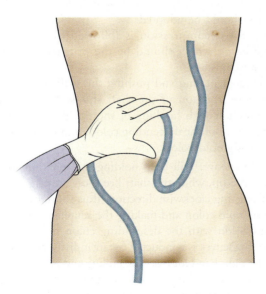

Fig. 5.21: The patient is turned on to the supine position from the left lateral position. Then the lower abdomen is palpated with the palmar surface of the left hand in order to identify the sigmoid loop. It is then gently pushed down by the left hand placed over the area of umbilicus, thus pushing the loop of the colonoscope downwards

of the colonoscope. If it remains standstill, then it has to be considered that the shaft is not straight and it has formed a large bend within the sigmoid loop forming N loop or alpha loop. Again the procedure is repeated to rectify the sigmoid loop as described before.

The clockwise half-twist of the shaft will only be effective if the shaft remains straight and the sigmoid loop is either small or has been pulled over the shaft like the sleeve of the shirt rolled over around the arm.

It has been shown that how the loop of the redundant sigmoid colon needs to be straightened over the shaft of the colonoscope. This is done by just hooking the tip of the colonoscope at the upper end of the sigmoid colon and then the shaft of the instrument is pulled back slowly, while keeping an eye upon the tip of the instrument, whether it remains still in position during this maneuver.

After rectifying all those technical problems, the shaft of the instrument is advanced forward and backwards, as described before until the tip reaches the acute angle of the splenic flexure.

In the same way, the tip of the instrument is hooked at the acute bend of the splenic flexure, and the shaft is gently withdrawn until it reaches to, say 50-60 cm. Gentle maneuver is very important, otherwise, the phrenicocolic ligament may be torn causing tear of the spleen.

It is also equally important to be sure that the tip has not been acutely angulated in the splenic flexure. A gentle bend is just necessary. However, air insufflation is done in order to visualize the internal anatomical feature of triangular mucosal rings. These are the classical landmark that would tell the endoscopist that the tip of the instrument is inside the transverse colon. Further advancement would be no more a problem if the procedure is followed.

If advancement turns out to be difficult, despite adopting all those maneuvers, the patient is turned on to the right lateral position. This will take away the pressure of the transverse colon from the splenic flexure. And the latter will move forward on its own, thus changing its angulation. The splenic flexure will lie in superior position facing downwards.

The procedure is recommenced in advancing the tip along the transverse colon. Once the problem has been overcome, the position of the patient is reversed to the previous left lateral position. In this way, the instrument is pushed towards the hepatic flexure, where the tip is turned down towards the cecum. If there is evidence of redundant transverse colon, the tip is hooked to the hepatic flexure and the colonoscope is slowly and gently withdrawn for about 30-40 cm in half-twisted clockwise direction. This will reduce the tension of the mesocolon and would straighten the transverse colon.

Examination of the Ascending Colon and the Cecum

The procedure for advancing the tip is recommenced as before, using the same maneuver. The tip will enter into the ascending colon. Suction of loose motion and air will bring the cecum higher up and shorten the ascending colon. Visualization of the ascending colon and cecum becomes quicker and easier. Total examination of the colonoscopy is then completed after reaching the cecum. Any evidence of abnormal bleeding vessels in this site would be suggestive of angiodysplasia.

When the colonoscopy seems to be completed, the tip is withdrawn, but it should not be done blindly. On the way back, the intraluminal features should be seen carefully. It provides a better picture when the tip is slowly withdrawn. All air must be sucked out at the same time in every stage. This will reduce the discomfort and the abdomen will return to its normal position.

This is a broad outline as well as a detailed description of the procedure involved in dealing with the overdistention, excessive sigmoid loop, and to get through the acute bend or anatomical flexures. Trainee will build the confidence and develop individual technique and skill on how to perform the total colonoscopy safely, comfortably and quickly. It is not possible to describe each and every technique to be used in dealing with each difficult problem in the clinical practice.

On the way back, biopsy is taken from the tumor or from the polyp. Several biopsy must be taken from the same lesion for histology. At the end, the tissue is sent in formalin for histology. Patient abdomen must be palpate in order to detect any peritonitis. If there is any suspicion of perforation, plane X-ray of abdomen should be arranged and an erect film should be requested in sitting or standing position, after the patient has fully recovered.

Complications of Colonoscopy

- Hypotension.
- Cardiac attack.
- Respiratory distress.
- Hypoxia in elderly patient.

All these medical emergencies are often associated with dehydration, electrolytic imbalance, and oversedation. Furthermore, overdistention of the colon and instrumentation may induce vasovagal reaction.

Complications Due to Faulty Techniques

a. Perforation through the diverticulum due to instrumentation or due to air pressure.

b. Perforation of the colon may be due to excessive force used and due to faulty technique.
c. Tear of phrenicocolic ligament and tear of the spleen.
d. Tear or hematoma in the serosal layer of antimesenteric border or in the mesentery.
e. Fecal peritonitis and emergency laparotomy.

Although these are broad techniques described in this book in order to assist the trainee surgeons, on how to carry out the colonoscopy, the trainee endoscopist should read other textbooks and attend the course for a practical training.

REFERENCES

1. Lauer JD, Carlson HC, Wollaeger EE. Accuracy of roentgenologic examination in detecting carcinoma of the colon. Disease Colon Rectum 1965;8:190.
2. Hamilton JB. The use of tannic acid in barium enemas. Am J Roentgenol 1946;56:101.
3. Fischer AW. Ueber die Rontgenuntersuchung des Dickdarms mit Hilfe einer Kombination von Lufteinblasung und Kontrasteinlauf (Kombinierte Methode) Arch klin chir 1925;134:209.
4. Boley SJ, Schwartz S, Lash J, Stern Hill V. Reversible vascular occlusion of the colon. Surg Gynec Obstet 1965;116:53.
5. Irwin A. Partial infarction of the colon due to reversible vascular occlusion. Clin Radiol 1965;16:261.
6. Schatzki R. Small intestinal enema. Am J Roentgenol 1943;50:743.
7. Saha SK. Unusual presentation of tuberculous colitis, Scarborough General Hospital, 2003.

6 Preoperative Preparation

FOR ELECTIVE SURGERY

Correction of anemia with the preoperative blood transfusion preferably with packed cell blood should be given two days before the date for the operation has been scheduled. Posttransfusion hemoglobin should be checked. It should be above 11 gm/dl.

In addition, correction of dehydration, assessment of renal function, correction of electrolytes depletions should be done. Blood sugar and urine sugar test should be done routinely in all preoperative cases and urine is tested in the ward for ketone, and acetone and it should be sent to the laboratory for microscopical, culture and sensitivity test for antibiotics.

Blood pressure, heart rate, respiration rate, ECG, and all maintenance drug therapy should be checked and rearranged in the drug sheet, in order to continuing taking those drugs, until they are discharged to home.

If the patient is on steroid or was on steroid therapy for sometime before coming to the hospital, he should be prescribed for intravenous hydrocortisone, 100 mg to be given 6 hourly for the first 24 hours and 12 hourly for the second day, and it is gradually tailed off within 5 days. The purpose of this supplement is to combat the adrenal crisis because of operative stress and injury.

Blood for grouping and retained serum or cross matching for 2 or more units should be arranged routinely in all major operative cases.

X-ray of chest should be done for exclusion of pleural effusion, enlarged heart and any other abnormality.

On the day of the operation, patient should have bed bath or a shower, as the case may be and a consent form is to be signed after full consultation. In this assessment, the site of the operation and site of colostomy, if indicated, must be marked with skin pencil. Prophylactic measures against the deep vein thrombosis should be adopted on the following conditions: These are overweight, above the age of 40, smokers, debilitating illness, dehydration and chronic obstructive airway disease, and high platelet counts.

The prophylactic measures are as follows: Graduated compression stockings in both the lower limbs from toes to mid thigh. It is known as thromboembolic deterrent (popularly known as TED, marketed by Kendall Company).

Three bottles of Dextran 70, should be given to the patient IV, one bottle (500 ml) before, one bottle during surgery and a third bottle within 24 hours after surgery. It acts against the platelets' adhesiveness.

Injection mini-heparin 5000 units should be given twice a day subcutaneously for 7 days or until the patient is fully mobile. The first injection should be given 2 hours before the operation is commenced. Statistics suggest that pulmonary embolism occurs more often after the patient is sent home, if prophylactic regimes are not followed prior to surgery.

Dehydration must be corrected, prior to operative procedure being undertaken. On the operating table, both heels must be rested on the soft rubber cushion or on the sand bag, thus keeping the calf above the mattress of the table. This would enhance a free venous return from the leg. In addition, both calf muscles are kept compressed by the pneumatic pump during operation.

POLICY FOR PARENTERAL FLUID INFUSION

Administration of fluid or drugs through any other routes outside the gastrointestinal tract are known as parenteral routes. In most instances, the routes used for therapeutic purposes are vein, intramuscular, subcutaneous and bone marrow.

The following fluid preparations are available for parenteral infusions:

- Blood, either whole blood or packed cell blood.
- 0.9 percent normal saline.
- 1.8 percent saline used for very low serum sodium.
- 5 percent dextrose.
- Dextrose saline (4.5 percent dextrose and 0.18 percent saline).
- Dextran 70, could be used for shock, and as a prophylactic measure against the postoperative deep vein thrombosis.
- Dextran 40 (low molecular weight) is used for renal perfusion.
- Ringer's lactate solution is used to combat the hypovolemic shock, until the blood is available.
- Mannitol 10 percent used for renal diuresis.
- Plasma (dried plasma made from 8-10 units of blood stored in a bottle freezed for many years) is used for many emergency conditions.

Fresh frozen plasma prepared within 4 hours is stored rapidly in the temperature of -20°C. This is done by immersing in solid CO_2 and ethyl alcohol. It is used for excessive bleeding due to platelets' deficiency, or due to abnormal coagulopathy (Serum albumin is used for low serum albumin in less than 20 gm/l).

CRYSTALLOIDS USED IN HYPOVOLEMIC SHOCK

Total parenteral nutrition (known as TPN) could be used in certain clinical conditions. They are prepared with 10 percent, 20 percent or 50 percent dextrose solution along with nitrogen and fat. Ideal TPN preparation should be made with 10 percent or 20 percent dextrose. Patient may require insulin therapy for a higher concentration of dextrose preparation added in the TPN. A higher concentration with dextrose solution may cause water retention in the tissues. Initially, it seems that patients have gained in body weight and they seem to be looking well-nourished, but these clinical features are misleading. In fact, this apparent appearance is attributable to water-log in the tissue.

Infusion of blood, plasma, saline, dextrose, combination of dextrose and saline and total nutrition is managed under a strict therapeutic regimen. Every clinician should be fully aware of the pros and cons of the therapeutic policy on daily fluid intake, and electrolytes' regimens.

SITES OF PARENTERAL INFUSION

In most instances, the following sites are preferably chosen for parenteral infusion: These are dorsal veins of the hand, radial vein over the wrist, any vein in the forearm or cephalic vein in the cubital fossa.

For babies, scalp vain is used. For CVP, and TPN, the central line is set up either through the subclavian, and external or internal jugular veins. During general anesthesia, anesthetist uses these veins for the insertion of central line. This central line provides an easy access for rapid infusion of fluid in acute hypovolemic or hemorrhagic shock.

In collapsed conditions, peripheral veins remain collapsed. This would delay the infusion of fluid in the management of shock. In this situation, alternative choice is to use the cut down of the long saphenous vein over the medial malleolus, but thrombophlebitis and deep vein thrombosis in the calf may develop. This site should only be used in emergency medical condition, if the clinician is not fully trained to set up a central line through the jugular or subclavian veins. And in rare condition, long saphenous vein may require to be explored by cut-down technique at the casualty department. This measure is necessary for a rapid infusion.

TOTAL BODY FLUID AND MANAGEMENT OF FLUID THERAPY

In a normal healthy subject, average total body fluid is 40 liters, but 25 liters of it lie in the cellular and 15 liters in extracellular fluid (ECF) compartment and the total blood volume is between 5 and 6 liters. The serum concentration of essential electrolytes such as serum Sodium (Na), Chloride (Cl), Potassium (K), Calcium (Ca), Phosphate (Ph), and Magnesium (Mg) is to be maintained within a narrow range in the management of everyday fluid balance. Depletion of the electrolytes from the permissible ranges would interfere with physiological function of the body. Of the total blood volume, 60-70 percent remains in the peripheral low pressure veins and in the splanchnic vessels.

In a state of shock, these vessels tend to go into vasoconstriction—thus transferring the peripheral blood into the heart. Spleen stores around 50 ml of blood. In hemorrhagic condition, body can cope with blood loss up to 10 percent. But patient starts sweating and having tachycardia when the blood loss exceeds 10 percent. In this emergency situation, blood transfusion is commenced.

HOW MUCH FLUID IS NECESSARY FOR A NORMAL HEALTHY PERSON?

Before assessing the daily fluid requirement, it is very important to know the concentration of the fluid to be administered. It is well-known that red blood corpuscles (RBC) remain unchanged in their shape and size in the plasma. It means that the osmotic pressure between the RBC and plasma is in a state of equilibrium. If they are suspended in the fluid, containing the osmotic pressure lower than that of the plasma, it will swell up and undergo hemolysis, liberating the hemoglobin. And if the osmotic pressure of the medium is greater than that of the plasma, then they would change in shape and size.

To avoid these changes, the osmotic pressure of the solution to be administered to the body must be consistent with that of the RBC and plasma. In all instances, hypotonic solution must not be used in transfusion or in any other therapeutic purposes, such as peritoneal dialysis, transurethral resection of the bladder tumor or prostate gland, postoperative bladder irrigation.

Pure water is hypotonic and must not be used in any therapeutic purposes. If it is used by mistake, it would lead to hemolysis of RBC. Hence the solution to be infused into the circulation must be isotonic to RBC. They are 0.9 percent NaCl known as normal saline, 5 percent dextrose, or 4.5 percent dextrose mixed with 0.18 percent NaCl. These are isotonic to blood. Any fluid greater than 0.9 percent NaCl or 5 percent dextrose does not cause hemolysis, but a higher concentration should be avoided if possible.

In a rare clinical condition, presented with hyponatremia, a higher concentration of saline, with 1.8 percent of NaCl in 500 ml is usually infused, thus sparing the cardiovascular system from being overloaded with normal saline. Overtransfusion in excess of daily requirement would be detrimental to the cardiopulmonary function and it would be detrimental to chronic cardiac failure. Although, the concentration at 1.8 percent of saline seems to be contrary to the physiology of the extracellular fluid compartment, it would not cause any detrimental effect to the RBC, after being diluted to serum. In this case, initially 500 ml is first infused slowly. Patient may need another 500 ml, if the serum sodium still remains below the normal range.

DAILY FLUID REQUIREMENT

In this section, only a limited aspect of daily fluid balance will be highlighted for the purpose of surgical care of the pre- and postoperative patients.

For an average person of 70 kg in weight, the daily intake of fluid would be between 2500 and 3000 liters. In other words, the best guideline for estimating the daily requirement of water to be infused to an emergency surgical patient should be 40 ml per kg of body weight, but it may vary in certain conditions. These are level of tissue hydration, age, status of cardiopulmonary function and renal function.

Furthermore, the above guideline may need to be evaluated by environmental conditions. These may be attributed to temperature, humidity, wind, clothes, and day-to-day individual activities (BMR).

For excessive sweating, the loss of sodium concentration in the water may be between one-third and half of the ECF. This excess sweating is due to combination of lot of moisture present in the atmosphere and high temperature, in excess of 37°C.

All subjects inhale dry air but expire moist air. During inhalation, the dry air is humidified with water in the upper respiratory tract by diffusion of water liberated from the lung tissue. The total volume may exceed due to hyperventilation, degree of moisture in the inhaled air and temperature. Average volume of water required for this vaporization is around 400 ml per day. In addition, there will be obligatory insensible loss of water through perspiration and respiration.

Daily loss of water depends upon the following conditions:

Total water lost for humidifying the dry air inhalation	= 400 ml
Total water lost through the skin perspiration	= 500 ml
Total urine output per day	= 1500 ml
Total water lost through feces	= 100 ml
Total loss of water	= 2500 ml

The insensible loss of water varies in many conditions. The important conditions are humidity, temperature and rate of respiration. Tracheostomy patient requires additional fluid of around 500 ml per day.

On the basis of the basic requirement, daily administration of total fluid could be worked out for an individual patient. Based upon the temperate climate, daily fluid requirement is as follows:

Pure drinking water (plane water, tea, coffee, etc.)	= 1200 ml
Total content of water in the solid food	= 1000 ml
Water derived from the oxidation	= 300 ml
Total estimated requirements of water	= 2500 ml

HOW TO EVALUATE THE DAILY REQUIREMENT FOR ELECTROLYTE?

Serum Sodium and Chloride

In the body, most important inorganic salts such as sodium, potassium, calcium, magnesium, chloride, phosphate and bicarbonate remain in solutions. They dissociate into ions. There are two kinds of ions; one are cations which are electropositive, and the other ones are anions, which are electronegative. Among the cations are sodium, potassium, calcium and magnesium. Chloride, phosphate, bicarbonate and sulfate are anions.

In the extracellular fluid (ECF), sodium remains the principal cation. Of the total body sodium content, 44 percent remains in the ECF, 9 percent in the intracellular compartment and 47 percent in the bones. More than half of the sodium stored in the bone is inactive and requires acid for its solution, but the remaining part of the sodium is water-soluble which are readily available to compensate the abnormal loss of sodium from the body.

The daily intake of sodium chloride varies for various reasons, but the average requirement per day ranges from 80 to 100 mmol. And a similar amount of NaCl is lost through the excretion of kidneys and sweating and a very little through the feces — thus, maintaining a balance between the daily intake and output.

These daily losses are replaced by daily intake with diets, thus maintaining the serum level of sodium within a permissible range between 137 and 147 mmol/l and serum chloride between 95 and 105 mmol/l.

It may drop below the normal range in certain conditions. It is referred to as hyponatremia. This results from restricted salt intake, inappropriate secretion of ADH from the carcinoma of the bronchus, or recurrent vomiting, gastric aspiration, ileostomy. Its serum level may drop in other clinical conditions, such as gastroenteritis, cholera, bowel preparation, diuretics therapy or continuous dextrose infusion.

Serum sodium may be elevated above the upper limit of normal due to over infusion of normal saline. It is referred to as hypernatremia.

In normal physiological condition, the daily requirement of sodium salts is around 80–100 mmol. And a similar amount is lost through the kidneys and sweating, thus a balance is maintained per day.

To maintain this equilibrium, patient needs fluids and electrolytes. This could be provided by a combination of either 2 liters of 0.9 percent of normal saline (1.8 gm) and 1 liter of 5 percent dextrose solution or 1 liter of 4.5 percent dextrose combined with saline (0.18 percent) or by a combination of 2 liters of 5 percent dextrose and 1 liter of normal saline that depends upon the level of tissue hydration and status of serum electrolytes.

Serum Potassium

Potassium unlike sodium is the intracellular cation, but only a small fraction which is around 2 percent, remains in the ECF. Its storehouse is in the skeletal muscle, thus holding around 75 percent of the total load. In catabolic state, skeletal muscles provide endogenous proteins for the purpose of energy. During the metabolic activities, potassium and nitrogen are mobilized. A part of the potassium gets into the ECF; but a major portion is excreted by the kidneys, thus maintaining the balance in the plasma. The daily intake of potassium that comes from the fruits and food is between 60–75 mmols per day. Normal serum potassium is between 3.5 mmol/l and 5.5 mmol/l.

In addition, kidneys also excrete potassium around 60-75 mmols per day. If the patient is not eating or drinking, the replacement of this obligatory loss of potassium has to be compensated. The recommended daily dose for KCl should be 60-75 mmol. in divided dose. This supplementation is to be considered if there is a good renal function and there is evidence of low serum potassium, but this is unnecessary if the patient can swallow food or can drink milk and fruit juices, which contain plenty of KCl.

In surgical patient, presented with hypokalemia, potassium chloride 20 mmol (1.5 gm) should be added to one liter infusion bag of 0.9 percent saline or 5 percent dextrose solution. In other cases, supplementation is necessary, if patient remains on infusion therapy all along for more than 3-4 days. For the safety, this dose should be added to alternate infusion bag. This manual addition remains a risk of error and breach of sterility of the infusion.

To avoid this risk, commercially prepared normal saline or dextrose solution, containing 0.2 percent of KCl is available for intravenous infusion. This dose is printed on the plastic bag. If this preparation is used for the patient, no other drug could be added into this infusion bag.

TREATMENT OF HYPOKALEMIA

Serum potassium may drop below the normal range, known as hypokalemia. In this biochemical change, H^+ ion and Na^+ move into cell in exchange of K^+ ions into the extracellular space—thus causing intracellular acidosis and extracellular alkalosis. As a result, kidneys excrete excess potassium and acid urine. It may result in paralytic ileus and cardiac arrhythmia. Patient feels lethargic, and develops slurring speech.

In the first postoperative day, serum sodium is held back by the corticosteroids, because of response to injury after operation; but in contrast, serum potassium is liberated from the tissue injury in catabolic phase that occurs immediately on the first postoperative day, but, unlike serum sodium, it is excreted through the kidneys, on the first postoperative day and this excretion is continued for the first 3-4 days after operation. Supplementation of potassium is unnecessary until the 4th postoperative day, in most instances.

Hypokalemia may be encountered within certain clinical conditions. These are continued diarrhea, oral purgatives, villous adenoma of the rectum, ileostomy, continued vomiting, continued gastric aspiration, metabolic acidosis, diuretic tablets with frusemide, and diabetic coma treated with insulin.

It is equally important to remember the primary diseases that may produce hypokalemia. These are ulcerative colitis because of persistent discharge of loose motion, diversion of ureters into the colon resulting in metabolic acidosis, pyloric stenosis causing repeated episodes of vomiting.

In cases with chronic hypokalemia, daily KCl supplementation may be given orally. The oral dose varies but it should be commenced with 600 mg of slow releasing potassium chloride three times per day. The maximum oral dose could be increased up to 6 gm in divided dose per 24 hours. It is advisable to give it after dissolving in water. If KCl tablet is swallowed, it may cause perforation of the small intestine.

In acute condition, infusion of KCl in a liter of dextrose or normal saline solution could be commenced; but one gram of KCl must not be given through the intravenous route in less than one hour. ECG monitor should be maintained concomitantly with the infusion of KCl in saline or dextrose solution. Overdose may cause cardiac arrest, if it is given too rapidly.

In normal postoperative care, 20 mmol of KCl is added to per liter of saline or dextrose solution on the fourth postoperative day, provided the hourly urine output is at least 40 ml per hour.

TREATMENT OF HYPERKALEMIA

If the blood result shows that the serum potassium is in excess of the normal range, this is known as hyperkalemia. It may rise due to cardiac failure, renal failure or in diabetic ketoacidosis. It may also be elevated after blood transfusion, if the blood stored in the blood bank was kept in excess of 3 weeks.

It is more often associated with high blood urea (3.5-6.5 mmol/l), elevated serum creatinine (>176 mmol), metabolic acidosis or respiratory alkalosis and hypocalcemia.

The immediate treatment for this acute condition is to inject insulin in case of diabetic patient. For nondiabetic patient, infusion of 50 ml of 50 percent dextrose solution along with insulin is given through the vein in the fore arm. This would transfer the KCl into the cells, because, insulin induces the increased permeability of the cell membrane.

Injection of frusemide at a higher dose may reduce the serum potassium. In this medical emergency, the drug must be injected intravenously slowly. In case of chronic renal failure, hyperkalemia is treated with peritoneal or hemodialysis.

HOW TO DEAL WITH DAILY FLUID BALANCE

If the urine output drops due to dehydration, or poor renal function, a special care is then taken. Despite the fluid challenged is made, and despite giving injection of frusemide, the urine output per hour may not be improving over 6 hours, then hourly infusion rate should be restricted comparable to the hourly fluid loss. This is measured by a combination of obligatory urine output and the insensible loss of water through the lungs and skin.

In this case, the daily infusion should be the total insensible loss of 900 ml and obligatory urine output of say 600 ml. The total volume of fluid should not exceed 1500 ml per day, but in this equation, the amount of fluid derived from the oxidation is around 300-400 ml. This amount needs to be deducted from the daily requirement which should be 1500-300 = 1200 ml. Again, any amount lost through the gastric aspiration, feces or fistula has to be added to the above figure.

HOW TO WORK OUT THE RATE OF INFUSION TO BE GIVEN PER HOUR?

Nurses should be instructed on the daily fluid balance chart about the rate of infusion to be continued per hour. It could be instructed in various ways.

If the infusion tube is regulated by the electrical pump, the rate of infusion is set up on the pump clock. In normal cases, it should be 125 ml per hour. As a result, one liter bag will take 8 hours to finish.

Alternative to the above procedure, the infusion rate could be set up by the count of drops of fluid per minute. For instance, one liter of fluid will take 8 hours at the rate of 30 drops per minute, 6 hours at the rate of 45 drops and 4 hours at the rate of 60 drops per minute.

The rate of infusion per hour is judged by the age of the patient, cardiac condition and level of tissue of hydration.

It is advisable that the infusion rate per liter should be restricted; if there is evidence of poor cardiac reserves, short of breath, raised jugular venous pressure in supine position, and pitting edema to the dorsum of the feet. To support the clinical judgement, X-ray of chest should be taken. In the film, pulmonary edema would be evident by the opacities, similar to features of cotton ball or by the pleural effusion or basal consolidation.

In addition, central venous pressure (CVP) should be measured in supine position of the patient. And the manometric reading is taken either at the level of midaxillary or at the level of suprasternal notch. The CVP for the former should be between -5 and +15 cm of H_2O, and it should be between -2 and +10 cm of H_2O for the latter.

It provides a guideline, but it is not reliable, and may provide a misleading reading in those cases, in which, the serum albumin is very low. Fluid will continue leaking from the vascular bed, thus revealing the negative CVP on the scale. Experiences show pulmonary edema and gross tissue edema, despite recording the CVP at -2 cm of H_2O. This was recorded in an elderly lady, whose serum albumin was less than 25 gm/l.

The pressure reading reflects the pressure at the right atrium, and does not provide advance warning about the pressure of the pulmonary arterial tree. By the time a high pressure reading has been recorded; it would be too late to stop developing pulmonary edema.

HOW TO SET UP THE CENTRAL VENOUS PRESSURE (CVP)?

Patient must be lying on supine position with the foot-end of the bed raised. Skin preparation is carried out with antiseptic solution. Sterile drapes are laid down all around the chosen site. The site is chosen by palpation and is infiltrated with 1 or ½ percent lignocaine injected into the subcutaneous plane for the insertion of the cannula.

If internal jugular vein is chosen, the landmark for inserting the cannula is 3-4 fingers above the sternoclavicular joint and the cannula is inserted along the anterior border of the sternomastoid muscles. It is directed downwards towards the suprasternal notch. Once the cannula is inside the jugular vein, the needle is next pulled out of the plastic cannula, leaving behind the latter *in situ*. A suitable catheter is negotiated through the cannula right down into the superior vena cava and the cannula is next pulled out.

The position of the plastic catheter is checked by X-ray of chest. The tip of the catheter must be in the right atrium. Alternative to jugular vein, subclavian vein could be used for setting up the CVP.

It is not without morbidity. During insertion of the cannula, there could be perforation of the apex of the lung, producing pneumothorax, and hemothorax or it may puncture the vein through and through or through the adjacent artery. This may develop hematoma around the vessels.

If the central line is kept in position over a few days, it may cause bacteremia, form clot at its tip and may run a low grade elevation of temperature. Therefore, a new CVP line should be set up every seven days and the catheter with clots stuck to its tip is sent for culture. Central line could be used for TPN or for chemotherapy.

HOW TO DECIDE HOW MUCH FLUID IS TO BE GIVEN PER DAY?

It is most difficult medical condition. By and large, the daily fluid load should not exceed three liters. But it should be around two liters if the patient is above 70-year-old, or has cardiac problems.

Administration of intravenous fluid requires slight alteration that depends upon the total output through the nasogastric aspiration (via Ryle's tube), output through the ileostomy, bile leaks, purulent peritoneal discharge, concentrated urine (strong color) with specific gravity of greater than 1.020 or diarrhea.

Final adjustment of the infusion has to be made based upon the clinical features of dehydration, daily urine output or daily fluid loss through the various sources and guided by the daily result of serum electrolytes.

These are broad outlines and a guidance to the clinician that how much fluid is to be given to the surgical patients per day. These guidelines may need to be reviewed everyday on the merits of the previous fluid balance chart, urine output, tissue hydration, chest condition, daily gastric aspiration, flatus, and daily results of serum sodium, potassium, urea, creatinine, and general appearance of the patients.

INTERPRETATION OF UNUSUAL AND CONFLICTING RESULTS OF SERUM ELECTROLYTES

1. The normal level of serum urea is between 3.5 mmol and 6.5 mmol/l, but if the serum sodium is reported to be less than normal range and serum potassium is normal.

   The most likely explanation would be that the low serum sodium may be attributable to any one of the following conditions:
   - Reduced salt intake (over hydration by drinking plain water).
   - Diuretic drugs therapy such as frusemide.
   - Continued infusion of dextrose.

   This could be confirmed by low PCV level and low level of hemoglobin.

2. a. If the serum sodium is very low, blood urea is elevated say above the 15 mmol/l level and it is associated with raised serum creatinine; but the serum potassium is within the normal range, in this case, these features are suggestive of dehydration.

   b. If the serum potassium is above the normal range, then the possible cause is:
   - Acute renal failure.
   - Glomerulonephritis.
   - Cardiac failure.
   - Obstructive uropathy.
   - Transfusion of old blood.

SERUM CREATININE (NORMAL VALUE 75–150 MMOL/L)

It reflects the normal tubular function, but its elevation may be affected by prerenal, intrarenal and postrenal conditions. The prerenal conditions are dehydration, cardiac failure, shock, and hypotension. Intrarenal conditions are glomerulonephritis, diabetes, renal artery stenosis, or renal hypertension. It has to be evaluated with the results of serum potassium, blood urea and urine specific gravity.

Postrenal conditions are obstructive uropathy, leading to bilateral hydroureters and hydronephrosis.

EVIDENCES OF DEHYDRATION

- Feeling of thirst (indication of cellular dehydration).
- Sunken eyes and face.
- Dry lips, dry and coated tongue.
- Dry skin, loose skin and lack of skin elasticity.

- Delayed venous filling rate.
- PCV (in dehydration, it may be elevated but it may be misleading if the patient has very low hemoglobin).
- Acetone smell in the breath.
- Ketone in the urine.

EVIDENCES OF REHYDRATION

This is assessed by the evidence of moisture noticed in the tongue and lips, but in some cases dry mouth may be present. This could be due to breathing through the mouth.

Patient stops feeling thirsty and this is the evidence of intracellular hydration.

Evidence of elasticity of the skin is measured by pinching the skin fold between the thumb and index finger. It would be difficult to pick up the skin fold in good hydration and in good nutritional state. If the skin fold returns quickly to its position, after releasing it; this suggests a good tissue hydration.

A good venous filling and venous return in the limbs is another sign of tissue hydration. In the state of dehydration, the subcutaneous veins remain collapsed.

Urine output per hour and per 24 hours, and its specific gravity – If the latter is below the normal range, it refers to a poor renal function, losing its power of reabsorption of water through the distal renal tubules. If it is above the normal range, it implies the concentrated urine due to tissue dehydration.

Jugular venous pressure is assessed clinically. If it is markedly prominent and appears to be dilated even in supine position, it may result from congestive cardiac failure and overtransfusion. And this is measured by inserting the catheter into the right atrium either through the subclavian or jugular vein. This is known as CVP. This is an invasive procedure and used in certain acute medical condition in the theater or in the intensive care unit. It reflects on the function of the heart, but the reading above the normal measurement indicates either overtransfusion or cardiac failure.

EVIDENCES OF OVERHYDRATION

- Short of breath, sweating and dusky skin color.
- Raised jugular veins.
- Rales and crepitation at the base of the lungs on auscultation.
- Dull on percussion in both sides of the chest.
- Pitting edema on the dorsum of the feet and over the medial malleolus of the ankles.
- Edema on the dependant part, in particular over the sacral area.
- In this context, blood results are reviewed on hemoglobin, PCV, serum electrolytes and blood urea.
- X-ray of chest should be reviewed for any evidence of cardiomegaly, basal congestion and pulmonary edema.

A BROAD GUIDELINE FOR BLOOD TRANSFUSION

Many resident doctors have a very little understanding about the volume of whole blood contained in the plastic bag. One unit of blood stored in a sterile plastic bag contains 540 ml. It is stored in a solution of 75 ml of anticoagulants at a temperature of 2 and 7°C.

The chemicals used in the anticoagulant solutions are, 2.2 gm anhydrous dextrose, 2.2 gm disodium citrate monohydrate, 800 mg citric acid in 75 ml water. Infection will be transmitted to the recipient, if the blood is stored at a higher temperature for 2 hours. And hemolysis will take place, if it is stored below 2°C.

INDICATION AND PREPARATION FOR BLOOD TRANSFUSION

For the purpose of blood transfusion, patient's blood is sent for grouping and cross-matching. It takes around two hours to get the cross-matching completed. Blood should be collected before any infusion is commenced, in particular before the solution of Dextran 70 is infused to the patient. The latter may cause problem in grouping and cross-matching due to formation of rouleaux of the red cells.

Until the blood is available, patient should be treated with other crystalloids in order to maintain the tissue hydration, and blood pressure. In emergency condition such as hypovolemic shock, Dextran 70, saline or plasma could be infused to combat the hypovolemic shock. In certain surgical emergency, such as leaking abdominal aortic aneurysm, blood with group 0, Rhesus D-negative should be used to meet the emergency crisis.

Blood transfusion is unnecessary, if the hemoglobin is below 10 gm/dl. But for a major surgery, the hemoglobin level should be above 12 gm/dl. In this case, preoperative blood transfusion should be given. In most instances, packed cells are preferred in anemia, aged patient, cardiac diseases, and small children.

Blood transfusion is also unnecessary in those circumstances in which the blood loss is between 10 to 20 percent of the total blood volume. Body can cope with this amount of blood loss by the peripheral vasoconstriction and by shifting the blood from the spleen. This may be one of the causes of hemodilution after a few hours. Pulse rate is the most sensitive indicator whether or not the total blood volume has dropped because of acute hemorrhage. It begins to rise due to persisting hemorrhage that could affect the total blood volume. Apart from the pulse rate, blood pressure may drop, if the blood loss in hemorrhage exceeds 20 percent.

In general, blood transfusion is given slowly and its average duration is four hours for each unit of blood, but for cardiac or elderly patients, it should be longer than four hours. In some cases, diuretic could be prescribed at the completion of transfusion.

ADVERSE EFFECTS OF BLOOD STORED IN THE BAG

Stored blood liberates potassium to the serum of recipient, white blood cells are rapidly lost in the blood and blood platelets lose their functional value after 72 hours.

Blood that has been stored over 3 weeks should be avoided, if several units of blood transfusion are indicated. Recent study suggests that the incidence of mortality may be worse, if the blood stored over 2 weeks is transfused to the patient. Red blood cells lose their metabolic capacity to release oxygen to the tissues immediately after the transfusion is given, but it regains its capacity within 72 hours in the recipient. It is recommended that blood should be transfused at least 2 days before the operation is due. In emergency condition, blood stored for less than 7 days should be used for transfusion.

Blood transfusion should be delayed if the patient is grossly dehydrated and shows gross electrolytes imbalance and elevated plasma urea and serum potassium. In this case, the tissue hydration should be improved first with 0.9 percent saline, until the renal function seems to be reasonable. Repeat blood test may reveal a different blood picture, in that previous level of hemoglobin may drop and all other parameters may appear to be reasonable. Blood transfusion should be commenced a few hours after infusion of normal saline has finished.

INSTRUCTION TO THE NURSES

During transfusion, nurses are instructed to record the temperature, pulse rate, blood pressure, and urine output per hour. In some cases, patient may reveal rise of temperature, tachycardia, skin reaction (rashes or urticaria), rigors and no urine output. These abnormal features may be attributable to incompatibility of grouping and cross-matching, presence of pyrogens in the storage bottle, malarial parasites, and allergic reactions due to repeated blood transfusion. Blood transfusion must be stopped straightaway and the remaining sample of blood is sent back to the blood bank for necessary investigation.

Other complications are disseminated intravascular coagulation. This may be attributable to massive blood transfusion in major emergency operation. As a result, platelet count and fibrinogen level may be very low.

Of all the adverse reactions, incompatibility due to wrong blood being transfused is the most serious medical condition. This may result in agglutination and hemolysis of the donor cells. It may lead to acute tubular necrosis and renal failure. Delayed complication would be serum hepatitis, HIV, TB, and malaria.

7 A Broad Outline for the Surgical Treatment

At the conclusion of all investigations, all the results are assembled together in order to review the patient and to make a definitive diagnosis. On the basis of clinical examination, supplemented by the results of investigations and tissue diagnosis, if available, a thorough consultation is made with the patient, prior to admitting him/her for a definitive operative treatment.

A plan for the curative resection of the colonic or rectal tumor is set up for the patient. It is influenced by the Dukes tumor staging (Fig. 2.4). Dukes classified the tumors in three groups, known as Dukes stages that depend upon the local invasion and lymphatic involvement. They are Dukes A, for the tumor confined to the rectal wall, Dukes B for the tumor found extended beyond the rectal wall but not invaded to the lymphatic nodes and Dukes C for the tumor found invaded to the lymphatic nodes.

The patient presented with carcinoma in the cecum, ascending colon or hepatic flexure will require right hemicolectomy and end-to-end anastomosis, if it is resectable and if it is either Dukes A or Dukes B. The tumor with Dukes C stage could be included in this procedure, if it is mobile. Similarly, left hemicolectomy with end-to-end anastomosis is undertaken, if the growth is located in the left colon, and it is either Dukes A or B.

Palliative resection could be done in some cases, if the lymph nodes are found to be enlarged along the major colonic vessels, where wide area of lymphatic clearance would be difficult without sacrificing the major colonic blood vessels. In particular, it would not be possible for the tumor located in the right side, if the superior mesenteric vessels are surrounded by the cluster of enlarged lymph glands.

In this situation, the feces should be diverted, by bypassing the tumor. The procedure for bypassing the obstruction is side-to-side anastomosis between the ileum and the transverse colon. Alternative procedure is cecostomy, colostomy, or ileostomy. This depends upon the site of the colonic obstruction. They are also regarded to be palliative measures to relieve the obstruction.

Anterior resection of the rectum is recommended for the carcinoma in the upper-third of the rectum or in the rectosigmoid region. In this decision, exact location of the tumor from the anal verge needs to be identified by the sigmoidoscopic examination. Again, it varies from one surgeon to another.

The indication for low anterior resection of the rectum is related to the position of the tumor from the anal verge, and related to mobility and Dukes tumor stage. The skill of the surgeon is also important. However, this approach is used in those cases in which the tumor appears to be mobile, Dukes A or B are located at the level above 6 cm away from the anal verge.

Alternatively, abdominoperineal resection of the rectum could be carried out for those cases in which the tumor is located below the level of 10 cm from the anal verge. This is a broad outline for the operative treatment for the colorectal cancer. A detailed operative technique for the tumor in the respective anatomical site has been described in the appropriate chapter.

In advanced cases, postoperative chemotherapy is given, but its benefit is limited to a small number of cases that depend upon the Dukes tumor staging and the histological report.

If there are findings of two primary colonic tumors, one is located in the right side and the other one in the sigmoid colon, or the tumor developed in the sigmoid colon has invaded the cecum or *vice versa*, the operative approach is total colectomy, and ileorectal anastomosis, provided both tumors are resectable, and with no evidence of liver metastasis or the spread of the tumor is localized.

PRINCIPLE OF OPERATIVE PREPARATIONS

Skin Preparation

In all operative procedure, skin surface is made sterile with antiseptic solution. These are povidone-iodine (bethidin) in alcohol, chlorhexidine in alcohol, ether and cetrimide (Savlon).

Alcohol-based preparations that provide effective bactericidal tools are preferably used in most cases but it should be allowed to let it dry in air, instead of wiping it out from the skin surface. This alcohol-based preparation carries a risk of skin burn, if diathermy is used where a pool of this solution is present, nearby. This inflammable product tends to accumulate in the skin fold, umbilicus, groin, or under the buttock. Therefore, necessary precaution should be taken to stop such accident. In certain anatomical sites, water-based solution such as water based chlorhexidine and bethidin solution or cetrimide should be used. These sites are oral cavity, penis, scrotum and perineum.

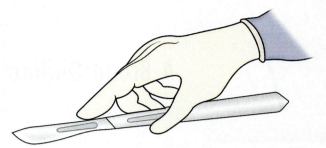

Fig. 7.1: Shows how to hold the scalpel before the skin incision is made

TECHNIQUE FOR HOLDING THE KNIFE

Incision is an important part of the surgical skill. It makes the scar neat and enhances rapid healing. In most operations, incision should be made along the line of skin crease, but in certain operations, a different line of incision may require to be adopted. The cut edge of the skin must be perpendicular to the skin surface. A bevel type of skin cut is undesirable. It leads to ugly scar. Infection may creep in due to necrosis of the epidermis along the beveled skin cut.

To avoid bevel cut, the blade has to be held firmly perpendicular to the skin surface. For avoiding the tilting of the blade, the handle of the knife is firmly held between the thumb and the middle finger, and tip of the index finger should rest upon the upper edge of the handle. This will keep the blade firmly down, while the skin is cut through and through (Fig. 7.1).

The handle of the knife should not rest upon the web between the thumb and the index finger. For a delicate dissection, the knife should be held like a pen.

Before the incision is commenced, a plan has to be drawn up, as to the site and size of incision to be made. Next the blade is firmly placed exactly on the proposed site that needs to be firm and smooth without any puckering of the skin.

Therefore, the incision should be made between the left thumb and index finger that keeps the site of incision firm and smooth. These two fingers move concurrently forward, with the blade that continues cutting the skin further down and away from those two fingers.

Once the skin cut is made perpendicular, it is continued for every few centimeters at a stroke, preceded by the change in position of the left thumb and index finger. The cut should be deep in one stroke and it should include the subcutaneous fat in one attempt. The process is repeated in order to cut the wound further deep. After the skin has been cut deep, the bleeding vessels are picked up by the artery forceps with a view to stopping the bleeding either by putting ligature around it or with electrocoagulation. Some surgeons change the blade after cutting the skin, and some surgeons use the cutting diathermy after initial skin cut is made with the knife.

Diathermy should not be used to stop oozing or spurting vessels, coming from the subcutaneous fat. Every precaution should be taken to avoid thermal burn to the skin edge.

BASIC PRINCIPLE AND TECHNIQUE FOR THE WOUND CLOSURE

Closure of the abdominal wound seems to be simple but it requires acquiring skill and understanding of the basic principle on the etiology of wound dehiscence, wound hematoma or infection. All thist morbidity is preventable if the wound is closed with due care and meticulously. First, a good relaxation is necessary and there should not be distention of the gut during closure of the peritoneum.

Therefore, a good relaxation is usually provided by the anesthetist. Surgeon should not struggle in bringing the peritoneal edges together and loops of small intestine should not be allowed to pop-up through the wound, while closing the peritoneum.

If the peritoneum is closed under tension, sutures may cut out, or there could be splitting of the peritoneum transversely. These torn areas may need to be closed with interrupted sutures. Eventually, omentum may protrude through the gaps, thus giving rise to abdominal wound dehiscence and incisional hernia in some cases.

It seems to a race between two teams, in that competition, one team would be busy in reversing the patient from anesthetic effects, before the abdominal wound is closed and another team, by contrast, would like to see more relaxation in the closure of the peritoneal wound. Without the help of the anesthetist, satisfactory peritoneal closure would be impossible; but too much relaxation may lead to delay in recovery that is not desirable. While maintaining balance, experienced anesthetist treats the patients differently that keeps every team happy.

However, the peritoneum should be closed without tension by a continuous vicryl, dexon, or polydioxin suture material. Silk or nylon should not be used under any circumstances. Chromic catgut sutures are not suitable for the closure of the laparotomy wound. They produce inflammatory reaction and their tensile strength loses in a week. Furthermore, it is no longer available in surgical practice, since mad-cow disease has been identified in the firming industry.

In the past, surgeons used to employ a large curved hand needle with a big eye. These are no longer used but one should know the adverse effect to the peritoneum. It makes a large puncture wound. Therefore, atraumatic curved (35 mm) needle should be used in closing the abdominal wound.

To avoid tension of the sutures, the spacing between the two sutures should not exceed 1 cm and the sutures bite should not be too far away from or too close to the cut edge of the peritoneum or the rectus-sheath. In the former case, there would be tension of the sutures and in the latter case, the sutures may cut out. To compromise between the two devils, the suture bites should be between 0.5 cm and 1cm away from the cut edge of the peritoneum or the rectus sheath. In this method of wound closures, the tension would be uniformly distributed to all those sutures and there would be no wound gap between the two sutures and between the cut edges of the peritoneum. In my experience, there was not a single case of incisional hernia or burst abdomen found in my surgical practice.

Continuous suture through the cut edges is the established surgical procedure; but junior assistants are abdicated to close the wound, while surgeons could be busy in writing the operation notes, or surgeons close the wound in a hurry, leaving behind a large space greater than 1 cm between the sutures. The implication of these methods of closing the wound was not fully understood, but instances of burst abdomen or incisional hernia would be very high.

When the sutures are tied at the end, the cut edges tend to buckle-up because of pulling of the thread at the conclusion of the closure. In other cases, the peritoneal cut edges tend to get apart between the two suture bites. This may lead to intraabdominal tension and it may occur only if the gap is in excess of 1cm, between the two suture bites holding the two cut edges together. The intervening sutures remain in undue tension, exerted by the postoperative paralytic ileus. Furthermore, these tissues could not remain relaxed anymore, once the effect of anesthesia being worn off. In this situation, patient tends to remain lying side ways, bringing the knees towards the belly.

As a result, the cut edges of the peritoneum tend to stay apart between the sutures, thus producing a wound gaping with a configuration of diamond shape between the sutures. This may exert undue tension upon the sutures that tend to keep holding the two cut edges together, but in some instances, a few of them may cut out of the tissues or snap off, at the time of recovery from the anesthesia or in the postoperative period.

After the patient has been transferred to the recovery room, in some cases, patients tend to cough violently due to irritation in the throat, at the time when the endotracheal tube is withdrawn. And at other times irritation in the throat may bring the cough in the postoperative period. If the burst abdomen seems to be eminent, there will be serous discharge through the wound that would be early signal, a few days prior to burst abdomen is imminent, and it has been noticed that it occurs usually 10-12 postoperative days and usually after taking lunch.

The risk of wound dehiscence would be much less or not at all, in those cases in which the laparotomy wound is closed in line with the above principle in all elective and emergency abdominal operations.[1, 2]

Hence, undue tension of the sutures should be avoided, and this could be done, if the sutures are inserted with equidistance from each other and without leaving too much gap between the sutures, thus sharing the total tension among these sutures. For the uniform distribution of the tension among the sutures, the cut edges of the peritoneum should be closed by the continuous suture that should be 1cm apart from each other and between 0.5cm and 1 cm away from the wound margin.

For the closure of the rectus sheath, same principle should be followed. Chromic catgut should not be used and the size of the suture should be no.1. And each suture bite should be between 0.5 and 1 cm away from the cut edge of the rectus sheath and 1 cm apart between the two sutures bites. For the closure of the rectus sheath, a loop of prolene suture or polydioxin sutures should be used, instead of other absorbable suture materials.

Mass closure of the midline wound involving the peritoneum and the rectus sheath is safe, without compromising the principle of suturing the wound. But every attempt should be made to exclude the rectus abdominis muscles in the mass closure, although in many instances, mass abdominal wound closure includes the rectus abdominis muscles. No adverse effect has been noticed but there remains a theoretical risk of ischemic change to the muscle by this method of mass closure.

It is also recommended that dead space between the rectus sheath and skin wound should be closed with continuous or interrupted absorbable sutures, using a 35 mm atraumatic curved needle. Collection of serous fluid or blood in the space between the fatty wound, particularly to the lower dependent part, keeps the two fatty layers apart under the skin wound. This exerts tension upon the sutures, inhibits primary healing, and causes pain because of tension, built up within the wound.

In addition, therapeutic level of antibiotic was found far less in the serous fluid, thus enhancing the bacterial colonization in the pool of inflammatory fluid. But closure of the dead space takes away undue tension of the sutures applied to the rectus sheath or the skin wound. Many surgeons do not comply with this principle. One should not hurry in closing the wound; instead, it should be closed methodically with due care.

Tension sutures for the major abdominal operations used to be common practice, but these did not prevent the wound dehiscence. On the contrary, it may cause necrosis around the sutures port and ugly scars, like tattoos would develop later after the patient has been discharged. It is now rarely used in the wound closure, since the technique of wound closure has been changed and since the synthetic suture materials are available in closing the wound.

Skin wound could be closed by various ways. For cosmetic result, skin edges are apposed closely by subcutaneous continuous sutures. Fine white dexon or Vicryl suture (2/0 or 3/0) should be used. Alternatively, 2/0 prolene suture could be used. The prolene suture may not glide smoothly under the subcutaneous tissue, when it needs to be pulled out. In some cases, it may be snapped off, leaving behind a residual segment under the skin wound.

Therefore, thicker thread should be used, or this should be avoided. If Vicryl or dexon suture is used, it may cause hypertrophy scar or roughness of the scar in some instances. For breast and facial surgery, this possibility has to be highlighted to the patient.

Skin wound could be closed with interrupted prolene, Vicryl, or dexon sutures, but they should be removed in 5 days for small wound, and 10 days for laparotomy or larger wound. Other alternative material is the autosutures. These are very quick to finish the job and are removed as and when necessary.

For thyroid surgery or closure of the skin wound in the neck, platysma is apposed together with interrupted absorbable sutures, the skin wounds are closed with metal clips, but they are removed on the second day.

Silk sutures should be avoided. It induces inflammation and ugly sutures' mark over the skin. Despite all these principles being followed, hypertrophy or ugly scar can develop in certain anatomical sites and in certain cases. Keloid is prone to develop among certain people or in certain anatomical sites, such as around the face, neck, chest and the joint areas. These delayed complications should be discussed with the patients.

■ Types of Skin Sutures

- Interrupted Suture (Fig. 7.2A).
- Interrupted Mattress Suture (Fig. 7.2B).
- Continuous Suture (Overlapping of the skin edges should be avoided) (Fig. 7.2C).
- Continuous Mattress Suture (Fig. 7.2D).
- Continuous Blanket Suture (Fig. 7.2E).
- Continuous Subcutaneous Suture (Fig. 7.2F)

In this technique, either monofilament nylon (2/0) or Dexon/Vicryl (white and 2/0 or 3/0) is recommended. Nylon or similar type of material is pulled out of the wound after 5 days. There remains a risk of snapping of the thread while

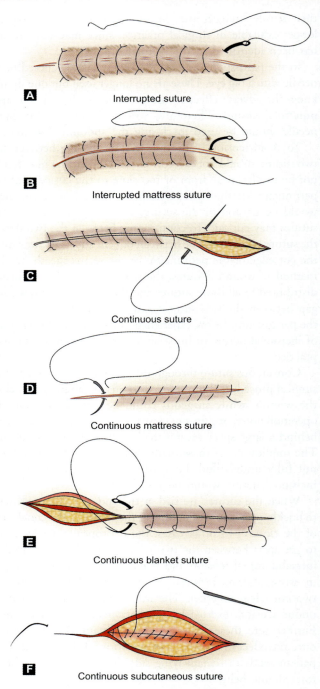

Figs 7.2A to F: Types of skin sutures

an attempt is made to remove it. And the risk would be greater, if fine thread (3/0) is used.
- Autosutures using clips.

PRECAUTION IN SUTURING THE SKIN WOUND

Overlapping of the skin edges should be avoided, in those cases in which, interrupted or continuous sutures are employed.

Sutures must not be too tight. All knots should be placed along the side of the skin edge and must not be left across the skin edges.

CLOSURE OF BURST ABDOMEN

Burst abdomen seems to be the sequel of poor surgical technique used in the closure of the abdominal wound. In most instances, it tends to occur among the emergency laparotomy undertaken, in those cases in which, patients were in poor state of health, and tissue perfusion remains inadequate. Furthermore, generalized tissue edema may develop in postoperative period due to over transfusion, cardiac or renal failure and hypoalbuminea. Other contributing factors are persistent chronic chest conditions, acute pulmonary edema, poor oxygen saturation, cough, wound infection, diabetes, and other debilitating health conditions.

Furthermore, emergency operations are usually carried out in hurry and by the trainee surgeons in unsocial hours. They may not be fully experienced or may be exhausted in the middle of the night while undertaking the complicated surgical procedures. Concentration may be lacking in closing the abdominal wound.

Disruption of the peritoneal sutures may occur when the patient is being recovered from the anesthesia. It may also occur during the postoperative period, when the abdomen tends to be distended due to swallowing of air, persistent paralytic ileus, or due to subacute intestinal obstruction. Intermittent vomiting, delayed flatus, and intraperitoneal abscess could cause undue tension upon the sutures. Serosanguineous collection, wound hematoma and local infections developed within the parietal wound are other incriminating factors for causing burst abdomen.

In the past, tension sutures were frequently used in the closure of the abdominal wound. In addition, many-tail bandage that goes around the abdomen was routinely used in order to provide additional support to the parietal wound. It was religiously believed to be a good prophylactic measure against the burst abdomen. This is a large thin cloth, fitted with several long tails along the edge of each side.

Each tail, measuring 2-3 inches wide and 12 inches long goes across the abdominal wound dressing and by turn it is overlapped by the corresponding tail bringing from the opposite side. It would look like a double breast and act as an abdominal corset. The end of each tail is held together by the adhesive tape or by safety-pin. In this way, all the tails are put over the abdominal wound.

But this did not make any difference in many cases; on the contrary, it seemed to have made an adverse effect upon the respiration, thus inhibiting the patient having cough or expectoration of sputum. It is now rarely used in emergency abdominal operation.

Although the instances of burst abdomen seem to have fallen, this improvement could be the result of combination of suture materials and the sutures technique used in the closure of the peritoneum and other parietal wounds. Closing the burst abdomen requires a greater skill.

It has been noticed that burst abdomen usually occurs after the sutures have been removed and after having lunch. It requires emergency repair; but patient needs to keep fasting for at least 6 hours, prior to general anesthesia being given and emergency theater may not be available for this procedure to be undertaken. So, prolapsed gut and the burst abdomen should be covered with sterile warm saline packs straightaway. This is again wrapped up by sterile towel until the theater is available.

Therefore, patient is kept nil by mouth and nasogastric tube is inserted into the stomach for emptying it and hourly aspiration should be continued. Parenteral infusion with saline and dextrose is commenced. Bladder catheter is to be inserted for recording the urine output and for fluid balance. Also the patient should be explained about the operative procedure to be taken, before a consent form is signed.

OPERATIVE TECHNIQUE FOR THE CLOSURE OF THE BURST ABDOMEN

Patient is placed in the supine position on the operating table. Usual skin preparation and sterile towellings are carried out around the wound. All packs are removed. If there were any sutures left across the wound, they are removed. More often, loops of the small intestine could be found herniated through a small area of the burst abdomen but the remaining healed skin edges should be broken apart from top to bottom of the wound.

In most cases, gut could be found lying under the healed skin wound. Therefore, it would be unwise just to close the small part of the burst abdomen without looking into the other part of apparently healed skin wound. All the skin edges, the rectus sheath and the peritoneum are opened up.

In the peritoneal cavity, small intestine remains matted together, and the peritoneum may be found receded or retracted away from the rectus abdominis muscles. And whitish fibrinous membrane could be found covering the loops of the gut or in between the loops of the gut. It should be removed without interfering with the loops of the gut. It would be wise, not to separate those adhesions, apart from freeing the fibrinous membrane.

There could be oozing or tear of the serosal wall of the gut, if they are attempted to be separated from the adhesions. Minimum attempt should be made in order to free the peritoneum from the nearby guts. And no attempt should be made to free the torn edges of the peritoneum and to bring the free-edge of the peritoneum closure to the midline of the wound, with a view to suturing them together. In fact it would cut out, if such an attempt is made.

Burst abdomen is closed in one layer, but before proceeding for the mass closure of the wound, it is important to be sure that there was no pocket of abscess or anastomotic leakage. Suspicion should arise if there is evidence of bile discharge or foul smell in the peritoneal cavity.

Loops of the intestine need to be freed from the surrounding peritoneal wound margin. This would be necessary to protect the gut from being injured, when the long curved needle would be inserted for the tension sutures across the peritoneal cavity. Once adequate room has been made by separating the loops of small intestine or the greater omentum, they are covered with a thin layer of wet swab. This is necessary to protect the gut from being injured by the needle. This is a temporary measure, and it would be pulled out after the tension sutures being laid down over the swab across the peritoneal cavity.

If there are necrotic sloughs present along the skin edges, these should be excised. It harbors bacterial colonization. Mass closure is the basic principle involved in the closure of the burst abdomen and that is done by tension sutures. Strong prolene or nylon suture with a long curved cutting needle is used. Each needle is used for each tension suture and it is inserted one inch away from the skin margin and is pulled out from inside the abdomen and it is inserted again from inside one inch away from the skin margin of the contralateral abdominal wound margin and it is pulled out from outside the abdomen. There should be a gap of two inches between the two tension sutures.

The tension sutures could be inserted in various ways. It could be passed across the wound margin, but the thread goes through the plastic tube that would lie across the skin wound, thus protecting the skin from direct contact and from the ugly scar. Alternatively, mattress suture could be used differently, in that it lies transversely over the skin one inch apart and one inch away from the wound margin, but the thread goes through the plastic tube, thus protecting the skin from being cut out or from the ugly scar. In this method, the skin margins are free from any tension sutures. However, there should be at least two inch gap between the two mattress sutures.

When the curved needle is inserted through the abdominal wall, the loops of the gut are protected by pressing down by the left hand under direct vision. Other free end of the tension suture that lies hanging outside goes through the nylon tube and is held by the artery forceps. The needle is pulled out from inside the peritoneal cavity and it is inserted again from inside through the contralateral abdominal wall, and pulled out from outside the contralateral abdominal wall one inch away from the skin margin.

The needle goes through the nylon tube before it is reinserted at the same horizontal level through the abdominal wall but one inch apart from the other suture. It is pulled out from inside the abdomen under direct vision. The same needle is pushed through the contralateral abdominal wall but there should be a gap of one inch away from the previous suture at the same horizontal level and it is pulled out through the abdominal wall and the needle is cut out. Both free ends are held together by the same artery forceps. In this case, both prolene threads remain inside the peritoneal cavity.

In this way, several mattress sutures are inserted across the peritoneal cavity leaving a gap of two inches between the each pair of mattress sutures. The swab is next pulled out after all mattress sutures have been inserted. Now the mattress or tension sutures are tied together one after another, making sure that gut is not caught between these sutures, before the skin wound is closed. Wound dressing is applied.

POSTOPERATIVE CARE

Routine care is carried out. Oral fluid should not be commenced until patient has passed wind per rectum. The skin sutures are removed in 10 days, but the tension sutures are removed in 14 days.

Incisional hernia may be the final sequel after many months.

BROAD OUTLINE FOR SUTURE MATERIALS

It is important to be familiar with the basic requirements in the plumbing works in gastrointestinal surgery. Cutting and suturing the gut remain the important skill in this specialty. The basic instruments used in all instances are scissors, occlusion clamps, crushing clamps, artery forceps and the suture materials.

Although technology has moved forwards, the pathological lesions in the gut have not changed. Therefore, the basic skill that needs to learn remains the foundation upon which experience and confidence are built up. This would assist in adopting the new technology in the reconstruction of the plumbing works.

Among the basic skills, hand sutures will stay in the plumbing works and everyone needs to learn how to handle the needle, threads, and technique for suturing the gut and the application of ligatures. These could not be trained without going through the operative surgery but opportunity seems to be limited to the hands on tools. They need to gain this skill at the workshops or in the theater.

In the anastomosis of the two transected ends, a small atraumatic curved needle is used in all instances and the size of the absorbable thread used in the hand suture would be number two zero (2/0). Other important instruments are a needle holder, a pair of tooth and nontooth tissue forceps, two pairs of occlusion clamps and a pair of fine scissors.

In the depth of the abdomen or in the pelvis, these instruments should have a long handle, so that the operating

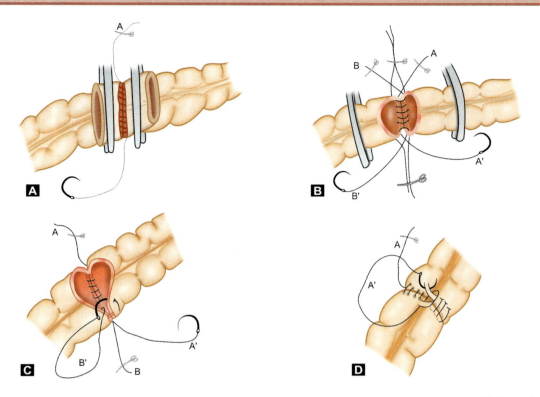

Figs 7.3A to D: Techniques for end-to-end anastomosis in two layers: (A) Continuous seromuscular suture; (B) Posterior anastomosis; (C) Anterior anastomosis; (D) Invagination of the anastomotic suture

hand holding these instruments would not obstruct the field of operation, while carrying out the delicate plumbing works.

PRINCIPLE OF ANASTOMOSIS

It has been the established practice that anastomosis between the two guts is carried out in two layers. The first layer of the anastomosis begins with a continuous suture that is inserted through the seromuscular layer of the two guts, when they are held together by two pairs of clamps.

The purpose of first layer of continuous suture is to support and conceal the second layer of anastomosis (primary anastomosis). It also helps to prevent the anastomotic dehiscence or leakage of the gut's content through the gaps left behind between the two sutures. This second layer of sutures, also known as primary sutures, goes through and through the cut edges of the two stomas, when they are apposed together.

Furthermore, at one time, silk sutures used to be employed commonly in undertaking the seromuscular sutures; but it is rarely used in the present day.

The practice of single layer anastomosis has been the popular choice, but it all depends upon individual skill and training on how he or she has been trained or developed the surgical skill during the residency. In this section, the methods of anastomosis in two layers have been demonstrated in the operative techniques in Figures 7. 3A to D. Figure 7.3A is the continuous seromuscular suture shown in the posterior wall of the two transected colon.

Figure 7.3B is displaying the inner continuous suture (primary anastomosis) going through the cut edges of the two adjacent stomas. Figure 7.3C is the continuation of the anastomotic sutures from Figure 7.3B. In this case, the needle has been shown to be passing from inside of one stoma. It will be pulled out from outside the same stoma and then it would be inserted through the serosal wall of the other stoma, until it is pulled out from inside the same stoma. When the thread will be pulled out at the end, the two cut edges will come close together. In this way, the anterior anastomosis between the two stomas will be completed. A clear demonstration of the technique used for the invagination of the two adjacent seromuscular layers by a continuous suture, thus concealing the primary anastomosis is shown in Figure 7.4.

The main purpose is to conceal the primary anastomotic sutures by the invagination of the seromuscular suture. This would not be possible if the seromuscular sutures are very close to the primary anastomotic sutures.

For single layer anastomosis, invagination is not necessary and the anastomosis is done by interrupted suture that goes through the full thickness of the cut edge of the stoma, when both stomas are brought together by the two pairs of occlusion clamps.

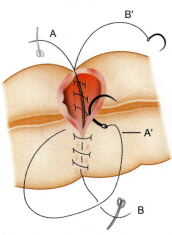

Fig. 7.4: A clear demonstration of the technique used for the invagination of the two adjacent seromuscular layers by a continuous suture, thus concealing the primary anastomosis. It requires the suture bites to be taken at least 0.5 mm away from the inner or primary anastomotic sutures' line

In undertaking the single layer anastomosis, the occlusion clamps should be applied an inch away from the transected ends of the stomas. And they should not be applied very close to the cut edges of the stomas; otherwise, it would be difficult to pass the sutures through the cut edges of the stomas. There should be spacing by 2-3 mm between the two stitches and the suture bite should be between 3-5 mm away from the cut edge of the stoma.

Alternative to the full thickness suture, the needle does not need to go through the full thickness of the gut wall, instead, it could be passed through the outer muscle coat sparing the mucosal layer of the gut wall; but each suture bite should be 5 mm away from the cut edge of the stoma.

STAPLING GUN

Stapling machine has been the new technology used frequently in the plumbing works. Although it has taken over the hand sutures in gastrointestinal surgery, it is very useful in those cases, where the access is limited, and where hand sutures would be difficult. Furthermore, it saves time but it is not cheap and is not 100 percent reliable, in that anastomotic dehiscence does occur in some cases, and anastomotic stenosis is not uncommon.

There are different varieties of autosuture. They are known as EEA (End-to-End Anastomosis) circular stapling, with different sizes ranging from 25 to 31 mm in diameters. It is used for end-to-end or end-to-side anastomosis.

On the other hand, GIA (Gastrointestinal Anastomosis) gun is used for side-to-side anastomosis with concurrent cutting of the anastomotic side walls, and TA (Total Amputation), ranging from 30 to 90 mm, is used for total amputation and suturing of the transected stoma.

One needs to judge the merits of this new technology in perspective, whether or not its benefits outweighs the overall cost and the risk of postoperative morbidity in certain cases.

ANASTOMOTIC CLAMPS

There are many named instruments designed for the resection and anastomosis of the gut. In the resection of the intestine, soft occlusion clamp which stops soiling of the feces and bleeding from the cut edge of the mucosa, is preferably used in all instances. But they should be applied away from the site of the transection or anastomosis.

Crushing clump used to be preferred decades ago, but it is heavy to handle and it devitalizes the tissues. Crushing clamp is used only to the transected segment of the diseased bowel that has to be removed and the main purpose for using the crushing clamp at the proposed line of resection is to stop spillage of the feces from the transected end of the gut waiting to be delivered to the bucket.

A pair of twin clamps known as Lain Clamp which has a locking device is used to hold the two segments of intestine side-by-side for side-to-side anastomosis. It is frequently used in Polya-gastrectomy and is very helpful to a single handed surgeon.

REFERENCES

1. Saha SK. A critical evaluation of dissection of the perineum in synchronous combined abdominoperineal excision of the rectum. Surg Gyne and Obstetrics 1984;158:33-8.
2. Saha SK. Efficacy of metronidazole lavage in treatment of intraperitoneal sepsis: A prospective study. Digestive Diseases and Sciences 1996;41:1313-8.

8. Principle and Policy for Postoperative Care

METABOLIC RESPONSE TO STRESS AND SHOCK

For the first few weeks after operation, metabolic response would lead to catabolic phase. During this period, patient continues to lose body weight due to excess loss of nitrogen in the urine. This loss of nitrogen is affected by the tissue breakdown. In addition, there would be excess secretion of hormones from the pituitary and adrenal glands, resulting in disturbance of water, and electrolytes balance. These changes are attributable to increased production of glucocorticosteroids, mineral corticoids, and antidiuretic hormone. After 2-3 months, excretion of nitrogen will be less in the urine; as a result, patient begins gaining in body weight. This period is known as anabolic phase.

In the immediate postoperative period, corticosteroid hormone reduces the excretion of sodium that may last for the first 2-3 days. As a result, sodium moves into the cellular space, in exchange of potassium ions that will move into the extracellular space. This exchange of sodium ions across the cell membrane is influenced by the mineral corticoids known as aldosterone hormone. In response to injury, reabsorption of sodium increases in the renal tubules and it occurs in exchange of potassium that is influenced by the aldosterone hormone. This explains the reason for reduced excretion of sodium in the urine for the first 2-3 postoperative days.

In contrast, there will be high concentration of urinary sodium and a high specific gravity of urine. This is due to reduced urine output, affected by ADH. The physiological disturbance will change after 2-3 days, when the urine output will increase and sodium excretion will return to normal.

The shift of sodium into the cells leads to intracellular hypernatrium and extracellular hyponatrium. During this shift, chloride will move along with the sodium in exchange for H^+ ions. This explains the mechanism for increased ADH secretion and increased excretion of potassium in the urine for the first 3-4 days.

POSTOPERATIVE STRESS TO INJURY

After the patient is transferred to the recovery room or to the ward, responsibility for the postoperative care lies with the resident surgeons. Their primary aim is to maintain the daily tissue hydration, urine output and fluid balance, oral feeding, relief of postoperative pain, prevention of chest infection, deep vein thrombosis and wound infection.

On the first postoperative day the urine output drops, despite adequate infusion of fluid. It ranges from 600 to 700 ml per 24 hours. It is called obligatory urine output. It is often referred to as obligatory oliguria. One needs to understand the basic physiology surrounding this reduced urine output. It is a response to stress, and postoperative shock, but it is attributable to increased secretion of antidiuretic hormone (ADH).

Apart from this hormone, other hormones such as corticosteroids, aldosterone, adrenaline and noradrenaline are secreted from the adrenal glands in excess, in response to trauma, stress or surgical shock. Their excess secretions are unavoidable. But they are directly attributable to pain, hypotension and tissue dehydration.

These mechanisms will be highlighted in short. First, pain causes peripheral vasoconstriction. This leads to tissue dehydration and increased rate of respiration, thus causing tissue hypoxia. As a result, it enhances increased ADH secretion.

In the study of postoperative pain relief, the urine output was found greater than 1000 ml per 24 hours on the first postoperative day after cholecystectomy.[1] This was due to maintenance of pain threshold level consistently throughout the postoperative period. This was in contrast to other cases in which the postoperative pain relief was managed by the conventional method, using 10 mg morphine sulphate or Omnopon given by intermuscular injection every 6 hours.

In those cases, patients were not completely pain-free and in some cases, they were in deep sleep and had low blood pressure. As a result, obligatory urine output was between 600 and 700 ml per 24 hours.

In contrast, continuous maintenance of pain threshold level with intravenous infusion of narcotics, blood pressure and respiration rate were maintained uniformly within the normal range. As a result, it is believed that secretion of ADH was relatively less in the postoperative period. This explains the reason how the urine output was over 1000 ml on the first postoperative day.[1]

Therefore, this physiological knowledge should be implemented in the management of infusion regimen and complete relief of postoperative pain.

POLICY FOR POSTOPERATIVE PARENTERAL INFUSION

Unlike the preoperative infusion regimen, postoperative infusion regimen would be quite different, in that saline should be given less, instead dextrose solution should be added more to the daily infusion regimen. The ratio should be one liter of saline and two liters of dextrose (1:2). After first two postoperative days, the regimen needs to be reviewed on the results of electrolytes and total output. In most cases, it should be 2:1.

SURGICAL PHYSIOLOGY OF THE GUT

Physiological function of the gut provides the basic guideline for postoperative feeding. It is well-recognized that inflammation, or injury to the tissues inhibits the normal function of the organ.

In gastrointestinal surgery, both segmental and propagative peristalsis is inhibited for a while after general anesthesia, resection of the gut or infection to the peritoneal cavity.

Return of bowel sounds does not imply that the gut has recovered from injury or infection, nor does it suggest that propagative peristalsis has passed across the line of anastomosis.

Bowel sounds, audible on the stethoscope are due to segmental peristalsis, which is irrelevant to the postoperative care, but functional state of the gut is recognized by the flatus passed per rectum and by the total volume of 24 hours' aspirate.

The successive reduction in 24 hour aspirates would relate that the gut has started absorbing the fluids. If there is an evidence of high output on successive aspiration, this would suggest that there is an evidence of mechanical obstruction or functional stasis of the gut. The former could be associated with the kinking of the dilated gut, or obstruction of the gut at the site of anastomosis. This could be due to edema, inflammation around the line of anastomosis.

The stasis of the fluid within the lumen of the gut would cause dilatation of the gut. This leads to venous and lymphatic congestion. As a result, there would be more exudation from the congested and edematous mucosa, instead of absorption of fluid and gas from the lumen. Despite this science, some surgeons encourage the oral fluids on the first postoperative day, contrary to the physiological function of the gut.

Furthermore, drinking of simple water may encourage peristaltic movements at some stage, but it would be encountered with the edema and inflammation developed around the anastomosis, and it may induce dehiscence of the anastomotic sutures. Wound healing of the gut is no different from the healing of the fractured bone. Furthermore, violent peristalsis inhibits localization of the purulent fluid. On the contrary, it enhances any leakage through the anastomotic line.

PHYSIOLOGICAL CHANGES OF THE POSTOPERATIVE GUT

On the immediate postoperative day, the small intestine remains silent due to paralytic ileus and becomes dilated. It would carry both air and water. The sources of gas collected within the lumen are from swallowed air, production of fermentation, and diffusion of gas from the gut wall. The gas contains around 70-80 percent of nitrogen, and the rest would be carbon dioxide and hydrogen sulphide.

Because of dilatation of the intestine, the thin-walled veins are compressed. The site of such impaction would be greater at the point of entry in the mesenteric border of the gut. As a result, there would be venous stasis within the wall of the gut. This venous congestion will lead to exudation of fluid into the wall of the intestine as well as into its lumen.

In normal physiological state of the gut, the total volume of fluid in the lumen would be around 8 liters, secreted by the pancreatic juice, bile and secretion of the small intestine. But in the state of paralytic ileus or intestinal obstruction, it would be greater than this estimated volume that would be sequestrated within the lumen of the gut thus causing tissue dehydration.

Hence, oral feeding would be contrary to the physiological function of the gut. Furthermore, patient would swallow air along with the drinking of water. All these actions contribute to further dilatation of the gut wall, leading to further venous stasis. As a result, there would be further exudation of extracellular fluid into the lumen of the gut, thus adding further distention of the gut.

The problem will not confine limited to the distention of the gut; it would cause elevation of the diaphragm and abdominal wall. All these conditions exert tension upon the abdominal wound and sutures, induce pain and inhibit the deep breathing. Because of distention of the abdomen, and inhibition of breathing, peripheral venous return would be inhibited by the intraperitoneal pressure. In these circumstances, patient will demand more pain-relief. As a result, analgesic requirement will continue rising. The adverse effect would be respiratory depression, sickness, poor oxygen saturation in the blood. The narcotic effect would delay the passing of flatus and induce further constipation.

CLINICAL APPLICATION OF NASOGASTRIC TUBE (RYLE'S TUBE)

Nasogastric tube is known as Ryle's tube. It is a long tube, measuring upto 105 cm in length. Its terminal end that is pushed down the esophagus is blind in which, a metallic ball is rested. It assists in advancing the tube, because of its weight and gravity, but there are holes, incorporated on the side wall proximal to the metallic ball. There are different sizes of bore available and it is marked with number that goes up to the size of 18 FG. For gastric aspiration, a moderate sized caliber, usually number 14 is used. For gastric feeding, a larger size should be preferred.

In the past, it was made with rubber. Now it is made with plastic which does not cause too much irritation or reaction to the tissue but it may cause discomfort to the patient and may produce inflammation to the upper gastrointestinal tract. It has several round markers at different level that would indicate the location of the tip of the tube in the stomach from the level of the nose. And there are round markers from one to four, printed around the tube. Each marker denotes the position of the tube from the level of the nose right down to the stomach.

The position of the distal end of the tube is identified by the number of round markers at the level of the nose. For instance, when a single marker reaches at the tip of the nose, it would indicate that the distal tip of the Ryle's tube is at the gastroesophageal junction (38-40 cm from the incisor of the teeth), two markers would suggest that the tip is inside the body of the stomach, three markers in the antrum and the four markers into the duodenum.

In this way, nurse would recognize whether the tip has reached at the exact location or proposed level down in the stomach or duodenum. The tube has a radiopaque material incorporated at its tip that will show in the X-ray of the abdomen, taken after the tube has been passed. This will confirm the exact position of the tip of the tube.

■ Technique for Advancing the NG Tube

Patient is explained about the benefit of this tube being negotiated into the stomach. Patient's cooperation is very important. He is asked to prop up in the bed with a pillow supporting his back. He should be asked for taking a deep breath as and when he would be advised to do so and this exercise is necessary when difficulty is experienced in advancing the tube.

KY jelly is put around the tip of the Ryle's tube. The tip is first passed through one of the nostril and it is advanced slowly, step by step and one step at one attempt. Patient should be given time to cooperate and to take a deep breathing, when it is pushed for a small part at one stroke. Never try to advance the tip very rapidly and in one go or by force or by pushing it in different direction. It will advance smoothly, if there is no nasal polyp or septal deviation within the nostril.

The first resistance may be encountered when the tip of the tube has reached the back of the throat. Patient may try to push it out through the mouth, by hiccup or by exerting resistance in the nasopharynx. This may be due to irritation in the back of the throat. At this moment of time, reassurance is necessary, and patient is asked to take a deep breath and to swallow a sip of water. This will open up the pharynx and would assist in advancing the tip further down because of peristalsis of the esophagus. Once it has passed beyond the level of oropharynx, advancing the tube through the esophagus becomes easier.

During this maneuver, air bubbles will be seen gushing out through other end that keeps hanging down outside the nose; but this end should be put into a small tray. Sometimes, patient is asked to keep holding this tray. The tube is stopped pushing further down through the nose, when the correct level of the markers has reached to the tip of the nose. To confirm whether or not the tip of the tube has reached in the antrum, a 20 ml syringe is connected to the proximal end of the tube and aspiration is attempted.

Bile or gastric contents will come out into the syringe, reassuring the nurse that the tube has been successfully put into the stomach. If nothing has been aspirated back in the syringe, resistance may be experienced while aspirating back, this may be due to blockage of the side holes by mucus plugs. Or it could be due to coiling of the tube in the lower part of the esophagus. To overcome this temporary blockage, a few ml of water should be pushed down by the syringe; but before proceeding with pushing water down through the Ryle's tube, it is very important to be sure that the tip of the tube has not entered into the upper respiratory tract.

Although, patient will experience respiratory distress, if the tube is inside the trachea, nevertheless, for the safe side, the other end of the tube is put into the glass of water. This will exclude whether or not the inner end is in the lumen of the esophagus or in the trachea. In the latter case, air bubble will be seen emerging from the glass of water.

In the absence of this evidence, it is now safe to push 5 ml of water through the tube that will dislodge the mucus plugs from the eyes of the side wall of the tube. At the second attempt, aspiration will bring back bile or gastric contents in the syringe. Once this experiment has satisfied the nurse, the NG tube is fixed to the tip of the nose by adhesive tapes. And the other end is either anchored to the cheek by another tape.

Final confirmation is made on record by taking a plain X-ray of the abdomen, whether or not the tip of the NG tube is in the correct level in the stomach.

In any difficult cases, lignocaine spray must not be applied to the throat. This may cause aspiration into the lung. In difficult cases, lignocaine jelly could be put inside the nostril a few minutes before the Ryle's tube is attempted to pass through the nose. If difficulty is encountered while passing through one nostril, other nostril should be tried.

It is not uncommon that Ryle's tube may slip out of the nose. This may be due to poor anchorage to the tip of the nose by a poor quality of adhesive tape or patient may pull it out.

At the end, the proximal end (outer end) of the tube could be closed by inserting a spigot in between the suction of the stomach contents or it could be connected to a bile bag for a free drainage. Any air swallowed by the patient will return into the bag or any reflux of bile and intestinal contents into the stomach will drain spontaneously into the bile bag in between the action of aspirations. In the latter procedure, patient will feel comfortable, but the weight of the fluid in the bag may drag the Ryle's tube out of the stomach.

Regular mouthwash should be carried out and any amount of water is allowed to swallow should be aspirated back. This keeps the oral cavity clean and moist. This mouthwash exercise will reduce the risk of causing parotidis.

PHYSIOLOGICAL VALUE FOR GASTRIC ASPIRATION

In the postoperative period, gastric aspiration seems to have been less popular. Among the many reasons, nurses are not dedicated in persuading the patient in accepting the Ryle's tube. It is true that it is uncomfortable, but it provides a considerable benefit to the care of the patients. These benefits need to be highlighted in perspective to the patient, before attempting to pass the Ryle's tube through the nose. Patient acceptance and then cooperation are very important in difficult circumstances.

First, patient does swallow air that induces dilatation of the stomach. In addition, swallowing of saliva and gastric secretions, which could be around 4 liters[2] would lead to gross distention of the stomach. As a result, patient would experience pain in the abdominal wound. Therefore, more narcotics would be needed for the relief of pain.

Furthermore, distention of the stomach along with the distention of paralytic gut will push the diaphragm higher up, thus interfering with the full inspiration and causing basal congestion of the lungs. If the patient needs more morphine for the continued pain, this would delay in passing the flatus. Distention of the gut will continue longer that would be detrimental to the venous return from the lower limbs. Patients would be less mobile and constipation will continue. Risk of deep vein thrombosis would be much greater.

All these problems could be reduced or avoided just by keeping the stomach empty. This requires hourly gastric aspiration and a free nasogastric drainage in between the hourly aspiration. Chest complication is more likely to be less and pain relief could be achieved with less analgesic drugs.

Furthermore, the potential risk of respiratory depression could be avoided, if the patient does not require too much narcotics for the relief of additional pain, arising from the abdominal wound. Apart from these therapeutic values, gastric aspiration will indicate whether or not the gut has recovered. This will be measured by the amount of daily aspiration which should be less by less on the successive days. On the merits of the 24 hours aspiration, a judicious decision could be taken whether or not oral feeding could be commenced.

Average daily secretion from the alimentary tract[2]

Sources of secretions	Volume
Saliva	1500 ml
Stomach	2500 ml
Gallbladder	500 ml
Pancreas	700 ml
Small intestine	3000 ml
Total	8200 ml

POLICY FOR ORAL FEEDING TO POSTOPERATIVE PATIENTS

To improve the situation, gut needs to be decompressed, air needs to be aspirated back and oral fluid has to be restricted. To achieve these objectives, regular aspiration through the nasogastric tube is necessary. Every hourly aspiration should be recorded on the fluid balance chart.

In the postoperative care, 25 ml oral fluid could be commenced on the first postoperative day, before hourly aspiration is carried out. It will moist the oral cavity and clean the mouth and esophagus, and the daily hourly regimen could be increased by 25 ml on the successive day, provided the hourly aspiration is getting less everyday, then the oral fluid may be commenced.

In this case, the rate of aspiration could be modified from hourly to 4 hourly that depends upon the volume of aspiration returned on the previous day. If the volume is becoming less on the successive days, it indicates that gut has started absorbing fluid and that there was no stasis in the stomach. This regimen should be continued until the patient could tolerate 100 ml of water, given 4 hourly and till the patient has passed wind per rectum.

Passage of flatus per rectum is clinically more important than listening to the bowel sounds with the stethoscope. Once the patient has tolerated free fluid orally, oral feeding with light diet could be commenced and the recovery would be much faster than other patients, if they were allowed oral feeding earlier.

A regimen for oral feeding should be consistent with the physiological function of the gut. This deals with the rate of aspiration and rate of oral fluids. If the total volume of aspirants per 24 hours comes down to less than 300 ml, and the patient has started passing wind per rectum, then it could be concluded that there is no mechanical obstruction and no physiological stasis of the stomach contents. In this way, the gut motility and healing of the gut anastomosis are evaluated.

In view of this evidence, NG tube is safe to be withdrawn. It is also safe to withdraw the drainage tube, provided the total discharge is less than 25 ml over 24 hours or there was no evidence of leakage of bile or feces through the drainage or suction tubing and no rise of temperature.

Therefore, cautious approach should be adopted. Some surgeons have a different policy and allow the patients to take oral fluids earlier than this regimen just described. The author believes: "If the patient waits for one more day, he gains a week in recovery from the operation".

In the gut surgery, it is well known and documented evidence that anastomotic leakage tends to occur usually on the fourth or fifth postoperative day. The reason for such complication is due to poor surgical technique, and poor vascularity. Therefore, it is very important to be careful until the fifth postoperative day has passed or until the patient has passed wind per rectum.

POLICY FOR ANTIBIOTIC THERAPY

In the past, prophylactic antibiotic therapy used to be a common policy, but it is now selectively used in some cases. Because the studies showed that it causes emergent resistant strains of bacteria.

But in certain surgical practices, prophylactic antibiotics are routinely used. These are vascular surgery, colonic surgery and orthopedic surgery. Among these specialties, colonic surgery is regarded to be infective operative procedures, despite undertaking all preventive measures against the wound contamination. It would be wrong to consider that the operative field is clean, once the colon is divided. Leakage of colonic gas, that contains intestinal bacilli, would technically contaminate the peritoneal cavity and even the environment of the operating theater.

Hence, prophylactic antibiotics should be prescribed before the patient is put in general anesthesia or placed on the operating table. Furthermore, prophylactic antibiotic should be prescribed in certain medical conditions, such as mitral valve disease, cardiac pacemaker, and prosthesis implanted in the body. Or it is prescribed if the patient needs implantation of the foreign body materials in the operative procedures.

In colonic surgery, it is advisable that combination of two different types of antibiotics should be prescribed. The reasons behind this policy are as follows:

a. In all instances, more than one bacterium is present in the infected wound. And anaerobes are one of them. It causes suppression of phagocytic function present in the wound. Hence, a combination of two antibacterial agents is usually used.
b. It reduces the risk of emergence of resistant strains.
c. Combination of two or three antibiotics provides a synergistic effect, which indicates that the bactericidal effect of two combined drugs would be much greater than that of one antibiotic, if it were used independently.

CERTAIN PHARMACOLOGICAL RESTRICTIONS

In the combination of antimicrobial therapy, it is also advisable against using a combination of bactericidal and bacteriostatic antibiotics. Such combination is incompatible. If such combination is used, it may encourage the emergence of resistance strains, but there are some exceptions that will be highlighted later.

It is also advisable against prescribing a very higher dose of antibiotic in the routine cases of colonic surgery. And it should not be used against the resistant strains.

It is well-recognized that benefit would be minimum, if the antibiotics are continued over 5-7 days. On the contrary, prolong use of the antibiotic therapy may cause mouth ulcer, known as thrush, or pseudomembranous colitis.

In the latter cases, broad-spectrum antibiotics destroy all commensal intestinal bacteria, thus allowing the multiplication of *Clostridium difficile*. As a result, patient starts having sudden onset of diarrhea that could be of a mild nature, but it could be worse, like cholera in certain cases. In some cases, acute mucosal inflammation may lead to ulceration, hemorrhage or perforation. In these cases, pseudo-membranous colitis should be suspected.

The exact pathogenesis is not clearly understood but it is probably due to destruction of the normal commensal intestinal organism, thus enhancing the resistant strains of *Clostridium difficile*. In healthy population, its incidence among the intestinal bacteria is 5 percent and it is an anaerobic bacilli and a member of the *Clostridium* family. Other bacteria of the same family cause tetanus, botulism, and gas gangrene.

Although it is a commensal intestinal organism, it remains under check by other healthy intestinal bacteria. If these healthy bacteria are killed by the antibiotics, the *Clostridium difficile* becomes virulent and produce two toxins which cause cellular damage of the intestine.

In this case, patient may develop hypovolemic shock, dehydration and electrolyte depletion, and hypotension. Clinically, abdomen will be noticed distended like paralytic ileus.

Obviously, intravenous fluid infusion is commenced to rectify the fluid deficit and to correct the electrolyte imbalance. In addition, intravenous hydrocortisone should be commenced in severe shock. Its purpose is to combat the shock. The recommended dose is 100 mg to be given intravenously every six hours, but a higher dose such as 500 mg every six hours for the first 24 hours could be prescribed. My experience supports the higher dose in dealing with the septic shock. The dose is reduced from the second day, and gradually tailing off everyday and it is discontinued within 5 days.

Other therapeutic measure is to discontinue the existing parenteral antibiotics, and instead, oral vancomycin and metronidazole are the choice of antibiotics to be commenced against the *Clostridium difficile*, but it would be sensible to prescribe the antibiotic which is sensitive to the bacteria reported on the stools culture.

Apart from stools culture, sigmoidoscopy should be attempted, if clinical condition permits. This local examination will reveal friable inflamed mucosa and whitish yellow plaques, which are regarded to be the clinical evidence of pseudomembranous colitis.

There is another variety of resistant strain of super bug, known as MRSA (Meticillins resistant *Staphylococcus aureus*). UK-NHS hospitals have been succumbing to the dreadful resistant bacteria. In the general population, 30 percent of the public are carrier of this dreadful bug in their skin surfaces. It does not produce any specific symptoms but it may cause deep abscess, septicemia, chest infection. It is difficult to eradicate with antibiotics. Major resources have been directed towards the eradication of these resistant bacteria. Isolation of the patient and cleanliness are the important measures to be employed in treating these patients.

In certain cases, certain drugs such as sulfonamides, tetracycline, gentamycin and metronidazole should not be given to pregnant lady and tetracycline must not be prescribed to newborn baby or children up to the age of 8 years old. This drug may cause brownish discoloration of their teeth.

INDICATIONS FOR ANTIBIOTIC THERAPY

- Evidence of postoperative chest infection, not responding to physiotherapy.
- Persisting temperature over two days and radiological evidence of chest infection.
- Evidence of wound discharge.
- Evidence of localized or generalized peritonitis.
- Evidence of urinary tract infection.
- Evidence of septicemia.
- Evidence of high white cell counts, and elevation of C reactive protein.
- Evidence of bacterial growth in the wound swab, or urine or blood culture.

Before commencing the antibiotic therapy, blood should be sent for WCC and CRP (C reactive protein). If the patient has an elevation of temperature, blood is also sent for culture and sensitivity test.

And at the same time, a sample of urine (MSU) should also be sent for both microscopical and culture and sensitivity test.

In the meantime, antibiotic therapy should be commenced. In the initial stage, broad-spectrum group of drug should be preferred and two types of antibiotics should be prescribed in order to cover both aerobic and anaerobic bacteria. And the dose for the drugs must be high enough to maintain the therapeutic level in the serum and in the tissue fluid.

The most common groups of drugs used are ampicillin, amoxicillin, gentamicin or cephalosporin group of drugs, but penicillin or amoxicillin must be avoided if there is any history of allergic reaction to penicillin. In most cases, a combination of metronidazole 500 mg and cephalosporin group of antibiotic has been found effective in controlling infection. But the clinician must check with the patients or their relatives whether there was any history of allergic reaction to a particular antibiotic. Some patients are allergic to penicillin and 10 percent of this group of patients may be allergic to cephalosporin group of drugs.

If there is any doubt, skin test should be done before the particular antibiotic is prescribed. Apart from this allergic issue, antibiotic should not be prescribed, if it is resistant to the particular bacteria, reported by the bacteriology department. Furthermore, the regimen of antibiotic should be changed, or discontinued; if the patient is not responding to the treatment or the temperature is persistently elevated for a few days without any obvious cause being known to the doctors.

It is advisable not to prescribe any expensive and strong bactericidal group of drugs at the very outset. If the temperature persists and patient remains toxic for a period of 2-3 days, antibiotic may need to be changed and it should be sensitive to blood culture report or wound swab culture report.

Nephrotoxic drug such as gentamicin (aminoglycosides) should be used with precaution. In this case, patient must have good renal function, normal urea and creatinine, and good urine output.

In severe infection, or cases with proven evidence of *Pseudomonas aeruginosa* infection, gentamicin (aminoglycosides) should preferably be used, but it tends to develop resistance strains very soon. To avoid this problem, tobramycin could be prescribed instead.

Aminoglycosides are bacteriostatic drugs that inhibit bacterial protein synthesis. It is used against the gram-negative enteric organism but it is not suitable against the anaerobic bacilli. Its plasma half-life is 2-3 hours. The dose to be prescribed should be related to body weight. It is 3-5 mg/kg of body weight per day and the total dose is given in three divided doses. Alternative to body weight, the recommended dose is 80 mg, but for elderly patient, the dose should be 60 mg. It is given either intravenously or intramuscularly every 8 hours.

Although, this antibiotic is bacteriostatic, it works effectively, if it is prescribed in combination with penicillin group of drug. In addition, metronidazole should be used in all cases.

If gentamicin is resistant to a particular organism, alternative antibiotic such as amikacin should be prescribed.

In all instances, gentamicin level in blood must be assayed and this test should be undertaken two days after the treatment has been commenced.

For this assay, two samples of venous blood, one collected one hour before and another one collected one hour after the injection of antibiotic has been given to the patient, are sent to the biochemistry department. The posttherapeutic serum level of gentamicin should not exceed 2.5 times of the pretherapeutic level (Average acceptable pretherapeutic (trough) serum level should be 2 mg per liter and posttherapeutic level (peak) should be between 5-7 mg/l).

Gentamicin is nephrotoxic and ototoxic. In most cases, it should not be used for more than five days. And it should be discontinued if the serum level of creatinine and urea has started rising or the patient is complaining of deafness.

Experiences show that discontinuation of antibiotic may bring the temperature down. This policy should be reviewed after a week. It has also been my experience that patient responds better with septrin, trimethoprim or augmentin in some cases, if the existing antibiotics appear to be ineffective in bringing the temperature down and in reducing the wound inflammation or wound discharge.

Response to antibiotic depends upon the therapeutic level of the drug in the tissue fluid and blood. And it also depends upon the sensitivity to the bacteria. Trimethoprim is also bacteriostatic antibiotic and it is commonly prescribed against most pathogens. Its oral dose is 200 mg twice a day. It could be prescribed in combination with sulphamethoxazole, which is commercially known as septrin (cotrimoxazole). These antibiotics are suitable in the treatment of chest infection and urinary tract infection.

In a suspected case of abdominal wound infection, where, the patient is having a mild elevation of temperature, with no obvious evidence of wound discharge, it has been my experience that temperature settles down spontaneously, since the antibiotic has been discontinued. And in other instances, it resolved since septrin (400 mg) was given twice a day for 3-5 days. This antibiotic contains trimethoprim 80 mg and sulphamethoxazole (400 mg). It was evident that a combination of two drugs was found more effective than relying upon either of the two antibiotics. This antibiotic is cheap and should be prescribed for a persistent temperature or a slight wound discharge, instead of relying upon the broad-spectrum antibiotics.

A NEW THERAPEUTIC APPROACH TO PRIMARY WOUND HEALING

There are two schools of thought in the treatment of infection. One school of thought prefers a policy of wait and watch for clean surgical cases. It recommends for antibiotic therapy if there is clear evidence of infection in the postoperative period. Another school of thought recommends prophylactive antibiotic therapy for gastrointestinal surgery and particularly in colonic surgery.

In gastrointestinal surgery, wounds are subjected to contamination, despite a meticulous care being pursued. Once the gut is open, its gas leaks and it is regarded to be mixed with both aerobic and anaerobic bacilli. Hence, the wound is contaminated. The incidence of wound infection ranges from 17 to 26 percent.[3] And in emergency surgery, it would be much higher. Since metronidazole has been used routinely in the antibiotic regimens, the wound infection has drastically reduced to 12 percent.[4] This varies from center-to-center.

Many surgeons claimed in the study that wound infection could be higher if perioperative blood transfusion has been given. In other retrospective study, a high incidence of wound infection was claimed to be attributable to advanced Dukes tumor staging.[5]

In sharp contrast, no such association was found in the prospective study, despite the fact that a high incidence of Dukes C rectal tumor was included in the prospective study.[6] Since this study was reported to the literature, no one had disputed the results of the study.

Pathogenesis of wound infection, in particular to gastrointestinal surgery is attributable to both anaerobic and aerobic bacilli. We were ignorant about the biological value of each group of pathogens present in the wound until 1978, when we recognized the significant difference in the result of treatment of tooth abscess with metronidazole. Since then, metronidazole has been routinely prescribed along with other antibiotics, sensitive to aerobic bacilli.

A new study with peritoneal lavage using a combination of metronidazole and cephradine was first published, but unusual tissue reaction was noticed in the parietal wound.[7] In the subsequent prospective study, no such tissue reaction such as oozing from the capillaries was evident in the parietal wound, since cephradine was excluded from the wound lavage. And it was encouraging that a better result in the control of infection was found consistently in all cases.[8,9]

The study revealed that anaerobes present in the wound inhibit the body's phagocytic function, thus encouraging the multiplication of the aerobic bacilli unopposed into the wound. This increased population of unopposed aerobic bacteria continues tissue necrosis, thus producing abscess in the wound.

To protect the body's phagocytic function, the anaerobic bacteria need to be eradicated completely, thus keeping the body's own phagocytic function unopposed. This will suppress the aerobic bacteria to be killed by the bactericidal antibiotics.[8,9]

Therefore, apart from the systemic antibiotic therapy, wound lavage is equally important in order to maintain the high level of metronidazole in the local tissue fluid or in the necrotic tissues where the systemic metronidazole cannot reach or it cannot maintain its therapeutic level in order to kill all anerobic bacilli harboring in the necrotic tissue, pool of infected fluid, hematoma or in the dead space within the peritoneal cavity and in the wound.

The wound infection was found in less than 2 percent in the second prospective study.[9] This lavage is carried out after the peritoneal cavity has been washed out meticulously with saline, that should be done at the completion of primary operative procedure undertaken.

The dose for metronidazole lavage varies according to the extent of infection. It would be 500 mg for appendicectomy, 1000 mg for major abdominal operation and 1.5 gm for fecal peritonitis. This IV commercial preparation should not be mixed with saline or dextrose solution.

The study showed that the phagocytic function of the blood that works against the aerobic bacilli is inhibited by the anaerobic bacilli.[9,10] As a result, aerobic bacilli may multiply in the blood and in the wound—thus causing tissue necrosis locally. This seems to be the mechanism in the pathogenesis of primary wound infection.

In achieving the primary wound healing, the aerobic bacilli are attacked by a combination of body's phagocytosis and by the bactericidal antibiotic such as cephalosporin drugs. Protection of local phagocytic function is believed to be the key issue in destroying the aerobic bacilli. Because of this reason, metronidazole is used routinely along with other antibiotics in all instances. And local application of the metronidazole was found to have no adverse effects to the body but it should be used judiciously in childbearing age group of patients, or it should not be used at all.

Reasons for persistent wound infection:
1. Drug may be resistant to the particular bacteria.
2. Therapeutic level of antibiotic in the tissue fluid may be below the bactericidal dose of antibiotic.
3. There may be dead space, collection of fluid or necrotic tissue within the wound cavity.
4. Uncontrolled diabetes.
5. Patient on steroid and immunosuppressive drugs.

In one study, the antibiotic level in the tissue fluid was found to be below the therapeutic range in 15 percent among the elective and 35 percent among the emergency operative cases, despite the fact that it was found normal level in the serum in both groups.[11] The reasons could be defined by the fact that systemic antibiotics may not reach the pool of infected fluid, blood or to the necrotic tissues in order to maintain its therapeutic level. It may also be attributable to poor tissue perfusion in the state of shock, dehydration, or peripheral vasoconstriction. This explains as to why the therapeutic level of antibiotic in the tissue fluid is worse in emergency operative cases. To overcome this problem, antibiotic lavage is recommended and metronidazole lavage was found effective in controlling the wound infection.

INDICATIONS FOR STOPPING THE ANTIBIOTIC THERAPY

- No elevation of temperature, no evidence of wound infection or peritonitis.
- No sign of chest or urinary tract infection.
- Resistance to particular organism, reported on sensitivity test.
- No evidence of bacterial growth in blood culture, or wound swab culture.
- Allergic reaction, such as skin rashes, urticaria, nephrotoxic, or ototoxic.
- Having diarrhea.
- Persisting temperature (Not responding to treatment).
- Leukopenia.

CLINICAL VALUE OF MAINTAINING THE TEMPERATURE CHART

In healthy subjects, body temperature varies between the morning and middle of the night. This is known as diurnal variation. It remains normal in the early morning; but it rises gradually as the day advances until 10 pm, and it begins to fall by the early morning. Again, temperature in healthy subjects varies with the exercise.

In all human beings, central body temperature is regulated within a narrow range and there are certain factors that enhance heat production. They are thyroid thermogenesis that controls the body basal metabolism, adenosine triphosphatase (ATPase) that acts as enzyme for the sodium pump of the cell membrane and the muscle activity which generates body heat during the day-to-day work. For maintaining the equilibrium within a very narrow band in the body temperature, all the heat is lost through various processes, known as thermostatic regulation. They are respiratory system, the skin and the blood volume.

For instance, the breathing loses body temperature in warming the inhaled air or heat is lost through expiration of warm air. In the body surface, the cutaneous vessels play an important part in both preservation and loss of heat. In this case, adrenergic autoregulation acts on the cutaneous vessels, where vessels may be constricted in order to preserve the heat or it may cause vasodilatation leading to sweating or perspiration through which body heat is lost.

The neural control is hypothalamus. It is the center of the regulatory process which is again feed back with the blood flow.

Recording of temperature among the healthy subjects is unnecessary, but body temperature is a sensitive indicator of our health. In clinical practice, it reflects early sign of the disease. It also reflects the progressive state of the systemic diseases or postoperative recovery. It assists in clinical diagnosis and indicates whether patient is responding to treatment. It is used as one of the prognostic tools in evaluating the therapeutic response to the disease and it also reflects a prognostic value of the clinical management. There are various features of temperature chart and each pattern carries a diagnostic feature. These are intermittent, remittent, relapsing or sustained types of temperature.

a. Intermittent temperature has a characteristic pattern, in which the difference between the peak and the lower reading is very large. The temperature falls to normal range everyday but it returns to very high on the same day. This indicates the presence of septic source somewhere and abscess and pyogenic collection should be looked for, somewhere in the body. In the absence of this pathological condition, lymphomas and military tuberculosis should be investigated.
b. Remittent temperature—It falls everyday but it does not return to normal level. It does not point to any particular disease.
c. Sustained temperature—It remains persistently high without any diurnal change. In this case, typhoid fever should be suspected.
d. Relapsing temperature—It may present in various pattern. The bouts of temperature recur at 2-3 day intervals of normal temperature. It may be associated with rigor. Malaria should be suspected.

A similar pattern known as Pel-Ebstein fever is suspicious of Hodgkin disease. In this case, the elevation of temperature persists for a period of 3–10 days, but it remains afebrile and asymptomatic for the subsequent 3-10 days. It may be repeated in cyclic order for many months.

This provides an overview about the characteristic pattern of a temperature chart that may assist in the diagnosis of the underlying diseases.

In clinical practice, temperature is recorded at regular intervals. This is done by putting the mercury end of the thermometer into the axilla under the garment, or under the tongue in the oral cavity. In certain cases, rectal temperature is recorded. There are a variation of readings between the axilla, oral and the rectal temperature. The difference would be one degree higher in oral and two degree higher in the rectal temperature, compared to the axillary temperature.

In surgical practice, a temperature chart is maintained from the day one since patient is admitted to the ward. Our clinical practice is limited to an acute surgical admission and postoperative care.

In other specialty, the temperature chart provides valuable information. For instance, the functional state of the ovulatory phase of the ovary could be assessed by recording the temperature everyday for a few cycles. A rise of temperature on a particular day would reflect the day of ovulation.

Hence, recording the central body temperature is regarded to be the good clinical practice, upon which subsequent changes may reflect progress and prognosis of the disease. In clinical practice, the body temperature is recorded at regular intervals, until the patient is discharged home.

The body temperature could be recorded from four routes and they are oral, external auditory meatus, axilla and the rectal. In addition, urinary temperature could be another source for recording the core temperature of the body. But it is not clinically practiced, because of inconvenience to the patient and micturition does not occur every hour.

However, there are three types of thermometers available to the clinical practice. One type of thermometer is used for recording the temperature either from the oral cavity or from the axilla and other variety is exclusively used for recording the transrectal temperature. And the third one is the electronic, that could be used either in the external auditory meatus, oral cavity or in the axilla.

In children, axillary temperature or rectal temperature is recorded. The temperature recorded by placing the thermometer in the axilla does not reflect the central body temperature and is 1-2 degree lower than the oral temperature or the rectal temperature.

In the case of children, it is not advisable to put the thermometer inside their mouth. They may break it down, by crushing between the teeth or gum. As a result, mercury may spill into the mouth and the broken glass may cause tissue damage or may be swallowed, if it is chewed, as if thinking of lollypop and it would be difficult to keep the thermometer under the tongue for two minutes.

To avoid these problems, rectal thermometer is used. And it is inserted into the rectum for recording the core body temperature.

For recording the core temperature, external auditory meatus provides an easy access and its temperature is registered within a second. In this case, the nozzle of the electronic thermometer is covered with a disposable plastic cover, before it is inserted into the external auditory meatus. This plastic cover is thrown out after the temperature is recorded. The purpose of using this protective disposable plastic cover is to prevent the transmission of infection from patient-to-patient.

After the body temperature is initially recorded, the recording is continued every hour for any sick and seriously ill patients. After the acute clinical condition has been evaluated, its recording pattern could be changed, that depends upon the clinical circumstances. In most cases, it is recorded every 6 hours.

The pattern of temperature recorded in the chart will reflect the clinical state of the disease. For instance, dropping of the reading reflects a good prognostic indicator. Successive falls of temperature implies that the patient is responding to treatment or antibiotics. During this observation period, patient should not be given soluble aspiring for bringing the temperature down. This may mislead the clinician.

In certain condition, where the temperature seems to have exceeded the critical level, then it would be absolutely necessary to get the body temperature down by other methods. These are soluble aspirin, body wash with wet towels across the forehead and to put on a table fan that would dry the perspiration and evaporation of skin temperature. In these clinical conditions, patient may lose a lot of sodium and water from the body.

If the temperature is swinging up and down, it is known as intermittent type that reflects that there could be a collection of purulent fluid in any part of the system or in the peritoneal cavity. It is a very reliable diagnostic indicator for the diagnosis of abscess. Successive elevation of temperature is a bad prognosis. Persisting of temperature at a constant level with a minor swinging indicates that patient is not responding to antibiotics. And it may drop like a steep fall after the abscess has been surgically evacuated.

If there is a recurrence of temperature a few days after the operation being carried out, suspicion should arise on the possibility of leakage from the anastomosis or development of abscess in the abdomen. In these cases, a thorough clinical examination should be done. These include inspection of the oral cavity, auscultation of chest, and examination of the wound and abdomen. These are palpation of the abdomen, whether there is any evidence of localized palpable lump, tenderness and guarding.

After clinical evaluation is completed, necessary investigation should be carried out in order to establish the etiology of a recurrence of temperature. Blood should be sent for WCC and Hb, culture and sensitivity test, CRP (C Reactive Protein) and ESR. MSU (Midstream Urine) should be sent for microscopical examination and for culture and sensitivity test. If there is evidence of sterile leukocytes in the microscopic examination of the urine and they are greater than 5 per cubic field, guinea-pig inoculation culture test should be done on three consecutive early morning specimen of urine. This will exclude TB kidney.

Ultrasound scan, plain X-ray chest in erect position, and X-ray of the abdomen should be arranged. If all these investigations seem to be inconclusive, CT scan should be done.

Plain X-ray of chest may reveal consolidation, collapsed lung or pleural effusion. X-ray of the abdomen may show a vague opacity in any part and may not show colonic gas in the distal colon or there could be some evidence of gas under the diaphragm. These findings in the plain X-ray are very helpful in establishing a provisional diagnosis.

In certain disease, evening rise of temperature is a classical diagnostic feature for tuberculous disease. A sudden high temperature is often associated with acute tonsillitis, or urinary tract infection. And if it is associated with rigors, then it could be associated with malaria, pyelonephritis or cholangitis.

If the patient is presented with an abrupt rise of temperature, when the patient is ready to be discharged, this clinical sign must not be overlooked. It is an early indication for intraperitoneal sepsis, or anastomotic dehiscence. In some cases, rise of temperature may be an early sign of pulmonary embolism, cerebral infarction or myocardial infarction. Patient should not be discharged, despite the clinical evidence of primary wound healing.

In day-to-day clinical works, temperature may be elevated in many other conditions. These are blood transfusion, long-standing indwelling catheter known as catheter cystitis, long-standing central line either in the subclavian or jugular vein, thrombophlebitis and hemodialysis.

There are many other diseases that may be associated with a rise of temperature, which is often referred to as a rise of temperature of unknown origin. Among many other varieties, hypernephroma, Hodgkin, non-Hodgkin lymphoma, acute leukemia should be suspected first for the rise of temperature of unknown origin. Further study on these diseases is advised.

POSTOPERATIVE PAIN RELIEF

Decades ago, relief of postoperative pain was badly managed. It was neglected. Lack of understanding and resources were the main reasons for this subject being left to the resident doctors at their discretion or at the responsibility of the ward nurses. The regimen for intramuscular injection used to be prescribed by the anesthetist from the theater, but he was not available for the next 48 hours to review the pain relief, whether or not the dose prescribed was adequate for the relief of pain.

In those years, the narcotic used to be given to the patients in every 6 hours. Although theoretically the dose was supposed to be calculated on the basis of body weight and age of the patients, but this was not taken into consideration, while prescribing the drug. As a result, patients used to go into deep sleep in some cases for the first three hours. The dose for this period seemed to be over dose; but three hours later, patients used to complain of discomfort or recurrence of pain. The dose for this period used to be regarded to be underdose that woke him/her up with pain. As a result, the cough reflexes could be inhibited, and there would be increased rate of respiration in excess of 28 per minute. This contributes to shallow breathing and poor oxygen saturation.

Of course, chest infection used to be the common sequel; but some clinicians would argue blindly that chest infection was probably due to the pain arising from the upper abdominal wound, thus inhibiting the full expansion of the chest movements. In fact, chest infection, atelectasis, and consolidation of the lung have been found in the postoperative patients. This resulted from the inhibition of the cough reflexes. As a result, the bronchial secretion will trickle down because of gravity that leads to the obstruction of the bronchioles, thus resulting in collapsed lung and then chest infection.

To overcome this problem, a new treatment has been designed, based upon the pain threshold level. It is an arbitrary level of consciousness that does not recognize any pain or discomfort. This level is established by a retrograde titration, using a narcotic that is infused very slowly until the patient experiences no more pain. This state of pain-free awareness is continuously maintained throughout the next 2-3 postoperative days. The pain threshold level is established by titration within half an hour after the patient has recovered from the anesthesia.

This pain threshold level is maintained continuously by topping up the dose that gets metabolized continuously from the pain neuroreceptors. This maintenance dose should be ranging from 1 mg per hour to 1.5 mg per hour for the first 24 hours that depends upon the rate of respiration. In this study, it was maintained between 16 and 22 per minute.

On the following day, the maintenance dose is reduced to between 0.8 and 1 mg per hour. In the prospective study, the patients did not develop chest infection nor did they go into deep sleep after operation. Furthermore, there was not a single case of obligatory oliguria. The average urine output for the first 24 hours was over a liter, noticed in postcholecystectomy patients. [1,12]

Since this new concept and regimen was reported in the literature, patient controlled analgesia, popularly known as PCA has become a popular choice. This does not require continuous nursing observation. On the contrary, patients feel confident psychologically that they can control their own pain relief, but in reality that has not been the case.

This expensive machine has provision of locking device that would prevent the patients injecting the drugs into the vein by touching the switch button, fitted with the machine.

Hence, the system cannot maintain the continuous pain threshold level, because of the fact that the serum level of narcotic that gets metabolized every second is not replenished by further infusion during the locking period.

As a result, the amount of narcotic what should have been topping up continuously through the pump remains deficit in the neurocenter that controls the pain thresold level.

The reason for not replenishing the deficit is due to locking device set up in the machine by the pain management team. As a result, the patient would experience pain and wanted further injection during the locking period. Therefore, complete pain relief is not possible by this approach. Because, the topping up of the narcotic that is necessary to be infused continuously in order to keep the serum level consistently at a constant level, is withheld deliberately by the locking device—thus lowering the serum level of narcotic during the locking period. Hence, the ideal purpose is not served by this approach.

Therefore, for a continuous relief of pain without affecting the central respiratory center, continuous infusion of narcotic with a dose ranging from 1 to 1.5 mg should be maintained through the pump but continuous observation is necessary monitoring the rate of respiration and to adjust the dose in accordance with the rate of respiration.

And a constant vigilance is necessary against the inappropriate use of the pump that may lead to overdose and death, if the patient pushes the syringe manually. This seems to be the practical manpower problem against the continuous infusion of narcotics.

COMPLICATIONS OF POSTOPERATIVE PAIN RELIEF

Vomiting, respiratory depression, perspiration, hypotension and reduced urine output are the clinical presentations with the overdose of narcotics. There have been such complications developed with the administration of narcotics, whether it is administered by PCA or by intramuscular injection.

Chest infection, collapse lung or consolidation of a particular lobe has been noticed in those cases, in which, pain relief has not been maintained adequately. Therefore, continuous observation is necessary in the management of postoperative pain relief.

TREATMENT FOR POSTOPERATIVE COMPLICATIONS

These are the potential risks of developing postoperative complications:
- Chest infection.
- Deep vein thrombosis and pulmonary embolism.
- Dehiscence of the anastomosis.
- Dehiscence of the abdominal wound.
- Urinary tract infection.
- Wound infection.

POSTOPERATIVE CHEST COMPLICATIONS

Predisposing Factors for Postoperative Chest Infection

- Smoking.
- Overweight.
- Chronic bronchitis.
- Diabetes.
- Age.
- Postoperative pain.
- Site of operation.
- Anesthesia.

Following recovery from the anesthesia, patient should be encouraged for active mobility, breathing exercise, assisted by pain-free and by physiotherapy.

In the ward round, patient is asked to give a cough that may reveal whether he is having upper respiratory chest infection. Temperature chart and any sign of wheezy chest should be looked for.

Initially, chest infection begins with dry cough with or without expectoration of sputum. Sometimes, they are unable to cough forcefully and tend to retain the expectoration because of pain in the abdominal wound and diminished cough reflex.

If this is not dealt with at the outset, this may progress to various forms of chest infection, such as bronchitis, atelectasis, bronchopneumonia, and lung abscess.

Initially there could be a viscid secretion from the upper bronchial tree. This may result from upper respiratory infection, initiated by a minor trauma from the intubations of the endotracheal tube. In the early postoperative days, patients find difficulty in maintaining deep breathing in and out. And they could not spit out the expectoration of thick mucoid sputum, due to inhibition of cough reflex or due to pain in the wound or due to trachitis; the secretion may trickle down particularly during sleep. Depression of cough reflex may be induced by the overdose of morphine sulfate, or due to pain. Restricted breathing due to distention of the abdomen may aggravate the cough reflex and breathing.

This viscid secretion may occlude one of the bronchioles, thus developing atelectasis of the involved lobe. If this blockage of the mucus plugs is not cleared off either by physiotherapy, or by the suction through the bronchoscope, this collapsed lobe of the lung will lead to consolidation and lung abscess (Fig. 8.1).

Apart from this pathogenesis, the base of the lungs may be squashed due to elevation of the diaphragm. The latter may be affected by the distention of the intestine, resulting from paralytic ileus, swallowed air, overdose of morphine sulfate,

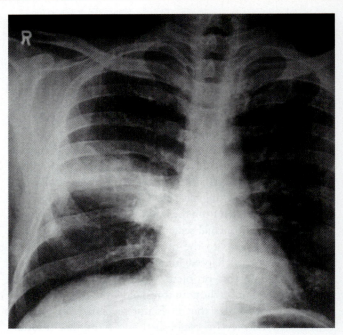

Fig. 8.1: Chest X-ray showing consolidation of the right middle lobe of the lung

and poor postoperative care. Mobility of the diaphragm may be inhibited by all those factors. These may lead to basal congestion and consolidation due to lack of full aeration of the basal lung. There may be reactionary pleural effusion and a secondary infection due to immobility and lack of physiotherapy.

In some cases, rapid infusion of fluid and overloading infusion may lead to cardiac failure, and pulmonary edema.

Clinical Features

Rise of temperature on the first postoperative day could be due to postanesthetic reaction, but on the second postoperative day, it would be pathognomonic. Patient may appear to be short of breath, produce dry cough or cough with expectoration of greenish or frothy sputum. Restricted breathing, tachycardia, rapid shallow respiration, associated with sweating and dusky skin color are evidences of chest infection.

On auscultation, there would be diminished breath sounds, ronchi, and dull on percussion on the affected side of the chest and restricted movement of chest wall. In addition, vocal resonance will be diminished on the affected lung.

Investigation includes sputum to be sent for culture, X-ray chest should be done. In the mean time, physiotherapy, postural chest drainage, and warm saline inhalation should be done. Appropriate antibiotic is commenced. In extreme cases, emergency bronchoscopy should be carried out in order to suck out mucus plugs from the bronchioles.

This procedure is normally done in the ward. If the patient is on ventilation, repeated aspiration of the bronchus should be done with a soft catheter. If no improvement is noticed, in that case, bronchoscope is passed through the endotracheal tube for the aspiration of the mucus plugs. This procedure may need to be repeated until evidence of aeration of the collapsed lung is noticed on a repeated chest X-ray.

Tracheostomy may be necessary at last.

MANAGEMENT OF WOUND DRAIN

There are various types of drainage systems. It may be employed at the conclusion of the operative procedures. The indications are:
- Drainage of residual pus or inflammatory fluid.
- Drainage of residual hemorrhage or clots.
- Drainage of peritoneal fluid, ascitic fluid or bile.
- To set up a track for the discharge of inflammatory fluid, or feces, if there is a potential risk of leakage from the site of anastomosis.
- As a prophylactic measure, drain is used in the wound, if there is a dead space left in the operative space, where there remains a possibility of collection of blood or blood stained fluid. In this sort of cases, drain is used in thyroid surgery, neck or groin block-dissection, breast surgery, and operation on the axilla, operation in the kidney, vascular reconstruction and in the orthopedic cases.

Types of Drainage Systems

A. Closed drainage
  i. No suction system.
  ii. Suction system.
B. Open drainage.

Types of Drainage

- Corrugated drain made with rubber or plastic or silicon material.
- Rubber or plastic tube drain of various calibers incorporated with or without multiple holes at one end.
- Vacuum drainage.

In the past, open drainage system was a common practice. In those days, rubber corrugated or tube drain was commonly used. Its purpose is to allow the blood, serous fluid to come out through the drainage tube or through the corrugated sheet. Its removal depends upon a few clinical criteria.

DAILY WOUND DISCHARGE

Open Drainage System

In the past, it was not a routine practice to record the volume of daily discharge through the drainage system and it was not possible to measure the volume, if corrugated sheet is used. In most cases, cotton pad is put around the drain and the decision to remove the drain or to start shortening the drain is made by a visual inspection about the size of the wet area, soaked by the blood or serous discharge in the dressing pad and on the pattern of temperature chart. Its removal is delayed, if there is evidence of foul smell or pus or feces in the discharge.

Abdomen and the wound should be examined, before the drain is removed. The purpose of this examination is to evaluate, whether there is any evidence of local collection, induration or swelling around the wound or in the abdomen and whether bile or feces are discharging through the drainage system. Its removal should be delayed until the temperature begins to recede and patient has passed wind per rectum or has opened the bowel.

Disadvantage of using a tube or corrugated drain is that it has no suction power and cannot drain all the collections or blood clots, collected in the dependent part of the wound.

Let us put an example in this aspect, in that how do you expect the water to drain from the bottom of a glass, if a corrugated sheet or a tube drain is put into the glass. Hence, the same mechanism follows in the open drainage system. Some residual collection or clots are expected to be left *in situ*, after the drain is removed. These clots or collection may cause adhesions or form an abscess.

If wound drain is considered necessary, it should not be removed without reviewing the previous collection or wound discharge, temperature and examination of the patient. Delayed wound collection is quite common and this residual collection may be the nidus for the bacterial growth. This could be the reason for developing wound infection or abscess after the drain is removed and even after the patient has been discharged home. In clean cases, wound drain could be removed after 2-3 days. But in gastrointestinal surgery, its removal depends upon many criteria.

Surgeon is the best person to decide when the drain needs to be removed. And he must be aware of the full consequent effect, after the drain is removed. If the drain is removed sooner, then there may be further delayed collection from the denuded surfaces. This delayed secretion may form an abscess. Hence, drain should be removed after a full assessment of the operative field, postoperative daily discharge and temperature chart.

After 5 days, the drainage tube or corrugated sheet is safe to be removed but it should not be removed straightaway. It is a common practice that a part of it is removed on the first time and shortening is continued everyday, until it comes out or it falls out. The purpose of shortening the drain everyday is to open a new track below the drain that may permit any further discharge, if there is some collection outside the track or some collection has been pent up outside the drainage tube. It also allows sealing of the dead space left behind after the particular segment of the drain has been removed.

A safety-pin is put across the tube or corrugated sheet after it is shortened. Its purpose of putting the safety-pin is to stop slipping of the tube into the peritoneal cavity. In case it has slipped back into the wound, X-ray of the wound or the abdomen will reveal the drain tube by this radiopaque safety pin. Nowadays, radiopaque marker is incorporated within the material used in the manufacture of the drain,

In colonic surgery, tube drain has other benefit. It forms a large track, even after it is removed. Feces or thick pus could discharge through the drainage track.

CLOSED DRAINAGE SYSTEM

Suction drainage apparatus is a closed system. It is incorporated with plastic tubing of various caliber connected to a reservoir, made with plastic bag, glass bottle (Redivac) or piggy bag. These reservoirs could be maintained with negative pressure that assists in sucking all blood or blood stained fluid from the depth of the peritoneal cavity or from the field of operation. In addition, a separate metallic trocker is supplied with other materials and it is connected to the drainage tubing, before the trocker is inserted from inside out through the parietal wall.

Nowadays, many types of drainage systems are available. In most cases, they are made with transparent plastic materials. The benefit in this closed system is to keep on sucking the residual blood stained fluid or serous collection from the depth of the wound. It is used in many operative fields. It could drain all clots and serous collection efficiently because of negative pressure in the glass bottle or in the plastic bag. It provides the opportunity to measure the total volume collected in the suction bottle for the last 24 hours and it would assist the surgeon to evaluate the clinical state of the wound inside the abdomen.

In case of discharge of blood, it would indicate whether there has been unusual bleeding from the field of operation. Other benefit is to evacuate all residual clots or serous discharge from the depth of the wound cavity. This is the distinct difference from the open drain, which cannot empty the collection from the depth of the wound.

In axillary surgery or in the block dissection in the groin, suction drainage tube could be left longer, if there is clear evidence of a lot of serous or lymphatic discharge collected in the bag or bottle everyday. Unlike the tube or corrugated drain, suction tube does not cause too much pain to the port of exit. It is removed if the total 24 hours collection is less than 25 ml.

MERITS AND MORBIDITY

In certain cases, suction drain system is not suitable if there is any risk of developing anastomotic dehiscence. It may cause damage to the gut and a small serosal wall may be sucked in by the end or by the holes of the tube, if the power of vacuum in the bottle is very strong and if the size of the drainage tube used in the Redivac bottle is greater than 3 mm in diameter.

The disadvantage with the corrugated tube is that it causes pain around the site of the drain. Complete evacuation of the serous or blood clots collected in the depth of the peritoneal cavity or in the wound is not possible. And open drain may add infection into the wound or it may cause pressure necrosis on the wall of the gut.

Delayed complication following removal of the drainage tube is the formation of fistula track, or herniation of the omentum. And omental band is stuck to the drainage wound inside the abdomen; it may induce adhesion that may lead to intestinal obstruction.

These are overviews of how the drainage system is dealt with. Apart from the drainage system, there are rare conditions where drainage system is not applicable. In these cases, the wound is packed with proflabin or with sofre-tulle. It acts as a pressure hemostat in order to stop bleeding or oozing from the large denuded wound cavity.

In the past, perineal wound used to be packed with a long and wide ribbon gauge in a plastic bag. In most cases, abscess cavity should be packed with wound dressing. Wound healing is achieved by secondary intention. It is a slow process of recovery. And wound packing is usually done initially daily and later it is done 2-3 times per day that depends upon the state and size of the wound.

MANAGEMENT OF CONSTIPATION

All surgical patients must be enquired during ward round whether they have passed wind per rectum and whether they have opened bowel in the last 24-48 hours. It is not unusual for them being constipated while staying in the hospital.

ETIOLOGY FOR CONSTIPATION

- Not having proper diet or remains nil by mouth for a few days.
- Not having physical exercise or staying in bed for a few days.
- Patient is on analgesic drug such as opiate group of drugs.
- Dehydration and or electrolyte deficit.
- Paralytic ileus or peritonitis.

In postoperative cases, bowel action is normally delayed for at least 4-5 days. This is due to postoperative pain, paralytic ileus, anastomosis of the gut or operation of piles.

CLINICAL RESPONSIBILITY OF THE DOCTORS

Resident doctors should examine the abdomen and the rectum. If abdomen remains soft, and not distended, and the rectal digital examination does not suggest impaction of feces, then wait and watch policy should be adopted, provided the patient is passing flatus.

If the rectal digital examination shows evidence of impaction of feces, oral laxative should be prescribed initially, and at the same time, glycerine suppositories should be inserted per rectum.

If no benefit is noticed with this approach, phosphate enema should be prescribed. Manual evacuation may be considered in rare cases.

Apart from these measures, patient is encouraged for taking oral drink, if not contraindicated.

Management of constipation among the postoperative patients should be handled differently and carefully. Rectal enema must not be prescribed to any postoperative patient or to any acute abdomen presented with peritonitis, or colonic obstruction. This may cause perforation of the colon.

Furthermore, glycerine suppositories should not be given even to the postappendicectomy patient for not opening the bowel after operation. This may cause blow-out of the appendicular stump due to spasm of the cecum.

There is a little difference in the treatment of constipation after hemorrhoidectomy has been done. In these cases, some surgeons rely upon diet and oral drinks for spontaneous defecation and in rare cases, phosphate enema with soap and water enema could be prescribed, if the rectal digital examination showed impaction of hard feces. In other cases, some surgeon prefers prescribing oral laxative such as liquid paraffin on the second postoperative day.

MANAGEMENT OF DEEP VEIN THROMBOSIS

Pathology of Deep Vein Thrombosis

Although prophylactic measures are adopted against the potential risk of deep vein thrombosis, pulmonary embolism has developed in certain cases. Of course, the primary cause is the deep vein thrombosis. It develops in the postoperative period and it usually occurs in a week but the potential period of risk remains up to one month. This is due to physical inactivity and delayed recovery at home.

The primary cause for deep vein thrombosis is the venous stasis or delayed venous return from the lower limbs. The possible etiological factors are dehydration, lack of physiotherapy, smoking, chest infection, prolonged paralytic ileus, distended abdomen and intraperitoneal collections. The commonest sites are in the leg (90%) and in the pelvic vein.

Thrombosis begins initially in one or two tributaries draining into the main vein, because of eddying flow of blood through the valves. Prophylactic TED stocking keeps these tributaries obliterated, thus preventing the formation of thrombosis.

It is presented with pain in the calf, swollen leg and thigh. In some cases, patient may not show any evidence of symptoms, apart from an unexplained rise of temperature and rapid pulse rate.

In addition, during routine ward round, clinician may recognize unusual unilateral swollen calf and pitting edema on the medial malleolus of the ankle. The skin color will appear shining around the affected limb.

On deep palpation around the back of the affected leg, tenderness may be elicited along the posterior tibial or peroneal veins and Homan's sign may be positive. Patient experiences discomfort in the back of the leg and in particular over the region of calf, when the foot is pushed towards the ankle (dorsiflexion) in flexion position of the knee. Because of dorsiflexion of the ankle, the tendo-achilles keeps pulling on the calf muscles that tend to press upon the posterior tibial veins.

This indirect pressure elicits discomfort in the calf of the leg in flexion position of the knee. In addition, tenderness may be elicited on deep palpation over the calf when the ankle is held in flexion position in extended knee. This clinical test is not always reliable but it should not be ignored.

Two distinct clinical presentations may be encountered. They are known as white leg –phlegmasia alba. It is associated with lymphangitis that would contribute further increase in swelling.

Other presentation is known as blue leg or phlegmasia caerulea dolens. This is due to extensive deep vein thrombosis involving the femoral and iliac veins. This may lead to a serious prognosis and gangrene of the leg would be the ultimate sequelae.

There may be dislodgement of smaller thrombi from the lower limb that may cause scattered small pulmonary embolism or there could be massive pulmonary embolism leading to sudden death. Average incidence of death due to pulmonary embolism could be between 5 to 10 percent among the postoperative patients.

Before patient succumbs into imminent massive pulmonary embolism, he more often asks for a bedpan, but, by the time the nurse brings the bedpan, the patient has already passed away. There is no explanation for this well known presentation, associated with the sudden death due to massive pulmonary embolism.

The following investigation may assist the clinical diagnosis. One is color Doppler scan of the lower limbs. And other one is the Doppler sonic-aid. The probe is placed over the femoral vein in the groin, this will transmit a venous hum, and it would be louder as if a roar. This suggests increased venous blood flow, when the squeeze is applied over the calf muscle but it would be absent if there is deep vein thrombosis developed in the femoral vein, causing obstruction of blood flow.

Venogram is no longer done, because of risk involved in this investigation. It may cause venous gangrene due to reaction.

TREATMENT FOR DEEP VEIN THROMBOSIS

Before anticoagulant therapy is commenced, blood test and coagulation screen must be done. Degradation of fibrogen products should be done.

Continuous intravenous infusion of heparin should be commenced straightaway. The recommended dose is between 5000 and 10000 international units (IU) every six hours given continuously through the pump fitted to the venous channel. It is continued for 7 to 10 days. For a long-term anticoagulant therapy, it is replaced by warfarin or aspirin.

Many clinicians believe that this therapy would be ineffective if the duration of deep vein thrombosis appears to be greater than 12 hours, but my experience suggests that effective therapeutic result has been noticed in those cases, in which the patient had presented unilateral swollen calf after 3-4 weeks.

Heparin therapy may cause thrombocytopenia. Hence, blood tests should be done daily. It may produce osteoporosis, if the therapy is continued over a year.

In some rare cases, platelets count may drop dramatically due to reaction to heparin. Patient may bleed excessively due to thrombocytopenia. In this situation, injection of heparin must be discontinued. And fresh frozen plasma transfusion should be commenced to stop hemorrhage.

For acute condition, intravenous infusion of heparin remains the first line of treatment. It reduces thrombin and fibrin formation. It raises the partial thromboplastin time up to 1.5 to 2 times of the control value.

Under any circumstances, aspirin should not be prescribed with heparin or warfarin. The pharmacological function of aspirin is to interfere with the platelets adhesive function. It should not be used if there is a history of peptic ulcer disease. If it is necessary to use aspirin, then other drugs dealing with peptic ulcer disease should be used concurrently.

Soluble aspirin 75 mg could be prescribed alone. There remains a risk of developing peptic ulcer if the aspirin is taken in empty stomach and the risk of perforation of the stomach or jejunum is greater if the patient swallows the tablet.

The dose for warfarin is 10 mg once a day for two days. It should be commenced two days prior to the heparin therapy that is intended to be discontinued. Prothrombin time (PT) is done after 48 hours and further drug therapy depends upon the results of PT. It should be between 1.5 and 2 times of the control value for surgical patients but this maintenance therapy remains under the supervision of the hematologist. Surgeon should not be involved in the maintenance therapy.

If there is acute episode of hemorrhage that is due to anticoagulant therapy, in this case, the treatment could be discontinued and is observed the clinical emergency. Alternatively, the PT could be reversed by giving injection protamine sulfate or by injecting vit. K.

REFERENCES

1. Saha SK. Continuous intravenous infusion of papaveretum for relief of postoperative pain. Postgraduate Medical Journal 1981;686-9.
2. Gamble JL. Cambridge, Mass: Harvard University Press 1954.
3. Kingston RD, Kiff RS, et al. Comparison of two prophylactic single dose intravenous antibiotic regimes in the treatment of patients undergoing elective colorectal surgery in a district general hospital, JR Coll Surg Ed 1989;34:208-11.
4. Saha SK, Robinson RF. A study of perineal wound healing after abdominoperineal resection. Br J Surg 1976;63:555-8.
5. Marks CG, Leighton M, et al. Primary suture of the perineal wound following rectal excision for adenocarcinoma, Br J Surg 1976;63:322-6.
6. Saha SK. Care of perineal wound in abdominoperineal resection. JR Coll Surg Edin 1983;28:324-7.
7. Saha SK. Peritoneal lavage with metronidazole. Surg Gynecology and Obstet 1985;160:335.
8. Saha SK. Peritoneal lavage with metronidazole, Joint Meeting of the Royal College PG Surgeons of England and Association of Surgeons of India, New Delhi, 1991.
9. Saha SK. Efficacy of metronidazole lavage in treatment of intraperitoneal sepsis: A prospective study. Digestive Disease and Sciences 1996;4(7):1313.
10. Ingham HR, Sissin PR, et al. Inhibition of phagocytosis in vitro by obligate anaerobes. Lancet 1977;2:1252-4.
11. Corbet CRR, Hollands MJ, Young AE. Penetration of a prophylactic antibiotic into peritoneal fluid. Brit J Surg 1981;68:314-5.
12. Continuous intravenous infusion strategy in anesthesia Edited by Walter S Nimmo and Graham Smith. Volume 2, Blackwell Scientific Publications, Chapter 76, page 1185.

9 The Colon

In all surgical practice, a good surgeon is judged by clinical acumen, vision for caring of the disease and operative skill. Among these criteria, merit of the surgical technique is evaluated by the uneventful postoperative recovery. Cutting and suturing are the bread and butter for every surgeon, but outcome of the operative procedures could not be the same among the patients, if the skill of a surgeon is not up to the scratch. In dealing with emergency surgical cases, a good clinician knows when not to operate upon the emergency case.

TECHNIQUES FOR ANASTOMOSIS

Anastomosis between the two resected segments of gut could be carried out in two layers or in single layer. In two layers anastomosis, there are a few confusing terminologies referred to in different textbooks. They are first layer. This is a primary anastomosis between the cut-edges of the stoma. It is also referred to as inner layer of anastomotic sutures.

The second layer is the seromuscular sutures used for invagination of the primary anastomotic sutures, or inner layer of anastomosis. It may be also known as outer layer of suturing. It goes through the seromuscular layer of the gut. This outer layer is to conceal the inner layer thus preventing any risk of leakage or dehiscence of the anastomosis. But the outer layer that invaginate, concealing the inner layer narrows the lumen at the anastomotic site and forms a shelf of anastomotic edge that projects towards the lumen of the gut.

In two layers of anastomosis, the terminal mesenteric vessels may be caught up in the sutures used in the second layer (outer layer or seromuscular layer) of anastomosis or they could be compressed from outside by the invagination of the seromuscular layer, thus affecting the blood flow to the cut edges of the stoma. This may lead to a risk of avascular necrosis or anastomotic dehiscence. In other uncomplicated cases the anastomotic shelf may delay the propagative peristalsis. Alternatively, a single layer anastomosis could safely be carried out with interrupted sutures between the transected ends of the stomas (Fig. 9.1).

The results are equally good, provided interrupted sutures are correctly applied, and vascularity to the site of anastomosis is good. Furthermore, the marginal mesenteric vessels are not subjected to be caught up in the sutures, if the seromuscular layer is not required to be invaginated. Recovery seems to be uneventful during 25 years of experience.

This single layer anastomosis could be done in two ways. In one school of thought the interrupted stitches are inserted only through the outer muscular coat, not incorporating the sutures through the mucosa. In this approach, the stitches are inserted 10 mm away from the cut edge. In this technique, the cut edges are inverted, when the sutures are tied together. But this has no consequent effect. No adverse result has been reported. The question could be highlighted whether there could be continuous oozing of blood from the transected edge of the mucosa.

Alternatively, the interrupted sutures are inserted through the full thickness of the stoma. And the sutures are inserted 3 mm away from the cut edge of the stoma. In this approach, the cut edges do not turn inwards, when the sutures are tied

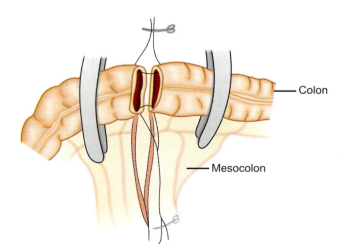

Fig. 9.1: Method of end-to-end anastomosis by interrupted single layer sutures

together. The results are equally excellent in all instances. This has been my common practice over the last 25 years and there has been not a single case of anastomotic leakage over the period of 25 years of surgical practice.

TYPES OF ANASTOMOSIS

Anastomosis could be done between end-to-end, end-to-side, or side-to-side of the two intestines. Difficulty may be experienced in those cases, in which there is a disparity noticed in the circumference of the two resected guts. End-to-end anastomosis seems to be a problem in this situation. But this disparity could be overcome by a number of choices available to the surgeon.

One of the choices is to rectify the shortfall of the circumference found in the smaller stoma. This is corrected by incising the antimesenteric border of the stoma, for a few centimeters at a time. To rectify the shortfall of the circumference of the smaller stoma, the antimesenteric border is incised longitudinally that has to be judged step by step when the cut edges are sutured with the corresponding site of the larger stoma until the disparity is corrected. But this corrective procedure should be done at the last moment after suturing the other areas of the stoma.

TECHNIQUE FOR END-TO-END ANASTOMOSIS (SINGLE LAYER)

Soft (noncrushing) clamp is applied a few inches away from the proposed line of resection. And the line of transection should be in line with the mesenteric vessels, supplying to the gut. Vascularity to the proposed site of resection must be satisfactory that is judged by the pink color of the cut edge. Dusky color, different from the neighboring gut wall is a sign of poor vascularity. If this is evident, further segment needs to be removed.

For the purpose of alignment, and to avoid twisting of the circumference of the stomas, stay sutures are applied between the cut edges of the two stomas, in that one stay suture is applied at the mesenteric border and other one at the antimesenteric border of the stomas, thus keeping each half of the stoma in equal alignment with each other.

The anastomosis begins with interrupted sutures. They are inserted through and through 3-4 mm away from the cut edges of the respective stoma. And it is commenced from the mesenteric border and is continued towards the antimesenteric border, where the stay suture has already been inserted. In the same way, the other half is carried out, commencing from the mesenteric border (Fig. 9.2).

For the purpose of secure anastomosis, there should be a space of 2 mm between the two stitches. And each stitch should go through the full thickness of the intestinal wall. Alternatively, the suture could pass only through the outer seromuscular layer without piercing through the mucosa of the stoma.

The positions of the stay sutures are changed in order to avoid any disparity. In that case, the stay sutures could be applied at 3 o'clock and 9 o'clock position. If disparity is noticed along the antimesenteric wall, between the two stay sutures, the antimesenteric border of the shorter stoma is incised by the scissors for a short distance. By trial and error method, the shortfall is corrected and sutured together with the corresponding part of the stoma (Fig. 9.3).

If the mucosa has pouted out between the stitches, it is pushed back with a nontooth tissue forceps. At the completion of single layer anastomosis, the soft clamp is removed from both sides, the ileum is milked out through the anastomosis

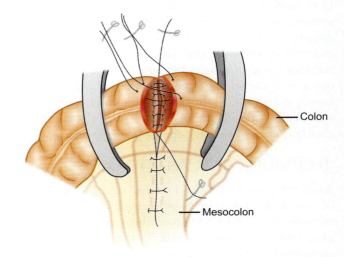

Fig. 9.2: Showing a single layer end-to-end anastomosis by interrupted stitches. It shows the interrupted sutures along the posterior layer of anastomosis

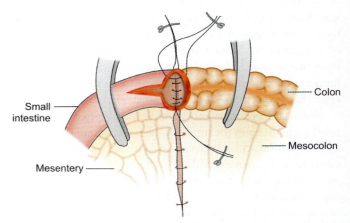

Fig. 9.3: Anastomosis between a larger and a smaller stoma of the colon, by interrupted single layer sutures. The antimesenteric border of the colon has been cut along its long axis in order to make it equal to the other stoma

towards the colon, if air bubble or liquid feces has not leaked through the anastomosis, it provides reassuring. Nevertheless, it should be covered with a thin layer of omental graft or with appendices epiploicae.

Finally, the gap between the two resected edges of the mesentery is closed. This is done either by interrupted stitches between the thin peritoneal walls without affecting the mesenteric vessels or by continuous sutures, commencing from the site of mesenteric attachment down to its root. Only the closure of the anterior wall is necessary. If the defect is not closed, herniation of the gut through this defect may occur.

TECHNIQUE FOR END-TO-END ANASTOMOSIS IN TWO LAYERS

After transection of the gut, both clamps are held together side-by-side. The first suture layer would be the seromuscular sutures of the two adjacent stomas (Fig. 9.4A). This should be referred to as outer layer or second layer of anastomosis. This would be a continuous suture that begins from the mesenteric border and is continued towards the antimesenteric border, where the remnant of the suture with needle is tucked under the swab for the time being, but it would be used to complete the remaining seromuscular suture along the other side. This suture line should be 1 cm above the occlusion clamps.

The next layer of anastomosis is better referred to as inner layer or primary anastomotic layer between the cut edges of two stomas. This end-to-end anastomosis is done by continuous or interrupted suture that is commenced from the mesenteric border and is continued all along until it is ended in the mesenteric border of the opposite side (Fig. 9.4B).

This anastomotic layer is referred to as inner anastomotic layer or it could be referred to as posterior and anterior anastomosis that depends upon how you want to as identify them. It is continued towards the antimesenteric border, where a few mattress sutures are inserted in order to bring the anterior cut edges of the stomas closer. The same continuous suture is continued towards the opposite site, i.e. towards the mesenteric border, where it is tied with the previous suture. This anastomotic layer is referred to as inner anastomosis or anterior anastomosis (Fig. 9.4C).

This inner layer of anastomotic sutures is to be invaginated by continuous seromuscular sutures. This suture bite is taken 1cm away from the inner anastomotic line and is commenced from the antimesenteric border, until it is ended at the mesenteric border where both ends are tied together (Fig. 9.4D). If the suture is inserted through the seromuscular layer closer or less than 1 cm from the inner anastomotic stitches, invagination of the seromuscular wall would be difficult or the sutures may cut out from the wall.

At the mesenteric border, invagination of the seromuscular wall around the mesenteric attachment is carried out by a few

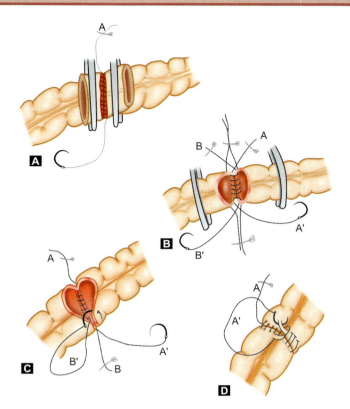

Figs 9.4A to D: Methods of anastomosis in two layers

interrupted stitches, but care is taken that the needle did not pierce through the terminal vessels. This site is a sorrow corner, known to the surgeon.

INDICATION FOR SIDE-TO-SIDE ANASTOMOSIS

This is a valuable approach. It could be used in many surgical conditions. It could be employed as a 'bypass' operation in those cases where the tumor is too advanced, causing mechanical obstruction. Resection is not possible.

In other conditions, continuity of the guts could be restored through this approach, or it could be used alternatively to end-to-end anastomosis, if there is wide disparity between the sizes of the bowels or the lumen of both bowels turns out to be small or contracted like Crohn's ileitis or atresia of the gut.

This may cause delay in postoperative recovery and bowel empty may be sluggish. In this situation, the transected ends of both guts are closed in two layers; but continuity of the gut is restored by side-to-side anastomosis with the closed end either facing in the opposite or in the same direction.

TECHNIQUE FOR SIDE-TO-SIDE ANASTOMOSIS

The proposed segment of the colon is picked up by two pairs of forceps. These tissue forceps, known as Babcock forceps are applied at the taeniae coli of the colon, which should be along the antimesenteric border. The size of the stoma between the two Babcock forceps should be 3 inches.

Assistant will keep holding these two forceps up. This would assist the surgeon to apply the soft occlusion clamps (Downs) below the tissue holding forceps. These clamps are applied along the long axis of the intestine and not across the mesenteric vessels. The contents of the bowel should be squeezed out, just before the clamps are applied.

The same two Babcock forceps are used again for the next bowel in the same way. A similar clamp is also applied to the corresponding site of the bowel. A judicial judgment is necessary while the clamps are applied. The continuity of the gut should be consistent with the isoperistalsis. The abdominal wound edges and peritoneal cavity must be protected from fecal contamination. Large wet packs are laid down around the clamps.

Anastomosis begins with a continuous suture, inserted through the seromuscular wall of the gut. It is commenced from one end and is continued up to the proposed level of anastomosis. The suture line should be 1 cm above the clamp. The seromuscular layer of the gut is incised by a knife and the incision should be made through the center of the taenia coli. The size of the stoma should be around 2-3 inches. The mucosal layer is next cut by the scissors (Fig. 9.5). Feces or lumps of feces are cleaned with wet gauze. Tissue forceps are applied to the outer cut edge, in order to keep holding the edges apart.

The anastomosis is carried out between the two cut edges. This is commenced from one corner and is continued towards the other corner, from where the same suture is used to be continued towards the opposite direction, thus suturing the other two cut edges together, until it reaches the previous site, where both ends are tied together. This is referred to as inner layer of anastomosis or primary anastomosis.

The needle goes through the full thickness of the respective bowel wall 2-3 mm below the mucosal edge. If mucosa has pouted through the cut edges and between the stitches, it is pushed back by nontooth forceps. These anastomotic sutures are buried or invaginated by a continuous seromuscular suture that was left from the other side.

After completion of primary layer of anastomosis, both clamps are released in order to carry out the second layer of anastomosis. The purpose is to conceal the primary anastomosis. It is also referred to as invagination of the primary anastomotic sutures. This is done by a continuous seromuscular suture, using the remnant of the previous seromuscular suture. The line of continuous suture should be 1 cm away from the primary anastomotic sutures. It is continued towards the opposite direction, until it reaches the previous site where both threads are tied together. If a generous room is not allowed, invagination would be difficult.

A few interrupted sutures are applied at both corners. These will take away the pressure on the primary anastomotic line at both corners. The anastomotic line is wrapped up by the omental graft. At the completion of this anastomosis, the mesenteric defect is closed.

ALTERNATIVE TO SIDE-TO-SIDE ANASTOMOSIS

Other option is to join the larger stoma with the side wall of the smaller gut, whose lumen is narrower than that of the other gut. In this case, the small stoma is closed in two layers or by autosuture. This is not a good option.

Apart from the hand sutures, anastomosis could be undertaken by autosuture that depends upon the aptitude and skill of individual surgeon.

RIGHT HEMICOLECTOMY

The operative approach to right hemicolectomy remains the same, whether the tumor is located in the cecum, ascending colon or in the hepatic flexure. For better understanding, the locations of the tumor have been shown in the barium X-ray films as well as in the drawings (Figs 9.6A to 9.8)

Double-contrast barium enema shows the typical filling defect of cecal carcinoma in Figure 9.6A. It appears like an apple bite on the lateral wall of the cecum. Further X-ray taken from the same patient shows a long stricture between the terminal ileum and cecum (Fig. 9.6B). This long tortuous filling defect is due to cecal carcinoma.

In another barium enema X-ray, done for another patient, a filling defect is present in the ascending colon, which is little below the hepatic flexure as shown in the barium X-ray (Fig. 9.8) In some patients, a similar filling defect could be found in barium X-ray which has been displayed in hand-drawn Figure 9.9.

Although, a broad outline in the operation of right hemicolectomy has been depicted in Figure 9.7, the resection of the right side of the colon includes mobilization of the terminal ileum, cecum, ascending colon and proximal half of

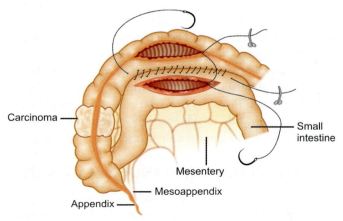

Fig. 9.5: Showing the technique for side-to-side anastomosis

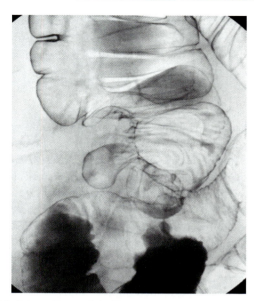

Fig. 9.6A: It is an X-ray of double contrast barium enema showing a filling defect in the cecum. It shows an apple-core filling defect in the lateral wall of the cecum and it is a classical radiological diagnostic feature for the carcinoma of the colon

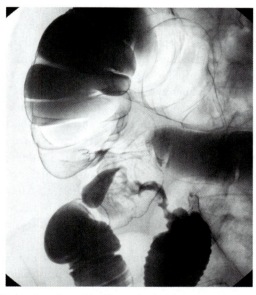

Fig. 9.6B: Another view of the X-ray of a double contrast barium enema, taken from the same patient. It confirms a persistent filling defect in the same area of the cecum and a string of long tortuous stricture between the cecum and the terminal ileum. This could be due to partial obstruction of the ileocecal valve by the invasion of the tumor

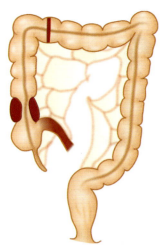

Fig. 9.7: This illustration shows the lines of resection for the right hemicolectomy to be carried out for the carcinoma of the cecum

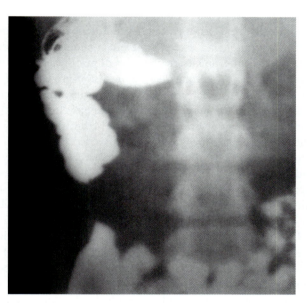

Fig. 9.8: An X-ray of barium enema of a separate patient, showing the filling defect in the ascending colon. It was carcinoma of the ascending colon. This was not a double contrast barium enema, thus highlighting the difference between this X-ray and the previous double contrast barium X-ray

the transverse colon up to the level that is supplied by the right branch of the middle colic artery.

Apart from the mobilization and resection of the colon, continuity is established either by end-to-end or side-by-side, or end-to-side anastomosis, between the ileum and the distal transverse colon. The anastomosis could be done by hand suture in single layer, two layers or by autosuture gun.

PREOPERATIVE PREPARATION

In most circumstances, anemia is the initial presentation, apart from other symptoms. Therefore, correction of anemia and any electrolyte imbalance has to be carried out. Among other investigations, USS, CT scan of abdomen and preoperative tissue diagnosis through the colonoscope should be done; but negative result does not exclude colonic cancer.

If the barium enema and/or small bowel enema suggests that there is a filling defect persistently present in every barium enema film, it is more likely to be a growth in the right side of the colon. In this case, laparotomy should be carried out.

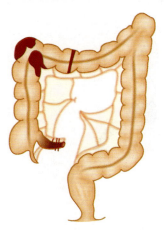

Fig. 9.9: Location of the tumor in the hepatic flexure and the area of the right colon to be resected

All other investigations, such as intravenous pyelogram, would be complementary.

During clinical examination, sigmoidoscopy must be done before barium enema is requested and it should be repeated a day before the operation is to be done. Purpose of this examination is to see that there is no rectal growth, and to see there is no residual inspissated barium or impacted hard feces present in the lower rectum, despite bowel preparations being carried out in the ward, a day before the surgery is scheduled. If there are lumps of inspissated barium in the rectum, these need to be evacuated before colonic surgery is undertaken. There remains a risk of anastomotic leakage because of lumps of inspissated barium, present in the distal colon, where they may cause partial blockage or may inhibit the propagative peristalsis.

Preoperative X-ray of chest, ECG, blood sugar, coagulation screen, and all other blood investigations should be done. For the purpose of operation, blood group and 4 units of blood cross match must be arranged. Urethral catheter must be inserted prior to surgery and the residual volume is recorded in the intake and output chart.

In the past, patients with colonic tumor used to be admitted 5 days for bowel preparation, but 24 hours bowel preparation is adequate, if there was no evidence of colonic obstruction. For bowel preparation, there are many commercial preparations available in the market. And they are oral purgatives.

Patient is asked to swallow the oral purgatives, a day before the operation and enema or rectal wash-out is given on the day of the operation. For this procedure, patient may be dehydrated. To combat this fluid deficit, intravenous infusion should be commenced on the night before the operation. On the day of the operation, antithrombotic prophylactic therapy is commenced, and antithrombotic stocking in both lower limbs must be put on. During induction, the patient must have parenteral appropriate antibiotics, covering for both aerobic and anaerobic bacteria.

Patient must be explained about the operative procedure, in which the question of resectability of the growth and palliative procedure has to be highlighted, if the tumor turns out to be too advanced.

OPERATIVE PROCEDURE

Skin preparation is done between the nipple and the groin. Sterile drapes are laid down all around the abdomen. Both legs must not be resting on the hard mattress. Abdomen is open through a midline incision. Initially, a small incision is made above the umbilicus. This incision could be extended down or upwards, after the initial finding of the tumor.

During internal examination, the tumor is palpated with a view to assessing its mobility and resectability that is judged by moving the tumor mass side-to-side. It would not be possible, if the growth is fixed to the psoas muscle, stuck to the second part of the duodenum, the gallbladder or the under surface of the liver.

Apart from these assessments, enlargement of the mesenteric lymph glands around the right colic and middle colic arteries are important consideration for right hemicolectomy. Despite these involvements, a limited resection could be carried out, provided the tumor is locally mobile and resectable.

Apart from these examinations liver, stomach, distal colon, rectum and bladder must be palpated. Bear in mind, there could be double primary colonic tumors, or there could be invasion of the cecal growth to the loop of the sigmoid colon that may lie in the right side across the pelvis. Such evidence is rare but it was evident in the cecum and in the sigmoid colon shown in Figures 9.6 and 9.10 of the same patient.

These two films taken from the same patient showed stricture of the sigmoid colon. It was annular carcinoma of the sigmoid colon. This patient had also developed carcinoma of the cecum (Figs 9.6A and B). It was rare incident that the same patient had developed two primary carcinomas in the colon.

Therefore, before requesting for barium enema, sigmoidoscopy must be done. X-ray films must be reviewed without reading the report of the radiologist. Sometimes, filling defect in the barium enema is reported that it may be due to lumps of feces or growth. In these cases, either barium enema should be repeated with a fresh bowel preparation or colonoscopy should be carried out. Despite these procedures being carried out, the tumor has been missed. Never trust upon other colleagues or their clinical findings and at the operation, every part of the colon and other organs must be palpated.

I have seen that the patient had right hemicolectomy done; but another primary tumor was left behind in the sigmoid colon. This was missed by the radiologist, because the patient did not have sigmoidoscopy, before barium enema was

The Colon

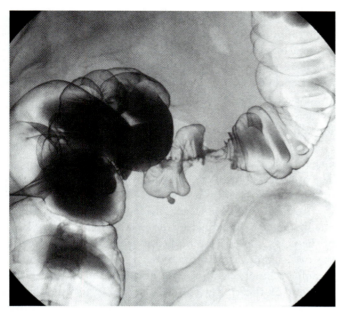

Fig. 9.10A: An X-ray of double contrast barium enema taken probably in supine position. It shows a stricture in the sigmoid colon and a rectal tube in the lower part of the rectum

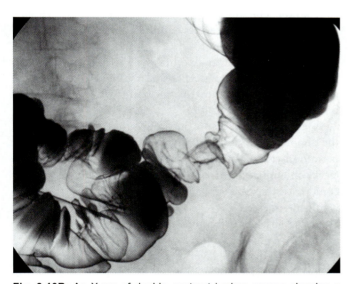

Fig. 9.10B: An X-ray of double contrast barium enema showing a stricture of the sigmoid colon, taken probably in supine or in erect position. The dark shadow proximal to the stricture is the air contrast in the sigmoid colon. A similar radiological feature was evident in other X-ray plates. This suggests that it was more likely to be carcinoma of the sigmoid colon and very unlikely to be a spasm of the colon

requested. And the surgeon relied upon the report of barium enema but he did not review the films and did not palpate the distal colon and the rectum. Because of these errors, these films are included in this section for being aware of rare pathology and for the importance of double check, review of the films, and a thorough examination of all organs in the abdomen.

PROCEEDING WITH THE SAME OPERATIVE TECHNIQUE FOR THE RIGHT HEMICOLECTOMY

During examination, tumor in the ascending colon or in the hepatic flexure could be found stuck to the second part of the duodenum, or with the right ureter. This revelation takes place after the tumor mass has been mobilized from the posterior wall. If the ureter is invaded by the tumor, but the growth has been mobilized from the psoas muscle, in this case, tumor could be resected, combined with right ureteronephrectomy, if the surgeon is competent and confident in undertaking this major procedure.

Despite the surgeon's confidence, this operation should not be undertaken without prior knowledge of the function of the left kidney. If intravenous pyelogram had not been done, this could be done on the theater table by injecting the contrast to the vein. Only one 15 minutes exposure is necessary to know whether the left kidney has shown radiopaque contrast in the renal pelvis.

For the double primary carcinoma of the colon, total colectomy should be the primary choice that depends upon the patient's age, fitness and Dukes tumor stage. If the tumor appears to be localized and resectable, it is preferable to carry out the total colectomy. It is then followed by ileorectal anastomosis.

If a compromise is contemplated, respective tumor could be resected separately with end-to-end primary anastomosis, like right hemicolectomy for the cecal carcinoma and left sigmoid colectomy for the tumor in the sigmoid colon. In this case, only a segment of the transverse colon will be left *in situ* but a few years later, further primary tumor may grow in the remaining segment of the colon.

In this case, the prognosis would be worse. There will be very little benefit in undertaking a selective resection for each primary growth, when there could be hidden multiple foci for the tumor to grow at a suitable time in any part of the remaining segment of the colon, which should be regarded to have a defective mucosa, like rest of the colon. In my experience, risk of recurrence of primary tumor would be much greater, if local resection for the double primary tumor is carried out.

TECHNIQUE FOR THE RESECTION OF THE GROWTH

After a thorough internal examination has been carried out, the abdominal wound is retracted by the self-retaining retractor. Parietal wound margins are covered with wet packs. Small intestine is pushed to one side and held back on the left side by a few large packs. Assistant will keep holding the cecum and the ascending colon, thus revealing the peritoneal reflection along the right paracolic gutter.

The parietal peritoneum is incised around the colon by the scissors. It is continued in both directions and its line of incision should be 2-3 cm away from the lateral wall of the cecum and the colon. The cecum and colon are lifted up from the posterior wall, by a combination of fingers, and swab or swab in swab holding forceps.

The cecum and colon will peel off from the posterior wall. The mobilization is continued upwards and along the hepatic flexure, where the greater omentum is resected either from the colon or from the stomach. In most cases, the greater omentum is separated from the colon or excised between the clamps and ligatures are applied around the respective clamps.

During this mobilization, the right ureter is looked for. Its wall moves like worms on touching with a tip of the finger. More often it remains in the fatty tissues surrounded by the ovarian vessels in female or testicular vessels in the male patients. If it is lifted up with the tumor mass, it is more likely that the ureter has been invaded by the tumor. If it is not densely adherent to the tumor, it should come off with a gentle swab mobilization.

Hydronephrosis is definitely a bad prognosis. In this case, nephroureterectomy has to be contemplated. Apart from the ureter, care is also taken that the testicular or ovarian vessels are not injured. Nevertheless, these vessels could be ligatured, if necessary.

The second part of the duodenum is next examined, whether the tumor is stuck to it. If the colon peels off smoothly from the duodenum, and then the prognosis seems to be promising. After this, the hepatic flexure is mobilized from the liver and gallbladder. In this area, gastrocolic omentum may need to be divided between the clamps and ligature is applied around each clamp. Rest of the transverse colon is separated from the greater omentum, in the same way as described with Billroth I gastrectomy.

At last, the terminal ileum is mobilized from the pelvic brim. Under direct light, the pedicle of the right colic vessels is identified. This could be done, if the assistant keeps holding the colon and cecum vertically up by both hands, the mesentery that will stand up like a screen will display the vessels running through the transparent fatty tissue.

Through the illumination, the roots of the right colic vessels could be seen going through the mesentery. Window is created on either side of the right colic vessels and they are then divided at its root between the two clamps. And strong ligatures are applied around the clamps. Similarly, the right branch of the middle colic artery is divided between the clamps and ligatures are applied to the vessels.

After mobilization of the colon, concentration is focused on the terminal ileum. The terminal ileum, which should be around 8-10 inches in length from the cecum, is next resected from the mesenteric vessels under direct vision.

After completion of the full mobilization, the smaller vessels arising from the arcades of the ileocolic vessels, which are the terminal branches of the superior mesenteric vessels are divided and ligatured by 2/0 absorbable thread. This delicate work is carried out using smaller artery forceps.

Resection is continued up to the mesenteric attachment to the small intestine. The terminal ileum is divided between the soft clamp applied across the proximal segment and a crushing clamp on the distal segment of the same intestine. The line of transection should be in line with the mesentery. The proximal stoma is cleaned with wet swab and is wrapped up by another clean wet swab.

The transverse colon is next divided in the proximal third, but it should be proximal to the middle colic artery. Color of the colon should be pink before it is transected between the two clamps, as before.

Soft occlusion clamp should be applied across the distal segment of the transverse colon and a crushing clamp, preferably the Peyer's clamp, is applied across the proximal segment of the same colon. The line of resection should be in line with the level of resection of the mesentery and with its terminal vessels. The whole resected bowel is put into the large bowel. The stoma of the transverse colon is next cleaned with wet swab several times, until all soft feces are washed away.

Now end-to-end anastomosis should be undertaken between the two stomas. Particular care is taken that the resected end of the ileum has not been twisted before it has been brought to the colon.

A few large wet packs are put around the stomas and around the abdominal wound. The main purpose is to protect the peritoneal cavity, small intestine and wound edges from the fecal contamination or from the leakage of colonic gas that could release aerobic and anaerobic bacteria, when the clamp would be released.

In the absence of acute or chronic obstruction, primary anastomosis should be done.

End-to-end single layer anastomosis could be done by interrupted Vicryl 2/0 stitches, or by continuous sutures in two layers, as described before. Alternatively, side-to-side anastomosis could be done in two layers, as described before. Continuity of the mesentery is restored as described before.

At the completion of anastomosis, the small intestine is laid down in right order. Normal saline washouts are given twice.

All water is aspirated back. It is followed by metronidazole lavage, using 1 gm intravenous preparation without mixing up with the saline. It is delivered in all areas of the peritoneal cavity with 20 ml syringe. It should not be aspirated.

Drainage tubing is left in the right side of the peritoneal cavity. Greater omentum is spread up covering the resected area. Abdominal wound is closed in layers or in one layer. The drainage tubing is left clamp on for 2 hours, but it would be put on suction later.

The patient is sent back to the ward or the high dependency ward for the postoperative care.

DEALING WITH THE PROBLEMS

During laparotomy, bowel preparation turns out to be inadequate, in that the distal colon contains solid lumps of feces. This needs to be manually evacuated or on table lavage. This may turn out to be a messy job.

In the case of fixed and not resectable tumor, side-to-side anastomosis between the ileum and the mid transverse colon remains the only option to the surgeon. But every attempt should be made for removing the growth, if possible. In most cases, the tumor could be mobilized from the surrounding tissues, if courageous approach is adopted with determination. For achieving this goal, the bowel should be mobilized all around first and handling of the tumor from its bed or from the surrounding attachments should be undertaken at last.

If the colon is grossly distended, proximal to the tumor and it is full of feces, mechanical evacuation is carried out. And it should be done through the site, which would be the proposed site for bypass anastomosis. This should be done through the midgut of the ileum.

In this case, a purse string suture is applied on to the antimesenteric border of the gut but large wet packs are laid down all around the small intestine and around the wound margin, as described before. In most cases, the bowel contains lots of gas and liquid feces. They will bubble up as soon as the intraluminal pressure is released by nicking the wall. Therefore, precaution must be taken in anticipation of this contamination.

Furthermore, a pair of soft clamp is applied across the intestine, on either side of the purse string suture, but they should be applied a few inches away from the purse string suture, before the proposed site is nicked with a small blade. These two occlusion clamps would stop any leakage of gas and loose motions when the suction tube, known as Savage's decompressor is inserted through the said puncture wound, made in the center of the purse string suture. Once this precautionary measure has been done, the proposed site of the intestine is nicked, through which, the suction tube, known as Savage's decompressor is inserted into the lumen of the intestine. The purse string suture is pulled tight around the tube and one of the occlusion clamps is released in order to permit the suction tube to be advanced to that direction.

The suction tube comprises of a combination of a cannula and a trocker. The latter is next withdrawn from inside the cannula and a cap is next put back to stop leakage of feces. The cannula has two short side channels, attached to the outer end, one is connected to suction machine and the other one, opposite to the previous one is left open but it is used to operate the suction. And this is done intermittently regulated by the right index finger that keeps the said side channel shut on and off, as and when necessary. In this way, suction is carried out when this side channel is shut with the tip of the index finger, thus maintaining the negative pressure inside the cannula.

The suction of the air and feces will start, thus collapsing the gut, if the air inlet is shut with the index finger, but the suction stops working if it is left open again.

This maneuver permits the surgeon to advance the suction tube further. It is moved towards the proximal, when the assistant keeps on milking the proximal gut towards the suction tube and the empty gut continues to glide over the suction tube up to its full length.

To change the direction of the suction tube, the air inlet tube is left open. The decompressor tube is next turned the other way round, towards the cecum, but the second occlusion is next released before the suction tube has changed its direction with a view to proceeding through the ileocecal valve. The assistant will keep on milking out the colon towards the cecum, for an efficient evacuation. After complete evacuation has been done, the instrument is withdrawn from the gut slowly but it should be done when the suction stops working, otherwise, the mucosa that has been sucked into the tube, could be damaged and it could be bruised.

During withdrawing of the tube, all the tiny holes of the said Savage tube should be kept wrapped up with a large towel all along. The purpose is to stop spilling of feces into the wound. The threads of the purse string are pulled out simultaneously by the assistant in order to close its opening.

For side-to-side anastomosis, a soft clamp is applied below the purse string suture and along the antimesenteric border of the small intestine. A similar clamp is applied across the colon. Side-to-side anastomosis is carried out as described before.

Alternatively, a similar evacuation could be done through the cecotomy, but there remains a risk of breakdown through the site of the cecal closure, due to the intraluminary pressure generated by the propagative peristalsis from the terminal ileum and by the reverse peristalsis, coming from the colon proximal to the colonic obstruction. This may lead to fecal peritonitis. Under these circumstances, cecotomy must not be contemplated. Instead, cecostomy could be undertaken either as a permanent palliative 'bypass' operation, or as an additional safety procedure.

RESECTION OF THE TRANSVERSE COLON

The incidence of the carcinoma in the transverse colon is rare. If the latter is involved, the tumor may invade the greater

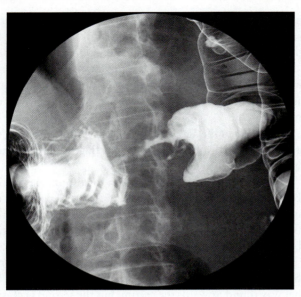

Fig. 9.11: Barium enema showing a stricture and apple-core appearance in the transverse colon. This is a classical feature of the carcinoma of the colon, and it was found in the transverse colon

curvature of the stomach, or the gastric tumor could invade the transverse colon. In either case, this may lead to fistula between the stomach and the colon. In the absence of local spread, the transverse colon has to be resected, combined with a wedge excision of the mesocolon. In this case, a large filling defect has been found in the middle part of the transverse colon. The filling defect in the transverse colon seems to have been all around the transverse colon, leaving a long narrow lumen in the center of the tumor. It is a stricture but the over-all radiological feature appears to be an apple-core filling defect all around the wall of the colon in the barium X-ray (Fig. 9.11).

OPERATIVE PROCEDURE

After a full internal examination, the transverse colon is separated from the greater omentum. Although, greater omentum is attached with the taeniae coli of the transverse colon, lymphatic spread from the colonic tumor does not occur but a direct invasion to the omentum is quite possible if the greater omentum is stuck to the colonic tumor.

In this situation, the greater omentum should be resected from the greater curvature, proximal to the gastroepiploic arcades. Reason for adopting this approach is to excise wider area of the greater omentum, in case it has been infiltrated by the colonic tumor by direct invasion. The omentum is divided between the clamps applied just above the gastroepiploic artery. Ligatures are applied around the clamps.

The level of resection should be consistent with the proposed line of resection of the transverse colon on both sides. In some cases, the transverse colon drops into the pelvis because of its long mesocolon being attached to the transverse colon. In this case, mobilization of the hepatic or splenic flexure may not be necessary for end-to-end anastomosis without tension.

Difficulty may be encountered, if the colon has a short mesentery. In this case, the hepatic and splenic flexures are needed to be mobilized. This is done by dividing the respective ligaments. To get the splenic flexure mobilized, the division of the gastrosplenic, gastrocolic omentum and phrenicocolic ligament has to be carried out separately, one by one between the clamps, but the left gastroepiploic artery must be preserved in this resection.

The distal one-third of the transverse colon and the proximal one of the descending colon needs to be mobilized either for resection of the tumor in the transverse colon or the tumor in the descending colon. Splenic flexure may remain adherent to the spleen. Meticulous care needs to be taken to protect the spleen from being torn while dividing the phrenicocolic ligament, gastrosplenic and gastrocolic omentum.

Therefore, under direct vision the splenic flexure is gently stretched down between the left index and middle fingers, in order to define the phrenicocolic ligament. The latter could be identified by blunt dissection and is divided between the clamps and ligatures are applied around the clamp, or it could be cut slowly with the tip of the scissors, thus mobilizing the splenic flexure away from the spleen.

In addition, the distal one-third of the transverse colon should be disconnected from the corresponding segment of gastrocolic omentum, which is divided between the clamps. And ligatures are applied around the clamps.

By bringing the hepatic and splenic flexure down, tension free end-to-end anastomosis is carried out.

In most cases, the tumor is located in the middle-third of the transverse colon. In this case, the mesocolon is resected in the form of 'V' shape, the apex of which is directed towards the root of the middle colic artery, which is a branch of the superior mesenteric artery. In this resection, enlarged lymph glands, if not closely adherent to the superior mesenteric vessels should be included in the division of the middle colic artery. The tumor along with a healthy segment of the colon of about 2-3 inches on each side of the tumor is resected en bloc with the greater omentum and the mesocolon.

If the tumor is located either to the right or to the left side of the midtransverse colon, then one of the branches of the middle colic artery could be spared, that depends upon the location of the tumor.

For the resection of the tumor, soft occlusion clamp is applied at the hepatic flexure, and crushing Peyer's clamp distal to this soft clamp. The colon is divided flush with the crushing clamp, but the line of resection should be with the line of mesentery. Similarly, a crushing clamp is applied across the colon distal to the colonic tumor or at the proposed line of resection and soft occlusion clamp is applied on the splenic flexure.

The colon is divided between these two clamps. The specimen is sent for histology. Both transected ends of the colon are brought closer together for end-to-end anastomosis. This could be done either by interrupted single layer or by double layer anastomosis using continuous or interrupted stitches, as described before in this chapter.

After completion of primary anastomosis, omental graft could be stitched around the anastomosis. Peritoneal saline wash-out is given and is followed by metronidazole lavage as described before in this chapter. A drainage tube is left near the site of anastomosis, before the abdominal wound is closed as described before.

RESECTION OF THE TUMOR IN THE SPLENIC FLEXURE

The tumor developed in the splenic flexure as shown in Figure 9.12 may invade the gastrocolic and phrenicocolic ligament. If it appears that the tumor has also invaded the hilum of the spleen, this presents a difficult task to the surgeon. The resection of the splenic flexure may involve the splenectomy along with the resection of the distal part of the transverse colon and proximal half of the descending colon, as delineated in Figure 9.12.

Resection of the splenic flexure requires skill and patience. In this case, the proximal part of the descending colon should be mobilized first from the parietal wall. This provides access to palpate the posterior wall of the colon and to examine whether the kidney or spleen are free from the invasion of the tumor. It also renders a greater mobility of the colon around the tumor. This mobilization commences from the left parietal wall and it proceeds towards the splenic flexure, where the phrenicocolic ligament needs to be incised under direct vision.

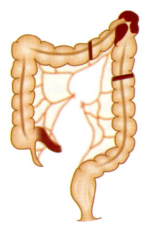

Fig. 9.12: This illustration shows the possible location of the tumor in the splenic flexure of the colon and it indicates the extent of the colon to be resected

Then the greater omentum is separated and excised—thus the distal half of the transverse colon would be free from the stomach and the greater omentum. The mesentery of the transverse colon should not be resected until the splenic flexure is mobilized from the spleen.

For the prevention of injury to the spleen, one wet pack is placed over the hilum of the spleen to be gently retracted upwards by the curved retractor and another wet pack is placed over the splenic flexure. To reveal the clear view of the phrenicocolic ligament, the left hand is placed over the splenic flexure covered by the wet swab and left index and middle fingers are placed on either side of the phrenicocolic ligament, which becomes well-defined when the splenic flexure is gently pulled down.

In some cases, the phrenicocolic ligament is divided between the clamps or it could be divided by a right-angled cutting diathermy. In addition, a part of the greater omentum attached to the splenic flexure is divided between the clamps. The splenic flexure will come down slowly.

Once the tumor of the splenic flexure has been free or mobilized from the surrounding attachments or from the spleen, the left branch of the middle colic artery is divided at the proposed level of resection. And in the same way, the left colic artery supplying to the proximal part of the descending colon and the splenic flexure is divided and ligated.

If difficulty is encountered in the separation of the splenic flexure from the spleen, the latter should be mobilized along with the tumor. In this case, the pedicle comprising of the splenic vein and artery is divided between the two clamps, but due care is taken against injury to the tail of the pancreas. In this case, the tail of the pancreas is first separated from the hilum of the spleen, before the clamps are applied across the vessels. The transected pedicle is ligated with silk or dexon.

After a complete mobilization of the colon along with the spleen, the resection is carried out in the usual way and end-to-end anastomosis between the two stomas is completed as described before. The defect in the mesentery is closed with interrupted sutures.

LEFT HEMICOLECTOMY

The colonic tumor in the descending or sigmoid colon presents with a change in bowel habit, anemia and loss of body weight. The incidence is much higher in this area than in the right colon. It is around 24 percent. Annular type of growth is present more often in the left than on the right side of the colon (Figs 9.10A and 9.17A and B) and the symptoms are often noticed by the patient, because of annular growth.

The routine investigations include flexible sigmoidoscopy or rigid sigmoidoscopy, barium enema, intravenous pyelogram and hematological profile.

PREOPERATIVE PREPARATION

Before the operation is undertaken, the following investigations are important: These are X-ray of the chest, ultrasound scan of the abdomen, and CT scan, if such facility is available. If there is evidence of low hemoglobin and abnormal serum electrolytes in the blood tests, these need to be corrected. Patient should be admitted a day before the surgery for bowel preparation, and for grouping and cross-matching.

In colonic surgery, both oral purgative and rectal washouts are the mandatory requirements for the resection of the bowel, but oral purgative should be withheld, if there is evidence of colonic obstruction. This needs to be confirmed both by abdominal palpation and straight abdominal X-ray.

If the oral purgative could not be given, several phosphate enemas, followed by soap and water enema should be given. At the completion of the rectal wash out, rigid sigmoidoscopy should be done in order to be sure that the lower rectum is free of old inspissated barium, and free of solid feces. Primary anastomosis would be inadvisable in the presence of incomplete bowel preparation.

Antithrombotic prophylactic therapy should be commenced and TED stockings in both legs should be worn before the patient is transferred to the theater. In the induction room, prophylactic appropriate antibiotics, covering for both aerobic and anaerobic bacilli must be given intravenously, and these should be continued for 5-7 days after operation. Urethral catheter must be inserted and residual volume is recorded in the intake and output fluid balance chart.

Patient must be told about all operative and postoperative complications. The question of colostomy or ileostomy should be discussed with the patient.

OPERATIVE PROCEDURE FOR LEFT HEMICOLECTOMY

If the tumor is located in the descending colon as shown in Figure 9.14 or in the barium enema X-rays as shown in Figures 9.15A and B if it appears to be mobile, left hemicolectomy should be done. After a mini laparotomy is done through the midline incision, the wound may need to be extended in either direction in accordance with the anatomical location of the tumor. A good exposure is the essence of a good postoperative recovery. The rate of wound healing remains the same, irrespective of the size of the wound.

The wound is retracted by the self-retaining retractor. All the loops of small intestine are pushed to the right side and tucked away under the several large packs. These are held back by the Kelley's or other suitable retractor.

The colon is lifted up by the left hand. This will display the peritoneal reflection on the left parietal wall. The peritoneum is incised an inch away from the colonic wall.

By combination of sharp and blunt dissection with the finger and swab stick mobilizations of the descending colon will be carried out from the posterior wall of the abdomen. As a result, the colonic tumor along with its healthy bowel could be swept away towards the center of the abdomen.

The left kidney, ureter and the duodenojejunal flexure are exposed. The position of the left ureter and testicular or ovarian vessels are looked for. If they are injured accidentally, they could be sacrificed by putting ligatures around them. Splenic flexure needs to be mobilized down. This could be done by dividing the gastrocolic ligament and by dividing the phrenicocolic ligament under direct vision. Injury to the spleen is possible during the mobilization of the splenic flexure.

Wet pack is put over the back of the colon to cover the retroperitoneal surface. Further mobilization of the colon depends upon the location of the tumor and the local lymphatic spread (Fig. 9.13).

Barium enema shows the stricture of the descending colon near the splenic flexure. The stricture in the descending colon has been shown clearly in the lateral view (Fig. 9.15A) and also in the anteroposterior view (Fig. 9.15B). Resection should include distal transverse colon and lower part of the descending colon. The anatomical distribution of the lymph glands has been shown in the Figure 9.14. A few of these glands may be found enlarged. This could be attributable to metastasis of the colonic tumor. Or they could be affected by the inflammation, developed in the ulcer of the tumor. Nevertheless, its prognostic value could be judged by the histological report. Hence, it is very important to palpate the lymph glands around the rectum, and along the inferior mesenteric vessels and around the abdominal aorta.

In the absence of local lymphatic spread, the tumor is resected along with a segment of healthy colon with a reasonable clear margin that should be between 5 cm and 10 cm away from the tumor. In this case, inferior mesenteric artery need not be divided from the aorta. Resection of colon along with its primary main feeding vessels is carried out. It is followed by primary end-to-end anastomosis.

If there are enlarged lymph nodes palpable, but there was no palpable liver metastasis, radical resection should be undertaken. In this case, the distal one-third of the transverse colon and splenic flexure are mobilized as described before and left hemicolectomy should be carried out. Primary anastomosis between the splenic flexure and the sigmoid colon is performed.

In this case, the inferior mesenteric artery is divided from the abdominal aorta between the clamps. Double ligatures are applied to the root of the vessel. The mobilization of descending colon is continued further down up to the pelvis. The safe level of resection would be 5 cm below the colonic tumor and 10 cm above the tumor.

The assistant will keep holding the descending colon vertically up which would reveal the left colic vessels. Division of the vessels is carried out between the clamps. The arcades

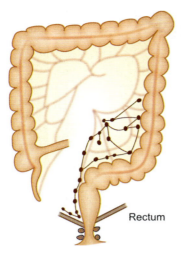

Fig. 9.13: Distribution of lymph nodes along the superior and inferior mesenteric vessels

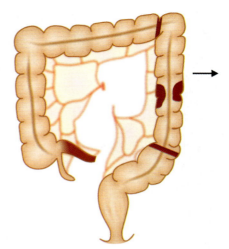

Fig. 9.14: This figure indicating the extent for the left hemicolectomy to be carried out for the tumor located in the descending colon

of the left middle colic artery must be preserved until the level of the resection of the descending colon is undertaken.

A soft occlusion clamp is applied to the distal colon, below the tumor, but it should be a few inches away from the proposed level of resection of the colon. A pair of crushing clamp is next applied at the proposed level of transection but a few inches above the soft clamp. The colon below the tumor is divided between the clamps. The distal cut end is covered with wet swab and the other end held by the crushing clamp is also covered with gauze that should be tied around. This safety precaution is necessary in case, the swabs fell down that may cause local implantation of the tumor and contamination of the peritoneum or parietal wound.

In the same way, the colon, proximal to the tumor is next transected between a soft clamp applied higher up and the crushing clamp applied below the soft clamp but at the proposed level of the resection that should be 10 cm proximal to the tumor. The whole specimen is sent for histology. Both transected ends are brought closer together for end-to-end primary anastomosis. This could be done either by interrupted single layer, or a continuous double layer anastomosis, as described in this chapter. The line of anastomosis is covered with appendices epiploicae, and/or with omentum.

The defect in the mesentery is repaired in the usual method. Routine regimen is followed for wound lavage as described before. A tube drain is left in the left paracolic gutter. All bowels are put back in order and in right place.

Abdominal wound is closed as described before.

HOW TO RESOLVE THE PROBLEMS

If the tumor has a local spread to the mesentery, it is debatable whether radical resection would make any difference to the prognosis and whether end-to-end anastomosis should be done. If the tumor appears to be advanced locally, terminal colostomy should be constructed.

If the tumor is not resectable due to invasion to the parietal wall, transverse loop colostomy should be done.

If the tumor is resectable but left ureter is infiltrated by the tumor, there are three options available to the surgeon. One of them is to excise the colonic tumor along with the segment of the ureter. The distal end of the ureter could be left alone but the proximal end could be brought out for cutaneous ureterostomy. In this case, surgeon need not know the other kidney function.

Alternatively, the proximal cut end of the ureter is ligated. This will lead to cessation of the kidney function. Or left ureteronephrectomy could be undertaken. In both cases, surgeon needs to know the function of the other kidney. If no such evidence is available, on-table IVU should be done as described in the section of right hemicolectomy.

If the tumor is resectable but it has caused colonic obstruction, leading to distention of the cecum, in this case, there are many options left to the surgeon.

These are:
a. Paul Mikulicz Technique: In this approach, the descending and sigmoid colon need to be mobilized from the left paracolic gutter. A double barreled loop is constructed by continuous seromuscular sutures between the two limbs.

   The total length should be around 3-4 inches in order to get through the parietal wound, made over the left lumbar region. After the abdominal wound is closed, the tumor is resected along with a segment of healthy bowel, thus leaving behind double barrel colostomies in place. This is rarely practiced.

Clinical Practice and Surgery of the Colon, Rectum and Anus

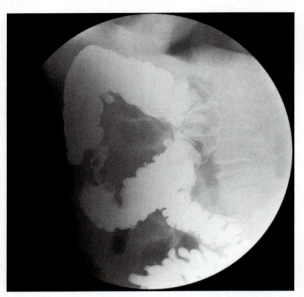

Fig. 9.15A: An X-ray of a barium enema shows a filling defect in the descending colon in lateral view and it is a stricture of the colon. This is due to the carcinoma of the descending colon

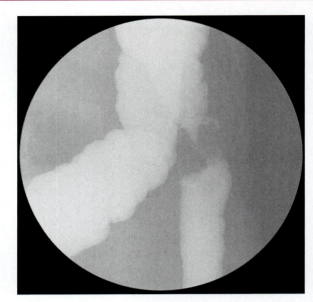

Fig. 9.15B: Barium enema showing a stricture of the descending colon near the splenic flexure. It was carcinoma of the descending colon

b. Mobilization of the descending colon and evacuation of the feces from the colon could be undertaken.

The same method is employed to evacuate the feces by the Savage's suction decompressor, inserted through a site that should be a few inches proximal to the colonic tumor. But this would be ineffective, if the colon contains solid feces. In this circumstance, either on-table lavage or manual evacuation of the solid lumps of feces could be carried out.

Therefore the left colon is mobilized along with the colonic tumor. It is followed by resection of the descending colon along with the tumor as described before. The occlusion clamp from the proximal colon is removed, and the stoma of the transected colon is put into the large bowel. The assistant will start squeezing the colon, thus evacuating lumps of feces slowly into the bowel.

Initially, the segment of the colon nearer to the stoma is evacuated first and later, the proximal segment is slowly milked out of all hard feces through the stoma. After this has been done, the manual evacuation from the sigmoid colon and the rectum is undertaken in the same way.

At the end of these procedures, both transected ends are brought together in order to find out whether there is any tension between the two segments of the gut. In most cases, the tension would be much less, due to emptying of the gut. If in doubt, the rectum could be mobilized from the sacral wall. Primary end-to-end anastomosis is carried out in single layer with interrupted sutures.

c. Evacuation of the feces through the midtransverse colon, using the Savage suction decompressor or by manual evacuation technique remains an alternative approach. This is followed by a simple transverse loop colostomy. The colostomy is normally constructed through the site of the evacuation of feces.

A few weeks later, resection of the tumor combined with end-to-end anastomosis should be done. Closure of colostomy is done later, provided, barium enema does not suggest that there was leakage of contrast through the anastomosis. It is a popular choice.

d. Alternative to all these procedures just described, cecostomy could be constructed. This is a simple and quick procedure that remains the choice of the surgeon, if the patient remains unwell. If the condition improves, resection of the tumor along with end-to-end anastomosis could be contemplated later. Closure of the cecostomy will be unnecessary after the resection of the tumor has been carried out. It will close slowly, if there is no distal obstruction.

RESECTION OF THE SIGMOID COLON

In some cases, barium enema may reveal a stricture in the sigmoid colon as shown in the double contrast barium enema in Figure 9.10A. The principle for the mobilization of the entire sigmoid colon remains the same as described in the mobilization of the descending colon. Figure 9.16 shows the extent of resection of the sigmoid colon, but due care is taken to protect the left ureter from injury during mobilization of the colon from the left parietal wall and pelvis.

In another case, patient was admitted with a colonic obstruction and a plain X-ray of the abdomen showed a gross gaseous distention of the small and large intestine up to the

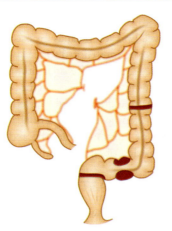

Fig. 9.16: The location of the tumor in the sigmoid colon and the line of resection for the sigmoid colectomy

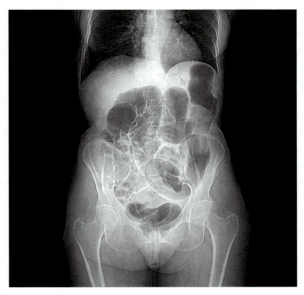

Fig. 9.17A: This is plain X-ray of the abdomen taken on emergency admission. It shows dilatation of the small intestine and the colon, but the exact site of obstruction is not clear in the plain X-ray of abdomen

level of colonic obstruction. There was no gas shadow in the rectum (Fig. 9.17A). Gastrograffin enema shows a total obstruction in the rectosigmoid junction as shown in Figure 9.17B.

To confirm the site of colonic obstruction, gastro-graffin enema was carried out, but it was not absolutely necessary when emergency laparotomy is necessary. Although, gastrograffin enema does not interfere with the emergency laparotomy, it may cause further pressure upon the preexisting distention of the colon and the cecum.

In view of the evidence of large bowel obstruction as shown in the plain X-ray (Fig. 9.17A), barium enema or gastrograffin enema is unnecessary. This patient needs emergency laparotomy, if general condition remains satisfactory. There remains a potential risk of perforation of the distended cecum, if gastrograffin enema is carried out. In this case, a serosal tear along the taeniae coli of the cecum may have already been developed due to overdistention of the cecum. Further pushing of fluid whether it is gastrograffin enema or barium enema would be detrimental to the site of existing seroral tear of the cecum.

To avoid the perforation through the existing serosal tear of the distended colonic wall, emergency laparotomy should be carried out, if the general condition of the patient permits.

In the emergency operation, patient could be treated either by transverse defunctioning colostomy alone or along with resection of the sigmoid colon and end-to-end anastomosis.

Alternatively, the resection of the sigmoid colon could be done and both descending colon and rectum could be brought out either separately for colostomy and mucus fistula of the rectum or both limbs of the mobilized segment of the descending colon and the rectum could be brought out, like a Paul Mikulicz type of double barrel colostomies in the left iliac fossa. After a few weeks, the continuity of the gut is restored by the closure of two colostomies like closure of colostomy.

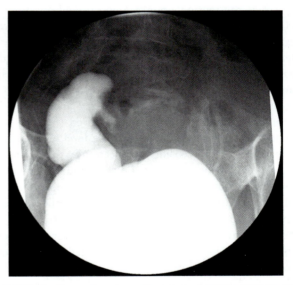

Fig. 9.17B: An X-ray of gastrograffin enema confirms stricture at the sigmoid colon and it was carcinoma of the sigmoid colon

In this case, end-to-end anastomosis is undertaken either by single layer with interrupted stitches or in two layers that depends upon the practice of the surgeon.

In elective operation, the sigmoid colon is mobilized along with the descending colon and rectum. In this mobilization, left ureter that passes across the left common iliac artery must be identified before dividing the sigmoid colon. In some cases, the ureter may be lifted up with the pelvic mesocolon and could be found attached with the posterior wall of the mesocolon. It needs to be peeled off from the mesocolon.

In some cases, the descending colon may require to be mobilized right up to the splenic flexure, where the phrenicocolic ligament needs to be incised under direct vision. For the prevention of injury to the spleen, one wet pack is placed over the hilum of the spleen to be gently retracted upwards by the curved retractor and another wet pack is placed over the splenic flexure. To reveal the clear view of the phrenicocolic ligament, the left hand is placed over the splenic flexure covered by the wet swab and left index and middle fingers are placed on either side of the phrenicocolic ligament, which becomes well-defined when the splenic flexure is gently pulled down.

In some cases, the phrenicocolic ligament is divided between the clamps or it could be divided by a right angled cutting diathermy. In addition, a part of the greater omentum attached to the splenic flexure may require to be divided between the clamps. The splenic flexure will come down slowly. This mobilization is necessary, if there appears to be short of length for end-to-end anastomosis to be carried out between the proximal transected descending colon and transected rectosigmoid junction. This mobilization of the splenic flexure will reduce the tension upon the end-to-end anastomosis.

The left branch of the middle colic artery and its arcades must be preserved up to the level of resection of the colon. After mobilization of the tumor along with a good length of the colon on either side of the tumor, the branches arising from the left colic artery, supplying to the sigmoid colon and part of the descending colon are divided and ligated. The superior rectal vessels are usually preserved (Fig. 9.13).

The mesocolon is divided up to the level of resection of the colon. Before proceeding for resection of the colon, large wet pack is laid over the denuded surface under the mobilized colon. Its purpose is to protect the field of operation from fecal contamination, when the colon is transected. A soft clamp is applied across the rectum and a little away from the level of resection. A crushing clamp is applied at the level of resection of the sigmoid colon. The latter is next divided from the rectum between the two clamps.

The distal transected bowel is covered with wet pack and the transected colon is covered with another swab and the latter is tied around the clamp. In the same way, the descending colon is transected between the clamps but due care is taken so that end-to-end anastomosis could be carried out without tension. The level of resection of the descending colon should be 10 cm proximal to the tumor. After resection of the descending colon, the sigmoid colon is sent for histology.

It is important to be sure that vascularity at the transected levels remains very satisfactory, with no evidence of dusky color at the mucosal level. The proximal part of the descending colon is brought down to be anastomosed with the recto-sigmoid section of the bowel. End-to-end anastomosis is completed. This could be done either by interrupted single layer or in two layers sutures as described before. The anastomotic line should be covered with omental graft. The defect in the posterior mesentery may be repaired. A tube drain should be left in the pelvic area around the site of anastomose. After peritoneal lavage with saline and with 500 mg of metronidazole, the abdominal wound is closed in layers, as described with other operations.

ETIOLOGY OF ANASTOMOTIC LEAKAGE

Anastomotic leakage usually occurs on fourth or fifth postoperative day. This is attributable to ischemic state of the tissue around the line of anastomosis, but there are other contributing factors. One of them is the postoperative trauma that may cause tissue edema due to inflammation, delayed lymphatic and venous drainage, and ligation of the marginal arteries to the stoma. Over and above, poor surgical technique for the anastomosis between the two stomas remains the important factor for the anastomotic dehiscence.

The important technical issues need to be highlighted further in this context. These are as follows:

- Poor vascularity at the level of resection. The ischemic state could be recognized by the dusky color of the mucosa and surrounding tissue at the transected level of the colon.
- Faulty surgical technique in the anastomosis of the stomas. In the anastomosis, the marginal arteries may be caught in the sutures applied at the mesenteric attachment to the gut and this is known as "sorrow corner" to the surgeon. It may occur during invagination of the inner sutures line.
- Other technical fault is the end-to-end sutures which may be very close to the transected end of the gut or there may be a wide gap between the two sutures bites.
- Continuous serosal suture line that is employed for invagination of the inner sutures (anastomotic sutures) may cut out, if this is inserted very close to the inner sutures line. Invagination may not be possible in this sort of situation.
- Capillary flow of the blood to the anastomotic tissue, particularly around the antimesenteric border of the gut may be affected adversely by the invagination of the serosal layer when continuous seromuscular sutures are inserted and it could be worse, if the marginal mesenteric vessels are caught in the sutures. As a result, edema may develop around the antimesenteric border where avascular necrosis may occur, thus breaking the anastomosis. This occurs usually on the 4th or 5th postoperative day. Because of this risk, oral feeding is usually delayed until the patient has passed wind per rectum.

10
The Rectum

PREVIEW OF THE OPERATIVE TECHNIQUES

The policy for the surgical treatment of the rectal carcinoma is decided by many criteria. They are location of the tumor from the anal verge, Dukes tumor staging and general health of the patient. It has been the consensus that anterior resection of the rectal carcinoma is undertaken for the growth presented with the tumor staging of Dukes A and B, and if it is located above the level of 10 cm from the anal verge.

Although, sphincter-saving low anterior resection has become a popular choice, because of the fact that patient does not need to carry the ileostomy or colostomy bag; merits of this technique need to be evaluated in perspective by the postoperative complications, morbidity, cumulative cost, quality of life, and a long-term survival rate. And it needs to be measured with alternative surgical treatment. This argument will continue among the surgeons.

Sphincter-saving low anterior resection has been used over many decades; it became popular, since the stapling gun has been devised. But the issue is yet to be decided on the merits of each case and for the benefit of the patients.

In the case of low anterior resection, the quality of life has been questioned whether the patient would be satisfied with a frequent defecation, urge incontinence or soiled bottom. These morbidities are attributable to many factors, but the continence of the anal sphincter depends upon the Dukes tumor stage, level of resection, postoperative complications and skill of a surgeon.

Furthermore, the anal sphincteric function is initiated and maintained by both anatomical and physiological factors. The anatomical factor is the longitudinal muscle of the rectum that lies between the internal and external anal sphincters. It keeps pulling and holding both anal sphincters in pari passu with the descent of the feces while having defecation. On the other hand, the physiological factor is the stretch receptors present in the puborectalis muscle and in the rectal wall that initiate the urge defecation. Therefore, the functional state of the anal sphincters may be affected, if these muscles are excised. This may contribute to urge incontinence, in some cases of low anterior resection.

Over the last decade, the issue of long-term benefit has been highlighted since lots of postoperative complications and delayed morbidity have been reported in the literature. The merits of these issues would be highlighted later with the operation of low anterior resection and that of abdominoperineal resection of the rectum. The choice remains with the patients.

At the outpatient clinic, patients are investigated to establish the rectal carcinoma. In this clinical diagnosis, the location and mobility of the growth are also noted. This is done by the rectal digital examination in most cases and by sigmoidoscopy. In addition, the diagnosis must be made before proceeding for establishing the tumor staging. These include X-ray of the chest, CT scan of the abdomen and MRI scan. These scans will reveal whether or not the tumor is invasive (Figs 10.1 to 10.3).

The CT scan (Figs 10.1 and 10.2) shows that the rectal tumor has invaded the bladder located anterior to the rectum. It provides an opportunity to the clinicians, whether this patient would be benefited from preoperative adjuvant radiotherapy or chemotherapy that has to be discussed with the oncologist. Eventually, the surgeon would take the final decision whether this tumor is resectable along with the excision of the bladder that could only be evaluated by palpation of the organs at laparotomy.

In the past, this sort of preoperative evaluation on the merits of prognosis was not possible for the surgeons.

The CT scan of the rectal tumor will assist in establishing the Dukes tumor stage, whether it is too advanced and whether it is suitable for preoperative adjuvant radiotherapy and/or chemotherapy.

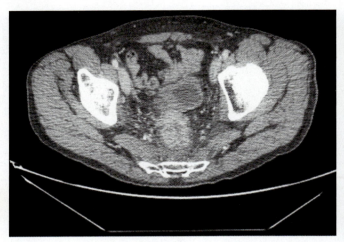

Fig. 10.1: CT scan of the pelvis shows invasive rectal carcinoma

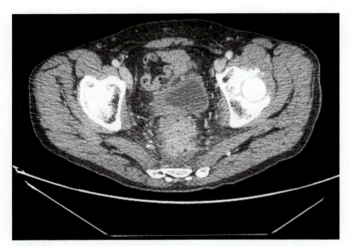

Fig. 10.2: CT scan of the pelvis, second plate from the same patient shows invasive rectal carcinoma (By *Courtesy* of Dr S Sinha)

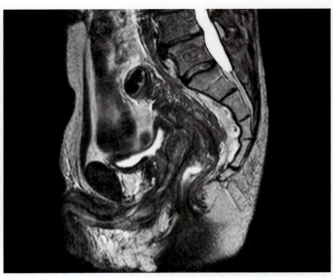

Fig. 10.3: Sagittal view of MRI scan taken from another patient. It shows the location of the rectal tumor with reference to the sacral vertebrae. It is situated at the level between sacral 2 and sacral 4 vertebrae and behind the prostate gland (By *Courtesy* of Dr S Sinha)

In some cases, the report may not be accurate that depends upon the experience of the radiologist. Despite these pitfalls in the investigation, surgeon must not be discouraged and should be fully aware of the inaccurate reports.

I have been misguided by the CT scan report on a few occasions. In one case, a middle-aged lady had sigmoid colectomy for colonic carcinoma two years ago, but the CT scan report indicated metastasis in the pelvic lymph glands. The radiologist was misguided by reading the past history of the colonic carcinoma quoted in the request form; but in fact, she had fibroid of the uterus that led to a wrong impression of enlarged lymph glands reported in the CT scan.

In another colonic tumor case, CT scan suggested pelvic abscess, but in fact there was inflammatory fluid collection in the pockets surrounded by metastatic lymph glands. In these cases, MRI scan in sagittal view (Fig. 10.3) could have provided with a better delineation of the rectal tumor.

Therefore, one should not be persuaded by one single investigation or one single report. To avoid all these errors or inaccurate reports, final decision about the future plan for the treatment should be taken by joint consultations in a multi-disciplinary team or among the oncologist, histopathologist, and surgeons.

After a full evaluation of the tumor staging, the initial decision whether or not the anterior resection of the rectum is feasible, depends upon the level of the growth and the Dukes tumor stage. Eventually, patient must be explained about the results of investigations, before the laparotomy is carried out.

CRITERIA FOR THE ANTERIOR RESECTION

Decision varies from one surgeon to another, but a final decision is taken on the operating table. The criteria for anterior resection of the rectum are as follows: The tumor should be above the pelvic peritoneal reflection and it should be above 10 cm from the anal verge. The growth would appear to be localized that is judged by mobility of the tumor mass on palpation. Furthermore, it is equally important to be sure that there is no evidence of enlarged lymph nodes along the inferior mesenteric vessels. Curative resection may not be feasible if the tumor appears to have invaded to other organs, the side-to-side movement of the tumor would be limited and the paracolic or mesenteric lymph nodes along the inferior mesenteric artery appear to be enlarged on palpation. Enlargement of some of these glands may not be invaded by the malignant cells, but they could be due to infection from the ulcerated growth of the rectum. In these cases, diversion of feces should be considered, alternative to anterior resection of the rectum.

PREOPERATIVE ASSESSMENT AND CONSULTATION

Prophylactic measures against the deep vein thrombosis, wound infection and bowel preparation need not be repeated in this section. Like any other colonic surgery, all preoperative treatment for anemia, electrolytes imbalance and grouping and cross-matching are taken care of. Preoperative tissue diagnosis must be recorded in the case note and is available at hand during consultation.

Patient should be explained that the final decision will be taken on the operating table, but the patient must be prepared to accept the burden of colostomy. Postoperative complication should be highlighted in this consultation. These are pelvic abscess, intestinal obstruction, wound infection, deep vein thrombosis, pulmonary embolism and fecal fistula. In some cases, re-exploration of the abdomen may be necessary for bleeding, wound dehiscence or breakdown of anastomosis.

TECHNIQUE FOR THE ANTERIOR RESECTION

Patient should be placed on the supine position, if the surgeon uses the hand sutures for primary end-to-end anastomosis, but the patient needs to be put on a lithotomy – Trendelenburg position, if the anastomosis is to be carried out by stapling gun. Indwelling catheter must be inserted per urethra in the theater and the residual volume is recorded.

Skin preparation is done between the costal margin and the mid thigh. Sterile drapes are laid down all around the abdomen and legs. The head end of the table is tilted down.

A midline incision is made between the umbilicus and symphysis pubis. The rectal tumor is palpated first and it is assessed to evaluate, whether it is resectable and above the peritoneal reflection. In this assessment, it is equally important to find out whether there are peritoneal seedlings in the pelvis or whether lymph nodes are palpable around the inferior mesenteric vessels. Examination of the liver and all other organs is carried out, like in all other cases.

The wound could be extended a little above the umbilicus, if the exposure is not adequate. All the guts are pushed up and tucked under the large packs. A self-retaining retractor is inserted to keep the wound margins wide apart and a center blade fitted with the retractor will keep holding the small intestine in the upper abdomen. The pelvis is now empty and well-visualized. The surgeon should stand on the left and the assistant on the right side of the patient. Initial mobilization of the sigmoid colon from the left parietal wall is easier, if the surgeon stands on the right side of the abdomen and later he could swap the position with the assistant. It depends upon the individual preference.

The sigmoid colon is lifted up by the left hand. This will demonstrate the parietal peritoneal reflection and a few omental or peritoneal adhesion between the sigmoid colon and the parietal wall. These are divided with the scissors. The sigmoid colon is mobilized by incising the left parietal peritoneal reflection. It comes off easily from the retroperitoneal wall. The mobilization of the rectum is continued down by incising the parietal attachment of the peritoneum.

The tumor is mobilized from the pelvic wall by putting the four fingers of the left hand behind the rectum. At this stage, the left ureter and the testicular or ovarian vessels are looked for. The ureter must be identified. If it is not coming off with the posterior wall of the mesentery or the rectal growth, the prognosis would be good. Normally, it passes over the common iliac vessels at the pelvic brim. Mobilization of the descending colon from the splenic flexure may be necessary, in order to avoid any tension at the site of anastomosis.

Resection of the rectum begins with the division of the left colic artery supplying to the sigmoid colon. The level of transection of the colon must be in line with the level of resection of the mesentery and the arterial arcades supplying the colon.

If the enlarged lymph nodes remain confined to epicolic and paracolic vessels, a limited resection is sufficient, but if they are present along the inferior mesenteric vessels (Fig. 10.4), then the origin of the inferior mesenteric artery is divided from the aorta between the two clamps. Double ligature is applied to the artery. The shaded area as shown in Figure 10.5 is resected.

In the absence of palpable mesenteric lymph nodes, the superior hemorrhoidal vessels are divided between the clamps. This division is normally done over the sacral promontory.

The rectum is further mobilized and is elevated from the sacral wall. This is done by inserting the fingers of the right hand behind the rectum. In this case, surgeon should stand on the left side of the patient. Mobilization from the sacral

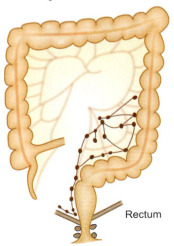

Fig. 10.4: Distribution of lymph nodes along the superior hemorrhoidal and inferior mesenteric vessels

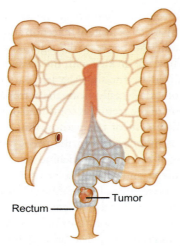

Fig. 10.5: The shaded area shown in the figure should be resected along with the specimen of the sigmoid colon and the rectum

wall becomes easier by standing on the left side. Initially, the distal part of the rectum may appear to be short in length. This apparent impression is due to attachment of the rectum with the curvature of the sacral wall but once the rectum is mobilized from the posterior wall, it loses its curvature and it becomes a straight tube and longer in length. Resection and end-to-end anastomosis will not be too difficult in most instances. And it becomes much easier in female than in the male pelvis.

Before proceeding with transection, a large pack is put behind the rectum. This will protect the posterior wall from fecal contamination, when it would be transected.

The rectum is divided between the clamps that should be 4-5 cm below the lower border of the tumor (Fig. 10.6).

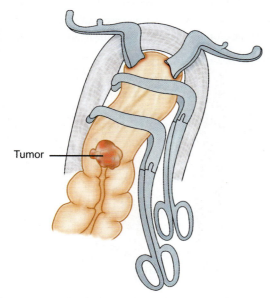

Fig. 10.6: Anterior resection of the rectum showing a level of resection of the rectum below the tumor between the two clamps

In this resection, soft clamp is applied far below the true level of resection and a crushing clamp is applied across at the true level of transection of the gut.

The transected end of the rectum is covered with a swab and the latter is tied across it. It is brought out of the pelvis. The proximal segment of the descending colon is brought down, in order to find out the exact level of resection without undue tension.

A soft clamp is applied across the descending colon, away from the proposed level of the transection and a crushing clamp is applied below the occlusion clamp but it should be at the proposed level of resection, which should be 10 cm proximal to the upper border of the tumor.

Vascularity to the colon must be checked before these clamps are applied. The colon is divided between the two clamps and the whole specimen is sent for histology.

The proximal stoma is brought down closer to the rectal stump. It should rest on the pelvis without any tension. The rectal stump is opened up by releasing the clamp and stay sutures are applied to the corners of the stump. The lumen of the rectum is cleaned with suction and with wet swabs.

Before end-to-end anastomosis is commenced, stay suture is inserted between the two stomas, one at the antimesenteric corner and another one at the mesenteric corner of the two stomas.

Between these two stay sutures, interrupted sutures are inserted between the two stomas and along the posterior cut edges, in that the needle is inserted from inside the proximal stoma, and it is pulled out from outside wall the same stoma.

The needle is next inserted from outside the rectal stoma and brought out from inside the rectal stoma. Both ends are held together. The procedure is repeated along the posterior anastomotic cut edges between the two stay sutures held by the artery forceps.

The sutures' line should be between 3- 4 mm away from the cut edge of the stoma and the intervening space between the two such sutures should be 2 mm.

At the completion of all sutures being inserted, they are tied one by one, and all threads are cut out leaving behind the stay sutures at the corners, held by the artery forceps. These corner sutures would assist the surgeon in carrying out the anterior anastomosis (Fig. 10.7).

In this case, the needle, unlike the posterior anastomosis, is inserted from the anterior wall of the proximal stoma to be pulled out from inside the same stoma. The needle is next reinserted through from inside the rectal stoma and it is pulled out from the serosal wall of the rectal stoma. In this way, all such interrupted sutures are inserted between the two corner stay sutures (Fig. 10.7).

It is not advisable to pass the needle through and through between the two stomas in one attempt. This may tear the mucosa, while trying to get the needle inserted through in

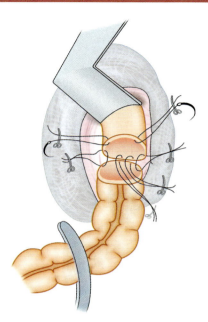

Fig. 10.7: Anterior resection of the rectum showing end-to-end anastomosis by hand sutures

one attempt between the two stomas. Each suture is held together by the artery forceps. The assistant will keep these forceps in order.

After completion of all interrupted sutures being in placed, between the two corners, each suture is tied one by one and their knots should stay outside the serosal wall. All threads are cut at the end. It is important to assess whether the serosal walls around the anastomosis turn out to be dusky, or bluish in color. This is a sign of inadequate blood supply to the area. If that occurs, the anastomosis needs to be redone by excising the ischemic segment of the stoma.

The proximal colon is milky down across the line of anastomosis in order to see any air bubble or feces emerging through the anastomosis. The swab packs are removed. The sutures line could be covered with omental graft or it could be put in the retroperitoneal space. In this case, the peritoneum is mobilized from the back of the bladder and from the parietal wall. It is anchored across the anastomotic line of the colon by interrupted sutures—thus covering the anastomosis. A tube drain is left in the pelvis by the side of the colon and its other end is brought out through a stab wound to be connected to a plastic bag. The tube drain is anchored to the skin by a silk suture and a safety-pin should be inserted through the tube. This would stop the tube drain slipped into the peritoneal cavity.

If some doubt creeps up in mind about the outcome of the primary healing of the anastomosis, or if the surgeon has noticed some dusky color in the tissues around the anastomosis, a defunctioning loop colostomy through the proximal part of the transverse colon could be constructed. This will be described later.

A thorough saline wash-out is given and all fluids are sucked out. It is followed by metronidazole lavage, which is used for parenteral therapy. The dose for this lavage would be 1 gm. It must not be mixed with saline and is squashed all parts of the peritoneal cavity. This is done by a 20 ml syringe. It must not be aspirated back. The retractors are removed. Small intestine is put back in the lower abdomen in sequence. Further solution of metronidazole is kept in the syringe to be used over the abdominal wound. It is equally important to be sure that instrument, needle or packs have not been left behind into the abdomen before the wound is closed in one layer, as described before.

ANASTOMOSIS BY AUTOSUTURE

Alternative to hand sutures is the anastomosis, performed by the stapling gun using EEA circular stapling. It is expensive and the results are no better than by hand sutures, but it saves time. Nevertheless, this technique requires learning and practicing.

First the stapling gun (TA55) is applied transversely across the rectum and it should be at least 3 cm below the tumor. A crushing clamp is next applied a little above the gun. The rectum is next divided just below the crushing clamp. The proximal stamp is brought upwards, above the pelvis.

The descending colon is next brought down to be divided at a suitable level that would permit for the stapling anastomosis without tension. It is divided between the two clamps applied a few inches above the tumor. The specimen along with the tumor is sent for histology.

At this stage, the patient could be changed to lithotomy position on the Lloyd Davies Table, (Fig. 10.8) by just lifting and abducting the legs supports in flexed position.

The gun (EEA) is passed through the anus (Fig. 10.9), and is advanced towards the pelvis, until it reaches the stapled stoma of the rectum. At this level, the spike is advanced through the posterior wall of the stapled rectal stump.

Next the proximal colonic stump is brought down and purse string suture is inserted around the edge of it before, it is glided over the anvil. The stoma is next firmly anchored around the central rod with the purse string suture, before the central rod is inserted into the cartridge.

Following this maneuver, a thorough inspection is carried out around the stomas, whether the appendices epiploicae has entered into the cartridge and whether the mesentery has been caught up in the space between the anvil and the cartridge. The colon is rotated at 90 degrees to the left so that the mesentery will stay on the right side.

By anticlockwise rotation of the knob, the anvil is brought down, until it is engaged with the cartridge and until the green line is in sight. The assistant dealing with the operation of the gun from the perineal stand is asked to fire the gun. When the

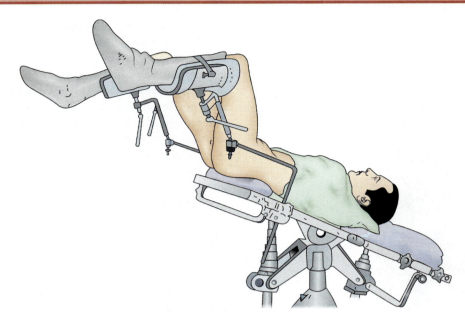

Fig. 10.8: Lloyd Davis Table. For the anastomosis with a circular autosuture gun, the patient is placed on this table

gun is fired, circular double row staples, made of stainless steel have inserted through—thus performing end-to-end anastomosis, and at the same time, a rim of circular gut wall is resected from each stoma concurrently. It is known as doughnut.

The perineal surgeon will gently unlock the stapling gun from the anastomosis. This is done by half twisting in anticlockwise direction, when a click is heard, indicating that the gun is free from the anastomosis. The gun comes out slowly by gentle half-twisting in either direction without dragging the rectum (Fig. 10.9). A pair doughnut could be retrieved from inside the instrument.

This confirms a complete end-to-end stapling anastomosis. The pieces of doughnut are sent separately for histology. The pelvic wash-out is given with saline and this will provide further clue whether any air bubble is leaking through the pool of saline left in the pelvis. After wash-out, metronidazole lavage is given as described before. The rest of the procedure is followed, before the wound is closed.

DEALING WITH THE PROBLEMS

If the tumor has invaded the ureter, or it is not resectable or there are peritoneal seedlings in the pelvic floor, these cases require transverse loop colostomy. Hartmann's procedure could be undertaken if the tumor is resectable despite the evidence of local peritoneal seedling being present.

TECHNIQUE FOR THE HARTMANN'S PROCEDURE

In this operation, the sigmoid colon and the rectal growth are mobilized from the pelvis. A limited resection for the rectal growth is undertaken, and the inferior mesenteric vessels are isolated from the sacral promontory and divided between the clamps. The superior hemorrhoidal vessels are isolated from each side of the rectum below the growth. They are divided between the ligatures.

The rectum is divided below the tumor between the two clamps. The distal rectal stump is closed either with interrupted or with continuous sutures. Alternatively, the rectum could be transected between the autosuture, using TA 55.

If the stump is closed by hand sutures, it is next invaginated with interrupted or continuous sutures. The sigmoid colon

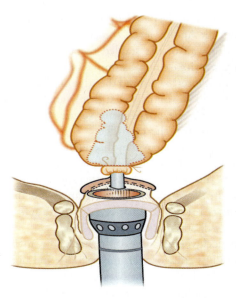

Fig. 10.9: Anastomosis by the autosuture, using a circular gun

is next transected at a suitable level above the growth. This resection is done between the two clamps. The specimen is sent for histology. The terminal transected end of the sigmoid colon is brought out for terminal colostomy.

PREOPERATIVE CONSULTATION FOR THE TERMINAL COLOSTOMY

For the construction of terminal colostomy, a suitable site should be identified, before the patient is taken to the theater. It has been a standard practice that a colostomy nurse explains the patient about the purpose of the colostomy and how to look after it, if it has to be constructed.

For the purpose of identification for a suitable site where the colostomy is to be constructed, patient is asked to find out the proposed site in the lower abdominal wall that would be comfortable to him or her and that would not have any affect on his or her day-to-day wearing of clothes. For this trial, he or she is asked to put on the colostomy appliance around the waist, and is instructed to move around in the ward with the colostomy bag, filled up with water, and fitted on the appliance.

By this trial, it would be possible for the patient to identify the suitable site in the pelvis that would not interfere with the day-to-day wearing of the clothes.

This trial requires adequate time for him to make up his mind and to identify the possible site for this colostomy to be constructed on the anterior abdominal wall. This preoperative trial gives confidence and understanding on what to expect from the operation and how to look after the colostomy bag.

Once the patient has identified the site to be used for the colostomy, it is marked with skin pencil.

Experiences show that many patients shut themselves out by not looking at the colostomy bag for a few days after operation. This is due to lack of confidence, and lack of preoperative consultation. Psychological trauma prevents them from going out because of the burden of colostomy. Over the last decade, things have improved.

If this has not been done, the usual site would be a little above the mid point between the anterior superior iliac spine and the umbilicus. And the preferable site should be over the rectus abdominis muscles, and it should not be constructed close to the anterior superior iliac spine. This guideline may not be suitable for a fatty and pendulous belly (Fig. 10.10).

OPERATIVE PROCEDURE FOR THE CONSTRUCTION OF COLOSTOMY

After completion of the primary operative procedures, surgeon needs to decide whether or not colostomy is to be constructed, and to determine whether he wanted to construct a loop or terminal colostomy, and where the colostomy is to be constructed, if skin mark has not been put on the site of the abdomen.

In the case of Hartmann's operation, terminal colostomy needs to be constructed in the left iliac fossa. For this purpose, a circular skin incision is made in the left iliac fossa (Fig. 10.10). Alternatively, a cruciate incision could be made over the proposed site and the corners of the skin are excised. The diameter of the wound should be around 1 inch. The subcutaneous fat is dissected out and held apart by the Langerbeck retractors. This will reveal the external oblique aponeurotic fascia or the anterior rectus sheath. This is incised by cruciate incisions.

The longitudinal muscle fibers underneath this fascia are split up by the strong scissors and they are then retracted by the Langerbeck. Sometimes, these muscle fibers need to be made wide open. This is done by inserting the two index fingers in the cleavage just made between the longitudinal fibers. The underlying posterior rectus sheath or the peritoneum is incised and the opening is made wide, so that two fingers can easily go through.

There should be adequate room within the colostomy wound for the colon and its mesentery to be brought out without being strangled by the contraction of the rectus abdominals muscle. The terminal end of the descending colon is pulled out through the said telescopic abdominal wound by the occlusion clamp or by the Peyer's clamp, inserted from outside through the colostomy skin wound. It is important to be sure that the terminal transected segment of the colon is not twisted before it is brought out.

The gap between the colon and the left parietal wall is obliterated either by interrupted or by a continuous suture. This obliteration should be done along the antimesenteric border of the colon which would be on the splenic side. The main purpose for closing this gap is to stop herniation of the small intestine that may occur from the splenic side.

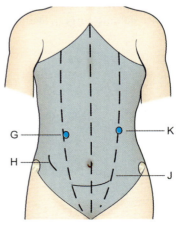

Fig. 10.10: Site for the construction of terminal colostomy. In this figure, G = site for ileostomy, H = site for the grid iron incision for appendicectomy, and K = site for terminal colostomy in the LIF

From inside the abdomen, the peritoneal edge is sutured with the serosal wall of the colon but the needle must not take a full thickness bite through the muscular wall that may cause fistula. For this purpose, 3-4 interrupted stitches are applied, without affecting the mesenteric blood vessels. Alternatively, the parietal peritoneum is elevated for creating an extraperitoneal space through which the terminal end of the descending colon is brought out for terminal colostomy. This is known as extraperitoneal colostomy.

From outside, the skin wound is retracted for putting sutures between the rectus sheath and the taenia coli. Four interrupted stitches are applied all around the colon. This anchorage will prevent the terminal colostomy from retracting down into the parietal wound. It also prevents the feces running back into the peritoneal cavity.

Before the Peyer's clamp is released from the stoma, the main abdominal wound is closed in the usual way and the skin wound is covered with dressing. This will prevent the wound from contamination of the feces, when the Peyer's clamp is open for suturing the stoma with the skin edge.

For suturing through the skin, cutting needle is used for anchoring the stoma with the skin edge by interrupted stitches. The edge of the stoma is everted, thus forming a spout around the skin edge.

For this purpose, the needle is first inserted through the skin edge, then it takes a serosal bite from the colon and finally it takes a full thickness bite through the edge of the stoma (Fig. 10.11). When the ends are tied together, the stoma would be everted (Fig. 10.12). The lumen of the colostomy is checked by inserting the index finger. This will reveal whether it is too tight to pass the finger through. A colostomy bag is put around the stoma.

POSTOPERATIVE CARE AND COMPLICATIONS

Postoperative care remains the same as in any other colonic surgery. And the risk of postoperative complications is no more different from other colonic surgery. Minor fecal discharge

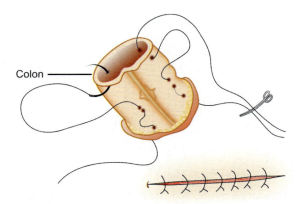

Fig. 10.11: Method of terminal colostomy in the LIF

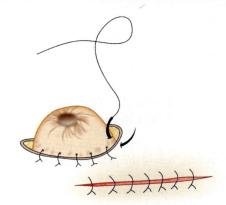

Fig. 10.12: The technique for the construction of terminal colostomy

through the drainage wound may resolve in three months time, if there is no general peritonitis and no distal obstruction. A colostomy bag could be put on this fistula track, until it closes by itself. But patient may need to go back to the theater, should there be any evidence of anastomotic dehiscence, pelvic abscess, intestinal obstruction, bleeding, burst abdomen or generalized peritonitis.

For septic shock and fecal peritonitis, preoperative resuscitation is necessary for the correction of fluid deficit, electrolytes imbalance, anemia and restoration of kidney function. Further consultation would be required for this emergency surgery. The question of colostomy must be highlighted with the patient and consent is to be obtained from the patient.

There could be additional complications with the terminal colostomy. These are retraction, cyanosis or necrosis of the colostomy, stenosis of the stoma, parastomal herniation, prolapse of the colostomy, and herniation of the small intestine through the parietal wall, lateral to the descending colon.

Surgical intervention may be required in dealing with the problems, as and when they cause concern to the patient and the surgeon. In some cases, emergency operation may be required for dealing with the gangrenous state of the colostomy. In other cases, elective surgery may be contemplated for stomal stenosis, parastomal herniation or prolapse of the stoma. In these cases, refashioning, or redone of colostomy may be necessary on a new site.

CONSTRUCTION OF THE TRANSVERSE LOOP COLOSTOMY

In emergency surgery, this is a life-saving operation. This is done in those cases, in which, the patient had presented with fecal peritonitis, or gross colonic obstruction, not suitable for definitive surgery. The purpose of loop colostomy is to prepare the patient for undertaking definitive restorative surgery at a later date, when the general condition of the patient has improved.

Closure of the colostomy is undertaken at suitable time after the second operative procedure being done, provided the postoperative contrast enema does not suggest any leakage through the previous anastomosis.

In elective surgery, colostomy is constructed with a view to protecting the anastomosis from being broken down. In other condition, it is done as a palliative procedure, if the tumor in the left colon is not resectable, provided there is no ascites, nor was there any widespread metastasis.

■ Procedure

After dealing with the fecal peritonitis or acute dilatation of the colon, the proximal transverse colon is isolated for 3-4 inches from the greater omentum. The latter is separated from its attachment to the antimesenteric border of the colon.

If the colon is grossly dilated, it may be associated with the serosal tear and the latter is more often seen along the taeniae coli. And the commonest site for serosal tear is over the cecum, decompression of the colon must be carried out in order to stop further tear, and the serosal tear is repaired with a continuous suture, using 2/0 polydioxin thread.

The procedure for such colonic evacuation has been described in the previous pages. The site for decompression should be proximal to the middle colic artery, so that this site could be used for colostomy. Therefore, it is important to select the site for colostomy that could be used for Savage decompression.

After the colon has been evacuated, a window is created through the mesentery without interfering with the right branch of the middle colic artery. And this is done by pushing the index finger close to the mesenteric attachment. A rubber tube is passed through this window. It is held together by the artery forceps.

The right edge of the laparotomy wound is picked up by the tissue forceps. The assistant keeps on holding these forceps, thus keeping the wound edge straight along the midline.

The site for the loop colostomy would be two inches away from the right costal margin, and 2 inches from the right wound margin (Fig. 10.13).

A transverse incision is made over the proposed site of colostomy. It is cut deep through the fat, until the anterior rectus sheath is in sight. It is also incised along the same line, but the opening of the rectus sheath should be made wider by cutting across its edge. The underlying muscles are split up between the fibers, and its opening is made wider by inserting the two index fingers, as described with the terminal colostomy. Under the protection of the large swab that is put inside the peritoneal cavity, the peritoneum is incised transversely.

The size of the colostomy wound is assessed by inserting three fingers through and through. If the wound is not wide

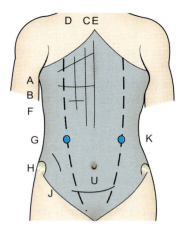

Fig. 10.13: The site for the incision over the right side of the upper abdomen has been marked with a letter F. It is the proposed site for a transverse incision to be made for the construction of a transverse loop colostomy

enough, the loop of the colon may be squashed by the contraction of the muscles that may not permit flatus and feces coming though the colostomy.

Through this wound, the ends of the rubber tube holding the transverse colon are pulled out through this wound. From inside, the loop of the transverse colon is gently pushed by the fingers, while the rubber tube is kept on pulling concurrently. Eventually, the loop of the transverse colon is brought out. Once it has been brought out of the wound, a rubber bridge is passed through the same mesenteric window that was made under the colon, before it was pulled out. This loop of the transverse colon will be resting on this rubber bridge that lies across the wound. Make sure that the loop of the colon is in line with the transverse colon (Fig. 10.14).

There are many types of bridge available for the loop colostomy or ileostomy. They are plastic tube, butterfly-shaped plastic flange, glass rod and thick rubber tube. One of them could be used as a bridge under the colon.

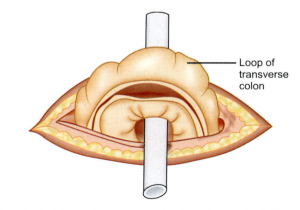

Fig. 10.14: A loop of transverse colon is resting on the bridge and a transverse incision has been made along the taenia coli with a view to constructing the transverse loop colostomy

Rubber tube or glass rod keeps the loop of the colon above the skin surface, and its position is maintained all along even after the bridge has been removed in 7 days time. This is due to adhesions of the colonic wall made with the surrounding wound. If the thin plastic flange is used alternative to the rubber tube, it does not interfere with the tight fitting of the colostomy ring around the bridge. In both cases, the ends of the rubber tube or the plastic flange are sutured with the skin. This will stop the bridge being disconnected from the skin or slipping into the peritoneal cavity.

The next question would be whether the colostomy could be opened straightaway or it should be done 2-3 days later. Both could be adopted that depends upon the convenience, but the tension of the abdominal cavity would be much less, if the colostomy is opened straightaway on the same operating table.

If the condition permits, it should be opened and in particular it should be done if there is evidence of colonic obstruction. Before the colon is opened, the serosal layer and the Taenia coli of the colon are sutured with the aponeurotic tissue. These are also sutured with skin edges by interrupted stitches. This anchorage that seals the space around the colon would stop the feces getting through the colostomy wound into the peritoneal cavity.

The added benefit would be that the colostomy is very unlikely to retract, after the bridge is removed sooner. After the colon has been anchored to the surrounding tissue, the laparotomy wound is closed first. And the skin wound is covered with appropriate wound dressing. This will protect the wound from fecal contamination.

The wound margin around the colon is protected by putting paraffin gauze, before the colostomy is opened. With a cutting diathermy needle, a longitudinal incision is made along the taeniae coli, taking a due precaution that the needle has not gone through the posterior wall of the colon. Initially, air bubble and loose motion will emerge through the tiny hole. It is next made wide by the scissors that would admit the index finger into the lumens lying by the side of the bridge.

The cut edges of the colostomy are sutured to the skin edges by interrupted stitches—thus everting its edges. At the end, the patency and its size of the lumen is examined by inserting the index finger. During this maneuver, air bubbles and loose motion may start emerging through the colostomy.

Alternatively, colon could be opened by a transverse incision made across the colon but suturing of the cut edges of the colonic wall to the skin edges may not be easy.

Decompression of the colon on both sides of the bridge is carried out by passing a suction tube. This mechanical evacuation will reduce the distention of the colon, thus taking away the intra-abdominal tension. As a result, patient will feel comfortable and there will be a less risk of wound dehiscence. A colostomy bag is fitted around the bridge.

Despite this benefit, there remains a risk of spillage of fecal fluid through the wound. On the other hand, suturing the colostomy wall with the skin edges would be unnecessary if the colostomy is opened 2-3 days later. For this work, anesthesia is not required, because of the fact that patient will not experience pain. The reason is that the bowel has no somatic nerve supply. Hence, it is a painless procedure that could be done in the dressing room of the ward. Only a diathermy set-up is required.

If diathermy pad is attached to the thigh, necessary precaution must be taken against the electric shock. Such precaution is not necessary for a monopolar diathermy set. The technique for opening the colostomy remains the same but the colon is opened transversely and the cut edges of the colon are not required to be sutured with the skin edges. And there would be no risk of running of the fecal fluid through the colostomy wound. Postoperative bowel adhesion with the skin margins will prevent the fecal fluid from entering into the peritoneal wound.

In this case, the bridge should not be removed in less than seven days. If removed sooner, the colostomy may drop down that may interfere with the objective of defunctioning of the distal colon. Such problem may not be encountered with the previous technique.

CONSTRUCTION OF THE PELVIC LOOP COLOSTOMY

In elective case, loop colostomy could be constructed in the left iliac fossa, where the loop of the sigmoid colon is brought out through a grid iron incision. This procedure is undertaken as a palliative measure, if the tumor is inoperable and causing colonic obstruction.

It is also indicated as an adjuvant measure to improve the quality of life, if the patient needs radiotherapy for the rectal or anal carcinoma, or patient has developed rectovaginal or colovesical fistula. Laparotomy is unnecessary in these cases. It should not be contemplated if there are widespread metastasis, with or without collection of ascites.

Procedure

For the construction of pelvic loop colostomy, the grid iron incision is made, medial to the anterior superior iliac spine. This exploration would be the same like the operation for appendicectomy, in which case, the peritoneum is opened through the gap created by splitting the external oblique aponeurosis and by splitting up the transversus abdominis and internal oblique muscle fibers.

In this approach, if the sigmoid loop is not accessible, or it is found stuck with the parietal wall by the peritoneum, mobilization of the colon would be necessary, in which case, the colon is gently pulled towards the umbilicus, by the

Babcock forceps. This maneuver would reveal the reflection of the parietal peritoneum holding the colon down.

The parietal peritoneum is incised with a pair of long scissors, thus allowing the pelvic colon to be mobilized forwards with a swab holding forceps. The mobilization is also continued in both directions, until a good length of the gut is mobilized with a view to bringing a loop of colon out through the wound.

In this blind procedure, care is taken against injury to the left ureter and testicular or ovarian vessels. To avoid this injury, the posterior wall of the mesentery is examined under direct vision, whether the ureter has been dragged along with the mesentery. If it could not be identified behind the mesentery, it is more likely that the ureter has not come up with the mesentery.

At last, the loop of the colon is brought out through the wound, where, a bridge is passed through the small window of the mesentery, just below the colon; but without damaging the vessels. The principle of opening of the colostomy remains the same, as described before with the transverse colostomy.

TELESCOPIC PELVIC LOOP OR TERMINAL COLOSTOMY

For the benign pathological conditions, as referred to above, pelvic loop colostomy could be constructed with the help of a colonoscope. In this technique, two sets of team are necessary for this procedure, in that one surgeon or the gastroenterologist will perform the colonoscopy, and another team will carry out the telescopic colostomy under general anesthesia.

Colonoscopy or flexible sigmoidoscopy could be carried out either in lithotomy or in left lateral position, but this procedure should be done under general anesthesia from the outset. The colonoscope is passed through the anal canal, when the patient is in the lithotomy position or lying in left lateral position. It is negotiated through the bends of the sigmoid colon until it reaches in the left iliac fossa.

If the initial colonoscopy is carried out in left lateral position, it is now necessary to turn the body to be placed on the supine position, and to turn the tip of the colonoscope anteriorly with a view to keeping it against the abdominal wall. The colonoscopic light could be seen illuminating through the skin in the left iliac fossa. The illumination would be brighter, if the main theater light is temporarily switched off. The operating surgeon must be ready for the next operating procedure.

CONSTRUCTION OF TELESCOPIC COLOSTOMY

Patient is placed in supine position on the operating table and the head end of the table is tilted down. A limited area is cleaned with antiseptic skin solution and is covered with sterile towel. A circular incision, measuring to about 2 inches, is then made exactly on the site of the illumination. The wound is deepened with a pen knife until the external oblique aponeurosis is in sight. This procedure is done under good light, but the tip of the colonoscope that continues to keep holding it in the same place firmly is next palpated by the index finger, before the peritoneum is opened.

The wound is held retracted by the two retractors, when the peritoneum is incised. The tip of the colonoscope is felt again by the index finger, and the colon is next picked up by the Babcock forceps. The colonoscope is withdrawn for a few inches down and away from the site of the colostomy. This would assist the surgeon to mobilize a limited segment of the colon from the pelvic wall, if it has a short mesentery. The loop of the sigmoid colon—once mobilized is brought out for a loop colostomy. The remaining procedure remains the same. At the end, the colonoscope is taken out of the rectum.

COMPLICATION OF THE PELVIC LOOP COLOSTOMY

This procedure is carried out with a limited access. It is a blind procedure. Risk of injury to ureter, testicular or ovarian vessels or small intestine could not be ruled out, while undertaking this procedure. And in some cases, the finding of the sigmoid colon may be difficult. In that case, patient may need a laparotomy.

It is also possible that the loop of the sigmoid colon may be twisted, when it is brought out blindly. As a result, the stoma may be constructed on the distal limb of the sigmoid colon, instead of constructing on the proximal limb.

COMPLICATION OF THE TELESCOPIC COLOSTOMY

Complication could be worse; if terminal colostomy is constructed instead of a loop colostomy being done. In this case, confusion may arise if the loop of the colon is transected inside the peritoneal cavity, by the autosuture using TA 30 or 55, where the proximal blind end is left behind in the peritoneal cavity by mistake and instead, the distal end is brought out with a view to constructing a terminal colostomy.

This gross error became apparent after 3-4 days when the patient had started complaining of distention of the abdomen, pain and vomiting. Plain X-ray will reveal the evidence of colonic obstruction. This needs confirmation by the gastrograffin enema. Of course, a second operation would be inevitable in this case.

To avoid this complication, colonoscope or sigmoidoscope should be inserted either through the anus or through the stoma. This will confirm, whether there was any error in the construction of colostomy.

SPHINCTER-SAVING LOW ANTERIOR RESECTION OF THE RECTUM

■ Preview of the Physiological and the Technical Merits of the Sphincter-saving Low Anterior Resection

This technique seems to be appealing to the patients, on the understanding that they do not need to carry a colostomy bag. The questions that remain to be scrutinized are whether it provides a good quality of life and whether the patients are benefited from the low anterior resection of the rectum. Preservation of the anal sphincter seems to be an emotional bargain for this technique to be used for those rectal carcinomas located between 6 and 10 cm from the anal verge.

Apart from this single criterion, Dukes tumor stage and accessibility to the growth has to be taken into a final decision. Dukes classified that only 15 percent of the rectal carcinoma were found to be Dukes A, where the growth remained limited to the rectal wall, Dukes B was 35 percent among the patients where it had invaded the extrarectal tissue but the lymph glands were not invaded by the tumor. The remaining cases were classified as Dukes C, where the tumor had invaded the lymphatic channels.[1] Apart from the lymphatic invasion, malignant cells do invade the extramural venous channels.

Therefore, only a small number of cases would be suitable for this technique; but over 50 percent of the cases would be unsuitable for this operation. This evidence is based upon the histology. But at laparotomy, it would be difficult for the surgeon to find out, whether the tumor staging of the growth which is in the extraperitoneal space is limited to Dukes A or Dukes B.

If the cases with advanced growth are included in this technique, these patients would be at risk of developing colonic obstruction due to recurrence of the tumor in the pelvis and around the anastomosis. Alternative to this approach would be the abdominoperineal resection (APR) that would not put the patient to the potential risk of second operation; if recurrences have occurred in the pelvis.

Furthermore, among the cases with tumor of Dukes A, it has to be judged in perspective about the anal sphincter function such as anal incontinence. It is imperative to evaluate the long-term benefit, in those cases in which the curative operation is to be carried out successfully and in those cases in which, the rectal tumor is below 6 cm from the anal verge. Goligher has found in his study that the physiological anal sphincteric function which provides a total continent is associated with the sensation, generated in the rectal wall.[2,3] Hence, the sphincteric function is expected to be impaired in some cases and in those cases, where the rectal wall has been excised.

Furthermore, the sense of urgency for defecation is also triggered off from the stretch receptors present in the puborectalis muscle. Clinical experience supports the physiological operation of the defecation that the initial stage for defecation begins in response to the limit of stretching of the puborectalis muscles and the rectum. This stretching is affected by the volume of the feces held in the rectum. And these muscles initially keep holding the rectum forwards, thus preventing the feces from further descent. It seems these muscle fibers act like a string of the bow. When they are stretched to their maximum limit, the stretch receptors present within these fibers and in the rectal wall are triggered off producing a squeeze around the rectum —thus pushing the lumps of feces further downwards. This gives a sense of urge to defecate and defecation becomes imminent. Eventually, defecation is completed by a combination of peristaltic contraction of the circular muscles of the rectum along with that of the puborectalis muscles.

The minimum volume of the feces that initiate to stretch of the puborectalis muscles from within the rectum is around 50 ml. This stretching effect gives rise to a sense of urgency. The mechanism of the anal continent cannot operate independently, in the absence of the rectal wall and the puborectalis muscles, despite the nerve supply to the sphincters being preserved.

PREOPERATIVE ADJUVANT TREATMENT

In certain cases, patient may require preoperative radiotherapy and chemotherapy that has to be determined at the combined meeting of the specialties, known as multidisciplinary team (MDT), where the results are discussed with radiotherapist, chemotherapist and pathologist. This has been a new policy in the management of cancer of the rectum. Benefit from the preoperative adjuvant therapy remains controversial, but there are evidences to support the argument.

Preoperative adjuvant radiotherapy to the advanced tumor does not alter the tumor staging or improve the prognosis, but it may transform from inoperable to operable tumor staging and enhances the prospect of surgical resection of the tumor.

Over the last decade, preoperative adjuvant chemotherapy and/or deep X-ray therapy have been a standard clinical practice. If the tumor is mobile and resectable, then debulking of the tumor by surgical ablation should be the primary aim, instead of relying upon the preoperative adjuvant therapy. The local surgical clearance of the tumor would be much quicker, and more effective than relying upon the adjuvant chemotherapy and radiotherapy. The therapeutic result will depend upon many factors. They are sensitivity of the tissue, dose of the drug or radiation, size of the tumor tissue and dose and duration of chemotherapy and radiotherapy. These are interlinked between the response and size of the tumor.

In some cases, adjuvant preoperative chemotherapy would be relatively less effective with the therapeutic dose if the tumor appears to be bulky. This is because, its penetrating power to the center core of the tumor mass would be less effective, where the vascularity remains very poor. Nevertheless, it would take much longer time, to reduce the bulky tumor mass to a bare minimum.

The efficacy of a therapeutic dose is dependent upon the total mass of the target tumor. Furthermore, the tumor cells will continue shedding via venous and lymphatic channels during the period of adjuvant preoperative therapy.

In fact, it would be more likely the case that chemotherapy would be more effective in treating the residual tumor mass, left *in situ*, after surgical ablation of the bulk of the tumor being carried out. Its therapeutic benefit would be widespread in those cases, in which, the tumor has deposited in the distant lymph nodes, liver, lungs, bones and brain. Nevertheless, preoperative adjuvant therapy seems to be a present trend in treating the colorectal cancer.

PREOPERATIVE PREPARATION

The preparation for this operation is no different from the anterior resection or abdominoperineal resection (APR). All the advices and the treatment protocol have been highlighted in the appropriate sections.

Preoperative adjuvant radiotherapy was not a routine clinical practice until 1978. It was initially recommended for advanced and bulky rectal tumor. The main objective was to see the effect of the deep X-ray therapy to the tumor which was previously thought to be radioresistant.

Dr Emmanuel, consultant radiotherapist (Sheffield) proposed, whether we could assist his research by referring cases with a rectal carcinoma for preoperative full dose external beam radiotherapy. In response to his guideline, we referred to him a few rectal carcinomas that appeared to be bulky by rectal digital examination and that may not be suitable for abdominoperineal resection.

But the results were excellent showing a complete resolution of the macroscopical appearance of the rectal tumor. The total dose used in those patients was 45Gy (4500 rad) delivered in divided doses over six weeks. There was erythema and redness around the perineum. Therefore, the operation for abdominoperineal resection was delayed for another 3-4 weeks.

At the completion of the operation, photograph was taken from the resected specimen of the rectum that was opened up along its full length. This showed that the previous bulky rectal tumor, present in less than 10 cm from anal verge, was found completely disappeared from the mucosal surface, as if the tumor had melted away and it was hardly recognizable macroscopically. This was the conclusive evidence of the preoperative radiotherapy before abdominoperineal resection of the rectum was done in 1979 (Figs 10.15A and B).

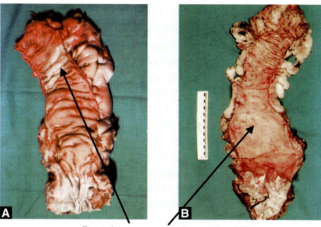

Rectal tumor melted away by DXT

Figs 10.15A and B: These two illustrations are from two patients, after the tumor was treated with radiotherapy, using a dose of 4.5GY (4500r). There was very little evidence of any residual tumor left *in situ*, after the treatment was given

We concluded beyond doubt that adjuvant radiotherapy had transformed the inoperable to operable tumor and it contributed to a radical resection, but my limited experiences did not suggest that it had altered the tumor staging and survival rate. Surprisingly, it did not affect in achieving primary perineal wound healing in all those cases treated with preoperative radiotherapy.

Since then, further study was carried out, and Swedish rectal cancer trial showed improved survival with preoperative radiotherapy in those cases in which the tumor was regarded to be resectable.[4]

It is now a routine practice to give a short course of preoperative radiotherapy and/or chemotherapy for sphincter-saving low anterior resection. The recommended dose for these cases would be 25Gy (2500 rad) in divided doses over one week. Of course, the policy for preoperative adjuvant therapy remains with the oncology department, the question could be highlighted in perspective whether the size of the tumor could be reduced with half the dose and within one week of the treatment completed; until such evidence is available, the views remain skeptical to the efficacy of this new mode of treatment.

The main objective for preoperative radiotherapy for the rectal tumor is to reduce the risk of local recurrence and to reduce the bulkiness of the tumor, but such beneficial effect is very unlikely to be achieved, in those circumstances in which viable malignant cells remain in the tumor bed of the rectum.

In the literature, so far no photographic evidence, like the previous one, was available that the size of the rectal tumor was found reduced in response to a reduced dose of radiotherapy, delivered in one week. It is presumed that it would not be equally effective in achieving the same objective, comparable to the result with a full dose of radiotherapy. Furthermore, it is equally important to know how effective it would be in less than two weeks using half of the therapeutic dose used in sphincter-saving low anterior resection. In my experience, the response to any regimen of therapy is related to therapeutic dose and total duration of treatment. Improved survival rate may be attributable to many contributing factors that could not be measured objectively, by a single factor.

It is equally important to be fully aware of the biological effect to the local tissue in response to a full dose. And it could be detrimental to the primary anastomosis; if sphincter-saving low anterior resection were carried out. Therefore, a reduced dose seems to be rational in avoiding a potential risk of postradiation proctitis, local vasculitis and anastomotic dehiscence. But these sorts of postoperative morbidities could be avoided if abdominoperineal resection is carried out instead. In view of these pros and cons, final decision should be taken with the full knowledge of the patient.

PREOPERATIVE CONSULTATION

Patient must be explained about the broad outline of the operative procedures, in that the need for temporary ileostomy has to be explained. And the risk of complications with the ileostomy has to be highlighted. Apart from this issue, the issues of anastomotic dehiscence in the pelvis and the question of further exploration for dealing with the anastomotic leakage, pelvic abscess or fistula require a thorough discussion and documentation in the case note. Patient should be provided with a printed leaflet about the merits of this operation.

Patient is advised that a suitable site has to be identified in advance for the loop ileostomy to be constructed in the right iliac fossa. This can only be done by the appliance set, fitted on the waist. And in this trial, the ileostomy bag, filled with water is fitted on to the appliance, as if the patient was carrying the true ileostomy bag that contains loose motion. This simulating experiment will reveal many unexpected problems, whether it causes any discomfort, or it drags down or the proposed site interferes with the day-to-day wearing of his or her clothing.

Colostomy nurse must be sitting with the patient, when this trial is conducted. The technical problem with the ileostomy bag could be the soiling of the clothes, if the ileostomy bag is pushed upwards in sitting position. If this seems to be the case in the trial, the appliance set needs to be fitted higher up.

This is the important part that needs to be sorted out when the trial is conducted by sitting as well as by walking in the ward. With these problems in mind, an appropriate site in the RIF has to be selected in order to obviate this embarrassing situation. Once this has been worked out, the site is marked out with a skin pencil.

It has to be reminded that the temporary ileostomy could be permanent if there is evidence of anal stenosis, stricture of the colorectal anastomosis, local recurrence or persisting leakage from the anastomosis, shown on repeated gastrograffin enema.

In other cases with uneventful recovery, frequency of bowel movements, urge-incontinence, or wet bottom should be ventilated to the patients.

TECHNIQUE FOR THE SPHINCTER-SAVING LOW ANTERIOR RESECTION

The patient is placed in the supine position on the main Lloyd Davis table and both lower limbs are left on the extended limbs on the Trendelenburg–lithotomy position, as described in the operation of APR. The skin preparation and layout of the sterile towels need not be repeated. After a thorough laparotomy has been completed, final decision is taken, on the following criteria: that the growth is mobile, there is no evidence of enlarged lymph nodes palpable along the vessels or in the mesentery, it is not bulky and above the level of 6 cm from the anal verge. If these criteria are satisfied, low anterior resection with the conservation of the sphincter should be undertaken.

The technique for the mobilization of the sigmoid colon and the tumor bearing area of the rectum remains the same, apart from the level of resection of the superior hemorrhoidal vessels. These are divided and ligated below the growth.

In addition, the descending colon and the splenic flexure may require to be mobilized, as described with the operation for left hemicolectomy. In this case, the inferior mesenteric artery, which arises from the abdominal aorta, is divided. The ends are ligatured. All other branches and vascular arcades are not disturbed. These vessels are expected to supply the blood right down to the level of anastomosis.

ANASTOMOSIS BY STAPLING GUN

The rectum is divided between the two pairs of clamps. They are applied across the rectum, but it should be applied at least 2 cm clear margin distal to the lower edge of the tumor. This is a new approach, but as to how this level of identification could be made on the operating table remains in question. But it is done by just palpation of the tumor mass from outside the colon.

The occlusion of the rectum could be done either by the autosuture TA 55 or by the right angled clamps that depends upon the availability of the instruments in the theater. After the rectum has been transected, the proximal rectal stump is brought up above the pelvis, but necessary precaution is taken so that the stoma does not slip out of the clamp or the blades of the latter does not come off. The technique for applying the stapling circular gun has been described in the operation of anterior resection.

Any bleeding from the sacral venous plexus or from the middle rectal arteries is controlled. This would be the most difficult task for the surgeon to reduce the venous oozing. Arterial bleeding could be controlled with coagulation, but venous oozing should be dealt with due care. Packing with the oxycel gauze (surgicel) will reduce the oozing. If no sign of improvement is evident, packing the pelvic cavity remains the only option for the time being. It should be left in place for 10 minutes. Fresh frozen plasma may require to be transfused if the platelet count is very low.

The sigmoid colon is next taken down to the pelvis with a view to undertaking anastomosis with the distal rectal stump. In doing so, the splenic flexure may need to be mobilized as described before and it is then brought down in order to avoid any tension encountered with the anastomosis.

After a proper assessment, the descending colon is divided between the two clamps, but a soft clamp should be applied across the descending colon a few inches above the proposed line of resection and crushing clamp is applied at the level of resection, below the soft clamp. The specimen is sent for histology.

If the autosuture gun TA 55 has been applied across the distal rectum, saline wash-out is given through the anus by the second assistant standing between the two thighs. The stapling gun of a suitable size which could be between EEA 25 and 31 is next negotiated through the anus by the assistant, until it reaches the distal stapled rectal stump. The assistant pushes the spike of the circular stapling gun, by clockwise rotation of the knob, fitted with the gun. This spike comes out through the posterior wall of the stapled sutures.

Next, purse string suture is inserted around the edge of the proximal colonic stump, before the latter is glided over the anvil and firmly tied to the central rod. The anvil is next fitted to the cartridge. Care is taken that the mucosal ends are not hanging outside or the mesentery or the appendices epiploicae has not been caught up in the cartridge. If they are caught up between the anvil and the cartridge, the staples would not be able to get through the wall of the stomas. This is due to the fact that the combined stomal walls would be much thicker that the length of the staples. As a result, there will be no stapled anastomosis in the particular site. Anastomosis will breakdown in the particular area.

Once this has been satisfied, the descending colon is rotated to 90 degree to the left and the mesentery remains to the right side. It is slowly withdrawn towards the cartridge, by anticlockwise rotation of the knob; until they are tightly held together and until the green line turns up (Fig. 10.16).

Assistant is asked to fire the gun, thus the staples made up with stainless steel are inserted in two rows between the two anastomotic ends and at the same time a rim of circular colonic edge is transected concurrently from the respective stoma.

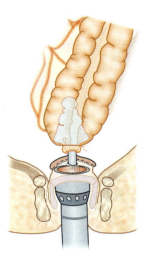

Fig. 10.16: Autosutures used in low anterior resection

The instrument is gently twisted in anticlockwise direction; until a click is heard, indicating that the cartridge is free from the anastomosis. The gun is eventually withdrawn slowly by half rotation in clockwise and anticlockwise direction until it comes out of the anal orifice.

A few interrupted sutures should be given around the anastomosis for a better security. The pair of the doughnuts is retrieved from the gun and they are sent separately for histology. This will confirm whether or not there was any evidence of malignant cells in either of the two doughnuts.

The anastomotic line could be covered with the parietal peritoneum and greater omentum; if available. There should not be any tension of the proximal colon.

All the small intestine is put back into the pelvis. The table should be put back in the neutral position. A redivac drain or a tube drain is left in the pelvis. At the end, construction of loop ileostomy is undertaken in the right iliac fossa. This will be described separately. The abdominal wound is closed in the usual way.

ALTERNATIVE APPROACH TO DEAL WITH THE RESECTION

To overcome this problem in a limited space, only one clamp could be applied, 2 cm below the tumor (Fig. 10.17). Although these technical problems could be overcome by many ways, question may be raised on how it is possible for the surgeon to be sure by external palpation that the distal rectal stump would be 2 cm clear from the tumor margin, before it is incised, and how could it be sure that tumor has not implanted in the line of anastomosis?

However, each case is judged by the palpation of the rectal tumor, before the rectum is divided. And in the limited space, it is divided with a right angled cutting diathermy needle. In

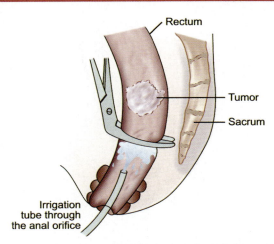

Fig. 10.17: Rectal wash-out with saline is given through the anal orifice. The purpose is to wash out any tumor cells dislodged from the primary tumor during handling and mobilization of the rectum. The rectum is transected below the clamp by a right angled cutting diathermy needle

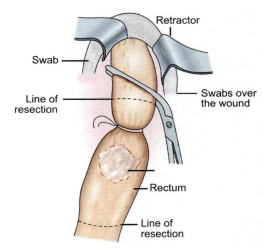

Fig. 10.18: A right-angled clamp is applied 2 cm below the tumor margin

this method, running suture should be applied around the cut edge of the distal stump. And this is done every time, a small cut is made. This running suture will control the bleeding and at the same time, it would act as a stay suture, it would keep holding the edge of the stump in position that would assist in undertaking end-to-end anastomosis by interrupted sutures.

Alternatively, a tourniquet could be applied around the rectum at a desired level below the tumor. This may stop spillage of the malignant cells during resection of the rectum. The distal part of the rectum should be washed out by a rubber tube or a Foley's catheter, passed through the anus, before a right-angled clamp is applied across the rectum below the said tourniquet. The rectum is divided at the level between the level of tourniquet and that of the clamp (Fig. 10.18). Having done this resection, the descending or pelvic colon is divided between the clamps and the level of resection should be at 10 cm above the level of the rectal tumor. The anastomosis between the proximal transected stoma of the descending colon and the distal rectal stump could be carried out by interrupted stitches or by autosuture.

Alternative to the techniques just described is the resection of the rectum between the two clamps applied below the safe level of the tumor, provided there is adequate room available for the two clamps to be applied across the rectum (Fig. 10.19).

If anastomosis is not done by circular gun, end-to-end anastomosis could be performed with interrupted stitches using the same technique as used in the anterior resection (Fig. 10.20).

To perform this hand anastomosis, a full length suture (2/0) for each stitch, a pair of long needle holder, a pair of long tooth forceps and a pair of long scissors must be used. The technique for end-to-end single layer anastomosis would be

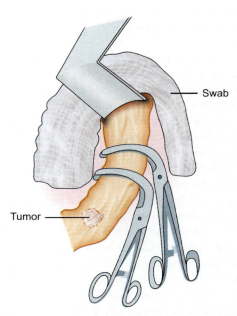

Fig. 10.19: Resection of the rectum between the two clamps applied 2 cm below the tumor

no different from other high anterior resection, despite working in the limited space.

Each suture bite is given between the two transected ends and they are separately held together by the artery forceps. No suture should be tied, until all interrupted stitches are applied around the stomas (Fig. 10.20). At the end the threads are ligated one after another. And they are cut out.

In this operative procedure, various alternative approaches to the resection of the rectum have been described, but a selection of a particular technique has to be made after evaluating the tumor, and surrounding space in the depth of the pelvis.

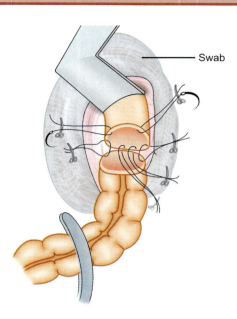

Fig. 10.20: Sphincter-saving low anterior resection showing the technique on how end-to-end anastomosis between the two stomas is carried out by hand sutures

A large pack is put in the peritoneal cavity under the proposed site of the incision, where the loop of terminal ileostomy is to be sited, as shown in the Figure 10.21.

A circular skin incision is made over the proposed site. The diameter would be 3 cm. The subcutaneous fat, aponeurotic fascia or the anterior rectus sheath is all excised in line with the skin incision.

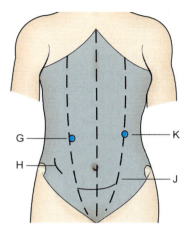

Fig. 10.21: The site of loop ileostomy is marked by G

At the completion of anastomosis, the anastomotic line should be covered by a patch of greater omentum and/or it is left in the extraperitoneal space. This is done by mobilizing the peritoneum from back of the bladder and side wall of the pelvis. It is sutured to the side wall of the rectum a little above the line of anastomosis. Pelvic cavity is thoroughly washed with warm saline at room temperature. Metronidazole lavage is given to the pelvis, like any other operation, as described before. A tube drain should be left in the pelvis near the site of anastomosis. All the guts and the greater omentum are put back in order, before a loop ileostomy is constructed.

CONSTRUCTION OF LOOP ILEOSTOMY

It is done in conjunction with the low anterior resection. It is a temporary measure against the potential risk of anastomotic dehiscence that may occur at the low anterior resection of the rectum. The main objective is to reverse the loop ileostomy at some stage after the result of gastrograffin enema that will show evidence of any leakage or dehiscence at the anastomosis.

The site for the construction of loop of terminal ileostomy is in the right iliac fossa. The skin surface should be smooth and away from the scar, the umbilicus and anterior superior iliac spine. This should be borne in mind at the time of construction, if the site has not been marked, before the patient is brought to the theater.

The skin edge is next held by the tissue forceps, by the assistant. The position of the laparotomy wound must be brought to the preoperative position by this gentle pull.

The underlying muscles are split up along its fibers. The posterior peritoneum is next opened by the scissors. The opening is made wide that could be sufficient for the loops of the small intestine to be brought out.

A small mesenteric window is created for the rubber or glass bridge to get through so that the loop of ileostomy can rest on the bridge for a few days. And it is made 8 inches proximal to the ileocecal junction.

To identify the proximal limb of the ileostomy, a suture marker is inserted through the serosal wall of the intestine. This should be an inch proximal to the mesenteric window so that the proximal limb could be identified when the ileostomy will be constructed.

This landmark would be necessary, when the ileostomy spout is to be constructed from the mucosal wall delivered from the lumen of the proximal limb of the loop of intestine and not from the distal limb of the same loop of the ileum. There should not be any ambiguity in the opening of the proximal limb. It is also equally important that the loop of the intestine that has been brought out has not been twisted.

The proposed loop of the terminal ileum is brought out through the ileostomy wound with the help of Babcock forceps. A rubber tube is next passed through the window of the mesentery and it would act as a bridge of the ileostomy. It is anchored with the skin.

The parietal space lateral to the distal limb is closed by a continuous suture applied between the distal limb of the ileostomy and the parietal peritoneum of the surrounding space. This is necessary to stop herniation of the gut.

The loop of ileum is anchored with the peritoneal edge of the ileostomy wound. This is done from inside the abdomen. In the same way, the serosal wall of the intestine is sutured from outside with the external oblique aponeurotic tissue. Four or five interrupted sutures are applied all around the wound.

The abdominal wound is closed and is covered with the dressing.

For the construction of the mucosal spout, the length of the loop of ileum should be 3-4 inches above the skin margin, but the proximal limb should be longer from the suture mark, compared to the distal limb.

The wall of the ileum is open transversely on the right side of the suture marker but the height of the opening should be 2 cm from the skin on the right side of the bridge and it should be 6-7 cm from the skin on the left side of the bridge.

Through this stoma, the mucosal wall of about 4 cm long is pulled out from the lumen of the proximal limb, by the Babcock forceps, thus everting the edge of the stoma of the ileostomy (Figs 10.22 and 10.23).

This everted mucosal edge is glided down across the serosal wall of the proximal limb and is sutured to the skin edge all around, but the cut edge of the stoma from the distal limb is sutured to the skin edge. The height of this stoma would be less than 2 cm and that of the proximal spout would be around 4 cm from the skin surface.

For the construction of spout, a small cutting curved needle is inserted through the skin edge first. It is then passed through the serosal wall of the intestine at the skin level. The same needle is then taken through another small serosal bite a little above the previous one and a little above the skin edge and finally it is next passed through the edge of the stoma in full thickness. Both ends of the thread are held together by the artery forceps.

The procedure is repeated and 5-6 such sutures are applied for the construction of spout that would appear like a nipple.

At the end, all individual sutures are tied. The everted edge of the stoma will remain sutured with the skin edge. The length of the spout of the proximal ileostomy should be 3-4 cm above the skin surface. In contrast, there will be no such spout constructed through the distal limb, but its edge will be sutured to the skin edge. The height of this stoma would be less than 2 cm from the skin level.

The index finger is inserted into both lumens in order to be sure that the lumen of the ileostomy is satisfactory. Ileostomy bag is fitted around the mucocutaneous edge snugly, without leaving any bare skin lying around the mucocutaneous junction.

For this reason, the opening of the ileostomy bag should be equal to that of the ileostomy at the mucocutaneous junction. A plastic flange could be fitted with the Koraya gum that will protect the skin margin from the contact of the loose motion.

CONSTRUCTION OF TERMINAL ILEOSTOMY

Terminal ileostomy is permanent. The criteria for the selection of the site are no different from that of a loop ileostomy. It is necessary if total panprocto colectomy, or total colectomy is to be carried out. The commonest pathological lesions that require this major operation are total ulcerative colitis, not responding to conservative treatment, multiple polyposis coli, Crohn's colitis, and angiodysplasia, not responding to conservative treatment.

There is not much difference in the technique for the construction of the terminal ileostomy from the colostomy. In previous preoperative consultation, the selection for the site of ileostomy, postoperative care and long-term morbidity has already been outlined.

After the definitive operative procedure being completed, the ileostomy skin wound is prepared over the proposed site. The size of the wound should be 3 cm, as described before. The cut end of the terminal ileum is brought out by a pair of Babcock forceps. In the peritoneal cavity, the parietal space,

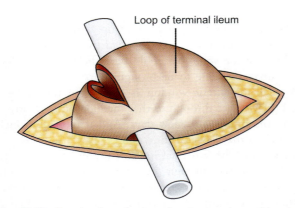

Fig. 10.22: Construction of a loop ileostomy, a loop of terminal ileum has been brought out

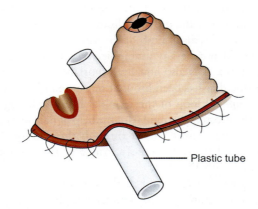

Fig. 10.23: The proximal stoma on the right side and the distal stoma on the left side of the bridge

lateral to the terminal intestine is closed by a continuous suture. And the free edge of the mesentery should be carefully sutured with the anterior peritoneal wall.

The length of the ileum should be 8 cm outside the abdominal wall. Therefore, in order to keep this length outside the skin surface, it is necessary to anchor the base of the said intestine between the serosal wall of the intestine and the aponeurotic tissue of the abdominal muscle, by a few interrupted sutures. This anchorage will stop the ileum returning into the peritoneal cavity. The boundary of the proposed site of anchorage needs to be defined by retracting the skin wound margin at one side and turning the intestine to the other side. A few interrupted sutures are inserted between the aponeurotic tissue and the serosal wall of the intestine using 2/0 dexon or Vicryl thread. These sutures must not go through the full thickness of the intestine. Otherwise, it would form a fistula.

For the construction of the mucosal spout, a pair of Babcock forceps is passed inside the lumen of the intestine. Its purpose is to hold a small segment of the mucosa with a view to pulling it from inside out when the Babcock forceps is slowly withdrawn. In undertaking this procedure, the edge of the stoma will be everted concurrently and it would slide down gradually over the serosal wall. Sometimes, the left thumb and the index finger are used in sliding down the stoma and mucosa over the serosal wall. As a result, the mucosa will stay outside the serosal wall of the intestine, and it would be inside out of the gut.

Ileostomy could be constructed in two ways. The simple approach is to anchor the everted edge of the stoma to the skin margin. Several interrupted sutures are inserted all around between the skin edge and the everted edge of the stoma.

Alternatively, a curved cutting needle with 2/0 Vicryl or dexon suture is first inserted through the skin edge and it is then pulled out from inside the said wound for a good length and then the same needle takes a first serosal bite at the same level with the skin margin. It is again pulled out from the serosal wall. After this bite, a series of a few small bites are taken from the serosal wall, until it reaches to the stomal end where the same needle takes a full thickness bite through the cut edge of the stoma, as shown in the Figure 10.24A. Both ends of the suture are held together by the artery forceps.

In this way, several similar anchoring procedures are carried out around the intestine. At the end, all these sutures are tied together one by one. The stoma will be everted in order to be sutured with the skin edge all around, as described in the Figure 10.24B. It is important to protect the skin around the mucocutaneous junction and it should be done with the fitting of the ileostomy bag snugly around the base of the ileostomy.

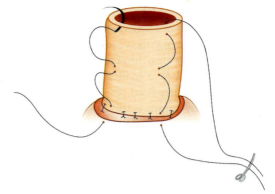

Fig. 10.24A: Construction of terminal ileostomy

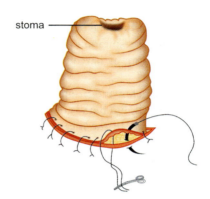

Fig. 10.24B: Showing the methods of everting the transected end of the ileostomy

POSTOPERATIVE CARE FOR THE LOW ANTERIOR RESECTION AND THE ILEOSTOMY

The average time required to complete this operation is over three hours. Patient remains in postoperative shock and requires continuous observation. Particular attention is given on the pulse rate, blood pressure, hourly urine output, temperature, respiration rate, perspiration, evidence of dehydration, and loss of blood in the drainage bottle.

Drop of hourly urine output below 40 ml may be attributable to pain, deficit of fluid balance, and shock. In normal cases, there will be an obligatory oliguria for the first 24 hours, despite maintaining a good blood pressure and pulse rate. Average total urine output is expected to be between 600 and 700 ml for the first 24 hours. But this clinical problem needs to be differentiated from the perioperative blood loss and deficit of fluid volume.

Hypotension associated with a rapid pulse rate and clammy feet or perspiration requires immediate attention. This could be due to hypovolemic shock, unless it could be due to the silent heart attack. Surgeon must look at the perioperative blood and fluid loss, whether there has been any deficit in that fluid balance during operation and how much these have been replaced.

Overtransfusion should be avoided. This may lead to cardiorespiratory embarrassment and pulmonary edema. Central venous pressure, jugular venous pressure and moisture of the tongue could provide clinical features of overtransfusion or dehydration. Therefore, a judicial assessment is necessary before pushing too much fluid.

Relief of pain may improve the oxygen saturation, if the patient is not on ventilation. It has been known that pain induces shallow breathing and increases rate of respiration that interferes with the oxygen saturation. And it also reduces the obligatory urine output per hour.[5]

If the patient is on PCA for postoperative pain relief, perspiration and hypotension may be attributable to respiratory depression. Again this has to be correlated to the rate of respiration per minute and the total dose of narcotics infused by the pump. If the rate of respiration drops to below 12 per minute, immediate antidote of narcotic should be infused through the vein.

In the mean time, further investigation should be arranged. These are blood gas analysis, full blood count, ECG, urea and electrolytes and chest X-ray. In the mean time, patient may respond well to replacement of blood loss and fluid challenge.

All prophylactic measures against the wound infection, chest infection and deep vein thrombosis must be continued until the patient recovers fully. After the first postoperative day, physiotherapy should be commenced and blood investigations are repeated. Further blood investigations on the successive day should be judged on the merits of the case.

On the 4th or 5th postoperative day, rise of temperature indicates systemic or local infection, if the chest infection could be excluded. The possibility of anastomotic dehiscence should be suspected. Collection of purulent fluid in the drainage bottle suggests pelvic abscess, whether or not it is attributable to necrosis or breakdown of the anastomosis. CT scan may reveal the source of infection. Patient may need to go back to the theater for the exploration of the abdomen.

POSTOPERATIVE COMPLICATION

Among the delayed complications, anal stenosis, and/or coloanal stricture anastomosis are expected to be present for various reasons. Disuse-atrophy is most likely the etiological factor, if the defunctioning ileostomy is not reversed soon. Other contributing factors are pelvic infection, preoperative local radiotherapy, ischemic condition, and local recurrence. It is difficult to treat this condition despite repeated dilation being carried out. Eventually many patients are contended with the permanent loop ileostomy but the whole objective would be defeated in this case.

Other morbidity would be a frequency of defecation, urgency and fecal incontinence, and loose motions that may lead to a debility condition and may discourage the patient going out in having a social life. Bladder dysfunction could be an added problem.

POSTOPERATIVE CARE AND MORBIDITY WITH ILEOSTOMY

Ileostomy does not work for the first two days. And for first few weeks, there will be a discharge of watery greenish motion in the bag. It needs to be emptied as and when necessary. To compensate the fluid deficit, intravenous fluid has to be increased. Color of the stoma should be checked. Contamination of the peristomal skin must be avoided. Bile is detrimental to the skin and it may cause skin excoriation.

Among other delayed morbidity or complications is parastomal herniation, prolapse of the stoma, ulceration of the mucosa, stenosis of the stoma, intestinal obstruction, vitamin B_{12} and folate deficiency, formation of gallstones, etc.

Therefore, the merits of the sphincter-saving low anterior resection must be judged by the following criteria:

a. Cumulative cost for the subsequent postoperative treatment per 100 patients.
b. Bed occupancy.
c. Anastomotic leakage.
d. Anal sphincteric dysfunction.
e. Anastomotic stricture and/or frozen pelvis due to infection.
f. Permanent ileostomy.
g. Local recurrence.
h. Overall 10 years survival rate.

The major postoperative complication is the anastomotic leakage. It ranges from 8 to 31.4 percent. It depends upon many factors. They are skill of the surgeon, faulty operative anastomosis, and anatomical position of the tumor and vascularity of the anastomotic sites.

The fact has to be highlighted that many authors do not wish to acknowledge the pitfalls of their own skill. They would analyze the results in various aspects, in order to divert the criticism. In one study, the results have been analyzed, based upon different criteria, included into several groups. These are curative resection, and palliative resection. In another analysis, the data have been distributed between the major and minor leaks or between the high and low anastomosis. But, all these are related to the operation. The true etiology for the anastomotic leakage is most likely to be avascular necrosis or ischemic change, if there is no mechanical defect, left at the site of anastomosis.

In the literature, it has been reported that the incidence of anastomotic leakage between the rectal stump and the sigmoid colon was found worse than between the rectal stump and splenic flexure of the colon and it was 31.3 and 14.4 percent respectively. Despite sacrificing a good length of a healthy left colon, the incidence of 14.4 percent seems to be very high.[6]

Many of these patients will suffer from intestinal hurry. This would be attributable to loss of absorptive power of fluid and loss of transit time of the feces. The question would be highlighted later whether there would be a further morbidity associated with anal sphincteric dysfunction.

It was obvious that anastomotic leakage was unavoidable in certain cases; inspite of the fact that a good length of healthy colon was excised and despite a defunctioning loop ileostomy had been constructed.

Obviously, the etiological factor for anastomotic leakage is primarily attributable to ischemic condition to the site of anastomosis. This also explains the reason as to why it takes four and six postoperative days, before the leak is clinically recognized. Peristalsis could not be the factor in this case, when ileostomy or colostomy has been constructed. It suggests that diversion of feces does not make any difference to the etiology of anastomotic leakage.

CLINICAL PRESENTATION OF ANASTOMOTIC LEAKAGE AND MANAGEMENT

However, anastomotic leakage is presented with peritonitis and septic shock. Routine assessment will reveal a rise of temperature, (swinging up and down) tachycardia, hypotension and dehydration. Abdominal examination will reveal a diffuse tenderness, marked guarding and rebound tenderness. In all postoperative cases, evidence of dull on percussion around the lower abdomen would be common. And it could be misleading in some cases. Rectal digital examination and proctoscopy must not be done. This sort of intervention may cause the anastomotic dehiscence.

After an initial assessment, patient first needs resuscitation for this septic shock. And then necessary investigations are arranged to establish the cause for developing peritonitis.

Apart from hematological investigation, other investigations include X-ray of the chest, USS, CT scan of the abdomen and gastro-graffin enema. In most cases, decision to reopen the abdomen is taken on the merits of clinical assessment. Gastro-graffin enema should be avoided at the initial stage. It may enhance the potential possibility into a full blown anastomotic dehiscence, because of back pressure by the contrast inserted from the anal canal. After a full clinical evaluation, patient may need further emergency laparotomy in order to deal with the peritonitis and pelvic abscess.

In other straightforward cases, defunctioning loop ileostomy will continue discharging the feces until further investigation has been carried out on whether there is any evidence of anastomotic leakage. This should be confirmed by the gastro-graffin enema, but this investigation should be arranged from the outpatient clinic, at least 6 weeks later, before reversal of loop ileostomy is undertaken.

But gastrograffin enema should be delayed longer than six weeks if the patient needs a second operation for pelvic abscess and for anastomotic leakage. If there is radiological evidence of stricture at the site of anastomosis, reversal of ileostomy is also delayed, until the stricture has been treated by regular dilatation.

If there is no evidence of any leakage from the site of anastomosis, loop ileostomy is closed. Patient is reviewed every six weeks for six months and then every three months for two years, but it could be extended to every six month after two years.

In this review, rectal digital examination, proctoscopy and sigmoidoscopy are normally carried out. And evidences of anal sphincteric function, number of bowel action per day, anal stenosis, local recurrence of tumor and appetite, body weight and liver metastasis are documented. Further investigation and treatment depends upon the patient symptoms, delayed morbidity or complication.

ETIOLOGY OF ANASTOMOTIC LEAKAGE

It is important to highlight the important aspects of blood supply to the rectum, and the lymphatic drainage from the rectal tumor.

Surgeon must recognize the physiological importance of the inferior mesenteric artery. Its physiological purpose is to supply additional blood flow to the left colon and the rectum. Unlike the blood flow to the right colon, the blood flow to the transverse colon has to climb through the middle colic artery against the gravitational force (Fig. 10.25).

Therefore, the total blood volume that eventually reaches to the left colon may be inadequate to meet the physiological demand of the distal colon and the rectum, despite the fact that a series of arterial arcades are preserved in continuity with those of the inferior mesenteric artery, supplying to the colon (Figs 10.26A and B).

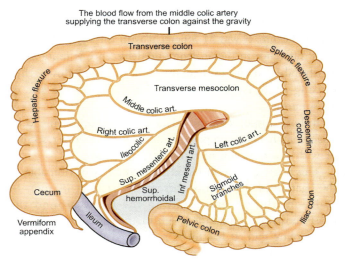

Fig. 10.25: The distribution of colonic vessels

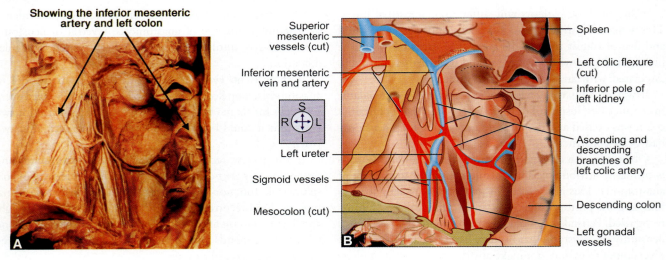

Figs 10.26A and B: The distribution of the inferior mesenteric artery to the descending colon and the rectum (*By Courtesy* of Human Anatomy. Second Edition, Page no. 4.43 Published by Gower Medical Publishing in 1990)

In healthy subjects, the purpose of the inferior mesenteric artery is to maintain additional blood flow to the descending colon, sigmoid colon, and the rectum (Fig. 10.26A). If the main supply of the inferior mesenteric artery is ligated at its roots, the supplement of additional blood flow would be cut off abruptly, resulting in acute ischemic effect to the tissues. Because of the fact, the amount of blood volume that passes through the arcades of the left branch of the middle colic artery would be insufficient for the immediate period to compensate the acute shortage of blood flow to the distal bowel. This explains the reason as to why ileostomy needs to be constructed, but it does not stop the anastomotic leakage.

This suggests that the etiology of leakage could be attributable to ischemic condition of the local tissue or it may result from the technical fault. Recent publication revealed that the incidence of anastomotic dehiscence was over 14 percent found among the cases of anastomosis done with the splenic flexure; it was 31.3 percent with the sigmoid colon.[6] This difference in the anastomotic dehiscence is more likely attributable to the immediate reduced blood flow—thus causing acute ischemia to the tissue around the site of anastomosis.

In both approaches, the incidence of leakage seems to be unacceptably high, compared with the high anterior resection or with the resection of right hemicolectomy.

This acute change in blood flow could be attributable to the ligation of the inferior mesenteric artery at its root. In addition, the ischemic state to the tissue around the anastomosis is compounded with the metallic suture used in the stapling gun. It has to be recognized that the operative technique must be consistent with the surgical anatomy and physiology of the mesenteric artery.

To overcome the ischemic state of the tissue and postoperative leakage, patient has to sacrifice a good length of a healthy bowel, thus reducing the transit time of the feces. And it reduces the total surface area that is required in absorbing the fluid and nutrients from the loose motion. These are contributing factors for causing the intestinal hurry.

In contrast, such cases of ischemic change in the left colon are very rare after the operation of the abdominal aorticaneurysm, where the inferior mesenteric artery is ligated. In this pathophysiological condition, the atheromatous plaque developed silently in the abdominal aneurysmal wall would gradually reduce the size of the osteum of the inferior mesenteric artery. As a result, a part of the blood flow would gradually be diverted through the superior mesenteric artery and then through the series of arterial arcades arising from the middle colic artery in continuity with those of the left colic artery.

As a result, the arterial arcades in the left mesocolon will get the sufficient time to increase the size and area of the capillary bed gradually over many years. This requires time to accommodate the increased blood flow slowly through those increased vascular bed. This is necessary to replenish the short falls of the blood requirement to the left colon and the rectum, but this is an on-going slow process that gives adequate time to the arterial tree to get adjusted and to increase its vascular bed; so that it can accommodate the extra load of blood flow.

Despite this evidence, it is not possible to predict which one would cause dehiscence after the operation. Hence, patient remains at potential risk of this complication and morbidity associated with the low anterior resection of the rectum.

Apart from these technical problems, it has been well-recognized that feces lose its transit time, if a part of the colon is resected. Patients would experience in having frequency of bowel movements more frequently and passing more loose motion compared to the resection of the colon from the other site such as right hemicolectomy. This is a physiological phenomenon that is due to a loss of transit time required for the motion to go through the whole length of the distal bowel.

In case of sphincter-saving low anterior resection, the transit time for the motion would be much reduced if a healthy segment of the descending colon has to be removed in order to avoid anastomotic dehiscence. And such evidence has been documented in the literature, in that the bowel movements had increased in all instances, whether the anastomotic level was at 3 cm or 6 cm from the anal verge.[6]

Incidence of Anastomotic Leakage[6]

These are the summary of the data from the same study. It was not fully understood whether the leakage was due to poor vascularity, or whether it was due to advanced Dukes tumor stage or it was due to inaccessible location of the tumor or due to poor surgical technique. In view of these inconsistent data, how a merit of a new operative procedure could be judged seems to be incomprehensible, particularly to those who are trainee surgeons.

    Curative resection = 15.88 percent
    Palliative resection = 22.45 percent
    Average resection = 17 percent
    Anastomosis with sigmoid colon = 31.3 percent
    Anastomosis with splenic flexure = 15 percent
    Twenty years experience from the same team = 12 percent[21]

Review of the Literature on the Anastomotic Leakage[6,18-22]

1994 Karanjia et al (*)	17.35 percent	(Br J Surg)
1996 Arbman et al	8 percent	(Br J Surg)
1998 Carlson et al	16 percent	(Br J Surg)
1998 Heald et al (1978-1997)*	12 percent	(Arch Surg)
2000 Machado et al	10 percent	(Br J Surg)
2003 Bulow et al	15 percent	(Br J Surg)

*The result published in 1994 seems to be inconsistent with that published in 1998 from the same institution.

Further study seems to be necessary to establish the fact, whether the patients are nutritionally depleted due to loss of transit time of the feces.

Summary of Etiological Factors for Anastomotic Leakage

- Ischemic change around the anastomosis.
- Postradiation vasculitis, if preoperative adjuvant radiotherapy was given.
- Effect of metallic sutures around the anastomosis.
- Faulty application of autosuture gun.
- Mechanical defect in the line of anastomosis, by the interposition of the appendages epiploic between the cut edges of the stomas, and or by the staples sutures failing to get penetrated through the full thickness of the stomas, because of shortness in length.
- Poor surgical technique.

Assessment of Delayed Morbidity

Anal stenosis has been noticed among many colostomy patients. This could be the result of disuse atrophy. The latter may result from the lack of urge defecation that is initiated by the stimuli from the stretch receptors, present in the rectum and the puborectalis muscles. In this circumstance, the sphincteric function remains suspended due to a lack of sensation, derived from the rectum and the puborectalis muscle.

The physiological function of the anal sphincters that maintains the continence of flatus and defecation of feces is operated upon in coordination between the tone of the sphincteric muscles and the stimuli generated from the stretch receptors.

It seems the technique of low anterior resection that removes the rectum and the puborectalis muscle appears to be in conflict with the physiological function of the anal sphincter. Hence, the total benefit from the preservation of the sphincters has to be measured objectively.

ANAL SPHINCTERIC DYSFUNCTION

It was claimed in the literature in 1992 that 208 cases of low anterior resection of the rectum were operated upon between 1978 and 1988, but anal sphincteric function was evaluated among those cases in which the resection level was either at 3 cm or at 6 cm from the anal verge. Among these two groups, 45 had resection level at 3 cm and 88 at 6 cm.

Among these 133 patients, those patients who had local recurrence or anastomotic leakage or died were excluded from the study. It seemed in 10 years period, only 68 (29%) patients were found suitable for reviewing the anal sphincteric function. The question could be raised as to why the anal sphincteric function was not evaluated sometimes after the reversal of ileostomy was carried out.

However, 65 cases were excluded from the study on various grounds. Among these cases, 50 patients died, 7 patients had either anastomotic leakage or local recurrence, and 8 lost to follow-up.[7] Therefore, this survey did not reflect the true prevalence of the postoperative sphincteric function associated with the level of resection and with the operative technique.

But it was claimed that all patients were reviewed every three months and their data have been compiled in the computer by a paid research assistant. Therefore, there was no reason for not relying upon those clinical data from the patients' case notes, and/or from the computer; when they were reviewed at the outpatient clinic.

It is presumed that patients' bowel symptoms were recorded and rectal examination was carried out at the follow-up clinic. Therefore, the question arises that why those clinical data were not or could not be retrieved from the computer with a view to analyzing the postoperative anal sphincteric function. It seemed that clinical data on bowel movements and sphincteric function were not documented for some reason or they were missing from the computer or from the patients' records.

Nevertheless, the postal survey that was carried out on a set of questionnaires may not transpire the true nature of morbidity or accurate information. However, this limited survey indicated that the anal sphincteric function related to frequency of defecation, flatus, and urge defecation or fecal soiling was found associated with the level of anastomosis.

And the sphincteric function was found worse at 3 cm than at 6 cm from the anal verge. Although these revelations were alarming, they should be regarded to be one of the criteria for measuring the merits of the operative techniques, quality of life and skill of the surgeon. If all other data were included in the analysis of the survey, it would have been a comprehensive study of the anal sphincteric function.

However, this limited study suggests that the incidence of incontinence of flatus, fecal soiling or urge defecation was 32 percent, 53 percent and 53 percent respectively, found among those cases in which the level of anastomosis was at 3 cm from the anal verge. In sharp contrast, the results were 24 percent, 11 percent, and 18 percent respectively in those cases in which the level of anastomosis was at 6 cm from the anal verge.[7] These incidences would have been much worse, if the cases with anastomotic leakage and local recurrence were included in the study. Nonetheless, many patients would remain 'housebound' or would be reluctant to going out for shopping, if they are encountered with these sorts of embarrassing situations, in day-to-day work.

Therefore, these are the contributing factors for anal sphincteric dysfunction:
a. Loss of transit time for the feces by the loss of a good length of the left colon.
b. Patients may experience with an intestinal hurry and loose motion. As a result, they may need to go to the lavatory frequently. This problem is related to the level of anastomosis from the anal verge. And bowel action would be worse, if the anastomosis is made with the splenic flexure than with the sigmoid colon. This is due to a sacrifice of the left colon, resulting in a loss of transit time of the feces as well as loss of absorption of the water and electrolytes from the feces.
c. Loss of the rectal Houston valves and puborectalis muscles in some cases.
d. Anastomotic stricture.
e. Anal sphincteric stenosis due to disuse action.
f. Frozen pelvis due to the effect of anastomotic leakage.

REVIEW OF LOCAL RECURRENCE

It was also reported in other study that the local recurrence was found associated with the anastomotic leakage. And it was 25.4 percent in five years follow-up and found directly associated with anastomotic leakage.[8] Other attributing factors are related to Dukes tumor stage, histological grade or differentiation, venous invasion, location of the tumor, level of clearance of the tumor and skill of a surgeon.

Hence, all these morbidities will affect the quality of life and cumulative cost for the treatment of the patient.

A SUMMARY OF THE POTENTIAL RISK FACTORS FOR THE LOCAL RECURRENCE OF THE TUMOR

- Curative or palliative resection.
- Bulky of the tumor mass.
- Dukes tumor stage—poor prognosis with the tumor Dukes C.
- Venous invasion.
- Distal resection margin clearance.
- Location of the tumor.
- Operative perforation of the colon or rectum.
- Extent of operative clearance of the distal resection margin.
- Mobility of the tumor.
- Operative technique.
- Experience and skill of the surgeon.

It has been well-established that the lymphatic spread of the malignant cells does not occur, 2cm distal to the lower margin of the tumor. It is therefore safe to divide the rectum with a clear margin of 2 cm, distal to the lower border of the rectal tumor. But there are many more questions to be answered than to recognise the theoretical benefit.

The fact has to be recognized that the boundary and in particular the lower margin of the tumors is not a straight clear border. In fact, more often, it remains very irregular in shape and its boundary and it appear to be friable and necrotic. They are vulnerable to be fragmented to a slightest trauma. It is very likely that local implantation of the malignant cells into the mucosa distal to the tumor may not occur by the lymphatic or vascular spread; but by spillage of cells from the tumor. Such evidence has been found in the rectum, where multiple daughter tumors had been grown distal to the primary growth (Figs 10.27A and B). And dislodgement of the tumor may occur during the mobilization of the rectum.

In *in vitro* study, viable cancer cells were found to have shed into the lumen of the colon.[9]

Recurrence of cancer at the site of anastomosis could be the result of local implantation of the malignant cells.

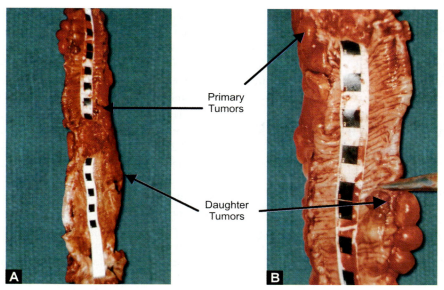

Figs 10.27A and B: Primary tumors, daughter tumors shown a little below the primary tumors

Furthermore, it has been claimed that a high incidence of local recurrence was found associated with the anastomotic leakage following a curative resection being carried out.

The incidence was 25.4 percent, compared with 10 percent found among the nonleakage cases in five years follow-up.[8] A similar association was found in other study, in which it was also evident that a higher incidence of death was found related to malignant condition.[10]

During my residency, on a number occasions, the bowel clamps were found to have accidentally come off or slipped out from the transected rectal stump due to a faulty application of the clamps or it has been noticed that the transected rectal stump had slipped out from the clamps, after the rectum has been transected between the clamps. In both cases, the pelvis would be contaminated with the feces and tumor tissues.

These sorts of accidents do occur in the resection of the rectum; but the physiology of the longitudinal muscle fibers of the rectum needs to be understood. They are smooth muscles and behave like an elastic coil. They tend to get stretched, when the surgeon tends to keep on pulling the rectum upwards during mobilization. This occurs when the clamps are applied across the rectum. As a result, the longitudinal fibers of the rectum start retracting from the clamps, when these muscle fibers are transected, between the clamps. As a result, the clamps are slipped out of the rectal stump in some cases. And the possibility of this sort of incident is more likely to occur in the operating table, if the tumor is bulky and clamps are applied close to the tumor. Such physiological phenomenon could not be ruled out in the low anterior resection.

In other cases, how these clamps could safely be applied below the safe level of the tumor by just external palpation of the tumor remains another technical and practical issue.

Although local wash-out is given with a view to clearing of all malignant cells from the denuded surfaces and from the lumen of the rectum, but reliability of this practice remains in doubt and in fact, wash-out of all those malignant cells from the denuded tissue are impossible. And such evidence could be substantiated by a high incidence of local recurrence, associated with the anastomotic leakage noticed among the potentially curative resection of the rectal growth.[8-10]

Other technical difficulty would be a limited working room and accessibility in the depth of the pelvis. If the tumor-free length of the bowel is believed to be around 6 cm from the anal verge, and the length of the anal canal is 4 cm, the remaining working space for the rectum to be transected would be no more than 2 cm.

Therefore, based upon this fact, how the rectum could safely be transected between the two stapling guns 2 cm below the tumor, seems to be incomprehensible and incompatible with those studies reported in the literature.

In 1930s, level of resection at 2.5 cm below the tumor margin used to be regarded to be a safe surgical practice;[11-13] but a high incidence of local recurrence was reported. To reduce the risk of recurrence, further study was carried out in that the resection level was 5 cm below the tumor margin. This study showed that the incidence of local recurrence was found much less in those cases.[14,15]

In contrast, the resection level at 2 cm distal to the tumor margin has been claimed to be safe.[16] Such views seem to be in conflict with the previous results in which a higher incidence of recurrence of the tumor was found in those instances in which the resection margin was at 2.5 cm.[11-13] In sharp contrast, much better results have been reported with the resection margin at 5 cm from the tumor margin.[14,15]

Nevertheless, the data reported from the same hospital[16] were found inconsistent with other literature.[8]

Despite all these conflicting claims, the merits of the new operative approach should be judged by the risk of local spillage, anastomotic leakage, local recurrence of the tumor and functional state of the anal sphincter.

WHAT IS THE SAFE LEVEL OF RESECTION?

Westhues = 2.5 cm	Leipzig: Thieme 1934[11]
Pannett = 2.5 cm	Lancet 1935[12]
Wangensteen = 2.5 cm	Surgery 1945[13]
Goligher, Dukes and Bussey = 5.0 cm	Br J Surg 1951[14]
Quer, Dahlin and Mayo = 5.0 cm	Surg Gyne and Obst 1953[15]
Heald = 2.0 cm	Lancet 1986[16]

The following incidences of morbidities or postoperative complications will speak for the merits of the new approach.

■ Contributing Factors for the Local Recurrence of Tumor[8]

Venous Invasion	Incidence of Recurrence
No evidence of venous invasion	9.7%
Evidence of venous invasion	21.6%
Dukes Tumor Stage	
Dukes A or B	4.1%
Dukes C	25.4%

These data suggest that the risk of these morbidities would be greater among the patients presented with Dukes C tumor.

■ Incidence of Local Recurrence Related to Anastomotic Leakage[8]

Operation	Incidence of Recurrence
Curative resection	8%
Palliative resection	15.8%
Distal Clearance of Margin	
Resection Level > 1 cm	9.9%
Resection Level < 1 cm	31.0%
Anastomotic Leakage	
No evidence of leakage	10.0%
Evidence of leakage	25.5%

This study has shown that there was a direct association of local recurrence with the anastomotic leakage. Hence, a curable disease turns out to be an incurable disease because of anastomotic leakage. The only explanation for the association of anastomotic leakage with local recurrence could be postulated that the tumor cells that remained dislodged within the distal rectal stump at the primary anastomosis had later got out of the rectum, when the anastomosis broke down.

Therefore, these data did not seem to be a realistic and safe surgical practice in undertaking the sphincter-saving low anterior resection of the rectum. "If I see a snake I will kill it but I will not hit it with umbrella stick; otherwise, it will hit me back." This should be the Philosophy in our surgical practice.

In 1920 Lockhart-Mummery developed a new technique for the rectal carcinoma. It was known as extended perineal resection of the rectal tumor. In those years, when the anesthesia was primitive, he used to employ this technique in the St. Mark's hospital. Dukes carried out a five year follow-up on the survival rate between perineal excision and abdominoperineal resection of the rectum.

Gabriel, who included the St. Mark's Hospital statistics in his book in 1948,[17] concluded that there was not much difference in the survival rate between the Dukes A and Dukes B groups, but the incidence of survival rate was 17.9 percent among the Dukes C group included in the perineal excision but it was found 31.0 percent in the same group included in the abdominoperineal excision of the rectum. Postoperative deaths were excluded from these statistics.

This study supports my view that the survival rate is related to the radical excision of the tumor. This old data exemplified that low anterior resection seems to be less promising to the patients, despite the fact that encouraging results were claimed in the literature. Argument may change with the passage of time, but rationality of the technique must be consistent with the tumor behavior and technical feasibility.

Consistency seems to be the integrity in the surgical practice, but inconsistency seems to be the apparent in the data reported in the literatures, published from the same hospital, despite the fact that the principal author was the coauthor in all studies. In one study it was claimed that only one patient had lost follow-up and the incidence of postoperative leakage was around 12 percent,[21] but the data included in the previous publication were quite different and much worse. Furthermore, the incidence of local recurrence was claimed to be 3 percent or less than 2 percent in curative resection, despite the fact that only one patient was lost to follow-up in 10 years follow-up, but in contrast 8 patients, representing 12 percent of the selected group was reported to have lost in the postal survey on anal sphincteric function.[7] This revelation would question the results in other studies reported in the literature.

REFERENCES

1. Dukes CE. The classification of cancer of the rectum. J Path and Bact 1932;35:323.
2. Goligher JC. The functional results after sphincter-saving resection of the rectum. Ann R Coll Surg Engl 1951;8:421-39.

3. Goligher JC, Duthie HL, Dombal ET, Watts JM. Abdominoanal pull-through excision for carcinoma of the middle-third of the rectum: A comparison with low anterior resection. Br J Surg 1965;22:311.
4. Pahlman L, Glimelius B, et al. Improved survival with preoperative radiotherapy in resectable rectal cancer-Swedish Rectal Cancer Trial. N Engl J Med 1997;336:April 3,part 14:980.
5. Saha SK. Continuous infusion of papaveretum for the relief of postoperative pain. Postgraduate Medical Journal 1981;57:686-9.
6. Karanjia ND, Corder AP, Bearn P, Heald RJ. Leakage from the stapled low anastomosis after total mesorectal excision for carcinoma of the rectum. Br Jl Surg 1994; 81:1224-6.
7. Karanjia ND, Schache DJ, Heald RJ. Function of the distal rectum after low anterior resection for carcinoma. Br Jl Surg 1992;79:114-6.
8. Bell SW, Walker KG, et al. Anastomotic leakage after curative anterior resection results in a higher prevalence of local recurrence. Br J Surg 2003;90:1261-6.
9. Skipper D, Cooper AJ, Marston JE, et al. Exfoliated cells and *in vitro* growth in colorectal cancer. Br J Surg 1987;74:1049-52.
10. Akyol AM, McGregor JR, Galloway DJ, et al. Anastomotic leaks in colorectal surgery: A risk factor for recurrence? Int J Colorectal Dis 1991;6:179-83.
11. Westhues H. Die pathologisch-anatomischen Grundlagen der chirurgie des Rektumkarzinoms. Leipzig: Thieme, 1934.
12. Pannett CA. Resection of the rectum with restoration of continuity. Lancet 1935;2:423.
13. Wangensteen OH. Primary resection (closed anastomosis) or rectal ampulla for malignancy with preservation of sphincteric function. Surg Gyne Obst 1945;81:1.
14. Goligher JC, Dukes CE, Bussey HJR. Local recurrence after sphincter-saving excision for carcinoma of the rectum and rectosigmoid. Br J Surg 1951;39:199.
15. Quer EA, Dahlin DC, Mayo CW. Retrograde intramural spread of carcinoma of the rectum and rectosigmoid: A microscopic study. Surg Gyne and Obst 1953;96:24.
16. Heald RJ, Ryall RDH. Recurrence and survival after total mesorectal excision for rectal cancer. Lancet 1986:1479-82.
17. Gabriel WB. Principles and practice of rectal surgery. 4th ed, London: HK Lewis, 1948.
18. Arbman G, Nilsson E, Hallbook O, et al. Local recurrence following total mesorectal excision for rectal cancer. Brit J Surg 2002;83:375.
19. Carlsen E, Schlichting E, Guldvog I, Johnson E, Heald RJ. Effect of the introduction of total mesorectal excision for the treatment of rectal cancer. Br J Surg 1998;85:526.
20. Bulow IJ, Christensen H, Harling O, et al. Recurrence and survival after mesorectal excision for rectal cancer Br J Surg 2003;90:974.
21. Heald RJ, Moran BJ, Ryall RD, et al. Rectal cancer: The Basingstoke experience of total mesorectal excision, 1978-1997, Arch Surg 1998;133:894.
22. Machado E, Goldman S, Jarhult J. Improved results in rectal cancer surgery—An effect of specialization? Colorectal Dis 2000;2:264.

11. Abdominoperineal Resection of the Rectum

Abdominoperineal resection (APR) of the rectum remains a popular choice in those cases, in which the rectal tumor is at or below 10 cm from the anal verge. In certain cases, where the tumor lies between 10 and 6 cm from the anal verge, sphincter-saving low anterior resection could be performed, because of autosuture gun. Despite its worldwide acceptance, merits of this approach need to be evaluated in perspective with reference to the operation of APR. And they have been highlighted in appropriate section.

The fact has to be recognized that APR is a radical operation for the rectal carcinoma, and provides a long-term good life, to the patients, presented with the Dukes A and B tumor. Unlike the low anterior resection of the rectum, abdominoperineal resection of the rectum removes the entire lymphatic channels as shown in the Figure 11.1.

The management of the rectal tumor should be decided at the MDT meeting, if such service is available. In addition to routine investigations, like all other colonic tumor, MRI scan and tissue diagnosis are necessary for assessing the prognosis, tumor staging and for preoperative adjuvant chemotherapy or radiotherapy. If the growth is in the lower rectum, a course of preoperative radiotherapy should be given.

In 1979, preoperative radiotherapy was a new approach to the rectal tumor present in the lower rectum. The purpose of this new adjuvant therapy was to assess the therapeutic effect, whether the tumor tissue was sensitive to the deep X-ray therapy. For this reason, a few of our patients were selectively referred to Dr Emanuel, for such adjuvant radiotherapy.

The criteria were that the growth would be less than 10 cm from the anal verge and it would appear to be bulky on rectal digital examination. The average dose used for these cases was around 4,500 rad. This was delivered from outside over a period of six weeks. At the completion of therapy, we noticed inflammation such as redness and excoriation of skin around the anus and over the perineal skin.

Because of this reason, APR was delayed for 3-4 weeks. This would allow the inflammation to resolve. It did not interfere with the primary perineal wound healing in those patients, treated with adjuvant preoperative radiotherapy; but such risk of delayed healing could not be ruled out in some

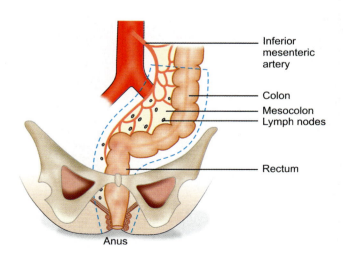

Fig. 11.1: Showing the area by dotted lines to be included in abdominoperineal resection of the rectum

cases; although excessive oozing from the perineal wound was evident.

The resected specimen showed that the bulky tumor had mostly melted away and was hardly recognizable in the rectal mucosa (Figs 11.2A and B).

Although preoperative adjuvant radiotherapy facilitates the resection of the tumor, it does not alter the tumor staging nor does it improve the survival rate after the operation.

Since 1908, abdominoperineal resection of the rectum (APR) has remained a popular choice, but it used to be done in two stages, advocated by Earnest Miles. In the first stage, pelvic colostomy used to be constructed and in the second stage, the rest of the sigmoid colon and the rectum including the anal orifice used to be excised through the perineal wound.

In the second procedure, the patient is turned on the left lateral position that helps the surgeon to carry out the excision of the coccyx along with the perineal resection of the rectum.

The perineal dissection entails excision of the anal orifice, levator ani muscle and whole distal specimen of the sigmoid colon and rectum. In those years, it was a routine procedure to pack the perineal wound with ribbon gauze soaked in proflabin solution. The aim was two folds; one of them was to stop bleeding and other objective was to encourage the wound healing by secondary intention. For these reasons, the wound packing was a common practice in order to stop bleeding from the denuded surfaces because of pressure and at the same time, it encouraged the wound healing slowly by the granulation tissue.

Since then the technique has evolved, in that the surgeons have started closing the perineal wound around a wide bore rubber drainage tubing.

Synchronous combined abdominoperineal resection of the rectum was adopted, since a new operating table was designed by Lloyd Davis in 1938 (Fig. 11.3). This procedure requires the patient lying on the Trendelenburg lithotomy position. This helps two surgeons working simultaneously, in which the abdominal surgeon is engaged in the resection of the rectum through the abdominal wound, and the perineal surgeon is involved in the perineal dissection of the rectum through the perineal wound. This reduces the total time in order to complete the operation, compared to the two stage procedures.

In mid seventies, further progress was made by adopting the primary perineal wound closure that had enhanced the primary perineal wound healing and quick postoperative recovery.[1-4] Despite this achievement, further work was carried out to avoid the risk of high incidence of bladder dysfunction reported in the literatures.[5,6] It was reported that retrograde dissection of the distal rectum and the anal canal undertaken by the perineal surgeon has resolved this morbidity.[2,3]

PREOPERATIVE CONSULTATION

In most cases, the prevalence of sexual desire seems to be much less among the patients over the age of 50. Nevertheless, it is the legal duty of the surgeon to highlight the problems before consent is obtained for this operation; despite the fact that the patient has no option left without this operation.

In female patients, possibility of the excision of the posterior vaginal wall and/or hysterectomy should be highlighted if they are found to have invaded by the tumor at the operation. Reconstruction of the posterior vaginal wall would be necessary if there is evidence of rectovaginal fistula. This may adversely affect their sexual function after operation.

Postoperative complications and morbidity must be discussed. These are injury to the ureter, bladder, or vagina,

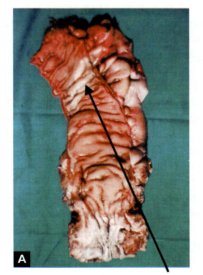
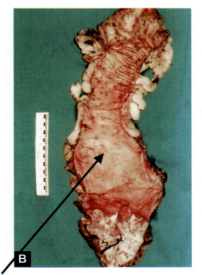

Rectal tumor melted away by DXT

Figs 11.2A and B: These were the two resected specimens of the rectum, after the rectal tumor was treated with preoperative adjuvant radiotherapy. It shows that the tumor mass has melted away from the mucosa of both rectums

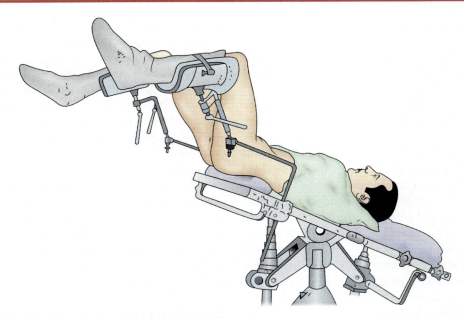

Fig. 11.3: Patient is on the Lloyd-Davis Table in Trendelenburg—Lithotomy position

prostate gland, urethra, hemorrhage, intestinal obstruction, deep vein thrombosis, pelvic abscess, wound infection and chest infection, or wound dehiscence. In the postoperative period, patient may require a long-term indwelling catheter, and there may be morbidity with the colostomy.

PREOPERATIVE PREPARATION FOR THE APR

Like other colonic surgery, preoperative bowel preparation is carried out with oral laxative and rectal wash-outs. The site of terminal colostomy is marked with a skin pencil in the left iliac fossa, as described before. Colostomy nurse should discuss with the patient several times about the care of the colostomy and other moral and social support, before the day of operation. This provides full confidence and reassurance how to look after the colostomy.

A full assessment is made about the general health. This includes bladder function, postmicturition residue, urine flow rate per minute, sexual function and nutritional state or fluid deficit. Correction of anemia, fluid deficit and electrolytes imbalance must be done. Grouping and cross-matching for six units of blood should be arranged for this operation.

Before the patient is transferred to the theater, indwelling catheter is inserted into the bladder and its residual volume is recorded in the fluid balance chart. Prophylactic antithrombotic measure should be contemplated, and for this purpose, TED (Thromboembolic Deterrent) stockings are put on in both lower limbs, but due care should be taken so that the stocking should not form any crease around the girth of the thigh or below the knee. These would act as a tourniquet, interfering with the return of the venous blood. As a result, there would be a venous stasis in the distal part, resulting in tissue edema around the ankle or on the dorsum of the foot.

In addition, subcutaneous mini-heparin is prescribed. Furthermore, prophylactic appropriate antibiotics covering for both aerobic and anaerobic bacteria are commenced in the theater.

TECHNIQUE FOR ABDOMINOPERINEAL RESECTION (APR) OF THE RECTUM

■ Patient on the Operating Table

Under general anesthesia, the patient is placed on the Trendelenburg–lithotomy position, in which both legs are rested on a leg support that is kept in semi-flexed and abducted position attached to the table. These supports are adjustable in all directions to suite the individual patient and the surgeons. These leg supports are kept apart away from the middle, thus allowing the perineal surgeon to carry out the perineal dissection, from the sitting position.

The buttock rests upon a soft rubber cushion or sand bag that lies transversely across the bottom edge of the table. The position of the coccyx should be at least 3 inches away from and outside the sand bag. This position must be checked by the perineal surgeon; otherwise, it would be difficult to carry out the posterior dissection of the anococcygeal region.

A perineal tray is fitted into the bottom of the table, so that necessary instruments could be kept on it. The head end of the table is tilted down. There should be two sets of instruments including diathermy forceps and diathermy pads. They are kept separate for the respective team of surgeons.

The abdominal surgeon stands on the left side and his assistant on the right side of the patient. One theater nurse will assist the abdominal surgeon and another one will assist the perineal surgeon.

A PRELIMINARY RECTAL DIGITAL EXAMINATION

Before proceeding with the operation, the perineal surgeon should carry out the rectal digital examination. This is important to find out whether the rectum contains lots of liquid or solid feces and whether the tumor is fixed to the vaginal wall or prostate gland or fixed to the sacral wall. This recollection of memory would guide the surgeon on how to avoid the operative injury to the surrounding structures.

It is wise to empty the lower rectum by a suction tube, instead of inserting the small swab inside the anal canal. The perineum should be cleaned again before a purse string nylon suture is inserted through the subcutaneous tissue around the anal orifice. A second purse string suture is also applied in order to bury the first one, and the ends of the suture are left long, so that it could be used as a retractor (Fig.11.4).

The purpose of closing the anal orifice first, before the abdominal surgeon begins opening the abdomen, is to stop soiling of the perineum and the sterile drapes that have already been laid around the perineum.

SKIN PREPARATION

The skin is cleaned with the antiseptic solution, covering the wider area between the costal margin and the midthigh including the genitalia. The perineal surgeon will clean the perineum. Both lower limbs are covered with a sterile trousers type drape. A large towel is put under the buttock and a large pad, preferably large gauze is put under the sacrum but over the sterile towel. To lay down these drapes, the buttock needs to be lifted up by the theater assistant. Sterile drapes are also laid down all around covering the chest, side of the abdomen and the genital area.

PROCEDURE FOR THE SYNCHRONOUS COMBINED APR

When every thing is ready, laparotomy is undertaken through a midline incision, commencing from the symphysis pubis and ending a little above the umbilicus. Internal examination is next carried out about the location and mobility of the tumor, evidence of enlarged lymph nodes along the vessels, and metastasis in the liver. If the tumor is mobile with no evidence of peritoneal seedlings, decision for the resection of the tumor is taken.

Surgeon should not be discouraged from this operation, if there is one or two metastases found in the liver, provided the rectal tumor remains mobile and resectable. Invasive rectal growth should not be attempted in undertaking this operation. If resectable, the secondaries in the liver could be dealt with later either by chemotherapy or by surgery. This decision should be taken after the patient has recovered from this operation and by further review in the outpatient clinics.

The quality of life would be much improved after excision of the primary growth, whether or not, it has invaded the ureter, or uterus or surrounding structures. The only doubt that may creep up in mind is whether the growth is resectable that could only be resolved by a courageous and judicious approach. This depends upon the skill and experience of the surgeon.[2,3]

After completion of the initial examination, the small intestine and the cecum are tucked into the upper abdomen, under cover of the packs. In this case, one pack is left in the area of splenic flexure, another one on the right side and the third one over the transverse colon. These packs will stop the small intestine entering into the operative field. The abdominal wound is retracted by a self-retaining retractor. A central blade is fitted for holding the small intestine under the cover of the packs, placed in the upper abdomen.

The loop of the sigmoid colon is next lifted up by both hands of the assistant and moved away from the left parietal wall. This will reveal the parietal peritoneal attachments or a few peritoneal bands holding the colon with the parietal wall. Once these bands are divided, the sigmoid colon will move further forwards, thus exposing the true boundary of the peritoneal reflection.

It is important to preserve the parietal peritoneum or the mesocolon before starting sharp dissection and mobilization of the pelvic mesocolon. Reconstruction of the pelvic floor will require this peritoneal reflection. Hence, it should be preserved, as much as it is possible, without compromising the radical resection of the tumor.

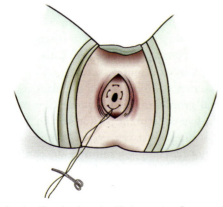

Fig. 11.4: Anal orifice is closed with two sets of purse string sutures applied around the anal orifice and a pair of long threads is left hanging to be used for the purpose of pulling the anal orifice in different direction as and when required in order to facilitate the dissection

Therefore, the true peritoneal reflection is incised with scissors, thus opening a cleavage and window to get into the retroperitoneal space. By gentle mobilization, the colon along with its mesocolon is mobilized further forwards. And the sharp dissection is continued downwards along the lateral side of the rectum, thus facilitating further mobilization and lifting of the rectum.

The anatomical position of the left ureter that lies across the bifurcation of the left common iliac artery is identified. The lateral cut edge of the left parietal peritoneum is gently lifted up by the two long artery forceps or Babcock forceps. This will reveal the location of the left ureter, but too much dissection should be avoided in order to avoid interference with the blood supply to the ureter.

The incision is next directed towards the bladder where the assistant will keep the bladder or the uterus retracted by a deep pelvic retractor (Fig. 11.5A). The incision is ended in front of the rectum above the rectovesical pouch or the rectouterine pouch.

Now the pelvic mesocolon is held up under the light. This will reveal the distribution of the left colic arteries supplying to the sigmoid colon. The mesocolon is opened distal to the left colic vessels and the dissection is continued up to the mesenteric border of the colon.

If there are no enlarged lymph nodes palpable, the vascular pedicle supplying to the rectum is next isolated. They are in fact the bunch of the terminal inferior mesenteric arteries, and known as superior hemorrhoidal vessels. In most cases, they lie over the sacral promontory and they are isolated by hooking around with the right index finger. This pedicle is divided between the two clamps and ligated, but the proximal stump is tied with double ligatures, using No.1 thread.

After division of these vessels, there would be minimum blood loss when the resection of the rectum is continued down, along the right side of the rectum. The next step would be the mobilization of the upper part of the rectum that is carried out by putting the right hand behind the rectum.

This approach allows the rectum to be lifted up from the sacral wall, thus defining the peritoneal attachment with the rectum further down. In this way, the sharp dissection is continued downwards until it reaches in front of the rectum, thus establishing a continuity of the dissection all around the rectum.

The sigmoid colon is next divided between the clamps using the Zachary Copes crushing clamps (Fig. 11.5B).

This division must be in line with the free edge of the pelvic mesocolon, thus preserving the lower left colic artery and its terminal branches.

The proximal transected end of the colon, held by the clamp, is covered with small gauze held in position by ligature. This will prevent from wound contamination, when it will be brought out through a separate colostomy wound for the construction of the terminal colostomy. This has been described in previous pages with the operation of the anterior resection of the rectum.

In the same way, the distal end, held by the other crushing clamp is also covered by a swab, and tied with ligature. This free transected end of the colon will assist the surgeon for further dissection of the rectum from the sacral wall. To identify the left lateral ligament, the rectum is lifted up from the sacral cavity and pushed towards the right side. A long and straight blade with a curved-shaped retractor as shown in figure 11.5C, should be used to keep retracting the bladder towards the symphysis pubis or laterally away from the field of vision.

A short band holding the side wall of the rectum could be seen. Under direct vision, this ligament is divided between the two long artery forceps. The ligament is ligatured. In the same way, the right lateral ligament is divided and ligated. In a narrow pelvis, demonstration of the lateral ligament is not easy. In that case, it could be divided by a long scissors and the bleeding vessels from the stump could be controlled with diathermy.

The mobilization of the rectum from the fascia of Waldeyer is continued deep down behind the rectum and behind the tumor until it reaches the anococcygeal raphe. The rectum is next separated from back of the bladder and the prostate gland or from the back of the posterior vaginal wall, known as pouch of Douglas.

In the meantime, the perineal surgeon has started on the perineal dissection (that would be described later) and at some point of dissection, he makes a contact with the abdominal surgeon, through the posterior perineal wound.

As a result, the proximal transected end of the sigmoid colon is delivered through back of the perineal wound. Having done this job, the abdominal surgeon starts reconstructing the pelvic floor, by freeing the peritoneal edges from the parietal wall of the pelvis. This is done by a finger mobilization. And this will assist in the reconstruction of the pelvic floor without tension. It would obviate the risk of ureters being caught up in the sutures; if they are identified and separated from the peritoneal edge. Having done this work, the neopelvic floor is reconstructed by continuous sutures.

This is commenced from back of the bladder and is ended over the sacral promontory. Meticulous care must be taken in suturing the free-edges of the peritoneum, in that the spacing between the sutures must not exceed more than 1 cm and there should not have any tension over the sutures and there must not have any defect or puckering of the free-edges or a hole between the sutures or in the peritoneum. This will be the potential risk of herniation of the small intestine.

The operating table is back to neutral position. The packs are removed. The small intestine and the cecum are put back in the pelvis in right order. No drain is normally required for

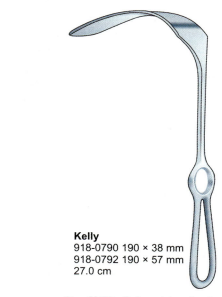

Fig. 11.5A: Kelly pelvic retractor

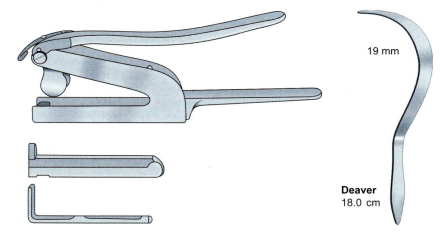

Fig. 11.5B: Zachary Copes retractor

Fig. 11.5C: Deaver retractor

the abdominal wound. The retractors are removed. After instruments and swab counts are done, the abdominal wound is closed in one layer as described before. The skin wound is next closed. After the wound is covered with dressing, the terminal colostomy is constructed at last, as described in the previous section.

All wet packs are weighed in order to work out the total loss of blood and fluid.

METHODS OF PERINEAL DISSECTION OF THE RECTUM

When the abdominal surgeon has decided that the tumor is resectable and the tumor has been mobilized, the perineal surgeon starts the perineal dissection, by giving elliptical incisions around the anal verge (Fig. 11.6).

The illustration shows a broad anatomical demonstration of the anal orifice and the surrounding structures of the anal orifice (Fig. 11.7).

THE LANDMARK FOR THE PERINEAL INCISIONS

First a curved incision is made on the one side of the anus, commencing from the center point of the transverse line drawn between the two ischial tuberosity and it is continued down around the anus, 2 inches away from the anal verge, until it reaches the back of the anal orifice.

After dealing with one side, a second curved incision begins from the same center point like the first one and it is continued down exactly in the same way around the other side of the anus, until it meets posteriorly with the other incision.

Each convex incision line should be 2 inches away from the respective side of the anal verge and then they are continued further down until they converge and meet just in front of the tip of the coccyx, felt by the tip of the left index finger, where the two incisions meet (Figs 11.6 and 11.7). The perineal wound would appear to be an elliptical shape.

The incision on each side is made deep and deeper initially and then by finger mobilization, the fatty layers are separated from the wall of the anal canal and the rectum. The major perineal vessels are ligated and then divided. Smaller bleeding vessels should be controlled with diathermy forceps. The surrounding wound is made deepened around the anal sphincters.

The medial skin flaps around the anal verge are held together by two pair of tissue forceps. And the lateral wound margin is retracted by the Langerbeck retractors. By finger mobilization, the anal canal is separated from the parietal fats, thus revealing the tributaries supplying to the external anal sphincters and the anal canal. These vessels are divided and ligated or coagulated.

The forceps holding the anal skin margins will keep on pulling the anal canal in different directions, as and when necessary, at the time of perineal dissection. The anterior wall of the anal canal is dissected from the transversus perineal muscles and the perineal body. To display the boundary of the transverse perineal muscles or the anterior wall of the rectum, the anal orifice is pulled down and the skin wound margin is retracted upwards or medially that will display the edge of the transverse perineal muscles. Although, these muscles could be sacrificed, it is not absolutely necessary in this operation and should be preserved, if possible.

This dissection could be undertaken in two ways. One of the techniques was described by Lockhart-Mummery in 1920.[5] In those years, anesthesia was primitive. The rectal carcinoma up to the level of 10 cm used to be excised through the perineal dissection. Since then, this technique remains popular, among many surgeons, despite its morbidity. The technique comprises of resection of the rectum all along around the anal orifice, anal sphincter, anal canal and the rectum. This dissection commenced from the perineal skin surface and ended into the pelvis, removing the anal verge, anal canal and rectum.

The dissection is carried out all along anterior to the rectum from the skin to the pelvis. Palpation and display of the bulbar and penile urethra are necessary to guide the dissection anterior to the rectum.

Figure 11.10 shows that there is a very little anatomical cleavage between the rectum and urethra or the vagina. To facilitate the dissection, transverse perineal muscles and perineal body need to be excised but it is an important structure for the urogenital diaphragm and it may bring the risk of severance of the neural plexus supplying the urethra and the urethral sphincters.[2]

The dissection behind the rectum is also carried out from the skin surface down into the pelvis, but there is an anatomical cleavage behind the rectum in the sacral cavity. The whole resected specimen is removed through the perineal wound.

In this method, initial communication is made with the abdominal surgeon through the opening made behind the rectum, this assists further dissection around the rectum and it is continued forward along the side of the rectum (Figs 11.8 and 11.9).

In sharp contrast, no such communication is possible in the anterior dissection until the specimen of the rectum is completely separated from those structures, lying anterior to the rectum (Fig. 11.10).

SAHA RETROGRADE DISSECTION OF THE RECTUM

By contrast, the anterior wall of the rectum and anal canal is separated from the back of the prostate and membranous

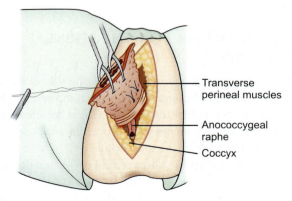

Fig. 11.6: Showing the line of dissection around the anal sphincters and anococcygeal raphe

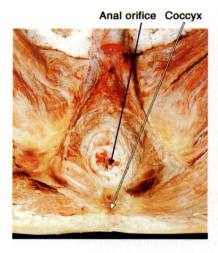

Fig. 11.7: The illustration displaying the anatomical features around the anal orifice. (*By courtesy* of Gower Medical Publishing in 1990 and reprinted in 1994 by Wolfe publishing from Human Anatomy, Second Edition)

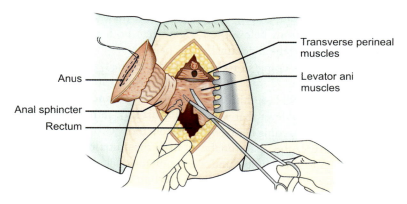

Fig. 11.8: Showing the perineal dissection and excision of the levator ani muscles under direct supervision and under the guidance of the left index finger as shown in the figure

urethra in male and from the posterior vaginal wall in female patient, by retrograde dissection. This anterior dissection is commenced from inside the pelvis towards the perineal skin surface anterior to the anal orifice. The direction of dissection of the anterior wall of the rectum is in opposite direction to that of the previous approach, described by Lockhart Mummery in 1929. Finding of the anatomical cleavage anterior to the rectum is not necessary in retrograde dissection. Therefore, it is not necessary to display the urethral tube in this approach.

Although, transverse perineal muscles are necessary to be sacrificed in the previous approach, it is not absolutely necessary in this approach and should be preserved, if possible.

This maintains the urogenital diaphragm and preserved the neural plexus present around the perineal body, bulbar urethra, and membranous urethra but excision of the perineal body and transverse perineal muscles may cause severance of the neural plexus, thus affecting the normal micturition.[2]

The perineal surgeon will next endeavor in the posterior perineal dissection. In the posterior perineal dissection, there is no technical difference from the previous approach, in carrying out the dissection of the rectum. During finger mobilization, the inferior hemorrhoidal vessels will be seen at the depth of the ischeorectal fossa, where the pudendal canal opens. They are divided between the clamps and ligated. The same method is used on the opposite side.

The posterior perineal dissection is continued deep in front of the coccyx, where the anococcygeal raphe is divided with a strong pair of curved Mayo's scissors. Once this has been divided, the anal sphincters and rectum move further forward, thus exposing the levator ani muscles and posterior wall of the rectum (Figs 11.7 and 11.8).

The tough whitish fibers known as fascia of Waldeyer could be seen just in front of the coccyx. It lies deep to the anococcygeal raphe. It is divided transversely in front of the coccyx. After this division being done, the presacral fascia and fatty layer is next opened up in order to make a communication with the abdominal surgeon. This fascia between the coccyx and the rectum is the fascia of Waldeyer.

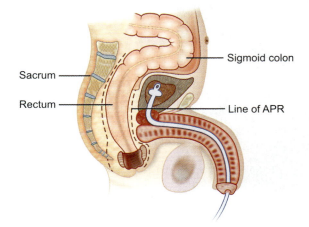

Fig. 11.9: Displaying the line of resection of the rectum and anal canal

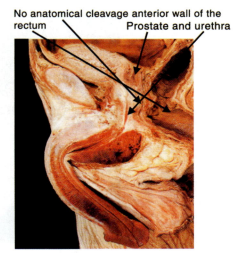

Fig. 11.10: Showing no true anatomical cleavage between the prostatic urethra and the anterior rectal wall. (By courtesy of Gower Medical Publishing in 1990 and Wolfe Publishing in 1994, for reproducing this illustration from the Human Anatomy)

The perineal surgeon could get into a wrong cleavage by elevating this fascia from the sacral wall, from below the perineal wound. It is safer if it is broken down by the abdominal surgeon but resistance may be experienced in doing so from the pelvis.

In this situation, the abdominal surgeon will keep his two fingers held down anterior to the fascia of Waldeyer that will direct the perineal surgeon, where to make an opening between two the fingers from below. To make sure, the abdominal surgeon pushes his two fingers through the said window and makes handshake with the perineal surgeon (Fig. 11.11A).

The window of the fascia of Waldeyer is next made widened further by the Mayo's Scissors. The levator ani muscles on each side of the rectum are next divided. It is commenced from the coccyx along each side of the rectum, and the levator ani muscles are cut with the scissor, lateral to left index finger that is insinuated in order to protect the accidental injury to the rectum (Fig. 11.8).

When the posterior perineal wound would appear to be wide, the abdominal surgeon would deliver the upper transected end of the sigmoid colon through the space made behind the rectum and then through the window made in the posterior part of the perineal wound (Fig. 11.11B). Once this has been done the proximal transected end of the sigmoid colon along with the clamp *in situ* is left hanging down over the perineal wound (Fig. 11.12).

The puborectalis muscles that keep holding the rectum with the membranous urethra or the vaginal wall is clearly seen around the rectum like a U-shaped sling (Fig.11.12). A plane of cleavage is created by pushing the index finger between the puborectalis muscles and the side of the rectum (Fig. 11.13). The fibers of the puborectalis muscles that run across the longitudinal muscle fibers of the rectum is shown clearly and these relationships becomes apparent in profile view when both ends of the rectum are held apart outside the pelvis.

In this maneuver, the perineal surgeon gets access to divide the puborectalis and then rectourethralis muscles under direct vision and a plane of cleavage is established.

In this way, retrograde dissection of the rectum is carried out from the back of the bladder, prostate gland and the urethra or from the posterior wall of the vagina. The plane of cleavage is maintained all along, provided the longitudinal muscles of the rectum are followed up in pari passu with the cutting of the transverse fibers of the puborectalis muscles (Figs11.14 and 11.15). This dissection is continued towards the anal orifice.

Once the sling muscle has been divided with a pair of fine scissors; the rectum starts peeling off gradually from the back of the prostate gland and membranous urethra or from the posterior vaginal wall. In this method of dissection, the membranous urethra is minimally disturbed and hardly comes into view. The whole specimen is removed. Bleeding vessels from the back of the prostate gland or from the cut ends of the middle rectal artery are coagulated.

If the tumor is located just behind the vaginal wall, it is advisable to sacrifice a small strip of the posterior vagina with the rectum. Reconstruction of the posterior wall is carried out by a continuous suture, thus bringing both cut edges together. If the cervix uteri are involved or a fistula has developed, then hysterectomy has to be included in the APR.

If the perineal wound is to be closed with a view to achieving a primary perineal wound healing, then two redivac drainage tubes are put inside the pelvic cavity. Each one is brought out through anterior part of the perineum, one on each side of the perineal wound and the tubes with multiple holes are

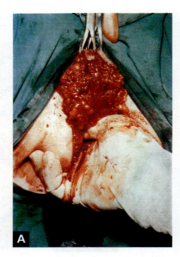
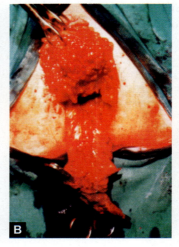

Figs 11.11A and B: (A) After the window is created by dividing the anococcygeal raphe and the fascia of Waldeyer, the perineal surgeon is making a contact (Handshake) with the abdominal surgeon and is attempting to grab the upper transected end of the sigmoid colon. (B) Delivery of the divided end of the sigmoid colon through the back of the anal sphincter

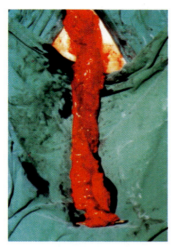

Fig. 11.12: In retrograde dissection of the rectum, the specimen of the rectum is left hanging down, but it is held by the puborectalis muscles

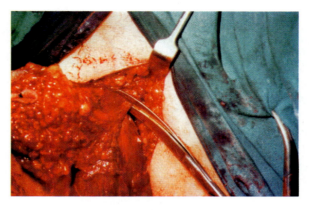

Fig. 11.14: An operative picture showing the division of the puborectalis muscles that was carried out under direct vision during the retrograde perineal dissection of the rectum

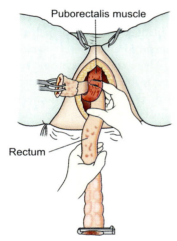

Fig. 11.13: This is an illustration, reproduced from the operative technique (Figure 11.12), displaying the anatomy of the rectum held by the puborectalis muscle and showing how to create a cleavage between the puborectalis muscle and the rectum. It is done by pushing the index finger from the inside that assists in the retrograde mobilization and dissection of the rectum from back of the prostrate and urethra and showing a clear cleavage created by inserting the right index finger between the puborectalis muscle and the longitudinal muscle of the rectum

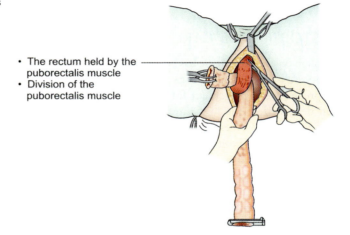

Fig. 11.15: Showing the technique on how the puborectalis muscle is divided by the scissors

left inside the pelvis. The perineal wound is closed in layers with interrupted stitches. This is followed by the closure of the skin with interrupted sutures (Fig. 11.16).[1-3]

In either method, the perineal wound could be closed by the wound packing, partial wound closure with tube drain or with primary perineal wound closure (Fig.11.16). In the case of partial wound closure, the drainage tube or corrugated sheet could be brought out through the middle of the wound margins (Fig. 11.17).

In case of primary closure of perineal wound, redivac drainage apparatus should be used. It can maintain an effective negative pressure within the glass jar. However, two suction drainage tubes, one on each side of the wound, are brought out through a puncture wound made from inside out, in the anterior part of the perineum, using a sharp ended curved metal trocker, fitted with a 2 mm sized plastic tube, and the site for this suction tube should be in the anterior part of the perineal wound and 2 inches away from the sutures line of the perineal wound (Fig. 11.16).

In rare condition, where excessive venous oozing has been coming from the presacral venous plexus, wound packing remains the only choice. In this case, the polythene bag is first inserted, covering the denuded surfaces of the perineal cavity, and a large and long gauze, soaked in proflabin is pushed inside the bag slowly and gradually, and until nothing more could be put in.

The polythene bag could be tied by the purse string in order to keep the ribbon swab inside the perineal wound. The wound surface is covered with large dressing pack, supported by the T bandage.

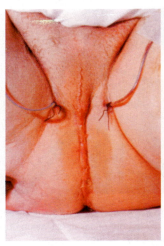

Fig. 11.16: This is a conclusive evidence of primary perineal wound healing after the perineal wound has been completely closed

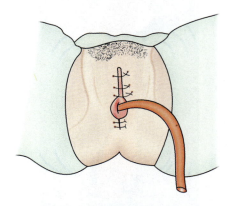

Fig. 11.17: Showing the drainage tubing passing through the middle of the perineal wound. Its anterior and posterior parts are closed by interrupted skin sutures

POSTOPERATIVE CARE

Although postoperative care has been described in other colonic surgery, it is no different from any other operation. And a comprehensive management for the postoperative shock has been described in the low anterior resection of the rectum. In addition, it is necessary to measure the volume of blood loss for the first 12 hours after the patient has been transferred to the recovery ward. Patients may need blood transfusion or colloids infusion for replacing the amount of blood lost or collected in the redivac bottles.

The average collection of blood in the bottle would be around 250-700 ml on the first postoperative day and it would reduce to 100-175 ml on the second day. This will continue dropping gradually every day, until it drops to 25 ml. Therefore, it is important to keep on recording the blood loss every day. It is equally important to make sure that the holes of the suction tube are not outside the perineal wound and that the vacuum is maintained in the bottle. They are removed after 5 days, provided the total collection in the suction bottle is less than 25 ml in last 24 hours.[1]

CARE OF URETHRAL CATHETER

In most instances, indwelling catheter is removed after 5 days, provided the patient is fully mobile and is taking normal diet. It is the duty of the nurse to record the volume of urine every time he or she has passed in the bottle. It takes 2-3 days to regain the normal urinary flow.

If the preoperative assessment revealed that the residual volume of the urine was in excess of 75 ml, it would be unwise to take the catheter out in less than 2 weeks. He may need transurethral resection of the prostate glands a few months later. In this situation, he may be discharged home with the indwelling catheter *in situ*, but arrangement should be made to replace the catheter every 4-6 weeks.

If the catheter is removed for trial, then daily output must be recorded and bladder needs to be palpated per abdomen whether it has emptied completely or it contains a large residual volume of urine. There could be chronic retention of urine. This could be due to bladder neck obstruction, bruising of the bladder wall or the urethra, or deenervation.

In these circumstances, a long-term indwelling catheter needs to be maintained, until further trial without catheter being carried out. If this condition is not dealt with, he may develop atony of the bladder due to over distention. He may need to be seen by urologist for definitive treatment.

If there is leakage of urine that soaked through the perineal wound or collected in the redivac bottle, suspicion should arise whether one or both ureters are caught in the stitches in the reconstruction of the peritoneal floor, or ureter has been damaged during mobilization of the rectum or the membranous urethra has been inflicted with the resection.

In these situations, necessary urological investigation is necessary. Therefore, intravenous pyelogram must be done as soon as possible. If it is normal, cystogram through the catheter should be done. At last, urethrogram should be done as a last resort and postoperative recovery would be quicker, if primary repair of urethral injury could be undertaken within 24 hours. In the latter case, patient needs a long-term indwelling catheter, after primary repair of the urethral injury being undertaken.

CARE OF COLOSTOMY

Colostomy starts passing flatus on 4th or 5th postoperative day. For a few weeks, it remains edematous and dusky in color. He needs to be taught how to change the bag and is encouraged in undertaking the care of the colostomy bag independently. Complications of the colostomy have been highlighted in the previous pages.

CARE OF PERINEAL WOUND

If the perineal wound has been packed from the theater, the first change of dressing should be done in the theater after 3 days. This change of dressing could be done without general anesthesia, if plastic bag containing the large gauze has been inserted into the wound, but general anesthesia should be preferable, if the wound has been packed with the dressing without the plastic bag being used. Furthermore, patient may need a blood transfusion in this case, if bleeding begins from the denuded surfaces. Therefore, necessary precaution should be taken in advance.

Subsequent change of dressing should be done every day for a few weeks. This could be extended that depends upon the progress. Local antibiotic lavage should not be done, unless a foul discharge is coming out from the wound.

If the perineal wound has a drainage tube through the center of the skin wound, this needs to be shortened, after five days, provided it stops draining. Perineal wound irrigation should not be done. This may add infection into the pelvis.

If primary closure of the perineal wound has been done, the redivac drainage tubings are removed after 5 days, and the skin sutures are removed on 12 days. Patient is advised against squirting for a few weeks and should sit on a soft cushion.

MERITS OF DIFFERENT TECHNIQUES USED FOR THE PERINEAL DISSECTION OF THE RECTUM

In the conventional approach, advocated by Lockhart-Mummery in 1920 and 1926,[5,6] the technical difficulties may be encountered with the dissection of the anterior wall of the rectum. This difficulty is due to finding of the anatomical cleavage, anterior to the anal canal and rectum (Figs 11.9 and 11.10). In fact, the dissection would be a blind procedure. Because of this reason, the transversus perineal muscles and the perineal body are required to be excised. Despite this excision, risk of operative injury to the urethra or posterior vaginal wall or to the rectum, could not be avoided in certain cases.[2]

A prospective study was undertaken in order to define the merit of the perineal dissection of the abdominoperineal resection of the rectum, between the Lockhart-Mummery technique[5,6] and Saha retrograde dissection of the rectum.[2,3]

To avoid bias, the first 20 consecutive patients (14 men and 6 women) were included in the former technique. It required 2 years to complete this study. In the subsequent three years, 42 patients (33 men and 9 women) were included in the latter technique. But three of this group were excluded from the results on the ground that one lady needed hysterectomy along with the resection of the rectal tumor, and among other two patients, the specimen of the rectum came apart through the tumor; but one of them had the rectal tumor invading the bladder wall and other one invaded the sacral wall. These three cases were not suitable for evaluating the merit of the retrograde dissection. And they were included in the former technique. Hence, 39 patients (33 men and 6 women) were included in the retrograde perineal dissection.

Among the 23 patients included in the former technique, operative injury to the anterior wall of the rectum occurred in five and that to the membranous urethra in one among 15 men. This represents 40 percent operative injury. And this was due to the lack of the anatomical cleavage or due to the former operative technique. Among the four female patients, operative injury to the rectum occurred in one and that to the posterior vaginal wall in another patient, operated upon by the former technique. Again, the incidence was 50 percent.

In sharp contrast, the incidence of operative injury to the anterior wall of the rectum was 6.25 percent among the 32 male patients and to the anterior wall of the anal canal (14%) in one of the seven female patients, included in the retrograde dissection. The operative injury to the female patient had resulted from the potential risk to the posterior vaginal wall. This comparative study suggests that the risk of operative injury to the urethra, or posterior vaginal wall would be much less with the retrograde perineal dissection of the rectum.[2,3]

In addition, the risk of injury to periurethral neural plexus is much less by this approach, in which, display or palpation of the urethral tube would be unnecessary in the retrograde mobilization of the rectum. And the experiences show that there remains a greater risk of severance of the fine neural plexus supplying to the membranous urethra, if it is necessary either to display or to palpate the urethral tube in the perineal dissection. Therefore, the display of the penile urethra would be detrimental to the bladder function, if operative injury to the urethra or the rectum is to be avoided. In the literature, a high incidence of bladder dysfunction, ranging from 24[7] to 59 percent[8] has been reported.

This morbidity is believed to be attributable to the damage to the neural plexus present around the urethra. Other sites of injury to the nerves could be at the exit of the pudendal canal, where the internal pudendal vessels and pudendal nerves could be inflicted at the dissection[2] or the injury could occur behind the fascia of Waldeyer.

In the literature of anatomy, the exact passage of nervi Erigentes, whose sacral roots are S_1, S_2 or S_3, S_4 remains unclear. These nerves are parasympathetic and lie behind the fascia of Waldeyer. In the textbook of anatomy, written by RJ Last, it has been highlighted that pelvic arteries lie anterior to and sacral nerves lie behind the fascia of Waldeyer. No structures pierce through this fascia. Furthermore, it has been noticed that parasympathetic nerves always follow the arterial vessels.

Like the vagus nerves, parasympathetic nerves to the bladder and the rectum should follow with the arteries. It could be a possible explanation that internal pudendal artery exits the pelvic wall in order to accompany the nervi Erigentes and pudendal nerves. Previous study supports this observation. In all the clinical experiences, in which retrograde dissection of the rectum was carried out, there was no evidence of bladder dysfunction in the results of those patients, operated upon by the same technique over 30 years.

Furthermore, there should have a consistency with the anatomical passage of other sacral nerves, whose root's value remains the same. In these cases, both nervi Erigentes and pudendal nerves have the same nerve roots S_1, S_2 or S_3, S_4 and have a common destination. Hence, they should follow the same anatomical route. In these cases, why the nervi Erigentes will follow a different route away from the pudendal nerves and away from the internal pudendal vessels seems to be incomprehensible.

There is no reason to believe differently and contrary to this rule in the distribution of the nervi erigentes in the pelvic and perineal structures. It is reasonable to believe that the nervi erigentes follow the internal pudendal vessels and pudendal nerves in order to reach to the penis, bladder and lower rectum (Figs 11.18 and 11.19). As a result, they are unlikely to be damaged during mobilization of the rectum from the fascia of Waldeyer.[2]

Retrograde dissection of the rectum through the perineal wound had prevented the risk of damage to these nerves, which are protected by the fascia of Waldeyer that lies anterior to the sacral plexus. The results of this study have been reported in the literature.[1-3]

In the literature, an alarming high incidence of bladder dysfunction has been reported and the results in bladder dysfunction have been compiled in table 11.1. In this respect divergent etiological factors have been postulated. These are a change in angulation of bladder neck with the urethra and division of the levator ani muscles,[4] or damage to the parasympathetic nerves.[5,6] It has also been claimed that bladder dysfunction was found worse in those cases in which the coccyx was not excised.[6]

But, experiences showed that damages of these nerves could delay the postoperative recovery. And the risk of injury to the nerves is much greater with the conventional technique, described by Lockhart-Mummery in 1920.[5] And the results were found worse with this technique, employed in abdominoperineal resection of the rectum.[7]

Dissection through the space, anterior to the rectum would be a blind procedure. There remains a further risk of injury to the rectal wall that allows the fecal contamination into the wound. As a result, primary perineal wound closure would be impossible. And the risk of local recurrence remains high due to perforation of the anterior wall of the rectum. All these operative morbidities are due to the fact that there is no true anatomical cleavage anterior to the anterior rectal wall.

By contrast, the retrograde dissection of the anterior wall of the rectum is done under direct vision. This permits the surgeon to define the anatomical cleavage by dividing the fibers of the puborectalis muscles along the side wall of the rectum by just following the longitudinal fibers of the rectum (Figs 11.12, 11.13 and 11.15). These longitudinal fibers are the best guideline to the perineal surgeon to follow the cleavage in order to get the rectum mobilized from the back of the prostate gland and penile urethra in male and from the back of the posterior vaginal wall.

Once the puborectalis muscle fibers are divided, the anterior rectal wall is slowly peeled off from the back of the urethra or posterior vaginal wall by the index finger. The risk of injuries to those structures or severance of the neural plexuses could be avoided. Separation of the anterior wall of the rectum is done safely without displaying the penile urethra.

And excision of the transversus perineal muscles and perineal body would be unnecessary in the retrograde dissection. Postoperative recovery remains uneventful in most instances.[2,3] By contrast, there was not a single case of bladder dysfunction found among those patients, operated upon by the retrograde dissection.[2]

POSTOPERATIVE BLADDER DYSFUNCTION AND MANAGEMENT

The dysfunction of the bladder is recognized after the urethral catheter is removed. The symptoms are recognized by chronic retention, incontinence of urine, difficulty in voiding urine or incomplete emptying of the bladder. In these cases, patient needs recatheterization and trial without catheter that varies from patient-to-patient.

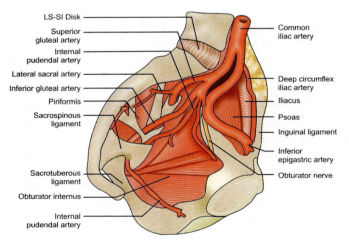

Fig. 11.18: Displaying the internal pudendal artery leaving the pelvis and entering into the perineum through the pudendal canal. (By courtesy of Prof RJ from his last book "Anatomy—Regional and Applied, Seventh Edition, Published by English Language Book Society and Churchill Livingstone Longman Group Ltd 1986)

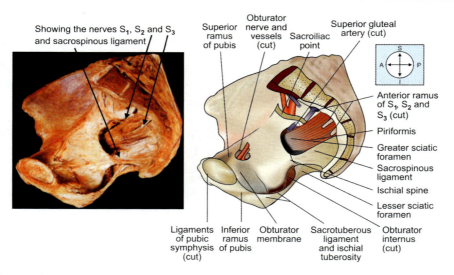

Fig. 11.19: True color photograph taken from the dissected specimen highlighting the anatomical distribution of the muscles and sacral nerves. (These illustrations were taken from the book Human Anatomy by courtesy of Gower Medical Publishers published in 1990 and later reprinted by Wolfe publishing in 1994)

Among the 62 patients, enlarged prostate was evident in preoperative assessment. He responded satisfactorily to TURP done three months later. Among other patients, indwelling catheter was necessary to be left *in situ* for other medical conditions, but difficulty in voiding was noticed in four of 15 female and six of 46 male patients, when the catheter was removed on fifth or sixth postoperative day. They required recatheterization on the same day. But apart from one patient, they recovered normal micturition, when the catheter was removed after 2-3 days.

The one who could not void urine after the second time had sustained urethral injury during perineal dissection. Obviously, he needed recatheterization that was kept for six weeks. He made a full recovery without further morbidity.

It was presumed that pain and inflammation could be the contributing factors for failing to pass urine in those cases, when catheter was first removed. And all 62 patients were included in retrograde perineal dissection.[2]

If the patients could not void after the second attempt, they would require indwelling catheter for a longer period. In the mean time, the tone of the bladder muscle needs to be improved by four hourly bladder drills. This means, patients are trained to keep the indwelling catheter clamped on by inserting spigot for every 2 hours interval for a few days and then every four hourly for several weeks, until it is withdrawn. If the enlarged prostate seems to be the cause for retention or incomplete emptying of the bladder, patient should be referred to urologist for urodynamic and for TURP.

Etiology of Bladder Dysfunction, Associated with Abdominoperineal Resection of the Rectum

a. Sites of severance or bruising of the neural plexus:
   i. Behind the fascia of Waldeyer.
   ii. In the perineal dissection, injury to the nerves may occur at the exit of the pudendal canal, or[2]
   iii. Around the periurethral space during dissection of the anterior wall of the rectum.[2]
b. Periurethral hematoma, bruising or infection around the urethra.
c. Bruising or injury to the membranous urethra or back of the bladder neck.[2]
d. Change in position of the bladder neck due to weight of the full bladder.
e. Enlarged prostate.
f. Open perineal wound packing.

The results of retrograde perineal dissection compare fovorably from other studies as shown in the Table 11.1.

Table 11.1: These are the data on the incidence of bladder dysfunction, retrieved from the literature		
Authors	Incidence	Source
Watson PC and Williams I	52%	Br J Surg p.19, 1952[4]
Rankin JT	24%	Br J Uro p.655, 1969[7]
Fowler JW, et al	59%	Br J Urol p.95, 1978[8]
Saha SK	0%	Surg Gyne Obstet p.33, 1984[2]

A STUDY OF POSTOPERATIVE SEXUAL FUNCTION AMONG THE MEN

To assess the sexual function after abdominoperineal resection of the rectum presented a difficult task, in particular to those who were over 50 years old. Sexual activity is related to many factors, but it would be difficult to assess after operation, if they were old, unmarried, or widower or they were psychologically depressed, because of the tumor. Nevertheless, this survey was undertaken in order to comply with the comment made by the editor of the journal.[2] Among the sixteen male patients, four had ceased their sexual activity before the operation, and one noticed some difference after the operation was done. He was not sure whether it was due to depression or due to operation. All of them were over 60 years old. Nevertheless, among the other 12 patients, 11 had retained the potency of sexual function.[2]

This study was extended among the younger age group patients who had underwent surgery for panproctocolectomy for ulcerative colitis. Although the number of cases was much smaller, there was not a single case of impotency found among these patients aged around 40 years old. In fact, one bachelor told me on the seventh postoperative day that he had noticed erection of his penis, in response to fondling by his girlfriend. This finding was reassuring, resolving the academic debate that nervi erigentes supplying the penile arterial vessels follow along the course of internal pudendal vessels. And this study supports my previous study reported in the literature in 1984.[2]

MERITS OF THE PERINEAL WOUND CLOSURE

Wound Healing by Secondary Intention

Perineal wound could be dealt with by various methods. It depends upon the experience and skill of the perineal surgeon.

Wound packing used to be acceptable practice 50 years ago. In a rare circumstance, where the bleeding from the sacral wall seems to be uncontrollable by coagulation diathermy, wound packing has to be done. And it is a life saving measure. This delays the postoperative recovery. Patients needed to stay in hospital for several weeks or months, until the wound appeared to be filled up by the granulation tissue that takes place slowly from the deep of the wound. Wound dressing is distressing and expensive.

The wound packing has been replaced by wound closure which could be either partial or complete perineal closure. In the former case, the front and back of the perineal wound used to be sutured together leaving behind a small gap in the middle of the wound through which either a large tube drain or a corrugated drainage sheet was brought out. Residual blood clots remain in the dependent part of the sacrum. In some cases, the residual clots may be infected, leading to formation of pelvic abscess. In this case, surgical drainage would be required.[1] In other cases, blood stained serous discharge may continue over several months.

REVIEW OF THE PRIMARY PERINEAL WOUND HEALING

Since 1970s, primary closure of the perineal wound has become a new approach. It resolves the question of residual blood clots being infected, and it enhances primary wound healing. This progress has been made possible due to a close suction appliance being available. Two suction tubes are left inside the pelvic cavity before the perineal wound is closed. Primary closure of the perineal wound requires a clean perineal wound, but study showed that contaminated wound could be closed, after the pelvic and perineal wound being lavage thoroughly with normal saline and then with metronidazole IV solution. The results are equally promising.[3]

In the literature, the incidence of primary wound healing was reported to be ranging from 45.2 to 100 percent. A profile of perineal wound healing is furnished in Table 11.2.

Table 11.2: A profile of primary perineal wound healing after APR		
Authors	Incidence	Year
Schofield PF	76.66%	1970
Hulton et al	75%	1971
Altemeier et al	92%	1974
Broader et al	69%	1974
Irving and Goligher	45.20%	1975[10]
Marks et al	56%	1976[9]
Saha and Robinson	88%	1976[1]
Saha SK	100% and 74% (*)	1983[3]

In a retrospective study from St. Marks Hospital, the etiology for the perineal wound infection was claimed to be attributable to Dukes C tumor present in their study.[9]

In 1976, the incidence of wound infection in our series was 12 percent. To resolve the inconsistent results in the perineal wound infection, a separate prospective study was undertaken; but no association was found in the results that wound infection could be attributable to advanced Dukes tumor staging.[3] In this study, metronidazole solution was used locally in the contaminated perineal wound. The incidence of primary perineal wound healing was found 100 percent in clean perineal wound and 74 percent in contaminated cases. In Table 11.3 and 11.4, there was no evidence to suggest that Dukes C rectal tumor had contributed to wound infection.[3]

Table 11.3: Dukes classification of the rectal carcinoma included in study

Tumor Staging	Clean perineal wound	Contaminated perineal wound	No.	(%)
Dukes A	-	-	-	-
Dukes B	7	6	13	(34)
Dukes C1	5	2	7	(19)
Dukes C2	7	11	18	(47)
Total	19	19	38	(100)

Table 11.4: Results of primary perineal wound closure after APR

Perineal wound	Clean cases	Contaminated cases	Total
Primary healing	19(100%)	14(74%)	33
Delayed healing	—	5(26%)	5
Total	19	19	38

CONTINUOUS PERINEAL WOUND IRRIGATION

In another study published in the Annals of the Royal College of Surgeons of England in 1985, the perineal wound was treated with a constant suction and irrigation with normal saline, following rectal excision for inflammatory bowel disease.[11] The main objective was to stop hematoma formation in the perineal wound. The merit of such treatment was questioned.[12] Because, there was no conclusive evidence to suggest that the wound hematoma developed within the pelvic cavity in those cases, in which, the perineal wound is closed completely, using two suction tubes for sucking out all blood stained fluid from the pelvic cavity.[1-3]

Although saline irrigation is not indicated and it is unnecessary, on the contrary, it would delay the primary perineal wound healing and would enhance absorption of the saline from the denuded tissue surfaces of the pelvis, thus affecting the fluid balance. And, it may cause overloading to the heart in certain cases. It would be detrimental to those patients who are known cases of congestive cardiac failure, chronic lung disease and suffering from hypertension.

Furthermore, patients would be needed to stay in bed until the irrigation is discontinued. Therefore, their mobility would be restricted. A constant nursing care would be necessary in order to look after the irrigation set, fluid balance, and change of wound dressing because of soaking of wound with seepage of irrigation fluid through the perineal wound. Despite all these disadvantages and detrimental effects, taking care of the patient would be expensive. This includes the nursing cost, irrigation cost, bed occupancy and wound dressing.[12]

MERITS OF THE PELVIC FLOOR RECONSTRUCTION

Alternative to the pelvic floor reconstruction, the small intestine could be left in the denuded surface of the pelvis. Although it saves a lot of operating time and it allows the surgeon to carry out a wide resection of the rectum along with the pelvic peritoneum, there remains a potential risk of adhesions among the loops of the intestine with the denuded surface of the sacral wall. If they are presented with the intestinal obstruction, the only feasibility for the relief of obstruction would be the intrasegmental bypass operation or loop ileostomy.

The author had experienced in dealing with 2 such cases, which required bypass operation that was carried out above the true pelvis. In this situation, patient may develop short gut syndrome and blind loop syndrome that may lead to a poor nutritional state of health. Therefore, reconstruction of the pelvic floor must be undertaken if possible.

MERITS BETWEEN THE SPHINCTER-SAVING LOW ANTERIOR RESECTION AND ABDOMINOPERINEAL RESECTION OF THE RECTUM FOR THE RECTAL CARCINOMA

Sphincter-saving low anterior resection seems to have generated interest among the patients and surgeons. It could be used for the rectal tumors present above 6 cm from the anal verge. Although this technique is not new, circular gun autosuture seems to have made the operative procedure much easier, compared to hand anastomosis. Whether the quality of life outweighs the total cost for this high-tech surgical approach has yet to be measured in perspective. All the studies suggest contrary to noble concept.

This technique carries a potential risk of anastomotic leakage, despite a loop ileostomy being constructed. The average incidence ranges from 14.4 to 31.3 percent that depends upon whether the rectal stump is connected to the splenic flexure or the sigmoid colon.[13,14] And it was over 14 percent found in the former and over 31 percent in the latter group included in the same study.[14]

In both groups, inferior mesenteric artery was ligated in order to bring the colon down to the rectal stump. This study supports the views that anastomotic leakage is attributable to ischemic condition and/or technical fault and not due to palliative resection, as claimed in the literature.[14]

In the literature, a correlation was reported between the anastomotic leakage and a high incidence of local recurrence.[13] In these cases, the curable tumor would turn out to be incurable.

However, reversal of loop-ileostomy done two or three months later does not assure a good quality of life in many patients, despite the fact that there was no evidence of anastomotic leakage or anastomotic stricture. And in certain cases, it may not be possible or may be delayed over six months, if there were evidence of leakage, pelvic abscess, stricture, or anal stenosis.

In one literature, of the 38 cases of anastomotic leakage, ileostomy was needed to be put back in 21 patients—thus representing an incidence of 37.17 percent.[14] Among these patients, thirteen had a permanent ileostomy. If those three postoperative deaths were included in the statistics, the incidence would have been higher. Although the true prevalence of permanent ileostomy is not known in the literature, thirteen patients needed permanent ileostomy, but true prevalence was not reported in the literature.[14] This seems to be in sharp contrast to the subsequent publication from the same research team, in that it was claimed that the temporary stomas was required in 73 percent.[15] It implied that there was not a single case of permanent ileostomy left *in situ* among his patients, operated upon over twenty years.

Among the cases of delayed morbidity, anastomotic stricture, and anal stenosis present a difficult task. It may result from disuse atrophy of the rectum and anal sphincter, because of diversion of feces for the first few months. Other attributing factors are preoperative adjuvant radiotherapy or postoperative inflammatory mass developed surrounding the anastomosis. The treatment for this condition is repeated dilatation under general anesthesia.

All these evidences suggest that patients are subjected to undue stress and uncertainty of the prognosis and many of them remain at risk of further operative procedures whether they are for the anastomotic leakage, pelvic abscess, and reversal of ileostomy or reconstruction of ileostomy, colostomy or for anal dilatation for anastomotic stricture, or anal stenosis. All the procedures are amounted to increased bed occupancy and cumulative cost.

Anal sphincteric dysfunction is another functional morbidity. It all depends upon the level of anastomosis. And it could be related to length of the colon being excised that may interfere with the absorption of water from the feces and that may lead to intestinal hurry due to loss of fecal transit time. According to published report, the overall functional morbidity would be worse off, if the level of anastomosis is at 3 cm compared to 6 cm from the anal verge.[16]

They are frequency of motion, incontinence of flatus, fecal soiling and urge defecation and their incidence were 32 percent, 53 percent and 53 percent, compared to 24 percent, 4 percent and 11 percent, respectively.[16]

From these evidences, one could draw a conclusion that many patients would remain 'house-bound'. And a curable disease may turn out to be incurable state in some cases, because of the fact that the risk of anastomotic leakage is much greater for the tumor located at or a little above 3 cm. And these cases remain at a greater risk for the higher incidence of local recurrence.

In the literature, many studies on low anterior resection of the tumor have been reported. And one of the reports claimed that the incidence of cancer specific survival at 5 years and 10 years was 68 and 66 percent respectively. It has also reported that survival rate was much higher found among the cases of curative resection. It was 81 and 80 percent at 5 and 10 years follow-up, respectively.[15]

Therefore, leaving aside all those prognostic factors, the merit of low anterior resection should be judged by the survival rate, quality of life, and cumulative cost. Although the Basingstoke studies claimed that the incidence of local recurrence rate was less than 2 percent among the curative resection, and survival rate among the curative resection cases was 81 and 80 percent at 5 years and 10 years follow-up respectively.[15] This was in contrast to 38 percent survival rate, published from Lyon, France in 1995.[23]

It has been found that data on various issues seem to be inconsistent with other publications from the same school of work. In one study, only one patient was reported to have lost from the follow-up, the incidence of anastomotic leakage was 12 percent and there was not a single patient requiring permanent ileostomy.[15]

These data seem to be inconsistent with other publications, in which eight patients were reported to have lost or not responded to postal survey,[16] and the incidence of anastomotic leakage was claimed to be ranging from 14 to 31.3 percent and 13 patients needed permanent ileostomy.[14]

Furthermore, if the survival rate among the 133 patients were reviewed, the survival rate was found to be much lower among the 133 patients operated upon over many years (1978-1980). It would be 56.4 percent, if lost follow-up cases were treated as being dead, or it would be 60 percent, if they are treated to be still alive.[16]

Although these data were not 10 years follow-up, the survival rate among these patients was no nearer to the results of 5 years and 10 years follow-up, published in 1998.[15] Furthermore, the data on missing cases between the two publications seemed puzzling and conflicting. And this sort of approach was not helpful in reviewing the outcome of the new operative procedure.[14-16] Nonetheless, it is not uncommon in any long-term follow-up.

CRITERIA FOR CURATIVE AND PALLIATIVE RESECTION

In the literature, curative and palliative resections are often referred to in order to define the outcome of the sphincter-saving low anterior resection of the rectum. Rationality has to be in agreement with consensus in deciding whether the cases with a palliative resection of the rectal tumor should be included in the operation for sphincter-saving low anterior resection of the rectum. There is no doubt that many of these patients would subsequently suffer from recurrence of the tumor or colonic obstruction. The latter may be attributable to anastomotic stricture or recurrence of the tumor either at the site of anastomosis or around the gut causing pressure from outside.

Many of these cases will require a second operation for a colostomy, if they develop colonic obstruction. Hence, it would provide a disservice to these patients, when the benefit from this operation would be short-lived. Therefore, true merit of this new operative procedure could not be measured by the inclusion of the palliative resection into the study.

Hence, it is important to define those criteria upon which the low anterior resection could be included in the treatment of the rectal carcinoma.

These are the criteria for the curative resection of the rectal tumor and for employing the sphincter-saving low anterior resection.

a. The tumor mass should be mobile on palpation.
b. Dukes Tumor Stage should be A or B.
c. A good distal clear margin below the tumor is achievable for end-to-end anastomosis.
d. The tumor has not invaded to the surrounding organs.

These are the criteria for palliative resection and not suitable for the low anterior resection.

a. The tumor stage is Dukes C, and mobile.
b. The tumor is adherent to the neighboring organ or to the parietal wall, but resectable.
c. Mesenteric lymph nodes are enlarged but within the field of palliative resection.

In those cases in which curative resection appears to be unsuitable, low anterior resection should not be undertaken, instead Hartmann's operative procedure, or abdominoperineal resection of the rectum should be undertaken.

MERITS OF ABDOMINOPERINEAL RESECTION

Although abdominoperineal resection of the rectum is universally regarded to be a curative operative procedure, it may also be regarded to be a good palliative procedure for the Dukes C rectal tumor, provided the rectum could be mobilized from the surrounding tissue. Adhesion of the tumor to the neighboring structures or posterior vaginal wall in women or to the back of the bladder or prostate gland carry a poor prognosis whether or not these patients are included in abdominoperineal resection, but such major procedure could be performed, if the tumor appears to be resectable on laparotomy and the surgeon is experienced in dealing with the extensive resection of the rectum from the surrounding organs.

In these cases, at least the patient will enjoy a good period of comfortable life and may not require a second operation due to recurrence of the tumor in the pelvis or in the perineal scar. And these recurrent tumors could be treated with an adjuvant therapy in some cases.

Furthermore, abdominoperineal resection compares favorably in many aspects, apart from the burden of terminal colostomy. And there would be no risk of spillage of malignant cells into the pelvis, in those cases in which the rectal tumor is Dukes A and B, unless accidental perforation has occurred during operation. Breaching of the rectal wall may lead to a fecal contamination and may open an access to the spillage of viable malignant cells, whether or not the tumor is Dukes' A or B.

Average postoperative bed-occupancy would be less than 2 weeks,[2,3] in those cases in which primary perineal wound healing has been achieved. It ranges from 56 to 100 percent that depends upon the skill of the operator and the operative technique used in perineal resection.[1-3,9] The risk of perineal wound contamination and bladder dysfunction could be avoided by the retrograde resection of the rectum.[2]

Although terminal colostomy rarely produces complication, it may present with parastomal herniation, prolapse of the colostomy or stomal stenosis. All these surgical conditions require further surgery. In addition, running cost for colostomy bag and appliances would be an additional financial burden upon the patient.

Unlike the previous technique, patients do not need to pay for those expensive autosutures and do not need to go to the theater for any other postoperative complications, despite developing local recurrence of tumor in the pelvis.

Therefore, selection of a particular technique must be judged on the merits of cost, morbidity and quality of life of the patients.

EVALUATION OF SURVIVAL RATE AFTER ABDOMINOPERINEAL RESECTION OF THE RECTUM

There are many crude factors that may influence in the prognosis of the survival rate. They are sex, age, location of the tumor and spread of the tumor, operative techniques used, adjuvant therapy and skill of the surgeon.

Dukes found in his study that five-year survival rate is relatively better in female than in male patients (Table 11.5).[17] This study was consistent with the report published by the Mayo Clinic and the difference between the two sexes was 5 percent.[18] No cause was identified in this difference.

Clinical Practice and Surgery of the Colon, Rectum and Anus

Table 11.5: Comparison fo five-year survival rate in men and women suffering form tumor		
Tumor stage	Men	Women
	Five-year survival rate	
	Crude/Corrected figure	Crude/Corrected figure
Dukes A	80.4 / 99.9%	81.8 / 93.8%
Dukes B	61.3 / 76.00%	71.60 / 82.00%
Dukes C	26.1 / 31.30%	29.10 / 32.70%

Table 11.6: Five-year survival rate related to level of the rectal tumor		
Level of the tumor	Lymph nodes	Incidence
0-5 cm	Dukes A and B	66.00%
	Dukes C	23.30%
	All cases	46.2%
6-10 cm	Dukes A and B	75.5%
	Dukes C	25.00%
	All cases	51.10%
> 10 cm	Dukes A and B	68.1%
	Dukes C	33.3%
	All cases	53.8%

The survival rate is also affected by the age of the patient. It states that the prognosis was found worse among the younger patients, below the age of 30;[17] but the result in Mayo Clinic was much better. This study was carried out by Johnson, Judd and Dahlin in 1959 between the period of 1925 and 1954.[19] Dukes concluded from his study that lymphatic spread was found much aggressive, among the younger patients, presented with the rectal carcinoma,[17] but radical excision of the tumor was regarded to be contributing factor in their results and no reference was made in this study whether or not there were evidences of lymphatic involvement in those cases of the rectal tumor.[19]

Apart from the sex, the survival of the patients is also influenced by the location of the rectal tumor.

This study was first undertaken by Gilchrist and David in 1947 and they reported on five-years follow-up and found that the prognosis following a combined excision of the tumor was worse in those cases in which, the rectal tumor was found in the extraperitoneal space than those in the intraperitoneal space. The crude five-year survival rate of the patients presented with intraperitoneal tumor was 65.4 percent, compared with 51.8 percent among the cases presented with extraperitoneal tumor.[20]

This result suggests that the prognosis for five-year survival was found much better after abdominoperineal resection of the rectum, among those cases in which the tumor was above the peritoneal reflection. And similar results were seen in other study, which showed that the survival rate was much better among those cases in which the rectal tumor was 6-10 cm or above 10 cm from the anal verge. This result was found associated with those cases in which there was no evidence of lymphatic spread.[21]

And the incidence of five-year survival rate among the cases with lymphatic spread (Dukes C) was found much better if the location of the tumor was above 10 cm from the anal verge (Table 11. 6).[21] This study was consistent with the previous report.[18] And all these studies exemplified that the prognosis of the survival is related to the radical excision of the tumor along with the wide clearance of the lymphatic spread.[21]

The results in 20 years follow-up were encouraging as shown in Figures 11.20A and B.[21]

Although the crude survival rate is affected by many other criteria, these include age, sex, Dukes tumor stage, histological grading, operative procedure and skill of the surgeons. The true or corrected survival rate is affected if there are concomitant or intercurrent diseases. To establish the corrected survival rate, all those factors need to be excluded from the statistics. The final figure could be referred to adjusted or corrected survival rate, which could be five-year, ten-year, fifteen-year or twenty-year follow-up. St. Marks Hospital has produced a corrected survival rate on those patients who were reviewed up to 20 years.

In the literature, it was claimed that the survival rate was not associated with the Dukes tumor stage, anastomotic leakage rate, level of the tumor from the anal verge.[15] This observation was in conflict with other studies in which it was reported that a good survival rate was found associated with the level of the rectal tumor included in the abdominoperineal resection[19-21] and the 5-year survival rate was found worse among the cases, in which, the tumor was at 0-5 cm from the anal verge, compared with those tumors, located higher up in the rectum. It was 66 percent, compared to 75 percent and 68 percent respectively. In all these cases, lymph nodes were not involved. And cases with palliative resection were excluded from the five-year follow-up.

Although the survival rate was found low among the cases presented with Dukes C, it was 23.3 percent, 25 percent and 33 percent in all three groups, there was no significant difference among the tumors located at 0-5 cm and 6-10 cm from the anal verge, despite the fact that lymph glands of both groups were infiltrated with the metastasis.

In contrast, the survival rate among other cases of advanced tumor (Dukes C), located above 10 cm from the anal verge was 33 percent. This suggested that a good and unrestricted access is very important in order to achieve a wider clearance of the mesenteric lymph nodes along with the radical excision of the tumor. This seemed to have contributed to a better

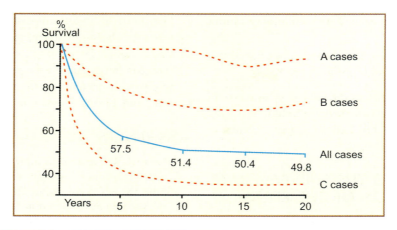

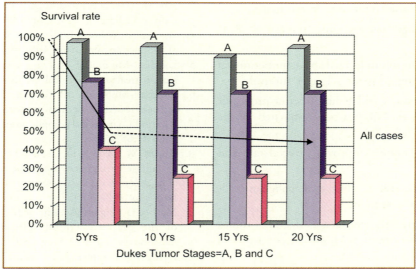

Figs 11.20A and B: Showing the survival rate among 2083 cases included in the follow-up over a period of 20 years

five-year survival rate,[21] but they were not comparable to those tumors of Dukes A and B. It seems evident that Dukes tumor stage as well as wider resection area provides a long-term survival rate.

If this was the evidence, then the prognosis would be worse in those cases in which Dukes C rectal tumors are located at 3 or 6 cm from the anal verge, whether or not low anterior resection or abdominoperineal resection is employed in the operation. The practical problem in the depth of the pelvis seems to be associated with a limited access to the tumor in the pelvis. And it would not be possible to see and look around the tumor under direct vision.

This exemplified that those tumors located at 0-5 cm from the anal verge, would carry a potential risk of operative morbidity and poor five-year survival rate. In view of these facts, low anterior resection would be inappropriate in these cases. And it would not be cost-effective in those countries, where health service is not free at delivery to the patients.

MERITS OF ABDOMINOPERINEAL RESECTION

a. All resectable tumors could be included in this technique.
b. There would be no risk of implantation or spillage of malignant cells locally, if the tumor staging is Dukes A and B and if there is no perforation of the rectum.
c. The question of anastomotic leakage does not arise in this technique.
d. Risk of developing bladder or sexual dysfunction could not be ruled out, but the bladder dysfunction is avoidable by the retrograde mobilization of the rectum is carried out under direct vision, as described in this chapter.[2]
e. Primary perineal wound healing is expected to be between 88 and 100 percent in clean operative cases.[3]
f. Bed occupancy is expected to be less than two weeks in straightforward cases.[2,3]
g. Burden of colostomy and its maintenance cost is unavoidable.

h. Delayed complications associated with colostomy cannot be predicted.
i. In most instances, further operation would be unnecessary if there is recurrence of the tumor in the pelvis.

Having known all the evidences and facts, conclusion could be made that the merits of the two operative techniques would be judged by the quality of life, bed occupancy cumulative cost and 10 years survival rate.

FACTORS AFFECTING THE SURVIVAL RATE AFTER THE RESECTION OF THE RECTAL CARCINOMA

Sex: Survival rate is worse in men than in women.[17,18]

Age of the patient: Younger patient under the age of 30 is worse prognosis.[17]

Location of the tumor: The tumor located above the peritoneal reflection has a better prognosis for a longer survival.[21]

Dukes tumor stage: Dukes A and B has a better prognosis than Dukes C stage tumor. This has been evaluated by the survival rate.[13,17]

Preoperative adjuvant therapy: Improves survival rate and reduces local recurrence.

Operative technique: The risk of spillage of malignant cells is greater in low anterior resection.

One has to recongnize that the prevalence of Dukes tumor stage varies from center-to-center. Such evidences have been cited in Table 11.7.

Table 11.7: Prevalence of the Dukes tumor staging reported in different studies			
Dukes Tumor Stage	A	B	C
Dukes CE (1940)	15%	35%	50%[24]
Saha SK (1983)	0%	34.2%	65.8%[3]
Karanjia et al (1992)	26.5%	39.7%	33.8%[16]
Bulow et al (2003)	23%	46%	30%[25]
Bell et al (2003)	25.1%	35.7%	39.2%[13]

It has been the consensus that the survival rate among the cases with abdominoperineal resection is influenced by the Dukes Tumor stage and local venous spread.[13,17] In the previous studies, it was reported that the survival rate for the Dukes C tumor would be less than 30 percent.[17,18] And it was also the consensus that the local recurrence would be much less among the cases of low anterior resection, if the distal resection level is around 5 cm from the lower edge of the tumor.[26,27]

Furthermore, the risk of spillage of malignant cells to the denuded tissue in the pelvis would be much greater, if the tumor is Dukes C. The risk could not be ruled out in other tumors of Dukes A and B, if the rectal wall is accidentally open in abdominoperineal resection.

The merit of abdominoperineal resection is also to be measured by the survival rate, quality of life and cumulative cost. And they are favorable in every aspect of all those criteria. The surgeons must examine the pros and cons of each operative technique with reference to the patient circumstance, tumor location and Dukes tumor stage.

REFERENCES

1. Saha SK, Robinson AF. A study of perineal wound healing after abdominoperineal resection. Br J Surg 1976;63:555.
2. Saha SK. A Critical evaluation of dissection of the perineum in synchronous combind abdominoperineal excision of the rectum. Surgery gynecology and obstetrics 1984; 158:33.
3. Saha SK. Care of perineal wound in abdominoperineal resection. J Royal College of Surg Edin 1983;28:324.
4. Watson PC, Williams I. The urological complications of excision of the rectum. Br J Surg 1952;40:19.
5. Lockhart-Mummery JP. Two hundred cases of cancer of the rectum treated by perineal excision. Lancet 1920;1:20.
6. Lockhart-Mummery JP. Two hundred cases of cancer of the rectum treated by perineal excision. Br J Surg 1926;14:110.
7. Rankin JT. Urological complications of rectal surgery. Br J Urol 1969;41:655-59.
8. Fowler JW, Bremner DN, et al. The incidence and consequence of damage to the parasympathetic nerve supply to the bladder after abdominoperineal resection of the rectum for carcinoma. Br J Urol 1978;50:95.
9. Marks CG, Leighton M, Ritchie JK, Hawley PR. Primary suture of the perineal wound following rectal excision for adenocarcinoma. Br J Surg. 1976;63:322.
10. Irving TT, Goligher JC. A controlled clinical trial of three different methods of perineal wound management following excision of the rectum. Br J Surg 1975;62:287.
11. Elliott MS, Todd I. Primary suture of the perineal wound using constant suction and irrigation following rectal excision for inflammatory bowel disease, Annals of the Royal College of Surgeons of England 1985;67:6.
12. Saha SK. Primary suture of the perineal wound using constant suction and irrigation, following rectal excision for inflammatory bowel disease. Letter to the Editor, highlighting the pitfalls of constant irrigation with saline into the perineal wound, published in the Annals of the Royal College of Surgeons of England, 1985;67:268.
13. Bell SW, Walker KG, et al. Anastomotic leakage after curative anterior resection results in a higher prevalence of local recurrence. Br J Surg 2003;90:1261.
14. Karanjia ND, Corder AP, Bearn P, Heald RJ. Leakage from the stapled low anastomosis after total mesorectal excision for carcinoma of the rectum. Br J Surg 1994;81:1224.
15. Heald RJ, Moran BJ, Ryall RDH, et al. Rectal cancer: The Basingstoke experience of total mesorectal excision 1978-1997. Arch Surgery August 1998;133:894.
16. Karanjia ND, Schache DJ, Heald RJ. Function of the distal rectum after low anterior resection for carcinoma. Br J Surg 1992;79:114.

17. Dukes CE. Discussion on major surgery in carcinoma of the rectum with or without colostomy excluding the anal canal and including the rectosigmoid. Proc Roy Soc Med 1957;50:1031.
18. Mayo CW, Fly OA. Analysis of five-year survival in carcinoma of the rectum and rectosigmoid. Surg Gynec Obstet 1956;103:94.
19. Johnson JW, Judd ES, Dahlin DC. Malignant neoplasm of the colon and rectum in young persons. Arch Surg (Chicago) 1959;79:365.
20. Gilchrist RK, David VC. A consideration of pathological factors influencing five-year survival in radical resection of the large bowel and rectum for carcinoma. Ann Surg 1947;126:421.
21. Waugh JM and Kirklin JW. The importance of the level of the lesion and the prognosis and treatment of carcinoma of the rectum and low sigmoid colon. Ann Surg 1949; 129:22.
22. Bussey HJR. The long-term results of surgical treatment of cancer of the rectum. Proc Roy Med 1963;50:494.
23. World Health Organisation International Agency for research on Cancer European Commission. Survival of Cancer Patients in Europe: The Euro Study. Lyon. France: IARC Scientific, 1995.
24. Dukes CE. Cancer of the rectum: An analysis of 1000 cases. J Path Bact 1940;50:527.
25. Bulow S, Christensen IJ, Harling H, et al. Recurrence and survival after mesorectal excision for rectal cancer. Br J Surg 2003;90:974.
26. Goligher JC, Dukes CE, Bussey HJR. Local recurrence after sphincter-saving excision for carcinoma of the rectum and rectosigmoid. Brit J Surg 1951;39:199.
27. Quer EA, Dahlin DC and Mayo CW. Retrograde intramural spread of carcinoma of the rectum and rectosigmoid: A microscopic study. Surg Gynec and Obstet 1953;96:24.

12 Prolapse of the Rectum

Prolapse of the rectum implies that the anal mucosa or the rectum has descended through the anal orifice. Prolapse of the anal mucosa alone is called a partial prolapse and prolapse of the full thickness of the rectum is referred to as a complete prolapse. In either case, it prolapses either on straining at defecation or on coughing.

PARTIAL PROLAPSE

Mucosal prolapse is referred to as partial prolapse that could be found localized or circumferential all around the anal orifice. It does not descend beyond 4 cm. When the descended part is palpated between the thumb and index finger, only mucous membrane and mucosa are felt and no muscular coat is palpable. It occurs either among the children, below the age of 4 years, or among the elderly people.

Complete prolapse does not occur among the children, but it is prevalent among the extreme age groups.

EPIDEMIOLOGY OF THE PROLAPSE RECTUM

Among the children, partial prolapse is prevalent within the first two years of age and its incidence declines after the age of five.[1] Furthermore, its incidence is greater among the boys.

Complete prolapse, by contrast, is prevalent frequently among the adult women, compared to men and its incidence is 84 percent.[2] Partial prolapse does occur in both sexes of adult groups.

ETIOLOGY

It has been found among the cases of partial prolapse that sacral curvature, that appears to be underdeveloped seems to be the predisposing factor for causing the partial prolapse found among the affected group of children. It reduces the resting support to the mucosal lining of the anal canal. Other etiological factors are diarrhea, whooping cough, and loss of body weight resulting in loss of fat in the ischeorectal fossa.

Partial prolapse is frequently associated with the third degree prolapsed pile, bladder neck obstruction, or urethral stricture that may occur among the adult subjects. In female patient, torn perineum at childbirth is the predisposing factor. Atony of the anal sphincter which is attributable to tabes dorsalis or tumor in the cauda equina is the causative factor in both sexes. Partial prolapse has also been encountered with the operation of the fistula-in-ano in which the sphincters have been divided.

Complete prolapse occurs in women more than in men and it seems to be affected by the parturition. In the literature, its incidence has been found higher among the multipara than among the childless women.[2,3] In women, complete prolapse is also associated with the prolapse of the uterus and hysterectomy.

SYMPTOMS

Among the patients with the prolapse of the rectum, the symptoms are discharge of mucus, bleeding from the exposed ulcerated mucosa, incontinence of feces and flatus. The latter is related to atony of the sphincteric muscles. It also soils the underclothes of the sufferers.

EXAMINATION

After abdominal examination, patient is asked to lie on the left lateral position bringing both knees together towards the abdomen. Inspection around the perineum is very important. To avoid embarrassment, patient pushes the rectum into the anus, before changing the clothes. Obviously, there would be no apparent sign of complete or partial prolapse to be seen outside the anus, but the abnormal feature around the anal orifice would be evident, and classical feature of anal verge would be absent. Instead, a patulous anal orifice, displaying the lax mucosa will be seen at first sight.

Before palpating the anus, patient is asked to strain down or to give a cough. This will demonstrate that anal mucosa or the rectum has prolapsed out through the patulous anal orifice. The prolapsed mucosa is next palpated in order to confirm whether it is a partial or complete prolapse. If it does not descend beyond 3-4 cm in length and if there is no musculature felt between the thumb and index finger, then the obvious diagnosis would be partial prolapse.

If the length of the prolapse is greater than 4-5 cm and palpation appears to be much thicker between the index finger, inserted into the lumen and the thumb placed on the outer surface of the prolapsed rectum, then it would be regarded to be complete prolapse.

After this examination, patient is asked to bear further down. The purpose is to see the total length of the prolapsed rectum and to see any evidence of loop of the small intestine in the pouch of Douglas present anteriorly at the mucocutaneous junction and to record ulceration over the surface of mucosa. Dilated veins could be seen in the submucosa of the prolapse during coughing or straining.

After this procedure, the anal mucosa or the rectum is pushed back into the anus. The tone of the anal orifice and power of contractility are tested, in that the patient is asked to squeeze the anal orifice without the index finger being placed inside the anal orifice. It would be evident that patient would be unable to close the anal orifice, which suggests lack of tone and lack of contractility of the anal sphincters.

Now the procedure is repeated, but in this case, the finger is held inside the anal orifice, it would confirm by the lack of tightness of the anal orifice felt around the surgeon's finger. This suggests that the sphincteric muscles have no power of contraction and in fact, have lost its muscle tone.

During this examination, the muscle tone of the anal orifice and that of the internal anal sphincter will appear to be deficient. It would show that the patient would not experience any discomfort and the surgeon would not encounter with resistance, when he will attempt to put the whole fist or at least 3-4 fingers through the patulous anal orifice.

Finally, proctoscopy and sigmoidoscopy are done in order to exclude any other lesion present inside the rectum. It is also important to exclude colonic tumor by barium enema and/or colonoscopy.

TREATMENT

Partial mucosal prolapse may descend up to 3.50 cm and children below the age of 4 years are vulnerable, but it is self-limiting condition. It responds to conservative measures. If it does not resolve, it is treated with injection of 5 percent phenol in almond oil, like treatment for the first degree internal piles in adults. The procedure would be the same but it requires general anesthesia.

Under direct vision through the proctoscope, phenol is injected in the submucosa above the anorectal ring with 1-2 ml at each site. Initially 2-3 places are injected in order to see the response to the treatment. The mucosa stops prolapsing within a week, thus inducing a fibrosis that tethers the mucosa with the muscle wall.

If it does not work, then Thiersch operation should be done, but thick chromic catgut, or dexon or similar type of suture, instead of silver wire or prolene is inserted subcutaneously around the anal sphincter. In most cases, no further treatment is required.

In adult patient, partial prolapse presents like a third degree internal piles but unlike the internal piles, it has broad based prolapsed mucosa and in most cases it occurs in a particular site.

It is treated with Goodsall double transfixation stitches with chromic catgut or Vicryl suture. Or the prolapse mucosa could be excised like prolapsed internal piles. In the latter case, by contrast to hemorrhoidectomy, there will be no skin bridge at the conclusion of the operation; but anal stenosis develops following wound healing. This may reduce the risk of recurrence of prolapse.

If the partial prolapse develops following the operation of anal fistula, or after the perineal tear during delivery of the baby, the operative results would be unsatisfactory. In these cases, prolapsed mucosa occurs through the affected site and it may tend to ulcerate and is often associated with incontinence.

In this case, submucosal injection of 5 percent phenol in almond oil may improve the conditions, but a larger dose (around 10 ml) should be used. Repair of the sphincteric muscles remains the option, or the tone of the muscles could be enhanced with perineal physiotherapy, and by electrical stimulation or with electronic implant to the sphincters. In extreme circumstances, temporary colostomy should be done, prior to local treatment being carried out.

SURGICAL TREATMENT FOR THE COMPLETE PROLAPSE

Complete prolapse of the rectum, by contrast, is a complete descend of the rectum through the relaxed or atony rectal sphincter (Fig. 12.1).

Elderly people and particularly women are affected with this condition. It is debatable whether it is a sliding hernia or intussusception. The etiology is unknown. Constipation and incontinence are two important clinical problems that may not be cured in many cases, after operative procedure being carried out.

Devadhar from Mumbai found in his study[4] that it is intussusception and that the lower part of the rectum has a thick wall compared to the upper part of the rectum.

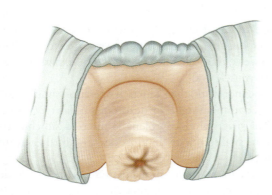

Fig. 12.1: It is a complete prolapse of the rectum

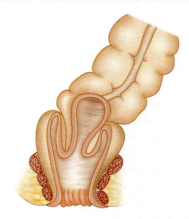

Fig. 12.2: Showing how the prolapse of the rectum begins

He had identified a 'crucial point' of intussusception at the junction between the two segments of the rectum. It has thick-walled peritoneum covering this crucial point, but surprisingly, by contrast, the prolapsed rectum does not carry the serosal wall or peritoneal covering with it, outside the anus.

The author believes that the thick-walled rectum, found in the prolapsed segment is the result of fusion of the two rectal walls that had prolapsed together over the years and that two serosal layers of the prolapsed segment of the rectum have fused together into one layer that covers the inner wall of the prolapsed rectum. And this could be the reason to find a thin-walled rectum, which is a normal rectal wall proximal to the prolapsed thick-walled rectum. The striking features in his claim that both anterior and the posterior length of the prolapsed rectum remains equal. Therefore, it could not be regarded as being a case of sliding hernia. And it appears to be rectostomy, similar to that of ileostomy (Fig. 12.2).

The rectal digital examination will reveal that the whole rectal tube has prolapsed and its wall would appear to be much thicker between the thumb and index finger, compared to partial prolapse of the rectum. Weak pelvic muscle tone or atony of the sphincteric muscles seems to be the major etiological factor for the complete prolapse.

The choices of surgical correction are as follows:
1. Thiersch operation.
2. Delorme's operation.
3. Anterior resection with or without rectopexy.
4. Rectosigmoidectomy operation.
5. Well's operation.
6. Rectopexy, using polypropylene mesh sling in the operation.
7. Devadhar operation.

Among these procedures, Thiersch operation provides a good result. It is a simple procedure, but it has other problems. Alternatively, Delorme's procedure could be undertaken. It is a relatively major procedure.

OPERATIVE TECHNIQUE FOR THIERSCH OPERATION

This technique was described in 1891 and silver wire was originally used in the technique; but nylon or prolene suture could be used instead. The purpose of using the silver wire was to induce tissue reaction that would produce fibrosis around the anal orifice in the subcutaneous plane, but no such tissue reaction has been found. Therefore, silver wire is less frequently used. Results are no different between the two approaches, but one is cheaper than the other.

PREOPERATIVE PREPARATION

Bowel preparation is very important and complete empty of the colon may not be achieved with one day laxative or with enema. Patient needs to be admitted a few days before the operation is intended to be carried out. Dehydration needs to be corrected, concurrently with the oral laxatives and enemas. Preoperative sigmoidoscopy should be done in order to exclude fecal impaction. Bladder catheterization should be done prior to the operation.

OPERATIVE TECHNIQUE

Patient is placed on the lithotomy position. Perineal skin is cleaned with Savlon or bethidin in water. Two small wounds are made with a fine knife, one at 6 o'clock and the other one at 12 o'clock position. The site of wound should be an inch outside the anal verge. A strong curved needle with an eye is inserted through the posterior wound and it is directed towards the anterior wound around the anal sphincter and through the subcutaneous plane. It is pulled out through the anterior wound. If silver wire is preferred in this procedure, it is threaded through the eye of the needle. When the needle is pulled out, this silver wire comes out with the needle. The other end of the wire is kept holding by the artery forceps.

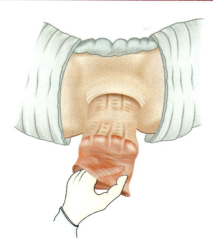

Fig. 12.3: Displaying the method of how the mucosa is separated from the surface of the prolapse of the rectum

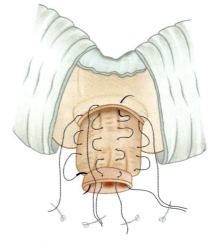

Fig. 12.4: Method of plication sutures inserted between the cut edge of the rectal mucosa and the cut edge of the mucosa around the anus

In a similar way, the same needle is reinserted through the same anterior wound and is directed towards the posterior wound around the other half of the anus. The needle is again pulled out through the posterior wound and the wire comes out with the needle.

Now both ends of the wire are pulled out in order to narrow the anal orifice, until it is tightly fitted either around an index finger or a large Hegar dilator, which one is available at hand in the theater. In most cases, assistant keeps the index finger inside the anal orifice, while this is undertaken. Both ends of the wire are needed to be tied, and this is done by twisting its ends several times, until the anal orifice is snugly fitted around the index finger. Ends of the wire are cut and buried under the subcutaneous wound.

It is important that these ends are not projecting out through the wound. Both skin wounds are closed with prolene sutures. And antiseptic dressing is applied over the wounds.

POSTOPERATIVE CARE

Patient should be given oral laxative from the first postoperative day. Rectal digital examination should be done at intervals in order to be sure that there was no fecal impaction inside the anal canal. Overflow incontinence may be noticed in many cases. To combat this problem, glycerine suppositories should be inserted into the anal orifice at times, if necessary.

Skin sutures are removed in 7 days.

COMPLICATIONS

Silver wire may ulcerate through. It may breakdown inside the wound. It may require to be replaced by a new one. If there is subcutaneous infection around the anal orifice, then reinsertion could be deferred for a few days.

DELORME OPERATION

It is technically a procedure for plication of the rectal wall. Under general anesthesia, patient is in the Trendelenburg lithotomy position and usual skin preparation is employed. Complete prolapse of the rectum is done by pulling down the apex of the prolapsed rectum. To reduce the hemorrhage some advocate using the adrenaline in saline (1: 300000) that is infiltrated in the submucosal space with a long spinal needle all around the prolapsed rectum. It will elevate the mucosa from the muscularis of the gut.

A circular incision is made all around the rectum, just distal to dentate line or one inch distal to the mucocutaneous junction and the rectal mucosa is dissected out from the rectal wall slowly all around towards the apex of the prolapsed rectum (Fig. 12.3).

The dissection is continued in reverse direction along the medial wall of the rectum, after arriving at the apex of the prolapse of the rectum, until it reaches near the anus or to the corresponding level of the outer circular incision, but care is taken that there would not be any tension when both cut edges of the mucosa would be sutured together.

The sleeve of the rectal mucosa is excised after reviewing those technical points just referred to (Fig. 12.4). If the mucosa is excised at the level with the apex, the result would be unsatisfactory, and if too much is removed, the anastomosis may breakdown due to undue tension.

Spurting vessels are controlled with coagulation. Now a series of purse string sutures like plication of the hydrocele of the testis are inserted, between the mucocutaneous junction of the anal orifice and the cut edge of the mucosa (Fig. 12.4).

The first suture, using polydioxin synthetic thread is commenced from the mucocutaneous cut edge and the curved atraumatic needle takes a series of bites at interval through the rectal muscular wall; until it goes through the cut-edge of the mucosa. Several similar sutures (around 8-10) are employed all around the anus.

Each one is ligated at the end. As a result, the apex of the prolapsed rectum will come to be sutured, like a circular collar around the anal orifice. All sutures are cut. Jelly net dressing is applied over the anus.

POSTOPERATIVE CARE

Patient should rest in bed for a few days until the edema and inflammation settles down. Parenteral antibiotics should be commenced and intravenous fluid should be maintained, until flatus has passed. Oral laxative should be commenced in the postoperative period. Incontinence or constipation may not be resolved completely. Dehiscence of the anastomosis may be encountered in the postoperative period. Stricture around the anal orifice is possible.

OPERATIVE TECHNIQUE FOR DEVADHAR OPERATION

This operative technique seems to be based upon the same principle of Delorme's technique, in that only difference is that the plication of the rectal wall is carried out through the peritoneal cavity.

Therefore, it would be a major operative procedure that is carried out under general anesthesia. Patient lies in supine Trendelenburg position. The rectum is approached through a lower midline incision.

The wound is retracted by self-retaining retractors. The rectum is mobilized upwards and crucial point of the rectum is identified by palpation, where a purse string suture using the silk or prolene is inserted along the anterior and the lateral wall of the rectum. This suture takes full thickness bite through the rectal wall without involving the mucosa; but it does not enter into the lumen of the rectum. When the rectal wall is invaginated upwards, the suture is tied. Three or four such sutures are inserted in the anterior wall of the prolapsed rectum in order to make it stronger wall, thus invaginating the anterior rectal wall into the lumen of the rectum.

This invagination is directed upwards and not downwards. Further sutures for placating the lateral wall are inserted, but the suture is commenced from above the 'crucial point' and it goes down as far as it is possible in the bottom of the pelvis. They are ligated producing a reef of the rectal wall.

The rectum would appear to be a rigid tube. Excess peritoneal wall may need to be excised, thus reconstructing the pouch of Douglas in female or rectovesical pouch in male pelvis. No recurrence was reported in 5 years follow-up.[4]

OPERATIVE TECHNIQUE FOR ABDOMINAL RECTOPEXY

If the patient has history of habitual constipation and at the laparotomy, there is redundant loop of sigmoid colon, in these cases, sigmoid colectomy may be required in addition to rectopexy, provided the general condition is permissible for these major procedures. Alternatively, a limited anterior resection of the upper rectum may resolve the problem because of postoperative adhesion that would keep the rectum adherent to the presacral fascia.

Abdominal rectopexy is an extraperitoneal anchorage of the rectal wall, using a strip of polypropylene mesh. The exploration of the rectum remains the same as described in the operation of the abdominoperineal resection of the rectum.

Patient remains in supine position with the head end of the table tilted down. Lower midline incision is used and the wound is retracted by the self-retaining retractor. All the small intestine is put in the upper abdomen. The rectum is separated from the left lateral wall of the pelvis in order to explore the presacral or retroperitoneal space.

To mobilize the rectum from the presacral space, the left and right parietal peritoneum needs to be incised along the side of the rectum; but the dissection of the anterior peritoneum covering the anterior wall of the rectum is not necessary in most cases.

The rectum is mobilized from the parietal wall and from the fascia of Waldeyer, right up to the coccyx, in that, the left hand goes around and behind the rectum, thus elevating the rectum from the fascia of Waldeyer. Lateral ligaments may need to be divided and the middle rectal artery needs to be coagulated.

Care is taken that ureters are identified and protected from accidental injury during the mobilization of the rectum. Once the rectum is fully mobilized from the pelvic floor, it is lifted up and held by the assistant, who may need to move the rectum in either direction that would allow the surgeon in stitching the propylene mesh to the back of the rectal wall as well as the presacral fascia.

Popylene mesh, measuring about 3 inches in length and 2 inches in width, soaked in providone iodine is anchored to the back of the rectum by several interrupted prolene sutures. This is commenced from the lower end of the rectum by suturing the lower transverse cut edge of the mesh to the back of the rectal wall. This anchorage is carried out by a series of interrupted prolene stitch (2/0) that goes through the muscular coat of the rectum and not through the lumen of the gut.

Next, the sides of the mesh are stitched with the corresponding side wall of the rectum by interrupted sutures, commencing from the lower corner of the mesh; until the upper corner of the cut edge of the mesh is sutured with the upper back wall of the rectum.

In the depth of the working space, it would be much easier to handle these stitches, if a series of stay sutures are applied between the mesh and the wall of the rectum commencing from below until it reaches the upper corner edge of the mesh, and then between the upper transverse cut edge and upper posterior wall of the rectum from one end to the other end. At the completion of all these stay sutures being done, each one is tied individually as well as cut from below upwards.

The next procedure is to anchor the upper transverse cut edge of the said mesh to the presacral fascia covering the sacral promontory. All these sutures are done by putting a series of stay sutures between the mesh and the presacral fascia. These stay sutures are inserted along the transverse cut edge of the mesh from one corner to the other end. Next, the stay sutures are tied individually and cut.

Hence, the posterior wall of the rectum is kept holding with the sacral promontory by the mesh that would be acting like a sling to the rectum. The rectum is next allowed to put back into the pelvis. The parietal peritoneum is closed. The abdominal wound is closed in the usual way.

OPERATIVE TECHNIQUE FOR WELL'S OPERATION

This is the same principle that requires the rectum being anchored to the sacrum by a sheet of polyvinyl alcohol sponge, known as Ivalon sponge operation. The technique of mobilization of the rectum remains the same. In the original technique, the rectum was anchored to the presacral fascia, in that the sheet measuring to 6 × 4 inches was first stitched with the presacral fascia with interrupted silk or prolene sutures.

It was next brought forwards all around the rectum to be anchored to the anterior wall of the rectum, thus covering the anterior wall of the rectum; but it produced a lot of fibrosis around the rectum, thus causing colonic obstruction. In those cases, this sheet needed to be removed. Over the decades the technique has been modified, in that the anterior wall of the rectum is not covered by the sheet, thus keeping the anterior wall of the rectum free. This would permit the feces and flatus to pass through without much problem.

CONCLUSION

In the literature, there are many operative procedures described but the end results are not very satisfactory. Surgeon must decide the best course of action to be adopted, on the merits of each case.

REFERENCES

1. Carrasco AB. Contribution a l Etude du Prolapsus du Rectum. Paris: Masson, 1934.
2. Hughes ESR. In discussion on rectal prolapse. Proc Roy Soc Med 1949;42:1007.
3. Gabriel WB. The Principle and Practice of Rectal Surgery 4th ed. London: HK Lewis, 1948.
4. Devadhar DSC. A new concept of mechanism and treatment of rectal procedentia. Dis Colon Rect 1965;8:75.

13 Emergency Admissions

CLINICAL PRESENTATIONS IN EMERGENCY ADMISSIONS

In most instances of emergency admissions, patients remain in a state of shock and dehydration. This results from many abnormal physiological conditions. Among them are body fluid depletion, poor oxygen perfusion and endotoxin shock. But in this section, it would be highlighted on the relevant pathology. To keep on maintaining the tissue perfusion requires a reasonable blood pressure and a reasonable cardiac output, but these could be affected by blood volume deficit.

In acute hemorrhage, peripheral resistance increases due to arterial vaso-constriction, thus shifting the peripheral blood to the heart. The cardiovascular system continues maintaining the blood pressure within a reasonable level, but it cannot sustain in a state of shock if the blood loss exceeds 10 percent of its total volume. The shock is manifested by acute hypotension, rapid pulse rate and perspiration. If the blood volume is not restored either by blood transfusion or by the infusion of crystalloids, the vital organs will suffer from poor tissue perfusion and anoxia. This may lead to irreversible state of shock and death.

The same sequence of events may occur in any other state of shock, resulting from the loss of extravascular fluid. In the state of hypotension, whether it is a manifestation of acute hemorrhagic or endotoxin shock, there is a clear difference between the two medical conditions.

In former condition, there will be peripheral arteriolar vasoconstriction that would be a physiological compensatory measure in response to acute blood loss. Its purpose is to shift the peripheral blood to the central vascular chambers.

In a state of endotoxin shock, there will be peripheral arteriolar dilatation. As a result, blood volume will be dispersed in the peripheral circulatory vessels, thus reducing the cardiac output and blood pressure. This will lead to reduced tissue perfusion to the brainstem and cardiac muscle, which will suffer from anoxia. Because of this reason, a high incidence of postoperative mortality has been encountered with fecal peritonitis, reported in the literature.[1,2]

In the past, many of my patients developed acute hypotension, after the emergency operation done for fecal peritonitis or strangulation of gut. In those years, the services of intensive care unit were not available in most district hospitals. And we were not fully aware of consequent effect of the emergency operation without adequate resuscitation of the shock, but all postoperative patients used to be looked after in the surgical ward, where the nurses were not fully aware that patient had developed hypotension. And when it was recognized, it was too late, by the time the resident doctors turned up to treat the patient. As a result, many postoperative patients died of a combination of postoperative and endotoxin shock.

Now every district hospital has intensive care unit and the old concept that sooner the offending material is evacuated from the peritoneal cavity better is no longer advocated. Instead, preoperative resuscitation becomes a mandatory measure in the management of hypovolemic or septic shock in all cases of septic abdomen. Nevertheless, similar physiological challenges are encountered either in the theater or in the intensive care unit. The pathogenesis for acute hypotension remains unchanged whether or not the patients are operated upon with or without resuscitation. But experience has taught us to understand the surgical physiology better in the etiology of postoperative hypotension.

A BROAD OUTLINE OF MANAGEMENT FOR ACUTE SURGICAL PATIENTS

Many emergency admissions in General surgery are related to pain in abdomen, vomiting, change in bowel habit or distended abdomen. It would be difficult for the general practitioners to recognize the actual pathological conditions that contributed to vague symptoms. Therefore, the task for unraveling the vague symptoms rests upon the resident surgeons.

In this section, the concentration will be focused on the large bowel pathology, despite the fact that all those symptoms could also be attributable to any of the surgical conditions, such as, peptic ulcer disease, pancreatitis, acute cholecystitis, small bowel obstruction, strangulation of the inguinal or femoral hernia, perforated colon, leaking abdominal aortic aneurysm, and acute appendicitis.

In emergency admission, patients may present with various clinical conditions, unknown to the family and initially unknown to the clinicians, until the patient is examined and assessed with the results of investigation. The primary concern of the clinician is to treat the shock first in order to protect the function of the vital organs. There are various types of shock. They are cardiogenic, hemorrhagic, septic, neurogenic, and traumatic shock.

In most instances, acute shock is presented with pale skin color, perspiration, cold and clamminess of the peripheral limbs, tachycardia, hypotension, dusky skin color, poor peripheral venous feeling and lethargy or loss of consciousness.

The following immediate measures should be taken, in order to be sure that airway is free, patient does not appear to be cyanosed, if so necessary measures are taken straightaway and in some cases, supplementation of oxygen via a plastic tube into the nose or through a mask placed over the mouth is commenced. In addition, foot-end of the bed is elevated. The next important issue is to find out the existing medical conditions, such as diabetic ketoacidosis, hypoglycemia, stroke, heart attack, and internal hemorrhage. Many of these informations could be obtained by asking the patient or patient's relatives about the medication and past medical history.

In the meantime, blood pressure, pulse rate, respiration rate and temperature are recorded. The next immediate care is to set up the lifeline for infusion of fluid. This would fill up the central vascular compartments that would improve the blood pressure, tissue hydration and kidney perfusion.

If peripheral vessels appear to be collapsed due to dehydration, and hypotension, difficulty may be encountered in inserting the cannula into the peripheral vein. In this emergency condition, central line must be set up either through the subclavian or jugular vein.

In this case, patient should be transferred to the intensive care unit where nursing assistant and equipments are readily available at hand for inserting the cannula into the wide bored vein. In most cases, anesthetist is involved in setting up the central line but resident surgeon should be trained how to insert the cannula into the subclavian or jugular vein and how to set up the central line for fluid challenge and for measuring the central venous pressure.

The next procedure is to insert the Foley catheter into the bladder in order to measure the hourly urine output and to record the residual urine volume; and urine is tested for sugar, ketone and blood. Color and cloudiness of the urine should be recorded. Concentrated urine will appear like a port wine, and it should not be confused with hematuria. Urine is sent for microscopy and for culture.

After all these measures being instituted, concentration is next focused on clinical examination and investigations, like any other medical conditions. If the shock seems to be attributable to peritonitis or septic condition, then broad spectrum antibiotics, covering for anaerobic and aerobic gram-negative bacilli are commenced. But patient's allergy to penicillin must be recorded and blood should be sent for culture first before antibiotics are given to the patient.

The next approach is to establish the diagnosis on the basis of the clinical examination and results of blood tests and other investigations, such as X-ray of the chest, X-ray of the abdomen, ECG and USS. After reviewing the clinical state of the patients, a broad outline is set up on how the patient is to be treated. This is a general principle in the management of acute shock.

After a period of four hours, hourly urine output is reviewed, whether or not the kidneys stop producing urine. This renal function should be evaluated along with blood biochemistry, blood pressure, and tissue hydration. Patient may have a gross fluid deficit that may contribute to anuria or oliguria. Sometimes, kidneys may stop functioning due to endotoxin shock.

In the state of renal shutdown, intravenous fluid management is to be carefully measured so that the patient is not overloaded. A detailed policy has been outlined in the section on fluid balance. If the condition has not improved and both blood urea and serum potassium are getting worse, renal dialysis should be arranged as a last resort.

CARE OF SEPTIC ABDOMEN

Background: The septic abdomen comprises of acute surgical conditions, presented with endotoxin shock, dehydration, and peritonitis. These conditions have resulted from many pathological conditions, leading to intraperitoneal sepsis. Among many surgical conditions are perforated peptic ulcer, empyema or perforated gallbladder, perforated or gangrenous appendix, strangulated gut and perforated colon. And a few of these cases are life-threatening and fecal peritonitis is one of them. It presents a difficult challenge to the surgeons, in those cases in which, the diagnosis could not be ascertained.

In a state of septic shock, blood pressure may not be recordable or low, pulse rate would be rapid and feeble, tissue hydration would be very poor and there may not be any urine output for the first few hours, and in some cases, patient will have perspiration. The patient may be in pain and is in a state of metabolic acidosis, septicemia, and confusion.

The primary care is to combat with the septic shock, and then to establish the diagnosis for the acute peritonitis; before contemplating the secondary care of the acute abdomen.

During the process of primary care, surgeons would be concerned when it would be safe to proceed with the emergency operation on the acute abdomen of unknown pathology. Septic abdomen carries a high risk of postoperative morbidity and mortality. The average incidence of morbidity and mortality could be very high, as high as 60 percent.

In view of these facts, his main priority is to deal with the surgical condition with a minimum risk of postoperative morbidity and with a reduced incidence of mortality, despite the fact that the patient remains at a critical state in which the outcome of the surgical care could not be predicted.

There is no clear guideline in the literature as to when the patient would be considered safe to be operated upon. One school of thought advocates that sooner the offending materials are surgically dealt with better, but this old concept is no longer in practice, because of the fact that a high incidence of mortality has been reported in the literature and it was between 36 and 60 percent.[1,2]

The present school of thought recommends for resuscitation of the shock, stabilization of the vital function and correction of tissue dehydration, before the operation is undertaken. Despite this measure being undertaken, the dilemma creeps up in clinical judgement on how long the resuscitation is to be continued. Here lies the conflict of judgement whether or not the operation should be delayed further after a period of short and sharp resuscitation. It is of paramount importance to understand the potential risk of physiological changes which may contribute to further hypotensive shock or multiorgan failure, if the patient is operated upon without full recovery from the shock and a complete restoration of the tissue hydration. It is also not clear in the literature about the prognosis of postoperative recovery, if the operation is delayed over a few more hours.

However, the decision to take the patient to the theater depends upon the following minimum criteria: These are hourly urine output at the rate of 40 ml per hour, hemoglobin over 11gm/dl and serum electrolytes within the normal range. These results do not reflect the true feature of tissue hydration. And it would not be possible to achieve a total rehydration in less than 12 hours, when the patient has developed this condition in more that 24 hours. It has been a clinical experience, projectile vomiting or repeated diarrhea drain the extra-cellular fluid volume very rapidly that could not be replaced with the same speed by a rapid infusion. Why this is not possible will be highlighted later.

These are the difficult clinical issues but surgeon may be confronted with a potential criticism for not operating upon the patient sooner after a brief period of resuscitation. Experiences showed that there would be a potential risk of developing perioperative hypotension, if the patient was operated upon without carrying out a full restoration of tissue hydration. The risk of mortality would be much greater among these cases, but it would be much less, if the operation is delayed, until the physiological state of the vital organs being stabilized.[3]

In a state of septic shock, patients remain on gross dehydration associated with poor renal function. In most cases, an emergency operation is undertaken after a brief period of resuscitation with the assumption that the patient is reasonably fit, but surgeons are in dilemma, pondering at times, whether it is safe to delay the operation. Fine clinical judgement is not always possible.

In most instances, patients recover from surgery, but many patients go through the turbulent postoperative recovery. A study was carried out in order to find out whether prognosis of the postoperative recovery would be worse or better if the operation is deferred?

It has been noticed in the theater that patient developed perioperative hypotension that seemed to have contributed to poor renal function. In this condition, rapid infusion of blood volume expander was carried out to improve the blood pressure (BP) and renal function, but risk of developing pulmonary edema and heart failure was not fully aware or not anticipated or was considered to be of lesser concern to the attending clinician at the critical moment of care and time. These physiological imbalances will be elaborated later.

In these circumstances in the theater, it becomes a pandemonium, keeping the anesthetist and other allied personnel busy in dealing with this difficult task, while the surgeons keep concentrating on dealing with the operative procedures without paying that much attention to what was going on at the top-end of the table. And a few of them may need ionotropic drugs; but they are not without problems. These drugs are adrenaline and noradrenaline, its main objective is to shift the fluid from the peripheral circulation in order to improve the blood pressure. This shift is the result of peripheral vasoconstriction, but it may cause reduced mucosal perfusion of blood that may lead to acute ischemia. This would interfere with the gut motility. Because of ischemic effect to the site of anastomosis, there could be a potential risk of anastomotic dehiscence. An increased metabolic acidosis is an added assault to the heart, lung and brain.

To overcome this acute physiological change and to avoid the unexpected crisis, the operation should be deferred until the tissue hydration and renal function are satisfactory. In many cases, the emergency operation was delayed on the ground of medical conditions. These include the electrolytes imbalance, low hemoglobin (<10gm/dl), high blood urea (>15 mmol/l) poor tissue perfusion (dehydration), low blood pressure, poor cardiac and respiratory condition. The postoperative recovery was found encouraging among these patients. This was a reassuring experience.

Contrary to old concept, repairing the puncture tyre would add a very little benefit, if the engine stopped working. And it is no point in cleaning the abdomen, when the whole system has already been flooded with billions of bugs, liberating huge load of toxins. This may lead to crippling the physiological function of the vital organs. There would be double assault to these vital organs, if emergency surgery being undertaken, without a full resuscitation is carried out.

Under these clinical conditions, a sufficient time must be allowed to correct the fluid deficit and to deal with the billions of bugs in the circulation, before the perforated colon is repaired and the abdomen is cleaned. Local clearance of infection and repair of the diseased gut will not resolve the systemic septicemia.

Hence, decision to operate upon the patient rests upon the patient's state of health, and outcome of resuscitations. The fear that the prognosis would be worse if the operation is delayed further was found unsustainable in those cases in which the operation was undertaken 24 hours later.

A PROSPECTIVE STUDY OF SEPTIC ABDOMEN

Among the 152 consecutive patients, operation was performed in 127 patients within 24 hours and the operation for the other 25 patients was delayed over 24 hours on the medical grounds (Tables 13.1 and 13.2). All patients received appropriate intravenous infusion, in addition to parenteral antibiotic therapy. This includes cefuroxime 750 mg and metronidazole 500 mg administered intravenously every eight hours.

Parenteral nutrition therapy (TPN) was only given if the operation was deferred or postoperative recovery was expected to be protracted. Supplementation of human albumin was also added at some stage, because of pitting edema present in the legs or ankles persistently over weeks, provided the level of serum albumin was below 20 gm/l and no benefit was noticed with diuretics.

EMERGENCY OPERATIVE PROCEDURE

A broad summary of the operative procedure is highlighted in this section. Definitive corrective procedure for the diseased organs has been described in appropriate place. At the completion of definitive operative procedure, the peritoneal cavity has been cleaned thoroughly with a warm normal saline. It was followed by adjuvant metronidazole peritoneal lavage, as described in the previous study.[3] For a localized abscess, due to appendicitis, the dose was 500 mg for the generalized peritonitis, the dose was 1 gm and for gross fecal peritonitis the dose was 1.5 gm, used in this study.

For uniform application, the said antibiotic solution, which is used for intravenous (IV) therapy, was squirted by a 20 ml syringe for uniform distribution in all areas of the abdominal cavity and 20 ml were left in the syringe to be used into the parietal wound, before the latter was closed. This IV solution must not be mixed with saline and it should not be aspirated back from the peritoneal cavity. If the intraperitoneal drainage tubing is inserted, this should be kept clamped on for 2 hours.

Abdominal wound is closed with a continuous PDS or prolene suture, which should be 1 cm apart from each suture bite and 1 cm away from the cut edges of the parietal wound. Furthermore, fatty layer should be sutured together in order to obliterate the dead space before the skin wound is closed.

OUTCOME OF THE OPERATIVE TREATMENT

Among the 127 cases, 15 patients developed perioperative hypotension and poor renal output, whether these complications were due to poor tissue perfusion, septicemia or both in combination could not be ascertained, but the operations were done sooner than 12 hours after admission to the hospital.

Among these 15 patients, fecal peritonitis was present in 6, acute intestinal obstruction in 4, gangrenous gallbladder in 3, chronic pyloric stenosis in 1, and gross purulent peritonitis in 1. Surprisingly, splenic artery aneurysm was an incidental finding at the laparotomy undertaken in one lady presented with strangulation of small intestine. In this case, splenectomy was carried out along with other procedure.

These patients required mechanical ventilation and developed gross pitting tissue edema, pulmonary edema and chest infection. All of them had low serum albumin (< 15 gm/l), but 3 of them were given human albumin that enhanced their quick recovery within 5 days.

Among other patients,[25] whose operation was deferred over 24 hours on the ground of medical conditions alone, fecal peritonitis was present in 10, but ovarian carcinoma with peritoneal seedling in the pelvis was found in 1, purulent peritonitis in 3, necrosis of the small intestine in 1, pyonephrosis in 2, Coloileovesical fistula in 1, multiple perforation of the small intestine due to a combination of previous surgery and postradiation ileitis in 1, coloileocutaneous fistula (umbilicus) in 1, colovaginal fistula in 2, retrocolic and pararectal abscess in 2, colonic obstruction due to carcinoma in 2, 1 located at the hepatic flexure and the other 1 at the cecum.

Among other things, the reasons for delaying the operations were abnormal serum potassium, elevated blood urea greater than 20 mmol/l, anuria or oliguria (urine <15 ml/hour) and congestive cardiac failure with or without atrial fibrillation. Apart from these conditions, the operation was deferred or considered at a greater risk of postoperative death in 6 patients, admitted under different teams, but an error of clinical diagnosis was found in 2 of them.

In the delayed group, infusion of human albumin was given to 4 preoperative and 5 postoperative patients, because of clinical evidence of pitting edema present in both legs, despite having supplementation of TPN over several weeks. These patients had serum albumin persistently low (<16 gm/l) over weeks, but it was encouraging to have noticed improvement with the elevation of serum albumin, since the latter was infused for 2-3 days.

Among these cases, a brief clinical presentation is worth highlighting in this section. One of them was a man aged 76, presented with acute septic abdomen. The initial diagnosis, based upon the CT scan and ultrasound scan was suggestive of septic aortic graft, despite the fact that his abdomen was full of purulent fluid and he was having swinging high temperature over a week. But he did not make any improvement with the conservative treatment that was continued for 8 days; until the emergency operation was done by the author.

In fact, the true diagnosis that was overshadowed by the scan reports was necrosis of the small intestine that resulted in subphrenic, paracolic and pelvic abscess. The total collection of pus was over a liter. Resection of midileum with end-to-end single layer anastomosis was carried out.

His recovery was uneventful, apart from a reactionary basal pleural effusion that was attributable to bilateral subphrenic abscess.

In another case, operation was delayed over 3 weeks on the ground of operative risk of death. She was an elderly lady aged 68 years, having discharge of feces through her umbilicus for several weeks. This was a long-standing coloileocutaneous fistula.

Her operation was delayed on the ground that her serum albumin was 16 gm/l, her hemoglobin and serum potassium were very low. And there was evidence of pitting edema in her ankles.

She was given supplementation of human albumin and blood, for 2-3 days, prior to undertaking sugery. At the operation, both large and small intestine required resection with a single layer anastomosis. Her postoperative recovery with primary wound healing was excellent, despite the fact that she had a frozen pelvis.

This was another case of old man presented with fecal peritonitis and colovesical fistula. The primary pathology was perforated diverticulitis. He was declared unfit for surgery by the emergency surgeon, but was treated by the physician with antibiotics, along with TPN for weeks. He also received infusion of human albumin prior to surgery.

In view of his improved health status, multiple operative procedures were undertaken in one seating that was carried out after 3 weeks. He had also made uneventful recovery from his operation.

This was an emergency admission of a lady aged 66 years, presented with pyonephrosis and anuria. She developed right sided pyonephrosis, associated with peritonitis. Her emergency operation was deferred on the results of blood investigation and renal function.

Her blood urea was 21 mmol/l, serum potassium 7.0 mmol/l, serum creatinine 400 mmol/l, and serum albumin 14 gm/l. She was badly neglected at home over 3 weeks. There was no gross pitting edema.

She was treated slowly with infusion over 3 days. At the operation, there was a lot of purulent fluid around the right paracolic gutter, right kidney and under the liver. The primary pathology was pyonephrosis that resulted from the impaction of a large stone in the pelvic ureteric junction. Eventually, she recovered from the operation done on the fourth day of her admission, and kidney started producing urine.

Unlike the previous group, all these patients did not present with hypovolemic shock during operation, nor did they produce pulmonary edema or gross pitting tissue edema, despite the fact that their operations were carried out between 2 and 30 days.

POSTOPERATIVE MORBIDITY AND MORTALITY

In this series, there was not a single incident of intraperitoneal sepsis and wound infection, but, there were five deaths (3.3 percent), three of them were from the immediate group (operation done <12 hours) and other two from the delayed group (operation done > 24 hours), thus representing an incidence of 20 and 8 percent respectively.

Of the three deaths, one 81 years old lady had perforation of the cecum. This was secondary to the colonic obstruction, caused by the carcinoma of the sigmoid colon. Her preoperative resuscitation was overlooked, because of the fact that she was admitted to the nonsurgical ward and clinically she was found dehydrated, when she was brought down to the operating room.

During operative procedure, she received 5 liters of blood volume expanders, in order to deal with the perioperative hypotension and poor renal output.

In the immediate postoperative period, gross dilatation of jugular veins, atrial fibrillation and breathing difficulty became obvious. She did not make any progress over 3 weeks, despite being treated with assisted mechanical ventilation. She died of multiorgan failure. Primary wound healing with no evidence of intraperitoneal sepsis was reported on the postmortem examination.

Another lady, aged 78 had developed chest infection after second operation done for the perforation of the jejunum. She died two months later.

The third patient was 59 years old man, presented with strangulation of the parastomal hernia. His resuscitation was shortened on the ground of strangulation of the hernia, but during operation, he needed massive infusion, in addition to ionotropic drugs, given for raising his blood pressure. At some stage, his blood pressure was not recordable and the urine output was very low.

In the postoperative period, he developed gross pulmonary edema and died of renal failure and chest infection.

Among the delayed cases, there were two deaths (8 percent), one of them was an elderly lady, aged 88 years, who died of congestive cardiac failure and atrial fibrillation. The other one was a man of 55 years old, presented with fecal peritonitis. This was due to multiple colonic perforations, because of ulcerative colitis. Although his immediate postoperative recovery was satisfactory following a total colectomy done for ulcerative colitis, he died of multiple medical conditions. These were bronchial carcinoma with metastasis in the adrenal gland, found only on postmortem examination. Other contributing cause was the pulmonary edema.

This patient was presented with fecal peritonitis but his operation was delayed for 5 days, due to abnormal serum potassium, high urea and poor kidney function. Although his serum albumin was 15 gm/l, there was no evidence of pitting edema in the tissue, nor was there any evidence of pulmonary edema. He made an uneventful recovery from the anesthesia but he started having difficulty in breathing, since TPN therapy was commenced on the fourth postoperative day, but he developed shortness of breath for which he was put on assisted mechanical ventilation on the 5th postoperative day. His whole body became logged with fluid, and a gross pulmonary edema became evident. This complication seemed to be attributable to 40 percent dextrose being added to the TPN preparation that seemed to have hastened his death.

SURGICAL PHYSIOLOGY IN EMERGENCY SURGERY

In preoperative assessment, blood pressure and hourly urine output did not always reflect on the outcome of the resuscitation or adequate tissue perfusion. Furthermore, the cardiac and the respiratory conditions among the elderly patients could not be assessed objectively. In fact, they are unreliable indicators of hypovolemia.[4]

In elective abdominal surgery, perioperative hypotension is a rare event but obligatory urine output in less than 700 ml is not uncommon among the elective operative patients noticed within 24 hours. This is a normal physiological response to trauma. But this would be worse in emergency surgery. It resulted from preexisting fluid deficit and perioperative hypotension. Among these cases, preoperative poor renal function is not uncommon and it is expected to be worse, and many of them require mechanical ventilation at least for 24 hours. Therefore, these patients require a greater care of preoperative resuscitation, so that their main vital functions reach to a state comparable to those cases of elective surgery.

In the state of shock, particularly among the aged patients, cardiac function may be subdued. It could be further depressed during general anesthesia.[4,5] Previous study showed that central venous pressure (CVP) and pulmonary artery wedge pressure do not register any abnormality, unless there is marked hypovolemia.[5,6]

In contrast, this situation is hardly encountered with major elective abdominal operation. This could be explained by the fact that tissue perfusion among the elective surgical patients remains better.

In contrast, tissue perfusion among the emergency patients remains poor. In these cases, the etiology of perioperative hypotension is more likely attributable to inadequate preoperative rehydration.

During emergency operative procedure, in some cases, patient develops acute hypotension. It seems that preoperative resuscitation was inadequate among these patients. And this hypotension is due to opening of precapillary sphincter, resulting from the anesthetic drugs. This permits the fluid entering into the third compartment—thus producing an apparent fluid deficit in the central vascular compartment. This seems to have contributed to sudden onset of hypotension.

In this hypotensive crisis, patient needs rapid blood volume expander, but it could not exceed the limit of mean pulmonary capillary pressure, which is around +7 mm Hg. In this situation, the driving force for the fluid to be leaked into the tissue spaces would be the combination of mean pulmonary capillary pressure and the interstitial fluid pressure, which could be as low as −16 mm Hg. The outcome would be gross pulmonary edema. In these cases, patient needs assisted mechanical ventilation.

To overcome this complication, the patients should be judicially hydrated slowly over many hours, before emergency surgery being undertaken. All the evidences suggest that adequate tissue perfusion could not be achieved in less than 12 hours, despite relying upon the CVP and pulmonary artery wedge pressure.

This study suggests that a risk of postoperative complications and death would be much less if the operation is delayed until the tissue perfusion has been achieved. And none of the patient had passed away prior to surgery by deferring the operation. On the contrary, postoperative mortality was found much less among this group of patients, despite delaying their operation.

How much fluid is to be given to fill-up the third compartment could not be measured by any parameter, and how to recognize at the outset that central vascular chambers have been correctly filled up is not possible in clinical medicine, despite relying upon the CVP.[6,7]

In my experience, CVP cannot measure the fluid deficit in the third compartment, which is regulated by the precapillary sphincter. Therefore, it is my view that the rate of tissue dehydration is equal to the rate of rehydration. This could not be compromised with short and sharp course of rapid transfusion.

In some cases, repeated vomiting, diarrhea, insensible perspiration and sequestration of intestinal contents or intraperitoneal exudation may contribute to extravascular fluid loss that could exceed in excess of 8 liters over a few hours, if not over 24 hours, but it would not be possible to compensate this amount of fluid loss within the same space of time. Otherwise, it would exceed the capacity of the cardiac output per minute.

If such an attempt is made, all the fluid will be logged in the cardiopulmonary vascular circuit that may lead to pulmonary edema, and congestive cardiac failure. This was the evidence, noticed in one of my postoperative patients who developed elevated jugular venous pressure, shortness of breath and pulmonary edema within an hour after she was transferred to the postoperative recovery. This cardiorespiratory embarrassment had resulted from infusion of 5 liters of crystalloids, given during the operative procedure, because of perioperative hypotension.

Although the plasma colloid osmotic pressure stops leaking the fluid from the capillary bed, the osmotic pressure in the capillary bed is more likely to be lower, due to hemodilution.

In this study, the serum albumin was found between 25 gm/l and 27 gm/l among the many postoperative patients; but it did not delay the postoperative recovery, in most instances. The Cohort studies estimated that the risk of death increases between 24 and 56 percent, for each 2.5 gm/l of serum albumin being lost.[8]

Many patients of this study were found to have serum albumin persistently very low (<16 gm/l), over weeks despite having supplementation of TPN. It has been reported that a high percentage of serum albumin leaked through the capillary bed in postoperative and septic patients. Although many contributing factors have been cited in the literature, the major factor is the increased capillary permeability.[9]

But contrary to the above report, it was found among our patients that serum albumin remained elevated persistently for a few weeks, after supplementation of human albumin was given. This observation was consistent with other study.[10,11]

It was also surprising that pitting edema had not been found in those patients, whose serum albumin was low, but it was evident among those patients who were on assisted ventilation and on supplementation of TPN.

It is presumed that overtransfusion of fluid could aggravate the situation, but the causative factor, among this group of patients, could be the positive pulmonary pressure that interferes with the venous and lymphatic return from the periphery. Furthermore, inactivity of the skeletal muscles of the limbs could be contributing factors for delay in lymphatic and venous return.

But many clinicians are less enthusiastic in prescribing the supplementation of human albumin to the surgical patients, with a fear of leakage of albumin into the tissue spaces, as reported in the literature.[9]

Although the therapeutic value for the infusion of human albumin has been questioned in the literature,[10] this therapeutic approach, on the contrary, seems to have reduced the pitting edema in all of them. At least no untoward effect had been encountered within those patients. These clinical experiences seem to be in conflict with the report.[9] On the contrary, our experiences are consistent with the physiological property of the albumin.

On the contrary, low serum albumin has detrimental effects. These are cardiac failure, reduced gut motility and delayed wound healing. These functional disturbances are believed to be attributable to edema in the tissue, thus interfering with the oxygen saturation and neurotransmission to the gut.

It has been observed that supplementation of the human albumin has enhanced flatus, thus reducing the risk of postoperative adhesions of the gut and it reduces peripheral tissue edema. Although, its half-life is about 3 weeks, it would be quite adequate for the patients to be on their feet by that time.

Therefore, the aim of delaying the operation is to give more time for correcting the fluid deficit in the third compartment, before surgery is contemplated; but rapid transfusion under the guidance of the CVP was found unhelpful in some cases, and it might have adverse effect on the interstitial tissue spaces, if the preoperative serum albumin remains very low.

For instance, an elderly lady, aged 80 years who had Billroth I gastrectomy done for pyloric stenosis, developed generalized pitting tissue edema, despite the CVP maintaining at −2 cm of water. In this case, she was not on mechanical ventilation but her serum albumin was 14 gm/l.

It was also evident that a few patients developed perioperative hypotension, after they were believed to be fully resuscitated. In retrospective observation, it became evident in many instances that the acute state of hemodynamic imbalance was encountered only with those patients who were rushed into the theater. And these sorts of perioperative encounters are quite common in the theater.

In sharp contrast, other patients, whose operations were delayed on the medical grounds did not present with similar problems in the theater.

In the state of hypovolemic shock, the precapillary sphincters remain shutting for a considerable period that would not permit the fluid to be dispersed into the third compartment, even after stabilizing the blood pressure. But these sphincters open up gradually as the time passes by or during general anesthesia.

The driving force for the sphincters to open up is believed to be the hydrostatic pressure of the arterioles, or by the anesthetic agents that induce relaxation of the sphincters, thus transferring the fluid into the third compartment. This seems to be the possible explanation for those patients, developing perioperative hypotension in the theater.

Hence, filling of the third compartment is of paramount importance before undertaking a major surgery, if such complication is to be minimized. And such physiological measure is very important, if the cardiorespiratory condition remains unknown to the surgeons.

Adequate preoperative tissue perfusion is also important for controlling infection and wound dehiscence. Previous study showed that the concentration of antibiotic level in the tissue fluid was found below the therapeutic range in 35 percent among the emergency and 15 percent among the elective postoperative patients.[12] This difference was attributable to poor tissue perfusion among the emergency cases.

In septic abdomen, normal saline lavage alone or with antibiotic is not a new modality.[13] Nevertheless, the incidence of wound infection ranges from 8 to 22 percent,[14-18] and peritoneal abscess from 11 to 38 percent among the parenteral antibiotic therapy; but it reduces significantly with antibiotic lavage (Table 13.3).

These patients remain at risk of further operation and harboring the deadly bacteria, known as Meticillins resistant *staphylococcus aureus* (MRSA) and *clostridium difficile*. Many studies reported that the wound infection could be attributable to perioperative blood transfusion, and advanced Dukes tumor stage,[19,20] but no such association was found in my studies.[3,21,22]

Why those studies showed a high incidence of peritoneal abscess and wound infection has to be examined in perspective. One of the factors could be a poor concentration of the drug in the tissue fluid,[12] but the primary etiology remains with the harboring of anaerobic bacteria.

The *in vitro* study showed that obligatory anaerobes suppress the phagocytic function of the body's defence, thus enhances the multiplication of aerobic bacterial growth, leading to tissue necrosis.[23]

Eradication of anaerobes enhances the body's own phagocytic function, thus suppressing the multiplication of the aerobic bacilli. This explains the reason as to why the intraperitoneal abscess was found 0 percent in all cases treated with metronidazole lavage.[3,24] The efficacy of this approach should be evaluated by the instances of intraperitoneal abscess, compared to parietal wound infection. Nevertheless, the incidence of parietal wound infection compared favorable in this study. This confirms the role of metronidazole lavage in eradicating the anaerobes from the peritoneal cavity in all instances. This study supports the explanation as to why the results in other studies were found less effective with a combination of parenteral antibiotic therapy.[15-18]

In my first series, the incidence of perineal wound infection among the clean cases of abdominoperineal resection of the rectum was 12 percent, in that metronidazole was not included in the antibiotic regimen,[25] and it was not available in 1970; but it was 0 percent in my second series, in which metronidazole was added to parenteral antibiotic regimen.[21] Further improvement was noticed among the cases with contaminated and infected wound, since metronidazole lavage has been used in the peritoneal cavity.[24]

In the first study in which metronidazole and cephradine were used in the lavage, the wound infection was 10.87 percent and the peritoneal abscess 0 percent. This encouraged me to set up further study, but cephradine was excluded from the lavage, on the ground that it was noticed that it induced tissue reaction, producing oozing of blood into the wound. This tissue reaction was no longer evident in the wound, since cephradine was excluded from the lavage.[3,21,22] This was the possible explanation for developing a high incidence of infection in the parietal wound in the first study.[24]

Further studies showed that the incidence of wound infection at zero rates was no longer a myth, since the dose of metronidazole was increased in the lavage for the fecal peritonitis. Other added benefit was that none of those patients had acquired MRSA. And this new modality has proved to be cost-effective, because of reduced bed occupancy, and no more cumulative cost for wound dressing.

Furthermore, the risk of intraperitoneal adhesions is expected to be much less, if the intraperitoneal sepsis that induces fibrinous adhesions between the loops of the gut does not recur. To achieve this objective, metronidazole has been uniformly distributed in all areas of the peritoneal cavity by using a 20 ml syringe. This new treatment should be used in all instances, in order to see whether the incidence of adhesion could be reduced drastically.

This study also showed that the incidence of mortality was found to be 20 percent among those cases, whose operation was carried out sooner than a full resuscitation. Although this result was worse, compared to the delayed group but it compares favorably to other studies, which showed that the incidence of mortality was between 36[1] and 60 percent.[2]

Therefore, the risk of postoperative mortality could be reduced considerably, if the operation is delayed until a full

Table 13.1: Demographic data of the patients included in the operations

Demographic Data	No.
Men/women	80/72
Age (M/F)	52/55
Localized purulent abscess	32
Intraperitoneal abscess	47
Fecal peritonitis	43
Acute intestinal obstruction	30

Table 13.2: Operative diagnosis of septic abdomen

A. Localized abscess	
Acute/gangrenous appendicitis	**32**
B. Intraperitoneal abscess	**47**
Perforation of peptic ulcer	3
Gangrenous gallbladder	7
Pyonephrosis	2
Diverticulitis	15
Perforated appendix	13
Strangulation of small intestine	5
Volvulus of sigmoid colon	2
C. Fecal peritonitis	**43**
Stab injury to the small intestine	2
Road traffic accident (perforation of colon)	2
Perforation of the diverticulitis of colon	16
Anastomotic dehiscence of the colon	2
Perforation of cecum due to Crohn's/ulcerative colitis	2
Intestinal fistula with bladder/vagina/umbilicus	5
Carcinoma of the colon	10
Volvulus of the sigmoid colon	1
Multiple perforation of colon due to ulcerative colitis	2
Anastomotic dehiscence of small intestine (postradiation case)	1
D. Acute intestinal obstruction	**30**
Carcinoma of the colon	19
Volvulus of the cecum	1
Strangulation of parastomal hernia/femoral hernia	2
Strangulation of small intestine	5
Carcinoma of the rectum	2
Ulcerative colitis	1

Table 13.3: Review of literature showing differences in results with antibacterial peritoneal lavage

Saline/Antibiotic Lavage	Wound Sepsis (%)	Peritoneal Abscess (%)
No lavage used[2, 26, 27]	36, 29.2, 27.2	24.8, 3.1, 8.1
Saline lavage[28]	24.1	2.00
Cephaloridine[27]	22.2	2.7
Ampicillin[29]	16.6	4.97
Tetracycline[26]	8.6	6.80
Metronidazole and Cephradine[25]	10.87	0
Metronidazole[3]	(*) 2.66, (**) 0	0, 0
Metronidazole (present series)	0	0

(*) = emergency operations, (**) = elective operations.

resuscitation has been achieved. It was evident in my 20 years experience that there remains a minimum risk of or no greater risk of postoperative death by delaying the emergency operation, until the tissue perfusion has recovered fully.

EPIDEMIOLOGICAL STUDY OF THE COLONIC OBSTRUCTION

Statistics from the Mayo clinics reported that the site of the carcinoma in the large intestine varies in accordance with the anatomical sites. It was reported that the incidence of the carcinoma was found to be 12 percent in the cecum and ascending colon, 2 percent in the hepatic flexure, 6 percent in the transverse colon, 2 percent in the splenic flexure, 4 percent in the descending colon, 24 percent in the sigmoid colon and 30 percent in the rectum.

In contrast, the statistics show that the left colon seems to be inflicted with colonic obstruction more frequently than that the right colon. And the tumor developed in the descending and sigmoid colon tends to present as an acute colonic obstruction more frequently than those tumors developed in the right colon. Its incidence was reported to be 44.6 percent, compared to 28.1 percent.[30]

The same report also suggested that the incidence of acute obstruction was 26 percent for those tumors developed in the transverse colon, 40.4 percent in the descending colon and sigmoid colon and 4.2 percent in the rectum.[30]

Although the statistics suggest that the rectum seems to be more vulnerable in the development carcinoma among the whole length of the large intestine, the incidence of colonic obstruction, by contrast, was found to be 4.2 percent and this is far less compared to the sigmoid colon and the cecum. On the other hand, the tumor developed in the sigmoid colon tends to develop colonic obstruction more frequently than those tumors developed in other anatomical sites. This worse prevalence is attributable to scirrhous type of growth that leads to annular type of stricture of the colon.

On the contrary, the incidence of colonic obstruction was reported to be 26 percent among the tumors developed in the transverse colon. This seems to be very worse incidence, compared to the prevalence of the tumor developed in the transverse colon. Its etiology is not known.

The only explanation for these differences in the prevalence of the colonic obstruction in the different anatomical sites would be that the cecum, ascending colon and the rectum has spacious room compared with the transverse colon, descending colon and sigmoid colon. And the cecum and ascending colon has a thin wall compared to other sites of the colon or rectum.

Because of this anatomical variation, the tumor developed in the cecum or ascending colon tends to cause obstruction much slowly, but it has a unique capacity to accommodate the back pressure due to distal colonic obstruction that may last for a longer duration, before the rest of the colon being affected, if the site of obstruction is in the distal colon.

This phenomenon could be correlated with the rubber balloon, where the distal part is dilated first before the rest of the balloon being affected with dilatation.

Large Bowel Obstruction could be of three varieties. These are:
a. Acute colonic obstruction.
b. Acute on chronic colonic obstruction.
c. Chronic colonic obstruction.

PRESENTATION OF ACUTE COLONIC OBSTRUCTION

In most instances, patients are admitted with colicky abdominal pain and vomiting, but these are the late symptoms of acute on chronic colonic or rectal obstruction that force the patient to be admitted to the hospital as an urgent medical condition. The spasmodic pain is mostly around the lower abdomen. This resulted from the obstruction in the proximal colon that may interfere with the ileocecal valves. The latter inhibits the propagative peristalsis and passage of gas. Frequency of vomiting depends upon the degree of dilatation of the small intestine but initially the jejunum may take the brunt of the back-pressure resulting the colonic obstruction. Episodes of vomiting occur later, when the dilatation of the small intestine has reached its limit.

In most cases, patient delays seeking medical advice, hoping that the present bowel symptom may resolve spontaneously. This is their ignorance, not recognizing the seriousness of the apparent symptoms such as colicky or spasmodic type of pain, nausea, anorexia, constipation or no passage of flatus. Sometimes, they do not reveal these symptoms to the family members, despite the fact that these symptoms were going on over a week. They initially rely on simple medication or oral laxatives. But in fact, the obstruction of the large intestine has begun a few weeks ago.

When the tumor has caused a total colonic obstruction, the proximal colon becomes a blind tube because of competent ileocecal valve. The back pressure falls primarily upon the cecum first, before the symptoms for a total colonic obstruction become apparent.

Hence, the distention of the abdomen continues without giving rise to symptoms of acute large bowel obstruction. In this situation, clinician has a responsibility to extract the underlying symptoms of chronic colonic or rectal obstruction. These could be retrieved by putting leading questions to the patient and the close relatives such as spouse, sons and daughters. To pin-point the duration of colonic obstruction requires the patient to answer to a question, when he or she had opened the bowels last or when he or she had not passed flatus per rectum. The answer to this question will reveal exactly when the bowel has been obstructed completely.

From this interview, classical symptoms of change in bowel habit, loose motion mixed with slime or blood or both, loss of appetite and body weight will emerge from the patients, but because of fear or ignorance, these symptoms were overlooked over many months before the acute symptoms developed. Therefore, patient needs to be examined thoroughly as described before. The distinctive obstructive presentation could be found from just visual inspection along with other abdominal and the rectal digital examinations.

In most cases, inspection will reveal the classical presentation of dehydration, dry and coated tongue. And the distention of the abdomen is more likely to be along the upper abdomen and along the flank; if the site of obstruction is in the sigmoid colon or the rectum. The distention of the lower abdomen becomes apparent, if the tumor is located in the cecum or ascending colon and if the ileocecal valve has given away due to retrograde colonic pressure.

In chronic and long-standing or neglected cases, inspection will reveal sunken eyes, and cheeks. Evidence of gross dehydration, coated and dry tongue would be noticed. In addition, loss of gross body weight will be apparent on the cheeks, supraclavicular fossa and around the chest wall, where the ribs will stand out and intercostal muscles will sink in between the ribs, what appears to be emaciated chest wall. There will be atrophy of the subcutaneous fat, resulting in loose dry skin around the limbs. Furthermore, the whole abdomen that includes the flanks, upper and lower abdomen will appear to be distended.

In chronic colonic obstruction, ileocecal valves will give way because of retrograde colonic pressure, thus resulting in distention of small intestine. Patient may experience with periodic colicky and spasmodic type of pain, associated with a periodic peristalsis and loud borborygmi that could be audible without putting the stethoscope on the abdominal wall. In some cases, the small gut will appear like step-ladder pattern associated with or without visible evidence of peristalsis. Serosal tear of the cecum and stercoral mucosal ulceration could be found at the emergency laparotomy.

Although all these symptoms would suggest acute on chronic colonic obstruction, other pathological conditions need to be borne in mind. These are diverticulitis, perforated colon, volvulus, and intussusception, small bowel obstruction, Crohn's ileitis, obstructed femoral or inguinal hernia. There would be very little difference in symptoms between these pathological conditions.

PALPATION OF THE ABDOMEN

Before proceeding with the abdominal examination, patient is first asked to empty the bladder in a bottle and the volume of urine is recorded. If the color of the urine turns out to be of dark brown color, it is an evidence of dehydration.

Next, the patient is asked to lie flat on the back but the head should rest on the pillow. After initial inspection of the abdomen, both groins and femoral canal are examined to exclude the strangulated inguinal or femoral hernia.

If there is non-tender lump palpable either in the inguinal ring or in the femoral ring, patient is asked to give a cough. If the impulse on coughing is transmitted through this non-tender lump, then this lump is more likely to be inguinal or femoral hernia. If the impulse is absent and the lump is tender, this lump could be obstructed or strangulated hernial sac. In some cases, chronic obstructed femoral hernia may not elicit tenderness. The feature may appear to be enlarged lymph glands.

In the absence of lump, then the diagnosis of inguinal or femoral hernia could be discarded.

Palpation of the abdomen is carried out, commencing from the left iliac fossa. Some vague lump could be palpated on deep palpation in this region, but it could be loaded lumps of feces. The palpation is continued along the left flank and then upper abdomen and finally it is ended in the right iliac fossa. Liver and spleen are attempted to palpate but it is very unlikely that they would be palpable.

On the right flank, it would be difficult to palpate any solid mass, unless the cecal mass is large enough to cause acute obstruction. In most cases, tenderness is not elicited on deep palpation. During this deep palpation, rebound tenderness is very unlikely to be noticed, when the hand is taken off from the site of deep palpation.

After palpation is completed, percussion and shifting dullness are carried out routinely. In some cases, there could be collection of some amount of free peritoneal fluid. This may result from exudation of serious fluid due to chronic distention of the gut or it could be malignant ascitic fluid. The latter may result from the secondary deposits in the greater omentum, parietal peritoneum or it could be attributable to other benign medical conditions, such as cirrhosis liver, congestive cardiac failure.

The most important examination is the rectal digital examination. A meticulous examination should be carried out along the rectal wall. It may reveal ballooning of the rectum, palpable mass either in the side wall or higher up in the rectum. It is also possible that a firm mass could be felt anterior to the rectum. This could be the tumor in the sigmoid colon that has dropped in the rectovesical or rectovaginal pouch.

During the rectal examination, if any irregular mass is felt on the finger, it is necessary to assess whether it is fixed to the side wall, whether it appears to be ulcerated, or cauliflower type and how much of the rectal wall has been encircled by the tumor, and whether its edges have been elevated or everted. At the end, the finger stall is looked for blood stain or mucus or friable greenish tissue. Under any circumstance, sigmoidoscopy should not be done. This will make the obstruction worse because of passing air beyond the obstruction.

Although the clinical presentations are strongly suggestive of colonic obstruction, concomitant abdominal aortic aneurysm should be excluded by palpation. This may reveal pulsatile and tender mass, usually located along the left side of the abdomen. At last, pulsations in femoral region and around the ankle should be recorded.

■ Investigations

Hematological Blood Profile

- FBC and hemoglobin.
- Serum electrolytes, urea, and creatinine.
- LFT.
- Blood sugar.
- ECG.

Blood hemoglobin may be reported to be disproportionately high. This would reflect the feature of hemoconcentration due to gross dehydration. This result needs to be evaluated with the clinical presentation and the results of blood urea, serum sodium and potassium. These results will reflect gross depletion due to vomiting and loss of fluid into the dilated gut.

PLAIN X-RAY OF CHEST AND ABDOMEN

Barium enema is contraindicated in acute colonic obstruction and it is unnecessary when the patient needs emergency laparotomy.

INTERPRETATION OF THE RADIOLOGICAL INVESTIGATIONS

The X-ray of the chest may reveal pleural effusion, enlarged heart and abnormal opacity or secondary deposits or TB lesion.

In addition, it should be taken on standing position of the patient. This may reveal gas under the diaphragm. If there is evidence of dark shadow under the left side of the diaphragm, it could be due to the perforation of the stomach or colon. One needs to be sure that the said dark shadow is outside the shadow of the fundus of the stomach. Its location is usually either lateral or above the shadow of the fundus of the stomach. Furthermore, the shadow of the fundus appears usually to be wide area.

In contrast, the free gas shadow, outside the fundus of the stomach would appear to be a thin streak, lying just under the diaphragm. For the perforation of the duodenal ulcer, the gas shadow lies under the right side of the diaphragm in the X-ray plate. In the perforation of gastric ulcer, gas shadows could be present in some cases under the diaphragm of both sides of the abdomen. These variations must be remembered, while reviewing the plain X-ray.

Nevertheless, suspicion should arise whether it is due to perforation of peptic ulcer disease or perforation of the diverticulitis. Colonic perforation due to carcinoma is rare. The differential diagnosis could be resolved by taking further X-ray of the patient lying in the right lateral position. In this case, a free gas shadow may be seen in the left lateral side of the X-ray plate.

Over and above, further review is carried out on the symptoms and abdominal examination. Pain in the lower abdomen associated with a localized tenderness and some degree of guarding and rebound tenderness would suggest that the clinical diagnosis should be perforated diverticulitis. Peptic ulcer perforation should be suspected if palpation reveals generalized peritonitis associated with cardboard rigidity of the abdominal wall.

PLAIN X-RAY OF THE ABDOMEN

It is taken in supine position. An erect X-ray is not recommended and not necessary. In rare clinical condition, a lateral film may be necessary to resolve the doubt in clinical diagnosis, whether or not there is any free gas in the peritoneal cavity.

In normal cases, the plain X-ray of the abdomen does not show any feature of small intestine, which suggests that there is no evidence of intestinal obstruction or paralytic ileus. In the area of duodenojejunal flexure, a few streaks of gas shadow could be seen in the plain X-ray of the abdomen. This is normal in most clinical conditions, but such finding should not be overlooked. In this case, perforation of the duodenojejunal flexure should be suspected if there is any history of blunt injury such as seat-belt injury, blunt injury while playing rugby, stab injury, or there was any history of swallowing either aspirin or potassium tablets.

In normal cases, the small intestine is not visible in the X-ray. Because water is not radiopaque, but in abnormal clinical conditions, such as paralytic ileus, or intestinal obstruction, both water and air or gas are held up within the segment of the dilated intestine. In this case, air would appear to be seen as black shadows in the plain X-ray of the abdomen because, air or gas is known to be radiopaque and multiple black shadows would be visible within the girth of the intestine. These shadows will float over the surface of the fluid and it would outline the girth of the small intestine, in those cases, in which the small intestine would appear to be dilated, holding both liquid and gas within its lumen. Evidence of such finding in the supine film of the abdomen would confirm that this finding is suggestive of mechanical obstruction or paralytic ileus. Further erect film is not necessary and it would not add any more information in order to establish the diagnosis.

Nevertheless, it is important to understand the reading of the erect film of the plain X-ray of the abdomen. In intestinal obstruction or in paralytic ileus, the plain X-ray of the abdomen taken on standing position of the patient would show multiple fluid levels in the X-ray plate. This means, the dilated lumen is filled up with both liquid and gas or air. And they are held up because of mechanical obstruction or paralytic ileus.

In standing position, the liquid will rest at the lower part and gas or air will float over the surface of the liquid, held within the girth of the dilated intestine. And, it would outline the upper circumference of the intestine. And in the X-ray, only the dark shadow will appear like a semilunar shape, the horizontal line of it is the demarcating level between the fluid and gas. The latter would appear dark shadow in the erect film, thus occupying the empty space above the fluid level and outlining the upper circumference of the intestine in a cross sectional view. This horizontal level is referred to as fluid level in the erect film, which would not be seen in supine film of the abdominal X-ray.

The pattern of gas present in the small intestine will be quite different from that of the colonic gas. In the proximal part of the small intestine, it would be recognized by its valvulae conniventes. The gas shadow will look like coils of wire markings with equidistant space between the wire markings that extend from one wall to the contralateral wall of the gut. In contrast, such features are absent or less prominent in the distal ileum. They would lie transversely. In some cases, all the characteristic features would be difficult to recognize due to over distention and due to overlapping one across the other.

INTERPRETATION OF THE COLONIC GAS IN THE PLAIN X-RAY

In normal cases, both colon and the rectum are full of gas. This will reveal as black shadows on the plain X-ray of the abdomen. These gas shadows are normally absent in the small intestine. In acute abdomen, clinician will conclude by the pattern of gas shadows in the colon, whether there is any mechanical obstruction in the large intestine.

Evidence of such shadows in the rectum suggests that there is no colonic obstruction. And absence of gas shadow either in the distal colon or in the rectum is a conclusive evidence of obstruction in the proximal part of the colon. Gas shadows present in the dilated loops may obscure the gas pattern and may conceal whether there is any evidence of gas in the distal colon or in the ampulla of the rectum.

Plain X-ray of the abdomen reveals gross dilatation of the guts. And it would be difficult to identify the level of obstruction, if the sigmoid colon is obstructed by the tumor. It will reveal gaseous colonic distention all along, right up to the level of the obstruction. It will show the characteristic feature of haustration folds that lie transversely from one intestinal wall to the other side, and it would appear to be a septum; but they are separated from each other with irregular space and may end across the lumen between the two contralateral haustration folds.

In advanced condition, small bowel may appear to be grossly dilated. This may result from the competent ileocecal valve or from the back-pressure of the proximal dilated colon transmitted through the incompetent ileocecal valve.

If the cecum is obstructed by the growth, distal colonic gas shadow would be absent but distention of the small intestine would be evident in the plain X-ray.

Barium enema should not be arranged, if the plain X-ray reveals colonic obstruction. It is unnecessary and it would be detrimental to the patient, if the patient needs emergency laparotomy.

Furthermore, barium enema or any rectal enema may trigger off cecal perforation because of added intraluminal pressure to the existing dilated colon. The fluid used in the preparation of enema will enter into the proximal part of the colon through the narrow lumen and it would not return because of paralytic ileus. Perforation may occur either through the tumor bed or through the pre-existing serosal tear of the dilated cecum. Furthermore, evacuation of the barium from the rectum may not be made possible successfully. Retained barium in the rectum will be obstructive element to the primary end-to-end anastomosis of the colon.

Gastrograffin enema could be arranged but it would be at risk of perforation. The addition of the water-soluble contrast per rectum would add further pressure causing further distention by the amount of fluid that would pass through the stricture or partially obstructed lumen of the colon. This contrast that would pass proximal to the obstruction will not return.

On the contrary, it may attribute to reflex spasm and cause further serosal tear on the surface of the distended colon. Gastro-graffin enema was done in this case, despite radiological evidence of large obstruction. The contrast did not pass beyond the stricture of the sigmoid colon. It was annular tumor present in the sigmoid colon.

Despite all these risks being known in clinical medicine, it may be recommended in some uncertain clinical diagnosis and rare condition such as pseudocolonic obstruction. Again, management of this condition is conservative for the initial stage. If it does not respond to conservative treatment, more often than not laparotomy should be considered and transverse loop colostomy remains the choice of operation.

PREOPERATIVE ASSESSMENT AND TREATMENT FOR DEHYDRATION AND CORRECTION OF ELECTROLYTE IMBALANCE

After reviewing these investigations, a tentative diagnosis is made and patient is prepared for correction of dehydration and electrolyte imbalance. A good renal function is restored. This is judged by the good urine output, which should be at least 40 ml per hour. These minimum measures are necessary, before considering emergency laparotomy. Intravenous infusion with normal saline should be commenced as soon as practically possible, before all investigations are arranged.

The next priority is to pass a Foley catheter No. 18FG per urethra. And the residual urine volume in the bladder is recorded after the bladder is completely emptied. This is done by pressing the lower abdomen. The hourly urine output will provide vital information on the renal function. All intake and output fluid volume are recorded.

Nasogastric tube should be inserted into the stomach for hourly aspiration. If the feculent fluid is aspirated in large volume, per nasogastric tube, then continuous suction should be commenced and at the same time, intravenous infusion with normal saline should be enhanced.

The deficit must be compensated by intravenous infusion. From the hourly chart, the total deficit could be estimated. In addition to the hourly urine output, and hourly stomach aspiration, around 800 ml insensible fluid loss is added to the fluid deficit per 24 hours. This volume of infusion of normal saline and dextrose 5 percent needs to be supplemented to the infusion regimen in divided dose every hour. After adequate tissue hydration, patient is prepared for emergency laparotomy.

But the decision for emergency operation has to be judged on the following points:
a. General state of health and tissue hydration.
b. Hourly urine output > 40 ml/hr.
c. Duration of the acute symptoms.
   i. If the strangulation of the gut is the tentative diagnosis and the symptom is less than 6 hours, sooner the laparotomy is done is better.
   ii. If the tentative diagnosis is colonic obstruction and the abdomen shows no evidence of peritonitis, the decision for emergency laparatomy depends upon the renal function, tissue hydration and duration of acute symptoms.

One needs to foresee, what would be the consequent effect during general anesthesia and after operation, if emergency laparotomy is carried out without adequate tissue hydration and without restoring the good renal function.

During anesthesia, the precapillary sphincter opens up that allows the fluid entering into the third compartment. This may cause apparent fluid deficit in the central circulatory compartment. As a result, hypotension and rapid pulse rate will be encountered in the theater, thus reducing the perfusion pressure to the renal tubules. Kidneys stop producing urine. In elective operation, these physiological problems are rarely encountered.

Out of apprehension, patient is overloaded with intravenous fluid challenge, preferably with colloids, thus exceeding the pulmonary capillary pressure (around 7 mm Hg) and stroke volume of the heart. The consequent effect would be cardiac and pulmonary congestion.

In this medical crisis, the driving force for the fluid to be leaked into the tissue spaces would be the combination of mean capillary pressure and the interstitial pressure, which is - 16 mm Hg. The end result would be pulmonary edema that may contribute to hypoxia. It would be a vicious circle. Patient would be at greater risk of developing heart failure, renal failure and gross tissue edema. This sort of clinical state of the patient is referred to as multiorgan failure or respiratory distress syndrome.

In these critical clinical conditions, patient needs assisted mechanical ventilation. Hence, to avoid the potential complications, patient needs proper tissue hydration, before major operation being contemplated.

To overcome this complication, the patients should be judicially hydrated, before emergency surgery being undertaken. But evidences suggest that adequate tissue perfusion could not be achieved in less than 12 hours, despite relying upon the CVP and pulmonary artery wedge pressure. This study suggests that a risk of postoperative complications and death would be much less if the operation is delayed until the tissue perfusion has been achieved.

How much fluid is to be given to fill-up the third compartment, and how to recognize at the outset of the sign of overloading to the vascular chambers, is a difficult clinical science.[31,32] In my experience, the rate of tissue dehydration is equal to the rate of rehydration. This could not be compromised with short and sharp course of rapid transfusion. If any such attempt is made to push fluid, beyond the capacity of the heart and lung, all the excess fluid will be held back in the pulmonary vascular compartment resulting in pulmonary edema and congestion of the right heart.

In most instances of chronic colonic obstruction, patient develops tissue dehydration over a week, but the risk of colonic perforation or gangrene would be greater, if the emergency operation is not undertaken sooner than usual. In this difficult dilemma, experience will guide the surgeon when to operate upon the patient.

PROCEDURE FOR EMERGENCY LAPAROTOMY

Acute abdomen is a mystery and is a musical box, but confidence and methodical approach is important in dealing with the emergency operation. Before taking him to the theater, patient must sign on the consent form and he or she must agree for defunctioning colostomy if such a procedure is necessary. Prophylactic antibiotic therapy must be commenced and prophylactic antithrombotic measures should be commenced, as outlined before.

On the operating table, both feet must rest on the soft cushion. Antithrombotic TED stocking is put on in both lower limbs from toes to midthigh.

After skin preparation, sterile drapes are laid down around the site of operation. Initially, a small midline incision is made below the umbilicus. If there is free peritoneal fluid, it is aspirated. Color and smell of the fluid will reveal whether it is of a purulent nature.

The cecum is first palpated; it will provide the first clue of the mystery abdomen. If it is found to be collapsed, then look for collapsed small intestine. It would be a case of obstruction of the small intestine.

If it appears to be dilated, then the obstruction could be anywhere in the distal colon. Next approach is to palpate the sigmoid colon and the rectum by inserting left hand towards the left iliac fossa and the pelvis.

If nothing is obvious, then the midline incision is extended towards the epigastrium. Further examination is carried out in order to identify the site of colonic obstruction. Handling of the colon must be dealt with gentle care. Serosal tear along the taeniae coli or on the antimesenteric border could be found during examination. Liver is next palpated for secondary tumor. Sometimes, benign cyst could be felt on the surface of the liver. No attempt should be made for taking biopsy from this lesion.

Operative procedure depends upon the site of the tumor, any evidence of secondary tumor in the liver and enlargement of regional lymph nodes. The latter could be attributable to secondary infection. Resection of the tumor depends upon the mobility of the tumor and experience of the surgeon.

If the tumor is mobile and is located in the right colon, the operative procedure would be right hemicolectomy. If it is not operable and liver is full of secondary tumors, then palliative procedure should be considered. It would be either side-to-side ileotransverse bypass operation or loop ileostomy or cecostomy.

If the tumor is located in the distal colon or the rectum, more often the tumor would be annular type and mobile.

Primary resection with an end-to-end anastomosis should be undertaken, provided the general condition of the patient is reasonable. Alternatively, a defunctioning transverse loop colostomy should be done.

If the tumor is in the rectosigmoid or further down, either Hartmann's procedure or pelvic loop colostomy could be carried out. In all procedure, distended colon or small intestine needs to be decompressed with Savage decompressor. This will permit more room in the peritoneal cavity and handling of the gut would be easier for any operative procedures to be undertaken. A detailed account of each operative procedure has been described in the subsequent chapters.

REFERENCES

1. Madden JL, Tan PY. Primary resection and anastomosis in the perforated lesion of the colon with abscess or diffusing peritonitis. Surg Gyne Obst 1961;113:646.
2. McKennan JP, Currie DJ, McDonald JA, et al. The use of continuous postoperative peritoneal lavage in the management of diffuse peritonitis. Surg Gyne Obstet 1970;130:254.
3. Saha SK. Efficacy of metronidazole lavage in treatment of intraperitoneal sepsis: A prospective study, Dig Dis and Sciences 1996;41(7):1996.
4. Price HL, Deutsch S, Marshall BE, Stephen GW, Bihar MG, Neufeld GR. Hemodynamic and metabolic effects of hemorrhage in men with particular reference to the splanchnic circulation. Circ Res 1996;18:469.
5. Mythem MG, Webb AR. Perioperative plasma volume expansion reduces the incidence of gut mucosal hypoperfusion during cardiac surgery. Arch Surg 1995;130:423.
6. Well MH, Shubin H, Rosoff L. Fluid repletion in circulatory shock. JAMA 1965;192:668.
7. Baek SM, Makabali G, Byron-Brown CW, Kusek JM, Shoemaker WC. Plasma expansion in surgical patients with high central venous pressure: The Relationship of blood volume to haematuria, CVP, pulmonary wedge pressure and cardiorespiratory changes. Surgery 1975;78:304.
8. Goldwasser P, Feldman J. Association of serum albumin and mortality risk. J Clin Epidemiology 1997;50:693.
9. Fleck A, Raines G, Hawker F, Trotter J, et al. Increased vascular permeability: A major cause of hypoalbuminemia in disease and injury. The Lancet 1985 (6 April);1:781.
10. Nilson E, Lamke LO, Liljedahl SO, Elfstrom K. Is Albumin therapy worthwhile in surgery for colorectal cancer? Acta Chir Scand 1980;146:619.
11. Wojtysiak SL, Brown RO, Roberson D, Powers DA, Kudsk KA. Effect of hypoalbuminemia and parenteral nutrition on free water excretion and electrolyte-free water resorption. Crit Care Med 1992;20:164.
12. Corbett CRR, Hollands MJ, Young AE. Penetration of a prophylactic antibiotic into peritoneal fluid. Br J Surg 1981;68:314.
13. Burnett WE, Brown RG, Rosemond GP, et al. The treatment of peritonitis using peritoneal lavage. Ann Surg 1957;145:675.
14. Drusano GL, Warren JW, Saah AJ, et al. A prospective randomized controlled trial of Cefoxin versus clindamycin Aminoglycosides in mixed anaerobic-aerobic infections. Surg Gynecol and Obst 1982;154:715.
15. Kirkpatric JR, Anderson BJ, Louise JJ, Stiver HG. Double blind combination of metronidazole plus gentamycin and clindamycin plus gentamycin in intraabdominal infection. Surgery 1983:215.
16. Lennard ES, Minshew BH, Dellinger EP, et al. Stratified outcome comparison of clindamycin-gentamycin vs chloramphenicol-gentamycin for treatment of intraabdominal sepsis. Arch Surg 1985;120:889.
17. Huizinga WKJ, Baker LW, Kadwa H, et al. Management of severe intraabdominal sepsis: Single agent antibiotic therapy with cefotetan versus combination therapy with Ampicillin, gentamycin and metronidazole. Br J Surg 1988;75:1134.
18. Mosdell DM, Morris DM, Voltura A, et al. Antibiotic treatment for surgical peritonitis Ann Surg 1991;214(5):543.
19. Marks CG, Leighton M, Ritchie JK, Howley PR. Primary suture of the perineal wound following rectal carcinoma for adenocarcinoma. Br J Surg 1976;63:322.
20. Tarter PI, Quintero S, Brown DM. Perioperative blood transfusion associated with infection complications after colorectal operations. Am J Surg 1986;152:479.
21. Saha SK. Care of perineal wound in the abdominoperineal resection. JR Coll Surg Edinburgh 1983;128:324.
22. Saha SK. A Critical evaluation of dissection of the perineum in synchronous combined abdominoperineal excision of the rectum. Surg Gyn and Obst 1984;158:33.
23. Ingham HR, Sissin PR, Selkon JB, et al. Inhibition of phagocytosis in vitro by obligate anaerobes. Lancet 1977;2:1252.
24. Saha SK. Peritoneal Lavage with metronidazole. Surgery, Gynecology and Obstetrics 1985;160:335.
25. Saha SK, Robinson AF. A study of perineal wound healing after abdominoperineal resection. Br J Surg 1976;63:555.
26. Stewart DJ, Matheson NA. Peritoneal lavage in appendicular peritonitis, Br J Surg 1978;65:54.
27. Uden P, Eskilsson P, Brunes L, Matzsch T. Clinical evaluation of postoperative peritoneal lavage in appendicitis. Br J Surg 1983;70:348.
28. Noon GP, Beal AC Jr, Jordan GL, et al. The Clinical evaluation of peritoneal irrigation with antibiotic solution. Surgery 1967;62:73.
29. Dellinger EP, Wertz MJ, Meakins JL, Solomkin JS, et al. Surgical infection stratification system for intraabdominal infection: Multicentre trial. Arch Surg 1985;120:21.
30. Goligher JC, Smiddy FG. The treatment of acute obstruction or perforation. With carcinoma of the colon and rectum. Brit J Surg 1957;45:270.
31. Well MH, Shubin H, Rosoff L. Fluid repletion in circulatory shock. JAMA 1965;192:668.
32. Baek SM, Makabali G, Byron-Brown CW, Kusek JM, Shoemaker WC. Plasma expansion in surgical patients with high central venous pressure: The relationship of blood volume to haematuria, CVP, pulmonary wedge pressure and cardiorespiratory changes. Surgery 1975;78:304.

14 Ulcerative Colitis

PATHOGENESIS OF ULCERATIVE COLITIS

Ulcerative colitis is a debilitating disease of the colon. It requires a life-long care, once the disease is diagnosed. Its etiology is unknown but there are many postulations proposed in the pathogenesis of this benign lesion. It could be associated with a family or genetic influence, or allergic phenomenon. Personal emotion or psychological element has also been correlated with the exacerbations of the disease;[1] but in other studies, this emotional behavior was found resolving after total excision of the colon has been carried out.[2] The question has been raised whether the psychological behavior is the cause or the result of the disease.

Despite a lot of studies being carried out, all studies have failed to establish the association of the ulcerative colitis with the bacterial assault, despite the fact that colon harbors all varieties of both aerobic and anaerobic bacilli. The fact that the ulcerative colitis develops in the rectum in 95 percent of the cases, and that rectum is the storehouse for the lumps of feces, before being defecated, provides some intriguing questions. The difficulty in establishing the bacterial assault to the mucosa is related to the lack of opportunity to catch the event, when the microscopical abscess begins. There was no other reason to form a microscopical abscess in the crypt of Lieberkühn, if bacteria cannot get harbored inside the crypts of Lieberkühn.

In the past, amebic or bacillary dysentery has been implicated in the etiology of ulcerative colitis, despite the fact that the pathological features in the colon were quite different from amebic colitis which has the normal appearance of the mucosa between the ulcers that is contrary to ulcerative colitis.

In those years, the pathological features of ulcerative colitis present in the mucosa of the distal colon or the rectum used to be regarded first to be amebic or bacillary dysentery, but subsequent changes such as pockets of suppuration and extension of mucosal ulceration were considered to be attributable to secondary infection, caused by the commensal organism.

But this argument could not be substantiated in the absence of *Entamoeba histolytica* in the feces or in the ulcerated mucosal lesions. Furthermore, all the literature indicated that none of those patients had initial episode of amebic or bacillary dysentery, before they had presented with watery diarrhea and hemorrhage, when they were investigated.

Recently, *Clostridium difficile* have been implicated in acute episodes of watery diarrhea, developed in postoperative patients, if they are on broad-spectrum antibiotics for a long time. The symptoms look like cholera or ulcerative colitis. These bowel symptoms have resulted from the emergent resistant strains of *Clostridium difficile* in the gut, in the circumstances in which the healthy normal colonic commensal bacteria have been killed by the broad-spectrum antibiotic.

And these normal commensal organisms are believed to be gram-negative aerobic group of bacilli. This implies that those commensal bacteria used to keep controlling the *Clostridium difficile* and any other anaerobic bacilli in the colon, but in their absence, one could postulate that the resistant strains of *Clostridium difficile* continue to have multiplication of its population, resulting in liberation of toxins which cause inflammation, and in some cases, cellular damage of the mucosa. These acute mucosal changes inhibit the water absorption; on the contrary, it increases the exudation of fluid and mucus, resulting in watery motions and hemorrhage. These symptoms are consistent with those of ulcerative colitis. And the end result of the mucosal injury would turn into pseudomembranous colitis, commonly present in antibiotic associated colitis.

These *Clostridium difficile* are member of the anaerobic group of commensal bacilli present in the gut, but its incidence is believed to be less than 5 percent among the commensal bacteria. It is rod-shaped and can multiply in the absence of oxygen, but it is not known whether its prevalence is uniformly distributed throughout the large intestine. It produces spores that allow them to survive longer in reduced oxygen environment.

The commonest commensal bacilli harboring in the colon are *Escherichia coli*, *Klebsiella*, *Proteus* and *Pseudomonas erogenous* and they are aerobic bacilli. There are also other varieties of bacteria that belong to anaerobic bacilli. They are bacteroides, *Clostridium welchii*, and *Clostridium difficile* and *Streptococcus faecalis*. Their physiological functions are not clearly understood.

In *in vitro* study, it has been shown that obligate anaerobic bacilli inhibit the phagocytic function of the body's defence.[3] This could influence upon the multiplication of aerobic bacilli that may cause tissue necrosis and suppuration, in the production of abscess or wound infection.[4] It is not clear whether the *Clostridium difficile*, although a member of the anaerobic bacilli act differently from other anaerobic organisms, but it has been found that they inflict virulently by liberating its endotoxins, causing cellular damage in the colonic mucosa, when its population exceeds its proportionate share among other healthy commensal bacteria.

However, in normal environment, these bugs remain under control by the dominant aerobic commensal bacteria, because of its negligible proportionate share of the bacteria, but its proportion share becomes offset, by its increased population. This is attributable to antibiotic therapy that kills other commensal organisms in the intestine. In this situation, its virulence would supersede the controlling power of the commensal organisms. Hence, its inflicting power seems to be related to its increased population that could exceed the proportionate share among the commensal organisms. It could be postulated from these studies that the pathogenesis of ulcerative colitis would be no different from the pseudomonas colitis associated with broad-spectrum antibiotics.

The only difference in ulcerative colitis in most instances is that it occurs in the distal colon and again preferably in the sigmoid colon or the rectum (Fig.14.1). And why the particular anatomical sites are preferred to be inflicted with mucosal ulceration, remains an enigma in medical science. Although in many medical conditions, etiology of the diseases remains unknown, nevertheless, they are believed to be associated with reasons and local factors.

We know that the distal colon and particularly the sigmoid colon becomes the site for the lumps of feces to be held back for a long period of time or it becomes the resting place between the actions of the defecation. And lumps of feces would be the ideal anaerobic environment for *Clostridium difficile* and other anaerobic bacilli to reproduce its population, beyond its proportionate shares with other commensal bacteria. It is presumed that the proportionate share of anaerobic bacilli could be much greater in this site than in rest of the colon.

It has been shown in *in vitro* study, that all the anaerobic bacilli inhibit the phagocytic function, thus allowing multiplication of aerobic bacilli within the mucosa. It could be postulated that in some circumstances, their concerted actions may inflict damage to the mucosa of the sigmoid colon or the rectum, which could be similar to those colitis caused by the *Clostridium difficile*.

In clinical medicine, this has never been postulated, although *Entamoeba histolytica* was at one time implicated in ulcerative colitis, but it was found that the macroscopical features of mucosal ulceration in ulcerative colitis appeared to be quite different from the amebic colitis and *Entamoeba histolytica* could not be isolated in the feces in those cases of ulcerative colitis.

It could be postulated whether these anaerobic bacteria could be regarded to be one of the etiological factors for the pathogenesis of mucosal ulceration in the selective sites of the colon or rectum, which are clinically regarded to be ulcerative colitis. The recent revelation of super bugs has raised this issue whether these anaerobic bacilli could be implicated in the etiology or pathogenesis of ulcerative colitis.

In figure 14.1, the mucosa from the midtransverse colon right down to the sigmoid colon has been affected by the ulceration and pseudopolyps, but the mucosa of the proximal colon remains unaffected. It suggests that the mucosa of this area seems to have been affected by bacterial assault.

It is also well-recognized among the public at large that the sigmoid colon and the rectum are the sites for the lumps of feces being crowded more often in the middle age group people, where the proportionate share of anaerobic bacilli, in particular to *Clostridium difficile* could be much greater within the anaerobic environment of the feces, in which they could survive longer and multiply its population. If this postulation could be established, then it is possible that anaerobic bacilli may acquire resistant strains in greater amount within the crowded lumps of feces.

If this hypothesis could be established, then it could be concluded that those anaerobic bacteria, in an unusual environment, produce a large amount of toxins in the sigmoid colon or the rectum that may lead to cellular injury and acute inflammation of the mucosal lining, which would be consistent with the ulcerative colitis (Fig. 14.1).

There is no other reason to believe as to why the colonic mucosa of a particular site could be inflicted selectively and spontaneously in the absence of any causative factors and why a small number of patients aged between 30 and 50 years are inflicted with ulcerative colitis, when all other members of the same family are not inflicted with this medical condition, seems to be in conflict with the concept of food allergy, psychological or genetic influence.

Despite this plausible argument, this hypothesis could be challenged in those cases in which the healthy rectal stump that has been left *in situ*, after total colectomy has been

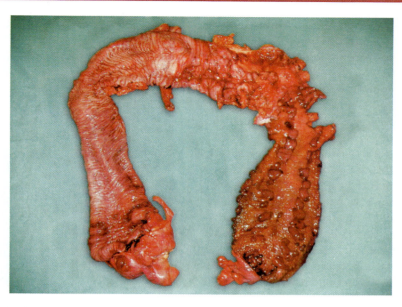

Fig. 14.1: Total colectomy for ulcerative colitis (By courtesy of Mr Dube and Medical library of doctors.net.uk)

performed or the feces have been diverted, has been found later inflicted with multiple mucosal ulcers and suppuration. But this issue could be overcome by the following facts.

After the operation, the rectal stump is regarded to be a blind gut which may not contain enough oxygen or air; and it could not be treated as being a sterile blind gut; on the contrary, small lumps of feces and colony of bacteria could be found scattered resting within the mucosal folds or on the Houston valves. Within this blind lumen, the environment would be ideal for the anaerobic bacilli to survive and multiply its population and they may acquire the resistant strains, if the postoperative patients were on broad-spectrum antibiotics. These resistant strains of anaerobic bacteria would continue damaging the rectal mucosa in due course, before the symptoms of proctitis being clinically evident.

Patient would experience discomfort and notice foul smell discharge, which could be a combination of mucopurulent fluid and blood that may start leaking through the anal orifice several weeks after total colectomy is done. These symptoms are due to scattered inflammation and multiple ulcerations which are classical features of proctitis. In these cases, swab material taken from inside the rectal stump should be sent for bacterial culture that may reveal evidence of colonic commensal bacteria.

EPIDEMIOLOGICAL STUDY

Women are more frequently affected and its ratio with men is 4:3. It affects the people between 30 and 50 years of age, but its prevalence is less frequent in second and sixth decades.[5] Its prevalence is much greater in England than Scotland, but American Negro children are rarely affected compared to white American children[6] or Maoris of New Zealand are less affected than European people settled in New Zealand.[7] These revelations support the genetic influence.

Furthermore, a consistent distribution of this disease has been found in the European countries, apart from England and Belgium.[8]

Instances per 10,000 hospital admissions:

Switzerland	5.8
Scotland	6.9
Finland	7.0
Denmark	7.8
Belgium	10.8
England	14.8

These distributions seem to be associated with climatic conditions, where both Belgium and England seem to be enjoying the same sort of climate, compared to other European countries.

PATHOLOGICAL FEATURES OF THE COLON

Ulcerative colitis does not follow a set pattern. Any part of the large intestine and the rectum or anus may be affected by this disease, but as a rule it develops initially in the distal colon, and gradually proceeds proximally.

Nearly in all instances (95 percent), the rectum and the sigmoid colon become the initial brunt of the ulceration. From these sites, it may proceed proximally. It may cease abruptly anywhere in the proximal colon. In advanced cases, the disease may implicate the whole colon and even to the terminal ileum up to a few inches. This is also referred to as ileitis, resulting from retrograde invasion like backwash, because of incompetent ileocecal valve. When the rectum is inflicted with the disease, it is referred to as proctitis and its incidence is 3.4 percent, found among the patients admitted at the Leeds General Infirmary (1955-63).

The ulcer develops in various sizes in the mucosa. And it may extend underneath the taeniae coli. It invades the submucosal layer later. Initially, the characteristic features are minute and discrete ulcer develops scattered in the mucosa. These minute ulcers coalesce together forming a sea of ulceration. This is attributable to pus collected in the crypts of Lieberkühn that burst into the surface.

The intervening mucosa between the ulcers becomes edematous and swollen. And the inflamed intervening mucosa may change to hypertrophy that is histologically known as pseudopolyp. In contrast, it is absent in amebic colitis, because of the fact that the mucosa in between the amebic ulcers remains normal. This is the distinct difference between the two pathological lesions.

The colon may appear to be spasm at the initial event, and it is due to the effect of the ulcers sitting over the taeniae coli. The spasm of the muscles may affect longitudinally as well as transversely. This is due to invasion of the ulcers into the muscle. This spasm may lead to a full blown stricture eventually, when intramural fibrosis develops.

There has been a debate whether the stricture of the colon in chronic ulcerative colitis is the end result of fibrosis. If so, then it would be an irreversible state, but this view has been disputed by Lockhart-Mummery who have claimed that the area of the apparent stricture is in fact attributable to hypertrophy or thickening of the muscle of the colon and it is reversible.[9]

Because of spasm, the colon loses its classical pattern of haustration on the barium enema (Fig. 14.2). It tends to be thickened and indurated or stiff on palpation that depends upon the severity of the disease. Such finding on palpation should be suspicious of malignancy in the affected segment.

From outside, the serosal layer remains unaffected at the early stage. It would look pale in color with evidence of increased vascularity. In acute stage, fibrinous plaques could be present on the surface, the gut wall would appear to be edematous and the bowel wall may be friable to touch during surgery. Mesenteric lymph nodes may be found to be enlarged and inflamed.

In the histological study, mucosa would be missing by the ulceration but a heavy infiltration of macrophages, lymphocytes, eosinophils and plasma cells have been found in the submucosa and polymorphonuclears in the crypt abscess.

Although ulcerative colitis is a benign disease, it may turn into malignancy after 10-15 years of follow-up. The risk of malignant change would be greater if the histology report suggests evidence of dysplasia in the submucosa. Pseudopolyps are not at risk of developing cancer. However, the incidence

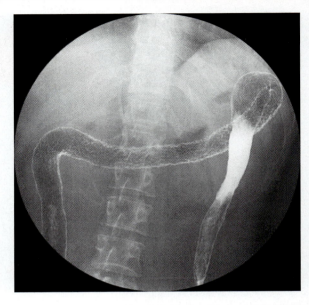

Fig. 14.2: Double-contrast barium enema shows a lack of colonic haustration and the transverse and descending colon appear to be straight due to spasm of the colonic wall. It also shows multiple superficial mucosal ulcerations in the full length of the colon. (By courtesy of Dr S Sinha)

of cancer is reported to be 5.8 percent at the 15 years follow-up in St. Marks Hospital[10] and 5 percent among the 2000 cases of ulcerative colitis at the Mayo Clinic.[11]

POWER OF HEALING

During remission of the disease, the cells from the depth of the surviving glands start regenerating, if the mucosal loss appears to be superficial, but in other cases, where the mucosal loss is complete, regeneration begins from the mucosa of the surrounding area or from the epithelial cells in islands of the surviving mucosa. Dukes reported that groups of epithelial cells are present in the submucosal layer of the colon, and they are not malignant cells.[9]

CLINICAL PRESENTATION

The symptoms very that depends upon the extent of the colon involved and the severity of the disease. At the beginning, patient overlooks the mild nature of bowel movement at least for a few months, despite the fact that he was having a slight loose motion, a few times per day and it is often associated with mucous and/or mixed with blood and pus. He becomes alert, when the symptoms are getting worse. Then he or she starts seeking medical advice.

The symptom that the frequency of loose motion is less than 5-6 times per day is regarded to be a less severing in clinical pathology. It is more likely limited to distal colon and the rectum what is commonly referred to proctocolitis or proctitis. But the striking symptoms of severity are watery diarrhea between 12 and 20 times per 24 hours. In these cases, the extent of the disease may have implicated the full length of the colon and the rectum, if not anus.

More often, patient passes mucous mixed with blood and/or mucopurulent motion. It may give rise to a feeling of tenesmus. Pain is not very common but discomfort at the perianal region may be experienced at times. Patient becomes dehydrated and emaciated due to loss of body weight. He may be bed-ridden due to weakness and anemia.

If the patient is having high temperature and distention of the abdomen, the clinical condition is a fulminating type and is a serious condition. These cases need hospital admission for the replacement of fluid, correction of dehydration and electrolytes deficits. Toxic dilatation of the colon would be the main concern to the clinician. This is a very serious medical condition and is a rare variety. In this case, the whole colon is more likely to be inflicted with the disease.

CHRONIC ULCERATIVE COLITIS

In the clinical assessment, a thorough examination should be carried out. For a milder variety and for ambulant patients, examination includes inspection as described before and palpation of the abdomen on supine position. Abdomen would appear to be unremarkable for the milder type of ulcerative colitis, but for the cases of acute exacerbation or cases of severe relapsing varieties, palpation may reveal gaseous distention, and tenderness along the sites of the colon and it would be marked tenderness with some degree of guarding or rebound tenderness particularly in the region of iliac fossa. No palpable mass or no evidence of generalized peritonitis would be elicited unless the colon is perforated.

Rectal digital examination would provide valuable information even at the early stage. There would be evidence of mucus, loose motions and blood on the finger stall. In advanced cases, perianal fistula, or abscess would be evident. In the anal canal and the rectum, stricture of the rectum or abnormal consistency along the rectal wall may be recognized, if the clinician is familiar with the pathological features.

PROCTOSCOPY

This examination must be carried out with an utmost care of gentleness because, the anal orifice may be found inflamed and the rectal mucosa may also appear to be inflamed and it may bleed to touch. In addition, it may be full of blood-stained and foul smelling loose motion or mucus or mucopurulent motions.

The severity of the disease could be divided into three categories. These are mild, moderate and severe.

In the mild variety, often after remission or at the first clinical examination, the mucosa will appear to be normal or slightly granular in appearance without evidence of normal vascular distribution. This change may be attributable to previous attack of inflammation or ulceration that has resolved, leaving behind a mild fibrosis. If there still remains an active state of the disease, contact bleeding would be obvious, but in the absence of contact bleeding, it is regarded that the chronic inflammation has resolved with treatment and the disease is in a state of remission.

In a moderate severe condition, the rectum may contain a small amount of fibrinous or mucopurulent exudates. On wiping out of these exudates, gently with a cotton bud or swabs, the granular appearance in the rectal mucosa associated with a contact bleeding would be characteristic features of proctitis.

In a state of severe variety, the rectal wall will be found full of blood-stained mucopurulent watery motion. Inspection through the instrument would be impossible without sucking those fluids out. The findings would be similar to the moderate variety but it would appear to be very inflamed and edematous. Biopsy is taken for histology.

SIGMOIDOSCOPY

Procedure for this examination remains the same but there should be certain instruments in hand. These are suction apparatus, biopsy forceps and swab holding forceps. All these instruments must have a long handle, so that its other end can get through beyond the end of the sigmoidoscope. The eyepiece of the sigmoidoscope should have a magnifying power for a better visualization of the rectal mucosa.

Minimum air insufflation should be used and the end of the sigmoidoscope should not rub against the rectal wall. This may cause contact-bleeding.

Through the instrument, the following cardinal macroscopical features are recorded, if anyone or all of them are present in the lumen of the rectum:
a. Blood-stained mucopurulent or soft or loose feces inside the lumen of the rectum.
b. Absence of classical pattern of submucosal vessels and lack of shining of the rectal mucosa.
c. Contact-bleeding.
d. Granular surface of the rectal mucosa.

These features are very important to make a tentative diagnosis, but they may not be present if the disease remains in a state of remission for some months. If inflammation is limited within the rectum, and the colonic mucosa appears to be normal, above the level of 15 cm from the anal verge, the diagnosis would be proctitis. If the inflammation is seen far beyond the level of the rectosigmoid region, then obviously, possible diagnosis would be proctocolitis.

At the completion of examination and visualization, biopsy must be taken, despite the fact that histology report may not be helpful.

Other investigations include cytology and stool examination for the exclusion of parasites, and for occult blood tests.

Merit of cytology remains in question, and histological examination must be done to confirm the clinical diagnosis and the cytology report.

HEMATOLOGICAL INVESTIGATIONS

- Blood for FBC, Hb, ESR, C Reactive Protein.
- LFT.
- Serum electrolytes, urea, creatinine.
- Barium enema and colonoscopy.

PLAIN X-RAY

X-ray of the chest and plain X-ray of the abdomen provide valuable clinical informations. In acute abdomen, X-ray of the abdomen may reveal the gross gaseous dilation of the colon and loss of haustration. This is a classical finding of toxic dilatation of the colon which is suggestive of acute exacerbation of ulcerative colitis.

And X-ray of the chest in erect film may reveal gas under the diaphragm and pleural effusion or basal consolidation. These findings are suggestive of perforation of the stomach ulcer, or colon. In other cases, these radiological presentations could be associated with other surgical conditions. These are acute peritonitis, acute intestinal obstruction, ulcerative colitis, or volvulus of the cecum or sigmoid colon.

Distention of the abdomen elevates the diaphragm or irritates the diaphragm that may contribute to basal effusion, or basal congestion. Similar radiological features in the X-ray of the chest could be associated with other medical conditions.

Barium enema is done in all instances at the outset of the primary investigation. A follow-up barium study may be requested in certain clinical conditions and it depends upon the discretion of the clinician.

Barium enema will show any one or all of the radiological features that would be consistent with the ulcerative colitis. These are:

a. Loss of haustration in a limited segment or whole of the colon. This will demonstrate whether the ulcerative colitis is limited to a segment or whole of the gut.
b. A similar feature could be present in ischemic colitis, Crohn's colitis.
c. Narrowing of the lumen or stricture of the gut or shortening in length of the gut.
d. Evidence of deep ulceration that has extended underneath the mucosa.
e. Gross irregularity of the bowel wall on a special view that depends upon the skill of the radiologist.
f. Multiple small irregular filling defects, if double-contrast barium enema is done. Colonoscopy is necessary to distinguish between the pseudopolyps and familial polyposis of coli.
g. Reflux of barium into the terminal ileum. This would suggest whether the terminal ileum has been inflicted with colitis by backwash.

From the repeated barium enema studies, all the evidences suggest that ulcerative colitis remains unchanged in clinical condition in 65 percent, it may progress further from the previous radiological finding in 24 percent and it may go into remission in 11 percent of cases.[12] And a similar conclusion has been made in another study.[13]

COLONOSCOPY

If the barium enema shows stricture, or multiple filling defects, which are suggestive of pseudopolyps, then colonoscopy is mandatory in order to exclude malignancy and to exclude either adenomatous polyps or familial polyposis coli. It should be done at a yearly follow-up, in order to review the response to the drug therapy and to record the extent and severity of the disease.

Despite its diagnostic value, this investigation should be deferred until all the barium is cleared off from the colon. The inflammation may relapse if oral purgatives are used for the purpose of colonoscopy.

■ Treatment

In most cases, patients presented with symptoms of ulcerative colitis are managed from the outpatient clinic, if the symptoms and results of investigations suggest that the disease is between mild to moderate type and limited up to the sigmoid colon. Hospital admission is only necessary for the treatment, if the whole colon is grossly inflicted with a relapsing fulminating ulcerative colitis or patient is not well for any acute symptom developed. These could be vomiting, rise of temperature and dehydration.

MANAGEMENT OF ULCERATIVE COLITIS

After a full investigation as outlined in the previous pages, patient should be reassured and advised to look for food allergy. In some cases, patient may be allergic to egg, milk, cheese or onion. Therefore, it is important to identify the food allergy.

This is done by omitting one particular item from the day-to-day diet for a few weeks. If no change in consistency or frequency of motion is noticed with the elimination of the particular food, then it should be put back to the diet, instead, any other item could be omitted from the day-to-day diet regimen. In this way, elimination continues by replacing one after another. Patient should be asked to record the body weight every week and to keep a chart about the frequency of the bowel movements per day.

Patient is also encouraged to take a high protein and carbohydrates diet but fatty food should be avoided. The response to any conservative treatment is measured by a number of bowel actions per day, consistency of the motion, and body weight. In addition, it is supported by regular blood tests and ESR. These tests should be done every 4-6 weeks.

In most instances, patients are treated from the outpatient clinics for ambulant and moderate type of diseases. Hence, drug therapy should be commenced with Salazopyrine or with Mesalazine capsule, commercially known as Asacol. Preference of a particular product lies with the clinician, but it could be replaced by the alternative one, in case it is found to be allergic to the patient.

The dose of sulphasalazine (Salazopyrine) or Mesalazine (Asacol) depends upon the severity of the disease.

If the general condition appears to be reasonable and patient is fully cooperative in having the treatment at home, the dose for Salazopyrine should be 1-2gm every 6 hours; and the dose for Asacol 800 mg every 8 hours per day. They are reviewed after 3 months.

If the frequency of motion has reduced to less than 6 times per day, maintenance dose for Salazopyrine could be reduced to 500 mg every 6 hours per day or for Asacol 400 mg every 8 hours. This maintenance dose must be continued for the rest of the life, despite the symptoms being in a complete remission over a year. Experience shows that the symptoms relapse at times and after the treatment has been discontinued. If the disease is limited to the rectum and the sigmoid colon, topical use of Salazopyrine or Asacol suppositories or retention enema could be prescribed.

For severe symptoms and the symptoms not responding to existing drug therapy, supplementation of steroid could be added. If the disease is limited to the rectum (proctitis) or both the rectum and sigmoid colon (proctocolitis), topical application of prednisolone enema 20 mg is prescribed. It is inserted in to the rectum once a day for 3 weeks.

In some cases, it could be given twice a day that depends upon the clinical assessment. Some trained assistant may be required for this treatment, but once the patient is trained how to do it, no such help would be necessary in future.

If the whole length of the large intestine is inflicted with the disease, in this case, prednisolone tablet is prescribed orally, and it should be taken after a meal. In some cases, patients are advised for both oral as well as topical therapy that depends upon the severity and extent of the bowel involvement.

The oral regimen varies according to the symptoms and among the clinicians, but it is recommended that patients are advised to take prednisolone tablet 15-20mg orally three times per day for two weeks, along with the Salazopyrine or Asacol medicine.

In most cases, the frequency of bowel movement reduces after a few weeks. And patient feels better. In view of this improvement, the prednisolone dose is curtailed to 30 mg in divided dose per day for the ensuing two weeks. In this way, the steroid is gradually tailed off every two weeks. Eventually, patient should continue taking 5mg tablet per day for a few more weeks. It is eventually slowly withdrawn over the next few weeks.

Prednisolone retention enema either once a day or twice a day is continued for 3 weeks; but in most cases, it would be unnecessary.

Patients are reviewed every 4 weeks in order to evaluate the response to the new treatment regimen. In this review, further blood tests, including ESR and C reactive protein are done. The response to treatment is measured by the gaining in body weight, number of bowel movements and consistency of the feces and a significant change in blood profile. Among the blood results, both hemoglobin and ESR is the indicator whether the disease has been responding to the treatment. If the level of ESR has dropped to near normal, it implies that the patient is responding to the treatment and the mucosal lesions such as ulceration, inflammation and secondary infection are resolving.

COMPLICATIONS WITH DRUG THERAPY

Salazopyrine may produce side-effects. These are nausea, vomiting, headache, anorexia, dizziness, diarrhea and skin rashes. Other complications are toxic hemolytic anemia, and agranulocytosis.

Asacol may induce a similar gastrointestinal reaction, headache and skin rash. It is recommended to review the literature of the manufacturers.

Oral steroid therapy may cause bleeding from the stomach and it may suppress the body immune systems if the treatment is continued longer than a few months. It may cause perforation of the gut due to friability and may render to pyogenic infection.

In severe cases associated with rise of temperature, systemic antibiotic therapy should be used with caution. It should be given parenterally, instead of oral therapy. Metronidazole in combination with broad-spectrum antibiotics is the choice of antibiotics for a week. It may cause monilial infection.

COMPLICATIONS WITH LONG-STANDING ULCERATIVE COLITIS

a. Pseudopolyps, its incidence is around 15 percent.
b. Fibrous stricture (6 percent) may develop at the anus or rectosigmoid region.
c. Carcinoma may develop after 10 years follow-up. Its incidence varies ranging from 3.5 percent to a higher incidence that depends upon the total duration of the disease. The risk of developing cancer is greater if the whole colon is affected by the disease, if the younger age groups are involved.

d. Toxic dilatation is encountered with relapsing fulminating type and its incidence is 1.5 percent.
e. Fistula is another distressing and pressing morbidity. It may occur between the colon and vagina or colon and bladder, and fistula-in-ano, its incidence is around 4 percent.
f. Other complications are ischeorectal abscess, chronic anal fissure or hemorrhoids.
g. Massive bleeding from the rectum (3 percent).

This chronic disease may affect skin, liver, joints, iris and kidneys. The liver may develop into cirrhosis due to hypoproteinemia and absorption of toxins via portal circulation.

SURGICAL INTERVENTION

Criteria for the Elective Operation

If the patients do not get better with the medical treatment, question may be raised about the operative treatment. The criteria for the elective surgery—

a. Recurrence of anemia despite repeated blood transfusion.
b. Emaciation due to loss of body weight.
c. Evidences of extensive involvement of the whole colon and the rectum or only entire length of the colon, not responding to the medical treatment and evidences of gross changes in the colon, confirmed by barium enema and/or colonoscopy. These are pseudopolyps, stricture, and severe dysplastic change on histology report.
d. Uncontrolled hemorrhage, and its commonest site is in the sigmoid colon or the rectum.
e. Local complications such as colovaginal fistula and colovesical fistula.
f. Systematic complications such as liver change, iritis, ankylosing spondylitis, skin lesion and pyoderma gangrenosum, erythema nodosum or arthritis.

In most cases, patients are confused by the conflicting medical treatment. Failure of maintenance drug therapy seems to be the major factor for the relapse of the disease. Repeated episodes of relapse due to lack of comprehensive medical therapy do not warrant for the operative intervention.

PREOPERATIVE PREPARATION FOR THE ELECTIVE SURGERY

It is important to prepare the patients for an elective operative procedure. Therefore, a full assessment on the nutritional state, tissue hydration, blood hemoglobin and renal function must be done.

Correction of blood hemoglobin and electrolytes deficits should be carried out a few days before the date of operation is due. If the patient appears to be emaciated and the serum albumin is less than 30gm/l and the hemoglobin remains below 10gm/dl, whole blood transfusion is preferable before the operation is undertaken.

In all other cases, packed cell volume should be given, if the serum albumin is within the normal range. Furthermore, blood transfusion should be given at least 2 days prior to surgery, in order to improve the oxygen saturation. If the serum albumin still remains very low, human albumin is supplemented in order to elevate the level of plasma protein above 30gm/l. To overcome the cardiac congestion in the middle of the night, frusemide 40 mg should be given orally, preferably before 6 pm.

In the consultation, patient must be told that total excision of the colon along with that of the whole back passage needs to be carried out. And for the discharge of feces, a permanent terminal ileostomy will be constructed in a suitable site in the right side of the lower abdomen. Patient's permission should be obtained on a consent form, if available.

The preferable site for the construction of ileostomy is determined by a trial and error on standing and on sitting position. It is determined by sticking an ileostomy bag, filled with water on the proposed site. Patient is advised to find out whether the ileostomy bag, fitted on a proposed site is causing any problem or discomfort in wearing the clothes. This trial should be continued for 2-3 days. Once the patient is contended with the particular site, it is marked with an indelible skin pencil.

From the technical point of view, the proposed site for the construction of ileostomy should be in the right iliac fossa, but it should be over the right rectus abdominis muscle, which provides a platform upon which the ileostomy is constructed and ileostomy bag appliance is placed around the ileostomy.

In this discussion, morbidity with the ileostomy and sexual dysfunction must be highlighted, although the risk of impotency, in particular to the man is much less compared with abdominoperineal resection of the rectum for the rectal carcinoma. Other postcomplications should be brought to the attention of the patient.

Mechanical bowel preparation is not necessary. Preoperative chest physiotherapy is encouraged.

TYPES OF THE OPERATIVE PROCEDURE

a. Total proctocolectomy and terminal ileostomy.
b. Total colectomy and ileorectal anastomosis.
c. Subtotal colectomy, preservation of the rectal stump and ileostomy.

Operative procedure will be described later.

MANAGEMENT OF ACUTE DILATION OF THE COLON

This is a relapsing fulminating colitis. It is associated with distention of abdomen and high temperature. There would be a history of watery and mucopurulent motions every half an hour to one hour, and it may be associated with a frank hemorrhage from the rectum.

After recording a full clinical symptom, patient is examined as described before. In one group of cases, patients would appear to be grossly dehydrated, emaciated and in moribund state of health. And in another group, general condition of health would appear to be less severe.

In the palpation of the abdomen, the following features are recorded in the case notes: These are evidence of distention, tenderness with or without guarding and rebound tenderness, and any palpable mass along the line of the bowel or in the iliac fossa.

Rectal digital examination and proctoscopy could be done with due care; but sigmoidoscopy examination should be avoided. This may cause further distention or perforation of the colon.

Investigations

Plain X-ray of the chest and abdomen must be done.

Blood profile, serum electrolytes ESR, LFT and coagulation screen are all done, as in any other colonic surgery.

The primary care is to resuscitate the patient, like any other acute abdomen as described before. Hence, intravenous infusion should be commenced as soon as possible. This is a top priority, replacing the fluid. Rehydration and correction of electrolyte deficit require a lot of experience of the surgeon. A Foley's catheter No.18FG is inserted per urethra for measuring the residual urine volume and for recording the hourly urine output. Nasogastric tube is inserted into the stomach for hourly aspiration. Patient must not be given any fluid or tablet orally.

Patient's temperature chart and pulse rate are recorded every hour.

After reviewing the blood results, second line of approach is to rectify the electrolyte deficits, correction of blood hemoglobin and to add parenteral antibiotic therapy, as outlined before.

In addition, patient should be treated with intravenous hydrocortisones and other supporting drugs such as Salazopyrine or Asacol therapy. The dose for Hydrocortisone varies from one clinician to another and upon the general condition of the patient. The minimum dose to be infused parenterally is between 100 mg and 500 mg every 6 hours. After 48 hours, the dose is reduced and it should be 1 gm per day in divided doses for the succeeding 2-5 days. This regimen should be continued until the patient could take the prednisolone tablets orally.

In the meantime, blood pressure, temperature chart, intake and output chart and level of tissue hydration are evaluated.

Among the results of serum electrolytes, serum potassium, sodium and chlorides are often found to be very low. Urea and creatinine are often found elevated.

Therefore, a judicious infusion policy has to be adopted. First clinical importance is to see the urine output per hour after a few hours. If there is evidence of total renal shutdown, then a fluid challenge could be contemplated at some stage of care. The next question would arise whether too much fluid infusion would be detrimental to the circulatory system, in the presence of anuria.

Injection of diuretic, such as frusemide 40mg should be given after adequate tissue hydration has been achieved. In some cases, the dose for the frusemide could be increased to 80 mg im. If the response is unsatisfactory, the infusion of saline or dextrose saline should be restricted and it should be no more than the total fluid loss as outlined before.

APPROPRIATE TIME FOR EMERGENCY LAPAROTOMY

If there is no evidence of colonic perforation, and no generalized peritonitis, conservative regimen should be continued for 3-5 days at the initial stage. If the clinical observation seems to be satisfactory, it could be continued for a few more days.

X-ray of the abdomen should be repeated, after 24-48 hours. Prognosis is expected to be good, if the patient has admitted that he has passed flatus per rectum and temperature chart and pulse rate appear to be either stable or coming down.

If the observations suggest that patient is not responding to the conservative regimen in 5-6 days, the decision needs to be taken for emergency laparotomy that depends upon other factors. They are correction of dehydration, hourly urine output (>50 ml), and level of hemoglobin (>11gm/dl), serum electrolytes and urea.

If the patient seems to be very toxic and is having hemorrhage which could not be controlled, or the patient is not making any progress with the specific drug therapy, patient needs to be taken to the theater for the major emergency operation. And the latter should be done sooner than previous policy. This change of policy has to be taken on the clinical and radiological evidences.

Although there is no argument against the emergency laparotomy, there could be a difference of opinion and a different line of action between the two schools of thought. One school of thought would recommend for an immediate intervention and would advocate that patient should be operated upon within a few hours after a quick and sharp resuscitation is completed, if there is evidence of perforation of the bowel, and toxemia.

In contrast, other schools of thought would prefer a delayed approach under the same clinical condition. My experience supports the latter.

This school of thought suggests contrary to the previous policy and recommends that the resuscitation must be continued until the tissue hydration and renal function seem to have been recovered reasonably satisfactorily.

Management of renal shutdown, resulting from acute perioperative hypotension would be much more difficult. This may add further burden to the patient. In this situation, pulmonary edema may be encountered with the rapid infusion that is carried out with a view to overcoming the perioperative hypotension.

On the contrary, all the evidences suggest that the risk of mortality would be no worse, by delaying the operation, but the risk of cardiac failure, pulmonary edema and poor renal function would be greater, if the operation being carried out prior to adequate resuscitation.[14]

All the studies reported that the incidence of postoperative mortality was around seven times greater than elective operation. These are the results compiled below.

A comparative result in postoperative death after proctocolectomy and ileostomy.

Authors	Year	Emergency Operation (%)	Elective Operation (%)
Lennard and Vivian[15]	1960	30.8	4.4
Brooke and Sampson[16]	1964	16.1	2.8
Hughes, ESR[17]	1965	14.3	6.0

Although the operative procedures were no different between the emergency and elective proctocolectomy and ileostomy, the only difference that could be apparent among the cases of emergency operation could be the level of tissue hydration, nutritional state, electrolytes and toxemia. But there would be not much difference in the operative procedure and postoperative cares between the perforated ulcerative colitis and perforated diverticulitis or cases with acute colonic obstruction in cancer of the bowel.

It would be an impressive argument that sooner the infective material is removed from the peritoneal cavity is better, but the bacterial pool in the circulatory system could not be eradicated by any other therapeutic measure, whether or not the peritoneal sepsis is cleared off within a few hours.

Apart from this difficulty, the tissue dehydration could not be rectified in less than 12 hours, before emergency laparotomy being undertaken. On the contrary, the precapillary sphincter opens up rapidly under general anesthesia, if emergency operation being undertaken without adequate tissue hydration.

As a result, the third compartment which is the center of fluid deficit is filled up with fluid, thus producing the fluid deficit in the main circulatory systems. This leads to gross hypotension while the patient is having emergency surgery. This physiological function does not occur in elective abdominal major operation.

In this physiological activity, time seems to be the essential factor in transferring the fluid into the third compartment, regulated by the precapillary shunt. The latter opens up slowly by the hydrostatic pressure, thus permitting the fluid entering into the third compartment.

Goligher in his study claimed that postoperative collapse was attributable to adrenal insufficiency. This could be one of the causative factors for a postoperative death in emergency operation for proctocolectomy and ileostomy, but my prospective study revealed that this postoperative collapse that resulted from hypotension is attributable to inadequate resuscitation and inadequate tissue hydration prior to emergency operations is carried out. In my study, mortality could be reduced if not possible to be averted, if the operation is deferred until a full resuscitation being carried out.[14] This physiological phenomenon has been highlighted in detail in the previous section.

CHOICE OF OPERATIVE PROCEDURE FOR EMERGENCY OPERATION FOR THE TOXIC DILATATION OF THE COLON

It would be another controversy on the operative procedures. Some will argue in favor of one stage operative procedure and others would advocate for two stage operative procedures. There are merits in supporting the both approaches.

The first stage operative procedure comprises of a total panproctocolectomy and construction of a terminal ileostomy. It is a major operative procedure that requires a confidence, experience and skill in undertaking this major operative procedure. Many surgeons will have some apprehension in this approach because of a poor state of health of the sick patient. This will be highlighted in detail later.

Alternative to this courageous approach is the two stage operative procedures. Of the two stage procedures, the first stage procedure is the emergency operation and the second stage procedure is the elective operation and is a continuation of the previous procedure undertaken as an emergency first stage procedure.

The first stage emergency operation has a few alternative choices. One of them is a construction of simple loop ileostomy, leaving behind the diseased colon *in situ* in the abdomen. This approach is adopted in a very frail and sick patient. Its objective is to divert the feces and to prevent from the risk of colonic perforation or other potential complications, but all the evidences suggest contrary to this perception.

In many studies, doubt has been expressed whether it would prevent the potential risk of perforation or hemorrhage from the acute dilatation of ulcerative colitis or from the rectum. Because of the fact, this diversion of feces cannot resolve the primary disease producing the acute dilatation of the colon. Hence, the rationality of this approach remains in question.

Leaving aside this debatable issue, additional procedure could be included; if the general condition of the patient permits. It includes total colectomy, and a rectal mucous fistula or total closure of the rectal stump. The risk of a high incidence of morbidity and mortality could not be ruled out in this emergency operation, whether or not a loop ileostomy or a combination of a total colectomy and a terminal ileostomy is undertaken.

The primary pathophysiological conditions, presented with dehydration, electrolytes deficit, high urea and creatinine and anemia do exist among these patients, whether or not the operative procedure is a simple loop ileostomy or a total colectomy or a panproctocolectomy and ileostomy. These patients require a full resuscitation before contemplating for any one of those operative procedures. Patient has to be prepared to combat against the surgical shock.

The second stage operative procedure is undertaken a few weeks later and it is an elective operation that could be a total colectomy, panproctocolectomy or excision of the rectal stump. It all depends upon what sorts of operative procedure was carried out in the emergency operation. There is no doubt that the general condition of the patient would appear to be much improved after the emergency operation being carried out in the first stage.

Apparently it sounds rational and sensible proposal in dealing with the acute dilatation of ulcerative colitis in two stages but a second stage operative procedure may appear to be much more difficult because of previous intraperitoneal sepsis and adhesion.[18]

In this debate, one needs to understand the physiological changes that may occur in the cardiovascular function during the emergency operative procedure. In surgical practice, such changes in vital function are less apparent, during and after the emergency operation is done, if preoperative resuscitation is not required. But it may be worse during and after the operation is done, if any form of emergency procedures is undertaken without a full resuscitation.

The full resuscitation implies that patient requires total correction of dehydration, electrolytes deficit, stabilizing renal function, blood pressure and correction of anemia. The experiences show that many of these patients develop acute hypotension during the emergency operation. This occurs due to opening of the precapillary shunt, thus transferring the fluid to the third compartment. Patient needs infusion of colloids in order to maintain the blood pressure and renal perfusion pressure. Complication of overtransfusion has been highlighted in other section.

This explains the reason as to why the incidence of mortality following a simple ileostomy would be no better, despite a better postoperative care being available in the intensive care unit. Nevertheless, the study has reported that the mortality in those years were worse. It ranges from 31.7 percent to 66 percent.[19-21]

This high incidence of mortality may be attributable to many factors in those years. But we understand the pathophysiological function better today than in those years, where the anesthesia was primitive and there was no broad-spectrum antibiotic available in the treatment of septicemia.

In sharp contrast, the general anesthesia has revolutionized over the last 4-5 decades. Better postoperative care is available because of intensive care unit, choices of antibiotics, physiotherapy and other facilities. Despite this progressive change in practice, controversy still exists whether there is any merit of undertaking the emergency operation, before the correction of fluid deficit and restoration of renal function have been achieved.

Many studies claimed that the emergency operative techniques would be no different from that in the elective operation. Many surgeons would advocate that in view of the poor general health, minimum operative procedure should be carried out in the first stage, as outlined in the emergency operative procedure.

This first stage is a temporary measure that would provide an opportunity to improve the general health with a view to undertaking the second stage elective operative procedure. It seems to be a powerful argument and advocacy. In the second stage, there are a number of options available, as outlined in the foregoing section.

One needs to examine the fact in perspective whether one stage procedure carries a greater risk of renal shutdown than with two stage procedures. The risk of perioperative and postoperative renal shutdown is often associated with the emergency operation, irrespective of the type of the operative procedures being carried out. It is due to sudden onset of hypotension developed in the theater. And it would be no different whether or not one stage or two stage operative procedures are carried out for cases with acute dilatation of ulcerative colitis. This risk of perioperative acute hypotension would be no worse, if total pan-proctocolectomy is included in the one stage procedure. Because of the fact, the resection of the colon and rectum is carried out without disturbing the posterior peritoneum or without mobilizing the mesentery. In fact, the bowel is resected close to the attachment of its mesocolon.

It seems to be the consensus that both terminal ileostomy and total proctocolectomy should be done in one stage, after a total resuscitation is done. Many surgeons advocate for subtotal colectomy and ileostomy; if the rectum remains unaffected by the disease. In this approach, the rectum is retained with or without construction of a mucous fistula.

The risk of blow-out of the blind end of the retained rectum is greater, if mucous fistula is not constructed through a separate wound. The reason for blow out of the blind rectal pouch is the collection of serous and mucous fluid within the blind pouch that may trigger off a retrograde peristalsis, thus causing dehiscence of the sutures inserted across the rectal stump. And it is also possible that the transection of the rectum that is carried out blindly may go through the diseased segment of the rectum.

Surgeon believes that this first stage procedure that could be undertaken very quickly may assist moribund patients to regain his health within a few months, before the second stage operative procedure being contemplated.

But such argument is unsustainable due to the fact that the time spent in the construction of a mucous fistula would be sufficient for the surgeon to complete the resection of the rectum and the anal canal. Furthermore, this resection would be much quicker and less traumatic, if the rectum is resected along its mesenteric attachment, leaving behind the mesentery and the fascia of Waldeyer intact over the sacral cavity. But the second stage operative procedure, either for the ileorectal anastomosis or resection of the rectal stump would be much more tedious and difficult. This will take much more time in mobilizing the rectum through the scar tissue.

However, in the second stage procedure, the operation comprises of reversal of ileostomy and restoration of the continuity of the gut by joining the ileostomy end of the small intestine to the rectal stump, provided the rectum still remains free from the disease. This operation is known as ileorectal anastomosis.

Furthermore, the ileorectal anastomosis may seem to be straightforward but it is not without problem. Since the rectal stump remains defunct over a few months, it may develop into disuse atrophy and may turn into a spastic change around the distal rectum and the anal sphincteric muscles. If due care is not taken, anastomosis may give way due to a resistance encountered with the rectal wall and the anal sphincters.

In contrast, other surgeon would prefer to do the same procedure in one stage. In this case, anastomosis would be simpler, easier and quicker, but ileorectal anastomosis would be contraindicated under the following conditions such as:
- Rectovaginal fistula.
- Rectovesical fistula.
- Perianal fistula.
- Chronic anal fissure.
- Perianal abscess.

In both approaches, the problems are unpredictable. Although apparently, the rectum appears to be healthy looking, the incidence of ulcerative colitis is around 90 percent in the sigmoid or left colon and the rectum remains in the close proximity to the primary site of the disease. The rectal stump may cause a great concern to the surgeon after the ileorectal anastomosis being performed. Regular sigmoidoscopic examination is necessary in every six months or sooner, in order to identify whether or not there is any evidence of recurrence of ulcerative proctitis or malignancy.

Patient will require further major operation after a few years. And operative procedure would be much more tedious and difficult due to adhesions and fibrosis, formed around the pelvis. And a long-term follow-up would be necessary over many years. The risk of cancer or recurrence of ulcerative colitis in the rectum could not be ruled out in a few years time.

Therefore, opinion will vary from surgeon to surgeon. One needs to analyze the pros and cons between the total proctocolectomy with terminal ileostomy and the ileorectal anastomosis done in one stage, before a final decision is taken in perspective whether it would be wise to deal with unpredictable disease, where the rectum remains at greater risk of developing the recurrence of ulcerative colitis in future.

REFERENCES

1. Grace WJ, Wolf S, Wolff HG. The Human Colon. London: Heinemann 1951.
2. Paulley JW. The emotional factors in ulcerative colitis. Gastroenterology 1956;86:709.
3. Ingham HR, Sissin PR, Selkon JB, et al. Inhibition of phagocytosis *in-vitro* by obligate anaerobes. Lancet 1977;2:1252.
4. Saha SK. Efficacy of metronidazole lavage in the treatment of intraperitoneal sepsis: A prospective study. Digestive Diseases and Sciences 1996;41(7):1313.
5. Watts J McK, de Tomball FT, Goligher JC. Long-term complications and prognosis following major surgery for ulcerative colitis. Br J Surg 1966;53:1014.
6. Bebchuk W, Rogers AC, Downey JL. Chronic ulcerative colitis in a North American Indian. Gastroenterology 1961;40:138.
7. Wigley RD, Maclaurin BP. A study of ulcerative colitis in New Zealand, showing a low incidence in Maoris. Brit Med J 1962;2:228.
8. Melrose AG. The Geographical incidence of chronic ulcerative colitis in Britain. Gastroenterology 1955;29:1055.
9. Lockhart-Mummery JP. Disease of the rectum and colon. 2nd edition, Bailliere 1934.
10. Dukes CE. The surgical pathology of ulcerative colitis. Ann Roy Coll Eng 1954;14:389.
11. Sloan WP, Bargen JA, Baggenstoss AH. Local complications of chronic ulcerative colitis on the study of 2000 cases. Proc Mayo Clinic 1950;25:240.
12. Rickets WE, Kirsner JB, Palmer WL. Chronic non-specific ulcerative colitis: A roentgenologic study of its course. Gastroenterology 1948;10:1.
13. Sloan WP, Bargen JA, Gage RP. Life histories of patients with chronic ulcerative colitis: A review of 2000 cases. Gastroenterology 1950;16:25.

14. Saha SK. Efficacy of metronidazole lavage in the treatment of intraperitoneal sepsis: A prospective study. Digestive Diseases and Sciences 1996;41(7):1313.
15. Lennard-Jones JE, Vivian AB. Fulminating ulcerative colitis: Recent experiences in management. Brit Med J 1960;2:96.
16. Brooke BN, Sampson PA. An indication for surgery in acute ulcerative colitis. Lancet 1964;2:1272.
17. Hughes ESR. The treatment of ulcerative colitis. Ann Roy Surg Eng 1965;37:191.
18. Crile G Jr., Thomas CY. Treatment of acute toxic ulcerative colitis by ileostomy and simultaneous colectomy. Gastroenterology 1951;19:58.
19. Rankin FW. Surgery for ulcerative colitis. Surg Gyne and Obstet 1939;68:306.
20. Cave HW, Thompson JE. Mortality factors in the surgical treatment of ulcerative colitis. Ann Surg 1939;46:79.
21. Cattle RB, Sachs E Jr. Surgical treatment of ulcerative colitis. J Amer Med Assn 1948;137:929.

15 Management of Ulcerative Colitis

OPERATIVE TREATMENT FOR ULCERATIVE COLITIS

The incidence of operative treatment for ulcerative colitis varies from center-to-center. It ranges from 16.7 percent to 36.3 percent.[1,2]

In elective cases, most surgeons prefer conservative surgery, sparing the excision of the rectum and anus. In this procedure, total colectomy and ileorectal anastomosis is done. This approach is particularly suitable to the women of the childbearing age and also male patients. Psychological and sexual disability present a difficult issue, and it would be highlighted later. Nonetheless, the long-term benefit with this approach is debatable, because of the fact that the symptoms may recur due to recurrence of ulceration in the rectum. This problem may also occur in the rectal stump, if the rectal stump is left *in situ* and instead, ileostomy is constructed for the time-being, with a view to rejoining the ileum with the rectal stump later at a suitable time.

Despite the feces being diverted, the risk of developing recurrence of ulceration, hemorrhage and mucopurulent discharge from the rectal stump could not be predicted, whether or not ileorectal anastomosis is carried out either at the same time or a few months later.

It has also been observed that the rectal stump that has been left behind *in situ*, with a view to considering for the restoration of continuity of the gut at a suitable time later has been found discharging the foul smelling mucopurulent liquid, sometimes mixed with blood from the rectum. Patient may experience with discomfort. In some cases, blood transfusion may be needed to correct the chronic anemia. The etiology for recurrence of symptoms is not known. These conditions are often referred to as proctitis.

The treatment for these cases is excision of the rectum like abdominoperineal resection of the rectum. The operative procedure in this case would be very difficult due to previous operation, or due to infection and friable nature of the rectal stump. Primary perineal wound healing may not be possible.

Apart from recurrence of disease in the rectal stump, there remains a risk of developing carcinoma within the rectal stump. Because of this risk, sigmoidoscopy and proctoscopy should be carried out every six months.

Alternative operative procedure is total proctocolectomy, often referred to as panproctocolectomy, and ileostomy that will eliminate all those potential risks.

For emergency operation, there are many choices available to the surgeon that depends upon the clinical conditions of the patients, and skill and confidence of the surgeon.

The choices are:
1. Simple ileostomy in the first stage, it is followed by the total colectomy, or proctocolectomy to be done in the second stage.
2. Total resection of the colon, followed by ileorectal anastomose in one stage.
3. Total excision of the colon, retention of the blind rectal stump and ileostomy in one stage and in the second stage, reversal of ileostomy and ileorectal anastomosis.
4. Subtotal colectomy, followed by ileostomy and rectal mucous fistula or sigmoid colostomy done in first stage. And in the second stage, reversal of ileostomy and reversal of rectal mucous fistula or reversal of colostomy followed by ileorectal anastomosis.
5. Total proctocolectomy and ileostomy done in one stage.

Total Proctocolectomy

This is a life-saving operation, when the ulcerative colitis did not respond to medical treatment. Total proctocolectomy should be undertaken despite the rectum being spared from the disease. Although ileorectal anastomosis could be carried out instead, there remains a potential risk of recurrence of disease in the rectum. Therefore, further surgery may be required for the excision of the rectum, and for the construction of a terminal ileostomy.

Those patients, whose rectum is left behind at the initial operation, require regular surveillance which may reveal the recurrence of proctitis, or rectal growth, whether or not ileorectal anastomosis has been done. In many cases, the rectal stump continues to pass foul smell and blood stained discharge. They may develop perianal fistula or abscess. Life becomes unbearable.

For cases with fecal peritonitis, or for acute dilatation of the colon, emergency operation may be undertaken, provided the patient is not in a state of shock. In all instances, they need resusitation before the major operation could be undertaken.

PREOPERATIVE TREATMENT

In many cases, they need blood transfusion and correction of electrolytes imbalance. Their nutritional state has to be improved by parenteral feeding with TPN, before surgery is undertaken in elective cases, if possible. If the patient was on steroid, this has to be continued. All other preoperative assessment and preparation remains the same as described in other colonic surgery.

PREOPERATIVE CONSULTATION AND PREPARATION

In this consultation, bladder and sexual dysfunctions are highlighted, despite the fact that the risk of sexual dysfunction is much less found among these cases. Because of the fact, the dissection of the rectum is carried out close to its wall, leaving behind the mesentery and parietal peritoneum *in situ*. All other complications and morbidities need not to be repeated in this section.

The preparation, and prophylactic measures against the deep vein thrombosis and infection need not be described in this section. This has been described in the APR. A Foley Catheter No.18FG is inserted per urethra and the residual urine volume is measured and recorded in the intake and output chart.

Prophylactic antibiotics such as metronidazole 500 mg and cephalosporin 750 mg IV should be commenced in the theater and these antibiotics are continued 8 hourly parenterally for 5-7 days. If the patient was on steroid in the past, injection of hydrocortisone 500 mg six hourly should be recommenced prior to anesthesia. This steroid is gradually tailed off within 3-4 days. He will not require any maintenance dose after the patient has fully recovered from the operation. The tablet Salazopyrine or Asacol must not be given after the operation. It would be unnecessary after the total disease has been surgically eradicated.

OPERATIVE PROCEDURE FOR TOTAL PANPROCTOCOLECTOMY

Patient is placed on a Trendelenburg–Lithotomy position on the Lloyd Davis table. Before proceeding further, the anal orifice is closed with purse string sutures as described in the operation of abdominoperineal resection. This will prevent spillage of loose motion into the perineum.

Skin preparation has been made with chlorhexidine in alcohol in both abdominal wall as well as around the perineum. Sterile drapes are laid down around the legs. They are also laid across the upper chest wall, along the flanks and across the suprapubic region. A separate drape is put under the buttock. The latter should be rested on a sand bag and beyond the edge of the table.

Before incision is made, it is important to be sure that the skin pencil mark made on the proposed site for ileostomy has not been wiped out. Abdomen is opened through a midline incision that is commenced from the epigastrium and is extended down through the umbilicus right down to the suprapubic region. The abdominal wound is retracted by a self-retaining retractor. A thorough internal examination is carried out. This includes palpation of the liver, gallbladder, pancreas, stomach, spleen and kidneys. The colon is handled gently and carefully, because its wall could be found to be edematous and friable.

The operative technique entails the procedures that included the resection of the right colon, transverse colon, left colon, and the rectum and anus. The operative technique for all these resections remains the same with those of colectomy, but the dissection of the colon would not be extensive. On the contrary, it would be close to its wall, in that the greater omentum need not be resected from the stomach and the mobilization of the rectum would be limited to its vascular attachments along its wall, without disturbing the posterior sacral wall and back of the bladder and the prostate.

After resecting the whole length of the colon from the cecum right down to the rectosigmoid region, perineal dissection is commenced by the same surgeon or by a separate perineal surgeon, as described in the section on abdominoperineal resection of the rectum.

For the perineal excision of the anus, synchronous combined approach would be appropriate in order to cut down the operating time. At the completion of the proctocolectomy, the terminal ileum is transected 12 inches proximal to the ileocecal junction. The whole specimen is sent to pathology department.

Terminal ileostomy is constructed in the right iliac fossa, as described in the previous chapter. Peritoneal cavity is washed with saline in room temperature several times. It is followed by metronidazole lavage (1gm) as described in the appropriate section. In the same way, the perineal wound is washed with saline and thereafter with metronidazole lavage. Both abdominal and perineal wounds are closed in layers, as described before.

POSTOPERATIVE CARE

As discused before, the same policy is adopted in the postoperative care, but patient may need nutritional support for few weeks until the oral feeding is commenced.

Postoperative complications have been described in the Chapter on abdominoperineal resection (Ch-11). Furthermore, complication and morbidity associated with ileostomy have been compiled in the section on ileostomy (Ch-9).

OPERATIVE PROCEDURES FOR SUBTOTAL COLECTOMY AND ILEOSTOMY

This procedure is undertaken in emergency operation, because of acute dilatation of the colon. This acute condition develops due to relapsing acute ulcerative colitis. Preoperative assessment remains the same, but it is the responsibility of the surgeon to highlight the merits, between the two stage operative procedures and additional burden in looking after the rectal mucous fistula or terminal sigmoid colostomy, if they are necessary to be constructed.

OPERATIVE PROCEDURE

In this case, patient lies on the back in supine position. Skin preparation and draping around the field of operation remains the same as described before. The abdomen is opened through a midline incision that goes through the linea alba. Unlike the procedure for proctocolectomy, the resection of the colon depends upon the extent of the disease. The level resection should be through the healthy segment of the colon that could be the lower end of the sigmoid colon or upper part of the rectum that depends upon the extent of the disease.

If the surgeon has decided to leave the rectal stump behind in the pelvis, then the resection could be carried out up to the level of healthy part of the rectum, where the latter is transected either by the autosuture gun, using TA 55 or between the Zachary Copes clamps. Before dividing the bowel, a good vascularity below the level of the resection must be preserved.

In the latter procedure, the transected end of the rectum is closed with hand sutures in two layers. This could be done either by a continuous or by interrupted sutures that go through the full thickness of the rectal wall. These sutures are invaginated by a second layer either by a continuous or by interrupted sutures that go through the seromuscular layer.

For the purpose of invagination of the rectal stump, the second line of sutures should be at least 1cm away from the first line of sutures. Invagination of the rectal stump could be difficult, if enough space is not left *in situ* between the first and the second line of sutures. In some cases, the sutures of the second line may cut out from the serosal wall, while undertaking the invagination of the first line of sutures. After completion of the procedure, the rectal stump is put back into the pelvis and it should be covered with a piece of the greater omentum or it should be put under the cover of pelvic peritoneum.

This depends upon whether this rectal stump will be used later for the ileorectal anastomosis at a second stage or it would be excised completely through the perineal dissection like the perineal resection of the abdominoperineal resection of the rectum. This second stage should be done after the patient has fully recovered. In this second approach, abdomen may not be required to be reopened and it is unnecessary in most cases; but the perineal dissection may turn out to be difficult in some cases.

If the rectal stump is to be brought out outside the peritoneal cavity, in that case, either the rectal mucous fistula or sigmoid colostomy could be constructed. In these cases, a longer distal stump would be necessary in order to bring out the transected end of the distal colon or the rectum through a separate skin wound like pelvic colostomy.

If the rectal mucous fistula is to be constructed, the rectal stump is first closed with the autosutures or with the Zachary Copes clamps (Fig. 15.1). This closed stump is brought out through a separate skin wound, made similar to that of the colostomy, in the lower part of the left iliac fossa or it could be brought out through the lower end of the main laparotomy wound. The risk of wound infection remains high in the latter approach.

If the transected end of the bowel is to be treated like a colostomy, and if the lower sigmoid colon appears to be unaffected by the disease, then a longer distal colorectal stump needs to be retained in order to construct a distal colostomy. In this case, the transection is carried out between the Zachary Copes clamps applied across the colon a little above the rectosigmoid junction. Alternatively, autosuture, using TA 90 could be applied for the same procedure but it would be expensive.

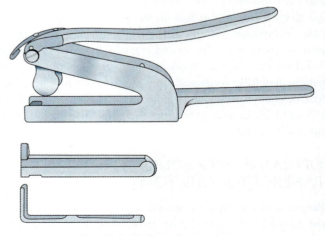

Fig. 15.1: Zachary Copes clamps

Alternatively, the same site could be transected between the two autosutures. The distal end is brought out through a colostomy wound as described before. If the rectal stump is not brought out through the extraperitoneal tunnel, the paracolonic gutter needs to be closed with a continuous or interrupted sutures inserted between the parietal peritoneum and the serosal layer of the colon. This will prevent herniation of the small intestine through the space lateral to the side of the colon.

If the rectal stump is brought out through the extraperitoneal tunnel in the first stage procedure, it would be a tedious job in the second stage procedure in order to get this rectal stump out of the extraperitoneal tunnel, when reversal of ileostomy is converted into the ileorectal anastomosis. All these problems must be known before contemplating all these techniques in the resection of the colon.

The procedure for removing the entire colon and terminal ileostomy remains the same as described before in the section on the proctocolectomy. If it is decided to keep the blind rectal stump in the pelvic cavity, a drainage tube should be left in the pelvis, near the blind rectal stump, before the abdominal wound is closed. The reason for putting a drainage tubing in the pelvic cavity is to let the infected fluid out of the pelvic cavity; in case the rectal stump blows out, discharging the infective feculent fluid into the pelvis. This is a safety measure against the potential risk of peritonitis.

Because of the fact, the rectal stump remains as a blind tube in which there would be a collection of mucopurulent fluid and air. This will build up a tension that may induce reverse peristalsis causing dehiscence of the closed rectal stump that may occur within 5 days after operation. There could be many causative factors for such dehiscence of the rectal stump, but the true factor is the resistance exerted by the anal sphincters at rest which is believed to be much greater than that of the sutures line of the rectal stump. As a result, the latter gives away. Because of this risk, many surgeons prefer the construction of rectal mucous fistula.

POSTOPERATIVE CARE

Management of Ileostomy

The fitting of the ileostomy bag is very important. Koraya Gum-commercially prepared paste, is put around the edge of the stoma up to the skin sutures, thus protecting the bare skin area from the contamination of bile mixed loose motion. This contamination may cause skin irritation and excoriation. The same material is also put around the plastic flange before the latter is pressed over the paste of the Koraya gum. This will seal the space between the plastic flange and skin of the ileostomy. This will stop leakage of the loose motions. This paste is left *in situ* for one week if possible. The plastic bag needs to be detached from the plastic flange, when replacement is necessary.

It is also important to be sure that the mucosal spout of the ileostomy which would look like a sausage is not ulcerated by the constant rubbing against the ring of the ileostomy bag.

FLUID BALANCE AND CORRECTION OF FLUID AND ELECTROLYTES DEFICIT

Ileostomy starts working after 48 hours. Accurate measuring of the loose motion is very important and it is done every time the bag is emptied. The concentration of sodium and chloride present in the loose motion is consistent with normal saline. Therefore, the total output per day should be replaced by the similar volume of the saline in most cases, but additional fluid is necessary to compensate other sources of fluid loss. These are insensible fluid loss, urine output and the daily nasogastric aspirates.

Despite this broad outline of the fluid balance, supplementation of potassium chloride should be added to the infusion of normal saline. The total dose per day is to be worked on the result of serum electrolyte. On an average, 13 m mol of potassium chloride, equivalent to one gram, could be added in each liter of normal saline or 5 percent dextrose solution per day, but the total dose should not exceed 6 gm of KCl per day and should not exceed the serum potassium level. Parenteral infusion should be continued, until oral feeding is commenced.

Within 2 weeks, the total volume of the loose motion may reduce to 400-600 ml per day. If it continues more than this estimation, patient could take codeine phosphate and/or Isogel orally. Patient is advised to identify any food allergy and should avoid those items that may induce loose motion. Fruits and vegetables are not suitable for certain patients. Iron tablets may improve the condition.

Care of Wound

Unlike any other abdominal operation, wound healing may be slowed for various reasons. No special care is necessary, but the wound infection should be dealt within the line of established practices.

Complications

- Complication of ileostomy.
- Complication of mucous fistula of the rectum or sigmoid colostomy.
- Complication of the rectal stump.

The problems with the mucous fistula, sigmoid colostomy and rectal stump have already been highlighted in the appropriate places. In this section, complication of ileostomy will be described. It could be divided into:
a. Immediate complication of ileostomy.
b. Delayed complication.

Types of Immediate Complication of Ileostomy

i. Leakage of loose motion.
ii. Ulceration.
iii. Necrosis of the mucosa or dehiscence of the mucocutaneous anastomosis.
iv. Dysfunction of ileostomy.

DESCRIPTION OF SPECIFIC COMPLICATIONS

Causes for Leakage of Ileostomy

It may occur through the space between the plastic flange of the ileostomy bag and skin wound margin. It could be associated with the selection of a site for the construction of ileostomy. If the ileostomy is constructed near the anterior superior iliac spine, or umbilicus or closer to the costal margin, water tight fitting of the plastic flange may not be made possible. As a result, there could be leakage of the feculent fluid through the gap under the plastic flange.

If the ileostomy has been constructed in the lower part of the right iliac fossa; as a result, the ileostomy bag may be pushed up or the plastic flange of the appliance may be lifted up by the right thigh being raised in flexion position. This may squeeze the bag that may cause leakage of fluid through the space between the plastic flange and skin surface.

The size of the spout is also an important factor for preventing the leakage. The ideal length of the spout should be between 1 and 2 inches. A flush stoma will cause leakage. On the contrary, a longer ileostomy stump may be rubbing against the inferior ring of the flange, thus producing ulceration or fistula in the inferior surface of the spout.

Causes of Ulceration of Ileostomy

This may result from rubbing of the mucosa against the plastic bag or plastic flange of the appliance. It may occur sooner or later that depends upon many factors. Immediate cause is the rubbing of the mucosa against the tight fighting of the plastic flange causing a constant rubbing with the mucosa. The commonest site for such contact is at the base of the ileostomy, which is around the mucocutaneous junction.

Other possibility is the recurrent disturbance of fitting of the appliance that may be lifted off from the skin surface when the thigh is brought in flexed position. This is related to the site of the ileostomy, as described before. In addition to leakage of feces, ulceration may develop, because of the same reason.

The same complication may be encountered with the prolapse of the ileostomy that takes a few weeks or a few months time to produce the prolapse of the ileostomy. It is regarded to be a delayed complication. In this case, the pathogenesis of the ulceration remains the same, but ulceration can occur in two places. A superficial ulceration can develop at the distal end around the spout. And another ulcer can develop at the proximal end near the mucocutaneous junction. In the former case, the etiology is the hanging of the ileostomy stump that gets a constant rubbing against the plastic bag.

The etiology for the ulcer developed at the proximal end is related to either tight fitting of the plastic flange around the mucocutaneous junction or the site of ileostomy was in the lower part of the right iliac fossa. As a result, the plastic flange is elevated from the skin surface during the sitting position or when the thigh is brought to the groin. All these factors continue to rub the mucosa leading to ulceration that may progress to fistula. In this situation, the site of the ulceration and fistula is located in the inferior wall or the undersurface of the ileostomy.

Apart from ulceration or necrosis of the mucosa, dehiscence of mucocutaneous anastomose may occur due to the disruption of the sutures between the skin wound margin and edge of the mucosa. This disruption may result from infection. This is attributable to leakage of feces into the mucocutaneous junction and due to a high concentration of bile salts which cause irritation to the tissue and necrosis of the skin.

DELAYED COMPLICATION OF ILEOSTOMY

a. Prolapse of the ileostomy spout.
b. Dysfunction of ileostomy:
   i. Parastomal herniation of the gut.
   ii. Stenosis of the ileostomy stoma that would not permit the little finger.
   iii. Skin necrosis or sloughing due to contamination of loose motion containing a high concentration of bile salts.
c. Stomal ulceration and fistula through the bed of the ulceration.

PROBLEMS OF PROLAPSE OF THE ILEOSTOMY

If the length of the spout is in excess of 3 inches from the skin surface, then it is regarded to be prolapse of the ileostomy. Surgical correction is necessary to prevent ulceration or leakage.

There are two types of prolapse:
1. One is a sliding type.
2. Other one is a fixed type.

In sliding type, the ileostomy protrudes out of the abdomen and keeps hanging down beyond the abdominal wall. It occurs on standing up or on straining. Its average length that remains projected outside the skin stoma is around 3-5 inches. The etiology is related to either faulty technique used in the construction of ileostomy or it may result from disruption of those anchoring sutures used between the serosal wall of the intestine (inner tube) and the rectus abdominis muscle or the rectus sheath all around, before the distal stoma (transected end of the intestine) is everted to be sutured with the skin edge. As a result, the inner tube moves in and out of the peritoneal cavity through the stomal (ileostomy) wound by gravity on standing or by intra-abdominal pressure on straining or coughing.

It may be ulcerated by rubbing against the wall of the plastic bag or against the plastic flange of the ileostomy bag. The ulceration that occurs at the site of spout is usually superficial and it is due to continuous rubbing against the plastic bag. It may also occur near the base that usually occurs on the inferior mucosal surface of the ileostomy. It should be dealt with sooner; otherwise it may lead to fistula, thus leaking the intestinal contents causing skin excoriation, if not properly protected by the Koraya-gum adhesive.

In a fixed type of prolapse, defective construction is believed to be the causative factor. At the outset, a longer segment of the transected intestine that is brought out through the ileostomy wound is left hanging outside the skin surface, before its serosal wall is sutured all around to the rectus sheath or the rectus abdominis muscles. The length of the intestine distal to the sutures line or distal to the abdominal wall could be much longer than the appropriate length to be required for the eversion of the stoma and construction of ileostomy spout. This length may be regarded to be very long and it has resulted from misjudgment, when the ileostomy is constructed. This error of measurement becomes apparent after the mucosal edge is everted and then it is anchored to the skin edge of the stoma.

In both varieties, there could be some degree of faulty technique, when the serosal layer of the intestine is anchored all around with the anterior rectus sheath or rectus abdominis muscles. A similar error may occur in inserting a few sutures passed between the everted mucosal edges, then through the serosal wall-like plication and finally through the skin stoma, but these sutures, inserted through the serosal wall should be at different level.

VARIOUS METHODS OF CORRECTION

a. Amputation and reconstruction of the ileostomy.
b. Refashioning of the ileostomy.
c. Relocation of the ileostomy.

AMPUTATION OF THE ILEOSTOMY SPOUT

It is not suitable for sliding type and not suitable for the fixed type of prolapse, if the duration of the latter is very short. Nevertheless, the technique is to amputate the spout at a correct level from the mucocutaneous junction. The procedure is similar to the technique used for prolapse of the rectum, in that, the rectosigmoid junction is resected and continuity is restored by end-to-end anastomosis. But in the correction of prolapse of the ileostomy, there remains a risk of necrosis of the everted mucosa, if the mesenteric vessels, supplying to the prolapsed ileostomy are divided, and ligated at the same level with the amputation of the prolapse of the ileostomy.

REFASHIONING OF THE TERMINAL ILEOSTOMY

A Short Description of Operative Procedure

First, the base of the ileostomy is detached from the mucocutaneous junction. This is done by a circular incision made around the mucocutaneous edge of the stoma. The everted mucosal layer is brought back to its previous position, by just reversing the outer tube. In other words, it is inverted again —thus bringing back to its original position.

The next approach is to assess the size of the skin wound, quality of the muscle and tissue around the skin stoma. If they are atrophic or wide, then a new site is to be chosen for the reconstruction of the ileostomy. Preferred site should be on the left side of the abdomen. In this case, laparotomy is necessary for resiting of ileostomy.

Alternative approach is to do the reconstruction of ileostomy at a different site on the same side or to repair the old wound. The size of the existing stomal wound could be narrowed by putting a few interrupted silk stitches. This may make the opening to be smaller, consistent with the size of the gut wall.

However, the serosal wall of the gut is anchored all around by interrupted silk stitches with the parietal wall of the stoma. These anchoring sutures are made between the rectus sheath or rectus abdominis muscle and the serosal wall of the gut. The correct length of the projected ileum is preserved after amputation of the excess in length. Reconstruction of ileostomy is carried out as described before.

If laparotomy is necessary, the ileostomy is separated from the surrounding of the stomal opening. It is withdrawn from inside the abdomen. The serosal layer of the gut is again anchored all around with the anterior peritoneal wall. The same procedure is also repeated from outside the abdomen and the serosal wall is anchored with the rectus abdominis muscle or the anterior rectus sheath all around the gut by several interrupted silk sutures. The ileostomy is reconstructed as before, but a correct length must be preserved before the reconstruction being carried out.

If the old stoma of the abdominal wall in the right side of the umbilicus appears to be wide and atrophic with poor quality of muscle, then it is wise to construct the ileostomy on a new site that depends upon the technical feasibility and anatomical site of the abdominal wall. A conservative outlook should be maintained. The same problem may recur from the new site.

DYSFUNCTION OF ILEOSTOMY

It could occur in the postoperative period or it may develop many months later.

The possible causes are:
a. Internal herniation of the small intestine.
b. Stenosis of the skin stoma.
c. Parastomal herniation of the gut.
d. Ileitis.

Patient may complain that he has not passed wind or motion through the ileostomy into the bag. In this situation, he may complain of spasmodic type of pain and distention of the abdomen. Clinically, abdomen would be tense and tender. Auscultation will reveal increased bowel sounds audible through the stethoscope placed on the belly. Evidence of guarding and rebound tenderness is suggestive of peritonitis which could be attributable to execration of acute intestinal obstruction or acute strangulation of the gut. Stoma should be examined whether it is present that could be evaluated by inserting the right index finger through the ileostomy. It may not be possible due to stenosis of the stoma, resulting from chronic scarring around the mucocutaneous junction or there could be tightness inside the ileostomy which could be due to inadequate opening made through the rectus sheath or abdominis muscles, when the ileostomy was originally constructed.

Apart from all other investigations, plain X-ray of the abdomen should be taken. If the proximal segment of the small intestine appears to be dilated, then it is more likely to be intestinal obstruction. In this case, the possible causes are adhesion between the loops of the intestine causing kinking of the gut or the omental bands causing strangulation of the gut.

If the X-ray shows that the small intestine is dilated right up to the site of ileostomy, the possible cause for dilatation of gut is either stenosis of the stoma or parastomal herniation.

MANAGEMENT OF THE OBSTRUCTION

The initial line of treatment is to adopt a conservative line of approach. In this case, nasogastric tube is inserted into the stomach for suction every hour or continuously that depends upon the volume of aspirate and intravenous infusion. And intravenous infusion with normal saline and 5 percent dextrose should be commenced.

In addition, glycerine suppositories should be inserted through the ileostomy, alternatively a large Foley catheter No. 24F could be inserted through the spout of the ileostomy for a good length. This may relieve the partial stenosis within the distal ileum by draining a few hundred liters of watery motions. If it is successful, then the catheter is left *in situ* or is reinserted every few hours. In some cases, it may not work due to blockage of the eyes of the catheter by the mucous plug or thick feculent materials. In this case, a few saline wash-outs could be tried. Or it could be removed, that depends upon the circumstances.

Patient is observed for 5-6 hours and further palpation of the abdomen should be done in order to evaluate the state of peritonitis. If there is evidence of less guarding and no rebound tenderness, conservative treatment should be continued. If no flatus has passed and patient is not getting better or pulse rate is getting worse, then emergency laparotomy should be considered.

If the gas shadow could be seen right to the entry of the ileostomy or around the right iliac fossa, palpation did not elicit tenderness, guarding and rebound tenderness; the possible cause could be paralytic ileus or ileitis. In this case, the treatment of choice is also conservative as outlined before.

In most cases, this condition may resolve spontaneously because of conservative approach. Edema within the ileal conduit or a tight stoma within the abdominal wall or skin stenosis around the base of the ileal spout are the possible causes for defunctioning of the ileostomy.

TECHNIQUE FOR SURGICAL CORRECTION OF STENOSIS OF THE STOMA

This may result from old technique that used to be employed in the construction of ileostomy. Its incidences are very high, ranging between 25 and 30 percent.[3,4] It has improved since the construction of ileostomy has been modified, in that the everted mucosa is sutured to the skin edge. Nevertheless, infection could be the primary causative factor encouraging the excess granulation tissue that may lead to fibrosis, around the mucocutaneous junction – thus reducing the size of the stoma. This is the mechanism how stenosis develops around the terminal ileostomy.

For the surgical treatment of stenosis, the scar tissue all around the mucocutaneous junction is excised and then the stoma of the ileum is mobilized and freed from the surrounding parietal wound of the skin and the surrounding subcutaneous tissues. Once a good length has been mobilized, refashioning of the ileostomy is done as described before.

OPERATIVE TREATMENT FOR PARASTOMAL HERNIA

Again, the same principle is followed in the exploration of the mucocutaneous junction. The ileostomy is dissected out from the surrounding adhesions and any loop of gut lying within the space between the rectus sheath and skin is mobilized slowly. It is pushed back into the peritoneal cavity. The defect in the parietal wound is closed. Refashioning of the ileostomy is to be done on a different and a new site, preferably on the other side of the abdomen. In this situation, laparotomy is necessary in order to deal with the hernia, to repair the weak parietal wall surrounding the stoma and to reconstruct the ileostomy in the left side of the umbilicus.

The treatment for stomal ulceration is to correct those causative factors as described before or refashioning of the ileostomy should be done.

Other Types of Colitis

Apart from ulcerative colitis, there are other varieties of colitis. They are Crohn's colitis, ischemic colitis, radiation colitis or proctitis and amebic colitis.

Crohn's Colitis

It is less frequently presented with bowel symptoms, compared to ulcerative colitis. Its etiology is not known.

Pathology

Its pathological features are quite different from ulcerative colitis. Unlike the latter, Crohn's disease implicates the full thickness of the gut. The classical macroscopical feature is similar to that of Crohn's ileitis. Multiple fissures are classical presentation on the mucosal surface of the affected segment. Eventually, cobble stone appearances become evident.

The barium enema X-ray as shown in Figure 15.2 demonstrates the transverse fissures in the transverse colon and the disease has involved the proximal segment of the descending colon. The spiky fissures have been filled up by the barium, suggesting deep mucosal fissures.

In the same colon, multiple segments may be inflicted with these features but the intervening segment remains normal, which is known as skip lesions. These sorts of skipping lesions could be noticed in the colon or rectum.

Because of these skip lesions; multiple strictures may develop in the large intestine. This lesion may not be present concomitantly in the small intestine. And both ulcerative colitis and Crohn's disease are not present in the same patient as a rule.[5,6] Like Crohn's ileitis, Crohn's colitis has a similar behavior, in that it tends to develop fistula with the small intestine or cutaneous fistula connected with the anal canal.

The histological evidence would be the sarcoid reaction in most specimens and, such evidence could be found in the mesenteric lymph nodes in some cases. Its incidence is 25 percent.[7]

Clinical Presentations

The symptoms associated with this disease are not different from the ulcerative colitis, but its severity is much less than the ulcerative colitis. It is also evident that patient deteriorates quickly. Diarrhea, mixed with blood and slime are common symptoms but less severe.

Palpation of the abdomen may reveal tenderness and colonic lump which is distinct from the ulcerative colitis.

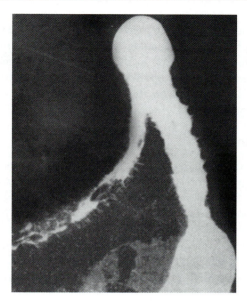

Fig. 15.2: Barium enema showing features of Crohn's Colitis in the transverse and proximal part of the descending colon (By courtesy of Lockhart-Mummery HE and Morson BC and by courtesy of the Gut 1964)

Rectal digital examination: In the anal canal, a large sized ulceration or fissure could be palpable. This is in sharp contrast to idiopathic anal fissure-in-ano, which is normally a crack or a sharp tear in the posterior anal canal.

On palpation, the rectal wall may appear to be rigid and cobble stone type mucosa or stricture may be found. These are not always evident on palpation.

Sigmoidoscopy may be normal in 50 percent of the patients and in some cases, mucopurulent or blood may be seen higher up. And in other cases, cobble stone type of rectal mucosa or patchy mucosal ulcer surrounded by healthy or edematous rectal mucosa may be seen through the sigmoidoscope. Biopsy should be taken for histological diagnosis.

Investigations

Although, clinically the symptoms are nonspecific, patient needs to be investigated with barium enema, small bowel enema and colonoscopy. In addition, all hematological investigations are carried out.

If the barium enema and colonoscopy suggests Crohn's colitis, small bowel enema should be done in order to exclude the Crohn's ileitis.

X-ray of the chest and TB screen should be completed in order to exclude TB colitis and USS of the abdomen may reveal mesenteric lymphadenitis. If facility is available, USS or CT scan guided needle biopsy from the mesenteric lymph gland should be done in order to exclude TB lymphadenitis. Author had resolved the longstanding misguided diagnosis in a young Asian cook. In this patient, a large well-defined raised granulation tissue was reported to have noticed in the mucosal surface of the ascending colon on colonoscopic examination. The lesion was localized in the cecum. Crohn's colitis was diagnosed by the histology. In fact, two years later, tuberculous colitis was diagnosed on the lymph gland biopsy that was carried out by the CT scan guided needle biopsy.[7]

Treatment

Crohn's disease has an unpredictable behavior. Conservative line of treatment is the primary aim. Medical treatment includes Salazopyrine and prednisolone. If the symptoms are not responding to these drugs, azathioprine is the next line of drug therapy to be considered in this sort of cases. It tends to recur from time-to-time. Surgical intervention is considered at last, if there is evidence of colonic stricture, abscess or fistula between the colon and small intestine or bladder. Recurrence of the disease is possible, after resection of the diseased bowel has been carried out and healing is another problem. Regular review along with the blood results and ESR should be carried out.

Treatment of anal fissure and anal fistula presents a difficult task to the surgeons. It is a difficult pathology that interferes with the primary healing. It tends to recur and in some cases, healing may not be possible, unless the Crohn's colitis is not treated.

LONG-TERM FOLLOW-UP

There remains a risk of further recurrence or stricture at the site of anastomosis, if resection of the diseased segment was carried out some years ago.

Patient may notice some degree of discomfort in the abdomen. This could be attributable to local recurrence that usually takes around 5-6 years. High-residue diet should be avoided. And other foods, in particular to those that are known to be allergic to the gut should be avoided. Further repeat of colonoscopy or barium enema should be done at every few years or when the symptoms are getting worse.

INDICATIONS FOR SURGERY

a. Medical treatment not working.
b. Stricture of the gut.
c. Evidence of internal or external fistula.
d. General health deteriorating rapidly due to diarrhea and bleeding.
e. Risk of carcinoma of the colon at the site of stricture.

A limited segmental resection with end-to-end anastomosis should be the primary aim in the surgical management. In extensive involvement or multiple colonic strictures, total proctocolectomy and ileostomy should be done.

Complications

1. Wound infection.
2. Anastomotic leakage.
3. Intestinal hurry or diarrhea, due to loss of transit time.

Other Types of Colitis:

1. Ischemic colitis.
2. Amebic colitis.

ISCHEMIC COLITIS

It is a rare presentation among emergency admissions, but suspicion should arise if elderly patients with a previous history of cardiac disease are admitted with acute pain in lower abdomen, vomiting, and fresh bleeding per rectum. Clinically, evidences of shock and pallor associated with tenderness in the suprapubic region or along the left flank are suggestive of acute ischemic colitis, unless proved otherwise. Barium enema in Figure 15.3 shows a classical feature of copper beaten appearances in the descending and sigmoid colon.

Ischemic colitis may be due to atherosclerosis in the main trunk of the inferior mesenteric artery. Other causes are thrombosis or emboli from the heart. In the operation of abdominal aortic aneurysm, inferior mesenteric artery is deliberately ligated, but acute ischemic change in the left colon is a rare event. This could be attributable to compensatory measures adopted by the middle colic artery and those arterial

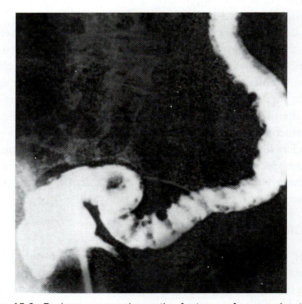

Fig. 15.3: Barium enema shows the features of copper beaten appearance. Its alternative name is often referred to as 'thumb-print' appearance in the sigmoid and descending colon. It is a classical radiological evidence of ischemic colitis. (By courtesy of Marston et al published in the journal Gut 1966)

arcades supplying blood to the left colon from splenic flexure right down to the rectum. These arterial arcades increase its vascular bed slowly and gradually with the passage of time.

This change in vascular bed is due to gradual occlusion of the osteum of the inferior mesenteric artery due to atherosclerosis formed in the wall of the abdominal aorta. Hence, acute ischemic change rarely occurs.

The commonest ischemic site of the colon is the splenic flexure and the lower in the sigmoid colon, after ligating the inferior mesenteric artery. It may present with frank gangrene of the colon, or slow ischemic change leading to mucosal ulceration and stricture of the colon. Patient presented with ischemic colitis should be followed up every 6 weeks and then every three months, either by barium enema or colonoscopy. The radiological review will reveal whether or not the size of the lumen has been changing, forming stricture. The latter could be the sequal of transient ischemia to the mucosa.

Apart from the routine investigations, sigmoidoscopy, colonoscopy and contrast CT scan may assist in establishing the diagnosis before contemplating for the definitive surgery. Barium enema may be arranged for persisting symptoms of pain and loose motion.

Surgical treatment for frank gangrene is the emergency resection of the colon, if the patient is in a state of shock. If stricture of the colon is causing persistent bowel problems, elective resection of the diseased segment should be carried out.

AMEBIC COLITIS

Dysentery is the common colonic disease in tropical countries. It could be bacillary or amebic dysentery. The *Entamoeba histolytica* are protozoa and harbor in the water. Furthermore, in developing countries, amebic colitis is a chronic disease, because of lack of sanitation and lack of proper sterilization of the drinking and cooking water. The mucosal ulcers develop diffusely in the entire colon but 75 percent of these ulcers remain confined in the sigmoid colon, like ulcerative colitis.

The symptoms are soft motion mixed with mucus or slime. Many patients may notice tiny streaks of blood in the stool. They need to go to the lavatory more than once, due to incomplete emptying of the bowel. Sometimes, the symptoms are suggestive of ulcerative or Crohn's colitis or tuberculous enteritis. They appear pale and emaciated due to chronic blood loss and indigestion. These patients are treated by general practitioners. Surgeons are involved in the differential diagnosis between the cancer of the colon or rectum and ulcerative colitis.

Apart from routine clinical examination, sigmoidoscopic examination will reveal the distinct difference between the ulcerative colitis and amebic colitis. In amebic colitis, multiple tiny ulcers and some punch-out or bottleneck ulcers are the classical macroscopical features, surrounded by normal mucosa, which are diagnostic features of amebic colitis. Unlike the ulcerative colitis, pseudopolyps are absent in amebic colitis. In some cases, chronic granulation tissue forming rectal stricture could be present and it may confuse with the rectal carcinoma. Despite this sigmoidoscopic finding, stool culture will confirm *Entamoeba histolytica*.

Consultation of textbook of medicine is encouraged for further information.

PROCTITIS

Proctitis is an inflammatory condition of the rectal mucosa, but in some cases, it can inflict the mucosa of the nearby colon or the anal canal. In fact, it is the local manifestation of other diseases such as ulcerative or Crohn's colitis. Nonspecific inflammation involves the lower part of the rectum and upper part of the anal canal. It is postulated that these sorts of inflammatory conditions may lead to a full blown ulcerative colitis at a later stage. Postradiation proctitis is a separate disease, resulting from the deep X-ray therapy.

Clinically, it could be divided into specific and nonspecific inflammation of the rectal mucosa.

Primary diseases affecting the rectal mucosa are:
a. Ulcerative colitis.
b. Crohn's proctitis.
c. Bacillary dysentery.
d. Amebic dysentery.
e. Tuberculous proctitis.
f. Gonorrheal proctitis.
g. Lymphogranuloma inguinale.
h. Postradiation proctitis.

Symptoms

In most cases, the symptoms are tenesmus, discharge of pus or blood stained soft feces. Patients are referred to the clinics because of frequent attempt of defecation or bleeding per rectum.

It has been found that similar symptoms, like proctocolitis have been reported after radiotherapy is given to the prostate gland, bladder, the cervix uteri or the rectum and anus. It is indistinguishable from other forms of proctitis. Postradiation proctitis presents the symptoms of frequent loose motion, rectal bleeding, tenesmus, and proctalgia and in some cases, constipation and pain in abdomen or mucus discharge. These postradiation symptoms may persist for many months and even years that depend upon the severity of the damage to the rectum. In some cases, stricture of the rectum may develop and sigmoidoscopy may not be possible.

Apart from the routine examination, rectal digital examination may reveal blood and pus on the finger stall. Proctoscopy and sigmoidoscopy may reveal contact bleeding, purulent fluids in the lower rectum, patchy acute inflammation on the mucosa of the rectum and the mucosa may appear to be granular, but ulceration of the rectal mucosa is very rare. These acute inflammatory features may be found higher up beyond the rectum. This finding would refer to the diagnosis of proctocolitis.

If there are multiple ulcers present in the rectal wall and healthy looking mucosa present between the ulcers, it is more likely to be amebic dysentery. In some cases, granulomatous lesion may be present as a soft tissue in the rectum that may appear to be rectal carcinoma.

For establishing the diagnosis, the tissue is scraped with a long-handle spoon and is sent straight to the laboratory for an urgent microscopical examination that will confirm whether or not it was amebic granuloma or carcinoma. For resolving the doubt, biopsy should be taken from this area for histological examination and at the same time, injection of emetine is given to the patient. This will discharge amebic cysts into the stool that should be examined under the microscope.

Apart from the stool examination, biopsy of the rectal mucosa should be taken from the different sites of the rectum for tissue diagnosis.

The initial diagnosis is made based upon the bowel symptoms, rectal examinations, blood test, stool examination and biopsy report. A detailed account of past history of lung TB, or gonorrhea would assist diagnosis and treatment to the patient.

Treatment

The treatment is conservative and symptomatic. This includes iron therapy or blood transfusion if the hemoglobin is very low. Specific treatment is considered if the pathology is related to ulcerative or Crohn's disease or amebic colitis. Both systemic drug therapy and prednisolone retention enema are prescribed in those cases in which the primary diagnosis is related to ulcerative or Crohn's disease.

If the disease is the complication from the radiotherapy, the treatment is empirical. If there are symptoms of constipation and cramp in abdomen, oral laxative at a regular basis could assist in relieving the symptoms.

If there are severe symptoms not responding to conservative treatment, and there is severe rectal stricture and/or rectovaginal fistula, pelvic loop colostomy should be performed, in order to alleviate the discomfort at defecation and constipation. Diversion of the feces would not improve the local inflammatory condition, if the primary disease is ulcerative or Crohn's proctitis. And it would not stop local hemorrhage.

Reversal colostomy may be reviewed after six months, but it may not be possible in certain cases. In extreme cases of bleeding from the rectum, where conservative treatment has not made any improvement or there is a long-standing rectal or anal stricture, further surgery may be necessary. In these cases, abdominoperineal excision of the rectum should be contemplated. In some cases, emergency rectal surgery may be necessary, if the rectal bleeding poses a life-threat to the patient.

REFERENCES

1. Waugh J McK, Peck DA, Beahrs OH, Sauer WG. Surgical management of chronic ulcerative colitis. Arch Surg 1964;88:556.
2. Watts J McK, de Dombal FT, Goligher JC. The early results of surgery for ulcerative colitis. Brit J Surg 1966a;53:1005.
3. Brooke BN. The outcome of surgery for ulcerative colitis. Lancet 1956a;2:532.
4. Counsell PB, Lockhart-Mummery HE. Ileostomy: Assessment of disability: Management. Lancet 1:113.
5. Lockhart-Mummery HE, Morson BC. Crohn's disease of the large intestine. Gut 1964;5:493.
6. Warren S, Sommers SC. Pathology of regional ileitis and ulcerative colitis. J Amer Med Assn 1954;154:189.
7. Saha SK. TB lesion in the ascending colon. Scarborough General Hospital, 2003. (personal experience).

16 Diverticula of the Colon

SURGICAL ANATOMY AND PHYSIOLOGY

Propagative movement of the semisolid feces in masses is initiated by the combination of intrinsic neural innervations and tone of the colonic muscles. Hence, volume of the feces is one of the important factors, for maintaining the tone of both circular and longitudinal fibers of the colon.

The study showed that a minimum volume is required for inducing the stimulation of the stretch receptors, present in the rectal wall and in the puborectalis muscles. It shows that around 50 ml of water in a balloon, placed in the rectum is required to induce the stretch receptors in order to produce urge defecation; but we know that overdistention of smooth muscle loses its muscle tone that may lead to atony of the gut.

On the operating table, we have found in the operation of habitual constipation that the sigmoid colon has been found loaded with a huge quantity of feces. This sort of condition is the effect of the drugs, prescribed to the psychiatric patients for the treatment of mental condition but these tablets cause relaxation of the smooth muscles of the gut. As a result, the patients do not feel the desire to defecate, despite the colon being loaded with solid feces. This dysfunctional event of the colon is the result of either lack of stimulation of the gut wall or atony of the muscle of the colon.

In dehydration among the healthy subjects, the colon tends to absorb fluid from the feces, thus reducing its volume and forming a pellet-like round dry balls of hard feces. As a result, lots of dry hard feces are necessary in building up the volume that keeps on maintaining the tone of the colonic muscles, but a reduced volume delays the response to the stretch receptors due to lack of the local tonicity of the circular muscles of the colon. Hence, in normal cases, bulky feces is the main factor for maintaining the normal tone that seems to be a primary factor for regular defecation.

An average time for the test meal to travel from the stomach to the cecum is 6 hours and from the cecum to the rectum is 6-12 hours. The transport of feces is much slower in the rectum by many factors, among which spacious capacity and Houston's valves may be the important factors for the delay in defecation, in some cases what is usually referred to as constipation in clinical practice.

As a result, accumulation of the small pellets-like round feces continues to be stuck up, one after another on the Houston's valves of the rectum. They are eventually overcrowded, causing stretching of the rectal wall and that of the puborectalis muscle. This induces urge defecation.

Unlike the small intestine, the longitudinal fibers forming a narrow strip, like a thin ribbon on the external wall of the colon do not cover the whole circumference of the colon. Instead, they are present along the three sites of the colonic surface. They are known as taeniae coli that support the circular muscles of the colon. They are shorter in length compared to the total length of the colon. This makes the girth of the colon much spacious, what is anatomically known as haustration. The taeniae coli begins from the base of the appendix and end at the rectosigmoid region; but the circular muscles, held together by the taeniae coli form sacculations or out-pouching in between the three sets of taeniae coli.

Unlike in the colonic wall, the longitudinal muscles invest all around the appendix and the rectum, thus supporting the circular muscles all around them. In sharp contrast, the circular muscles of the colon are stretched outwards, thus increasing its surface area and enhancing its absorptive power. Because of these reasons, they form sacculations along the colonic wall. Other anatomical variation is the position of the ascending and descending colon that remain in retroperitoneal space, but both transverse and sigmoid colon are held by the free mesentery and are not fixed to the posterior abdominal wall. As a result, these two segments tend to get elongated because of intraluminal pressure, generated by those hard feces held back in the rectum because of delay in defecation.

This may be the reason for the sigmoid colon being stretched along its longitudinal axis, thus forming several loops of the sigmoid colon in the pelvis. This explains how the lower abdomen would appear to be protuberant, like a pot-belly among the middle-aged people.

Because of intraluminal pressure, the colonic muscles continue working hard against those resistance exerted by those lumps of feces held in the rectum. As a result, both circular muscle and longitudinal fibers get hypertrophied up to a point.

PATHOGENESIS OF THE DIVERTICULOSIS

Constipation is the primary cause for the development of diverticula. This leads to increased intraluminal pressure of the colon. As a result, some of the pressure tends to get diverted through the weakest sites of the wall, which are the port of entry of the colonic vessels. Hence, the pressure pushes the colonic mucosa outwards through those ports of blood vessels—thus producing eventually mucosal pouches in the wall of the colon.

In fact, their commonest sites are along the attachment of the taeniae coli. Their main objective is to offset the increased intraluminal pressure. However, these pouches, known as diverticula lie by the side of those vessels (Fig. 16.1).

Through these routes, the mucosa starts prolapsing out, forming pulsion diverticulum (Fig. 16.1). In layman language, it is referred to as cul-de-sac, or pouch. In the clinic, patients are explained with this simple language. No such diverticulum passes through the taeniae coli and it is absent in the rectum. Furthermore, it has no muscular coat covering its wall (Fig. 16.2).

And these changes are more marked in the region of the sigmoid colon than in the ascending colon. This explains as to why the diverticula occur more frequently in the pelvic colon than in other parts of the colon.

If the constipation continues, the circular muscle of the colon loses its tonicity. This could be the reason for atony of the gut wall that may contribute to habitual constipation. Therefore, drinking of water is a major component for keeping the feces bulky that induces the increased tone of the gut, which in return enhances motility and regular defecation. Change in regular bowel habit should be treated with a great suspicion among the subjects above the age of 30 years.

Although the pathogenesis of diverticulosis seems simple, one needs to understand why is it absent in the appendix and in the rectum. The reason for this variation is related to the distribution and display of the longitudinal muscles all around the appendix and the rectum.

PATHOLOGY

Diverticulum is an acquired change in the wall of the colon but it could be congenital, in which cases, the commonest anatomical sites are in the second part of the duodenum and jejunum. The acquired varieties occur more in men than in women. The ratio is 2:1. The average incidence among the population above the age of 40 years varies from literature to literature; but it ranges between 5 percent and 10 percent. The commonest sites are the sigmoid and descending colon but it may develop in any other part of the colon (Fig. 16.3).

It is acquired over the years due to constipation and poor diet habit. The colonic mucosa that pushes out between the circular fibers eventually forms a blind pouch. Its opening could be of various shapes that could be either round or slit-like openings. They are found along the sides of the taeniae coli and by the side of the mesentery. Feces get stuck inside the diverticula where it gets inspissated and dried out. It remains stuck inside the mucosal pouch causing inflammation. Infection supervenes in the diverticula due to poor vascularity. This leads to pain and change in bowel habit. If this inflammation is not treated, it may lead to cellulites and peridiverticular abscess or it may perforate, causing local peritonitis or general fecal peritonitis that depends upon the state of the colon.

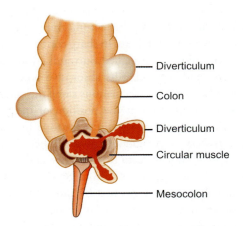

Fig. 16.1: The herniation of the colonic mucosa through the gap between the hypertrophic circular muscles of the colon

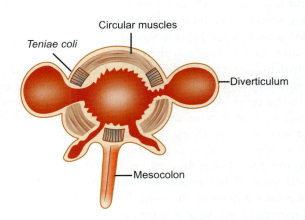

Fig. 16.2: The cross section of the colon displaying the prolapse of the colonic mucosa. It has no muscular coat but it is covered by the peritoneum

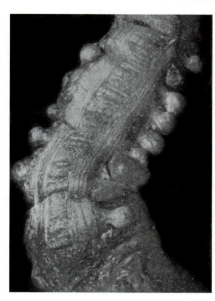

Fig. 16.3: (By courtesy of Lloyd-Davies, OV reproduced from Proc Roy Soc Med 1953). This is a photograph showing multiple diverticula along the side of *Teniae coli* of the colon

▪ Symptoms

- It may remain silent for many years.
- It may present as habitual constipation, associated with or without change in bowel habits, which would be similar to colonic carcinoma.
- It may present as acute pain in the left side of the lower abdomen. This could be due to acute diverticulitis.
- It may present as a chronic pain that could be recurrent now and then in the left iliac fossa or in the suprapubic region, associated with a change in bowel habit.
- It may present as urinary tract infection and passing of air bubbles and in extreme cases, feces may be discharged with the urine. These are referred to as colovesical fistula.
- It may present as fresh bleeding per rectum without any other symptoms.
- It may present as an inflamed swelling, localized in the left iliac fossa, associated with pyrexia and other bowel symptoms.
- It may present as large bowel obstruction or as fecal peritonitis due to perforation of the diverticulitis.

DESCRIPTION OF THE CLINICAL PRESENTATION

For years, patient remains symptoms-free, despite having diverticulosis in the colon. In fact, this pathological change in colon remains undiagnosed for many years, until they are having anyone of those symptoms, referred to above.

Although constipation is the striking habit of the patient, passage of pellets- like round solid feces are frequently present among many subjects over the age of 30. But, they do not consider being of any significant bowel problems. They adjust their way of life and begin to learn to live with this habit of constipation, until such time, when they start feeling uncomfortable in the belly because of incomplete emptying of the bowel. They may experience with aching in the left iliac fossa and/or suprapubic region. Eventually, the pathology of the diverticula continues worsening over the years.

In most cases, many patients are seen in the outpatient clinic for the change in bowel habit, discomfort or bleeding per rectum. They are examined and investigated, as outlined in the investigation of case with cancer in the bowel.

In the outpatient clinic, abdominal examination may reveal thickened colon in the left iliac fossa or along the left flank. Rectal digital examination would be unhelpful in this case, but proctoscopic examination may transpire piles, which may not be of any significance to the diagnosis of diverticulitis.

Sigmoidoscopy may be unhelpful, if it cannot be passed beyond the 12 cm in length from the anal verge. The source of rectal bleeding may not be obvious at this stage.

The next line of investigation is the double contrast barium enema, but it should not be requested, if there is evidence of diverticulitis or tender palpable lump in the left iliac fossa.

Once the inflammation has resolved clinically, barium enema should be requested 2-3 months later, if the symptoms are not suggestive of colonic carcinoma. In some cases, both pathological conditions could exist in the sigmoid colon. In the absence of barium enema, CT scan should be arranged in order to exclude colonic carcinoma.

Despite the radiological evidence of diverticulosis, colonoscopy should be carried out in order to exclude colonic lesion.

If the diverticulosis is inflamed, the following types of symptoms may be presented:

a. Pain in the suprapubic region, left iliac fossa and right iliac fossa. The discomfort in the right iliac fossa may be possible, if the loop of the sigmoid colon lies across the pelvis towards the right iliac fossa. Sometimes, it could be mimicking of acute appendicitis in this abnormal position of the sigmoid colon. This pain varies with its intensity and frequency that depends upon many factors such as inflammation, progressive constipation, and structural anatomical change of the gut.
b. Patient may also notice a change in bowel habits, which could be of various forms, such as softer motion, episodes of diarrhea followed by a period of constipation, pipe-stem type feces, or round hard feces like marble or pellets.
c. From time-to-time, fresh bleeding may occur during defecation. This is more often related to coexisting piles, but this could be attributable to venous congestion in the pelvis and the rectum.
d. Patient may complain of distended abdomen associated with vomiting and spasmodic type of pain if the inflammation of the diverticulum is getting worse.

i. In extreme circumstances, patient may be admitted with a fresh bleeding per rectum without any evidence of peritonitis.
ii. Patient may be admitted with septicemia.

PROBLEMS WITH THE DIVERTICULOSIS

Although the development of diverticulosis is the result of poor diet and inadequate drinking habit, this benign condition may lead to chronic clinical conditions. These are due to impaction of hard feces inside the diverticulum. As a result, either one or many of them may develop inflammation and pain. In most cases, a good length of the sigmoid colon is usually inflicted with this condition. The initial problem is the inflammation that may affect either a single or many of the diverticulosis.

If the inflammation remains untreated, it may lead to tissue edema, collection of infective or inflammatory fluid around the particular segment of the colon. Eventually, it may lead into abscess formation, forming a peridiverticular mass in the left iliac fossa or it may burst into the abdomen causing either localized or generalized peritonitis.

In some cases, patients may experience with recurrent episodes of inflammation and a spontaneous resolution of the symptoms along the sigmoid or descending colon. In response to every resolution of acute inflammation, chronic fibrosis may supervene around the diverticula and colonic wall, without implicating the colonic mucosa. These changes may lead to atrophy or peridiverticular fibrosis implicating the circular muscles. A segment of the colon may turn into narrowed, rigid lumen or there could be stricture (Fig.16.4).

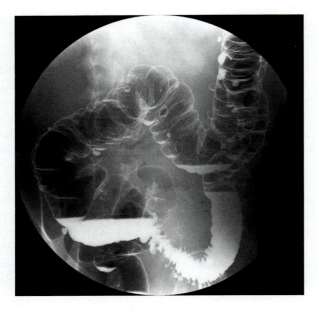

Fig. 16.4: A double-contrast barium enema shows multiple diverticula in the proximal colon and multiple varieties of various sizes along with classical 'rose thorn' pattern in the sigmoid colon

Patient may experience with flatulence, constipation, incomplete emptying of the bowel. All these symptoms may result from the stricture of the colon, but this stricture that involves a large segment of the colon is in contrast to the colonic tumor, which implicates only a very small segment of the colon.

In rare cases, fresh bleeding per rectum presents a diagnostic dilemma. It seems to be associated more frequently with diverticulosis than with the diverticulitis.[1] The incidence of rectal bleeding associated with the diverticular pathology varies from clinicians-to-clinicians. Its incidences are 29, 27 and 14 percent respectively.[2-4]

It has been found that the etiology of acute bleeding from the diverticula is the ulceration developed in the wall of the diverticulum or around its osteum, often referred to as neck of the diverticulum, where the blood vessels attached to the diverticulum tend to get eroded by pressure necrosis, because of inspissated feces being impacted in the diverticula.[5,6]

The colonic bleeding may present a diagnostic dilemma. The possible sources are from the diverticulosis, diverticulitis, ulcerative colitis, and carcinoma of the colon, polyps and angiodysplasia. Among these varieties, the incidence of acute mild or moderate colonic bleeding has been found to be very high in the cancer of the left colon, compared to diverticulitis or ulcerative colitis, but the incidence of massive rectal bleeding is reported to be higher among the cases of diverticulosis compared with the colonic carcinoma and ulcerative colitis[1] and a massive colonic bleeding could also be attributable to angiodysplasia.[7] The latter may coexist among the patients with symptoms-free diverticulosis.

In the literature, a distinct difference in etiology of the colonic bleeding was highlighted between 221 cases of moderate and 25 cases of massive colonic bleeding admitted over 5 years (1955-60) with various colonic lesions.[1]

	Moderate bleeding in 221 patients	*Massive bleeding in 25 patients*
Carcinoma of the left colon	33%	13%
Diverticulosis	20%	71%
Diverticulitis	8%	nil
Ulcerative colitis	18%	nil
Polyps	10%	4%
Carcinoma of the right colon	10%	4%
Sarcoma of the rectum	nil	4%
Miscellaneous	6%	4%

Other complication is the formation of fistula. It could be of internal or external type of fistula. In the former, it may develop between the colon and bladder. This radiological evidence has been shown in contrast barium enema which shows a gross sigmoid diverticula and a fistula between the sigmoid diverticulum and the bladder (Fig. 16.5).

This is another radiological evidence of colovaginal fistula. In this plate, barium has entered into the vagina from the sigmoid diverticula (Fig. 16.6). Fistula may also develop between the colon and small intestine. It may perforate in the peritoneal cavity (Fig. 16.7). In some cases, it could develop between the colon and parietal wall or umbilicus, known as colocutaneous fistula.

In cases with colovesical fistula, urinary symptoms are the initial presentation. It may be associated with pneumaturia. But sometimes, this vital information could be missing, unless the patient is asked with a leading question. In some extreme cases, cloudy urine could be seen if it is collected in a clean bottle. Apart from these findings, patient may experience with a dull aching in the loins or in the lumbosacral region.

Apart from urine culture, cystoscopy will show an area of patchy inflammation in the posterior wall or in the dome of the bladder. There could be evidence of fronds-like papillomatous lesion seen wavering in the bladder, in chronic cases. Biopsy from this site should be taken to exclude bladder tumor. The true fistula track may not be possible to be radiologically demonstrated either with barium enema, or with cystogram, but these two investigations should be done, if diagnosis is in doubt.

In other diseases, fistula may be found in Crohn's disease, commonly with Crohn's ileitis, carcinoma of the colon, postradiation colitis or ileitis, or bladder tumor.

Author was involved in the management of two cases of colovesical fistula; one of them was an elderly man, presented with fecal peritonitis and sloughing of the posterior wall of the bladder and other one was an elderly woman, presented with the discharge of feces and urine through the umbilicus.

In summary, the diverticular disease may present with any one of the following complications:
a. Chronic colonic obstruction due to stricture.
b. Localized diverticulitis with pericolic abscess.
c. Fecal peritonitis associated with septic shock.
d. Massive colonic bleeding without symptoms of acute diverticulitis.
e. Formation of either internal or external fistula.
f. Among the external fistulae is the colovesical fistula, colocutaneous fistula and colovaginal fistula.

MANAGEMENT OF DIVERTICULOSIS

a. Conservative approach.
b. Operative approach.

Operative Treatment

i. Elective procedure.
ii. Emergency procedure.

Conservative Approach

If the barium enema does not show any evidence of stricture, or gross narrowing of the lumen of the sigmoid colon, the line of approach would be conservative. Patient is advised to stay on high fiber diet and is encouraged to drink plain water and to cut down the consumption of the tea, coffee or coco.

Patients are reviewed every three months. If the barium enema shows gross multiple grapes-like diverticula in the sigmoid or descending colon and the colon appears to have shown a long narrow segment of lumen or stricture, resection

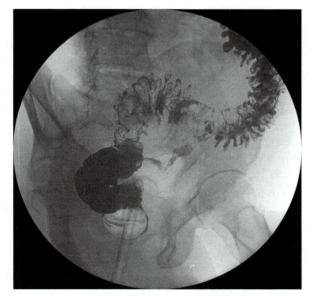

Fig. 16.5: It is a colovesical fistula. Double-contrast barium enema showing gross sigmoid diverticulosis and a fistula track of barium entering into the bladder

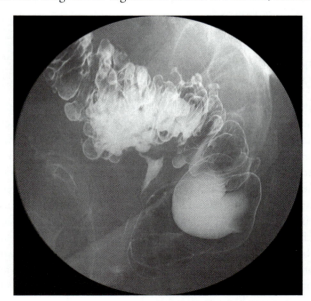

Fig. 16.6: Colovaginal fistula. Contrast barium enema showing gross sigmoid diverticula and a fistula track of barium into the vagina

Clinical Practice and Surgery of the Colon, Rectum and Anus

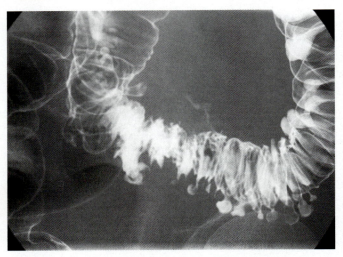

Fig. 16.7: Perforation of the sigmoid diverticulum. Double contrast barium enema of the sigmoid colon shows streaks of barium emerging from the diverticulum

of this segment may be considered that depends upon the age, general health and degree of abdominal pain and constipation.

If patient is having a recurrent painless bleeding at defecation and its cause is from the piles, then it could be treated with injection of 5 percent phenol in almond oil.

ELECTIVE OPERATIVE TREATMENT

Definitive operative procedure depends upon the pathological state of the colon. These are:
A. Colonic stricture– a. Sigmoid myotomy
b. Resection of the stricture
B. Colonic fistula—Multiple reconstructive procedures that depend upon the pathological state of the adjacent organs involved.

PREOPERATIVE ASSESSMENT OF THE PATIENT

Patients presented with a fistula remain grossly dehydrated, and results of blood tests may reveal electrolytes deficit, anaemia, hypoproteinemia, high urea and elevated serum creatinine. All these abnormalities need to be corrected with necessary measures, such as intravenous infusion, antibiotics, and blood transfusion. In addition, TPN (total parenteral nutrition) infusion should be commenced through the central vein for at least a week. And in some semi urgent cases, infusion of human albumin should be given in order to bring the serum albumin level above 30 gm/l. There are debates and controversies in the benefit of this treatment, but author has not encountered any adverse result, on the contrary, recovery becomes much more effective.

Patients with colonic fistula, need elective operative intervention. This procedure should be done, once the condition of general health and all other vital functions seem to have made a reasonable progress.

It is important to be sure that the hemoglobin level should be above 12gm/dl, and serum albumin level above 30gm/l, blood urea within normal range. Patient should be on high protein and low residue diet for a week, and rectal enema should be given everyday for 2-3 days prior to surgery being undertaken.

Sigmoidoscopy should be done. Its main purpose is to be sure that there are no residual hard inspissated feces, or barium enema in the sigmoid colon and the rectum. This mechanical clearance is important, if primary anastomosis is considered to be necessary.

Otherwise, anastomosis may breakdown, if there are hard feces or inspissated barium present in the distal colon or rectum. They may interfere with the propagative peristalsis.

When patient seems to be well-hydrated and has a good urine output per hour, he will be prepared for the laparotomy, but total bowel clearance is necessary. To achieve this objective, oral purgative with a double dose of picolax is given a night before the operation. Intravenous infusion with saline or 5 percent dextrose should be continued.

■ Operative Policy

The surgical correction of the colonic disease could be done in one stage, two stages and three stages; it all depends upon the general health of the patients, diseased state of the gut and confidence of the surgeon.

The three stage procedure comprises of preliminary diversion of the feces by constructing a transverse loop colostomy. A few weeks later, the diseased segment of the colon and/or internal fistula tract is resected. In the final stage, a loop colostomy is closed, a few weeks later, if the postoperative barium enema, done three weeks later shows no evidence of leakage of contrast.

The two stage procedure is the resection of the primary diseased colon along with a restoration of the continuity of the gut and repair of internal fistula. This is followed by the diversion of the feces through a transverse loop colostomy, constructed on the right side of the midline wound. The second stage is the reversal of the said colostomy, if the postoperative barium enema done three weeks later does not show any leakage of contrast through the anastomosis.

One stage procedure is to resect the diseased colon with end-to-end anastomosis and to repair the internal fistula without diversion of feces.

■ Operative Procedure

In the theater, Foley's catheter No.18FG is inserted per urethra prior to transferring to the main theater. Patient is placed on the lithotomy position for rectal digital examination and sigmoidoscopy. This procedure would reveal whether the rectum and the sigmoid colon have been adequately cleared of feces and residual barium. In some cases, tightness may be found in the anal orifice due to disuse atrophy or inactivity. This may provide some degree of resistance because of disuse functional state of the striated muscles of the anal sphincter, thus inhibiting the smooth passage of postoperative flatus. In these circumstances, there remains a risk of anastomotic dehiscence.

To eliminate this potential risk, anal orifice should be dilated up to three fingers and sigmoidoscopy would also assist in overcoming the spastic state of the rectum and sigmoid colon. It is like a preoperative physiotherapy. The author had never encountered with the postoperative leakage in all his patients, since this new maneuver being introduced to his patients.

At the completion of this procedure, patient is put back on the operating table in supine position. Both feet must be rested on a soft cushion. Skin preparation and sterile draping are laid down all around the operating area, as described before. The abdomen is opened through a midline incision that goes through the linea alba. Paramedian incision could be used; if the surgeon is trained for it, but it is rarely used nowadays. The only snug with the midline incision is the risk of developing incisional hernia.

The wound margins are held retracted by the self-retaining retractors and its margins are protected from fecal contamination. Hence, large wet swabs are put around the wound margins. All internal organs are examined and palpated. The diseased colon is examined in order to assess the total extent of the colon to be resected.

■ Sigmoid Myotomy

Sigmoid myotomy was originally borrowed from the concept of Ramstedt's pylomyotomy. The operation has been originally designed for the congenital pyloric stenosis found in the newborn baby, where the pylorus, which acts as a sphincter and an outlet of the stomach, has a thick circular muscle all around it. Its physiological function seems to be quite different from the colonic wall, made up with a thin circular muscle.

In sharp contrast, diverticulosis of the sigmoid colon is a long-standing acquired pathological development, involving the whole sigmoid colon. And the diverticulum develops scattered in between the circular fibers of the colon and it remains at irreversible condition and its surrounding colonic muscles turn into a permanent pathological change. The thickness of the taeniae coli is around 1 cm that supports the circular muscle of the colon on three different sites around the circumference of the colon.

Nevertheless, the original concept was to split up the muscle fibers of taeniae coli, present along the antimesenteric border of the colon and then to divide the circular muscle – thus permitting the colonic mucosa herniated through, in the early stages of development of diverticulosis, but by the time this operation is indicated, the disease has already advanced. In those circumstances, permanent pathological changes have developed around the muscular wall of the colon associated with a chronic inflammation and infection. The consequent effect of all these changes would be a subclinical fibrosis around the diverticula and under the taeniae coli.

In these clinical conditions, a true benefit remains in doubt, because of the fact that apart from splitting up of the longitudinal fibers of the taeniae coli along its long axis, the circular muscle needs to be separated from the undersurface of the taeniae coli, before they are divided in order to allow the colonic mucosa prolapsed through.

In this uncertainty, the first question would be whether it is safe to carry out this procedure. In technical term, the herniation of the colonic mucosa through the surgeon's made window would appear to be a man-made diverticulum. The consequent effect would be no different from true diverticula.

The final question is whether this procedure could offset the colonic pressure, and whether it could reverse the pathogenesis of the diverticulum. Relieving of intraluminal pressure of the colon could not be made possible if it appears to be technically difficult in separating the circular muscles widely from the under-surface of the taeniae coli, because of fibrosis developed between the two muscle layers.

Apart from the risk of potential complications, one needs to understand the physiological function of the colonic mucosa, prolapsed through the transected fibers of the circular muscles. There remains a doubt in the peristaltic function of the affected segment of the colon; because of the fact that colonic mucosa cannot play fully in the peristalsis without the muscular support. Furthermore, those feces stuck in the said herniated mucosal fold will stay inspissated like other feces in other diverticula.

Hence, there remains in doubt whether the transected fibers of the circular muscles could maintain a normal peristalsis, like other intact circular muscles. On the contrary, being smooth muscles, those transected circular fibers would remain retracted from each other. As a result, the lumen of the colon will remain contracted and defunct. In view of this physiological state of affairs, the Riley Myotomy seems to be in conflict with the surgical sciences.

In fact, it was found to be less effective and less safe procedure. However, further morbidity was experienced in some cases due to leakage of feces. Hence, it is no longer used. And it should never be referred to the surgical procedures.

In general, the instances of elective colonic resection for benign disease have dropped dramatically. This improvement is due to high fiber diet and drinking of plenty of plain water.

RESECTION OF THE STRICTURE

It is a difficult judgment between a major operative procedure and the pathological state of the colon. The balance has to be worked out between the benefit after resection and the potential risk of fecal peritonitis of the sigmoid colon without operation being undertaken. However, the procedure is no different from the left colectomy or anterior resection.

After a full laparotomy has been carried out, the sigmoid colon or the descending colon is mobilized from the left parietal wall as described before. In this case, the important precaution is to identify the left ureter, when the diseased descending and sigmoid colon has been mobilized from the left parietal wall. Minimum dissection of the colon is necessary and ligation of the left colic vessels are done close to the colon. But, end-to-end anastomosis should be done between the healthy lumen of the proximal and the distal transected end of the colon without any tension.

SURGICAL TREATMENT FOR INTERNAL FISTULA

Internal fistula may occur between the colon and any other structure. This could be between the stomach and transverse colon, between the sigmoid colon and small intestine or the cecum, between the sigmoid colon and the bladder, or between the rectum and the vagina.

The etiology for the fistula may be attributable to many conditions. The commonest condition is the tumor, invading to the adjacent organ that could be between the stomach and transverse colon. In this case, the tumor of the stomach may more often invade the transverse colon.

And there could be a fistula between the cecum and the sigmoid colon. This may be due to the tumor developed either in the cecum or in the sigmoid colon that may lie across the pelvis and may rest on the cecum. Crohn's disease or postradiation ileitis may cause fistula between the different organs, as highlighted in the previous section. In all these cases of unusual pathology, operative treatment has to be planned differently.

If the operative procedure is intended for the resection of diseased colon and fistula tract, then a detailed review is carried out in order to find out any evidence of adhesions, mobility of the diseased colon, any hidden abscess, or any other fistula with small intestine or bladder or rectum.

All other healthy intestine are put in the upper abdomen and covered with warm wet packs. Only the segment the bowel with a fistula tract is isolated by putting warm wet packs all around of the operative area. Before proceeding further, vascular tree supplying to the diseased colon and other structures are identified.

Mobilization of the colon is commenced from the adjacent viscus. After a good length of the bowel has been mobilized, its blood vessels are divided and ligated.

In the same way, other diseased bowel is mobilized. Soft clamps are applied across the proposed line of resection. And they are applied away from and on either side of fistula. The diseased segment is next transected between the two clamps, applied on the respective side, away from the fistula. Good bleeding points from the mucosa are noted.

The transected segment with the clamps applied on both ends, is next resected out either from the bladder wall or from the small intestine, as the case may be. Continuity of the gut is re-established by end-to-end anastomosis, either in two layers or by interrupted single layer sutures, using Vicryl or dexon sutures 2/0, as described before. The defect in the other organ is closed in the usual way.

COLOVESICAL FISTULA

Diverticulitis is the causative pathology for developing colovesical fistula. Crohn's ileitis and Crohn's colitis are also other etiological factors for ileovesical or colovesical fistula. Sigmoid colon is usually involved in this fistula. In the past, diversion of feces alone through the transverse loop colostomy did not heal the fistula tract spontaneously. If the fistula is with the bladder, then the bladder wall is excised along with the resected segment of the colon. The line of resection from the bladder wall should be consistent with the layout of its bladder muscle.

Between a few stay sutures inserted around the fistula, the bladder is opened by making incision around the colovesical fistula. Before proceeding further, both ureteric orifices are identified. Foley's catheter is also identified. Minimum resection of the bladder wall is required, but edematous tissue should be included in the excision of the fistula track. The excision of the bladder fistula track is carried out along with the segment of the colon or small intestine. Bladder is washed out with antiseptic solution. The bladder wall is repaired with interrupted sutures or in two layers without tension. The line of repair should be left in extraperitoneal space; if possible, alternatively, it should be covered with a piece of omental graft.

The segment of the colon, that carries a lot of diverticula or appeared to be narrow, contracted and edematous, needs to be resected. Continuity of the gut could be restored by a primary end-to-end anastomosis. In addition, defunctioning loop colostomy may be necessary in some cases. Alternatively, the two stomas of the resected segment of the colon could be brought out for double barrel colostomies, which could be constructed in the left iliac fossa. A few months later, continuity of the colon could be restored between the two stomas.

ILEOCOLIC FISTULA

If the fistula is with the small intestine, again the same principle is followed for resection and end-to-end anastomosis. Again, it could be done either by interrupted single layer or two layers of anastomosis. Care is taken that both transected ends do not contain edematous tissue, and has a good vascularity, and good mucosal perfusion.

If there is any doubt in the primary anastomosis of the gut, a transverse loop colostomy could be constructed on the right side of the midline, as described before. It is important to check that all instruments and swabs packs have been removed, before the wound is closed.

The abdomen is next washed out with warm saline several times. It is followed by metronidazole 1gm (IV preparation) lavage, (not mixed with saline and not aspirated back from the peritoneal cavity). Two drainage tubings are left, one on each side of the abdomen. Omental graft should be put around the repair sites.

Both drainage tubings are anchored to the skin by stitches, and they are clamped on for two hours. This will permit the metronidazole to kill all bacteria. At last, 20 ml solution of the metronidazole are added into the parietal wound, before the latter is closed in layers, as described before.

MANAGEMENT FOR EMERGENCY ADMISSION

Line of Conservative Treatment

If the patient is admitted with acute pain and vomiting, the management of the abdomen depends upon the clinical diagnosis associated with supportive investigations.

If plain X-ray of the abdomen and X-ray of the chest in erect position do not suggest gas under the diaphragm and the clinical features are suggestive of localized diverticulitis, the line of treatment would be conservative. This includes nil by mouth, intravenous infusion of fluids, antibiotics and intake and output fluid chart for 5-7 days. The area of tender palpable mass should be marked out with a skin pencil. If patient admits that he has passed flatus per rectum, it suggests a good response to the conservative treatment.

Despite this clinical evidence, conservative treatment should be continued until the tenderness has resolved completely and there is no palpable mass present in the left iliac fossa or in the suprapubic region.

Localized Peritonitis and Pericolic Abscess

If the patient has not responded to conservative treatment, and the area of local inflammation is getting worse, in that case, the abdomen is re-examined in order to find out about distention, spreading cellulites and evidence of generalized peritonitis.

Question may arise whether the tender palpable mass has extended beyond the previous skin pencil margin. And whether the overlying skin of the lump appears to be grossly indurated associated with cellulites, and there is a wide area of inflammation and marked redness, indicating fluctuation on gentle palpation, and pointing to an imminent burst, but all these clinical findings are limited to a particular area, which could be in the left iliac fossa, or around the suprapubic region. It is presumed that a paracolic abscess has developed; but it has been sealed off by the greater omentum from the rest of the abdomen.

Apart from these clinical findings, temperature and pulse rate are reviewed. Whether the temperature has been fluctuating up and down with a tendency to elevating and it is associated with a rapid pulse rate. In this situation, patient will appear to be toxic that should be assessed by the evidence of dry and coated tongue, and dehydrated body surface and lips as well as ketone smell in the breath. In addition, patient may feel nauseated or is having vomiting.

The following investigations should be done: Full blood count, Hemoglobin, C reactive protein, serum electrolytes, urea and creatinine.

X-ray of the chest and a plain X-ray of the abdomen.
USS over the inflamed area and CT scan.

Purpose of a plain X-ray of the abdomen is to see the gas pattern of the small and large intestines, whether they are grossly dilated, whether there is any gas in the rectum, or along the left paracolic gutter. These evidences would suggest that sigmoid colon has perforated, thus discharging colonic gas in the retroperitoneal space or along the left paracolic gutter. In some cases, surgical emphysema may be evident on palpation over the left lumbar region.

If the bursting abscess is not surgically drained, it may burst through the fluctuating inflamed skin, forming a colocutaneous fistula. Feces will be discharging through this abscess wound. Alternatively, the abscess may burst into the bladder or in the pelvis, forming either colovesical fistula or generalized purulent and fecal peritonitis.

To stop further deterioration, the abscess should be drained under general anesthesia in the theater. Deroofing of the abscess is carried out by making cruciate incisions over the fluctuating lump. After surgical toileting, colostomy bag is put around the skin stoma. Rest of the postoperative care should be followed in the usual way.

If the clinical examination suggests that the patient is in a state of shock due to generalized peritonitis, then resuscitation should be carried out before proceeding with emergency laparotomy.

During this management, evidence of colovesical fistula should be looked for. If urine report showed no evidence of gross infection, then colovesical fistula is very unlikely and further investigation should be done. This includes cystogram, barium enema, and cystoscopy.

If patient is presented with massive rectal bleeding then initially, blood transfusion should be commenced as soon as possible after a full investigation has been completed. In most cases, bleeding stops spontaneously with the infusion of 4-5 units of packed cell blood. In the meantime, further investigation should be done. These are sigmoidoscopy, colonoscopy, and selective angiogram and/or red cell isotope scan, if such facility is available.

If the clinical diagnosis is suggestive of localized diverticulitis, then conservative line of treatment along with blood transfusion and parenteral antibiotics should be adopted. Sigmoidoscopy and colonoscopy should be avoided. Emergency barium enema is also contraindicated. This may cause perforation of the diverticulitis. But CT scan with contrast could be arranged in order to exclude perforation and a local pericolic abscess.

COLONIC HEMORRHAGE

If the patient is still having massive bleeding, despite 4-5 units of blood transfusion being carried out over 12 hours and abdomen remains soft with no evidence of peritonitis, further investigation should be arranged to exclude angiodysplasia.

All the evidences suggest that the incidence of bleeding from the diverticular disease is far less in diverticulitis than with diverticulosis. In most instances, it stops spontaneously with conservative treatment and with intermittent blood transfusion. Anxiety may arise, if the bleeding appears to be massive and is not stopping despite necessary conservative measures being undertaken. In this case, selective angiogram, and red cell tagging with radioisotope should be done in order to establish the causes and site of active bleeding.

If the patient needs operation, then the question may arise how to identify the exact site of the hemorrhage at the laparotomy. There are various options available. These are:
a. On table colonoscopy or sigmoidoscopy to be carried out through the mid transverse colon. This may reveal the site of hemorrhage. If the cecum and ascending colon do not contain any blood, then the likely source of bleeding would be in the left colon and more precisely it could be in the sigmoid colon.
b. If definite source and location is not possible to be identified, the choice of operation is total colectomy and ileostomy or ileorectal anastomosis.

MANAGEMENT FOR THE PERFORATED DIVERTICULITIS

Fecal peritonitis is a serious surgical condition. It carries a high morbidity and mortality, if this is not treated surgically. This requires expertise in undertaking the judicious preoperative resuscitation before emergency laparotomy is contemplated. There are varieties of pathological conditions, which cause fecal peritonitis and septic shock. These conditions are as follows:
a. Perforation of the sigmoid colon diverticulitis.
b. Perforation of the cecum due to distal colonic obstruction either resulting from the sigmoid volvulus, or the tumor in the colon.
c. Perforation of the ulcerative colitis.
d. Stab injury to the intestines.

To combat the hypovolemic and hypotensive shock, these patients need first resuscitation that entails the stabilization of the blood pressure, control of systemic infection, restoration of the renal function, correction of dehydration and the electrolytes imbalance.

At the same time, necessary investigations are carried out to establish the general state of health and to establish the etiology of generalized peritonitis and the septic shock.

It is very important to bear in mind that the rate of dehydration would be equal to the rate of rehydration. Any attempt to rectify the dehydration with fluid challenge sooner than the permissible time, may lead to overload to the cardiorespiratory reserves and gross pulmonary edema. The incidence of postoperative mortality would be between 36 and 60 percent, if the emergency laparotomy is undertaken without proper resuscitation.[10-12]

Once the patient has recovered from the shock, arrangement is made for the laparotomy. The principle for preoperative care and consultations need not be repeated in this section. Patient must be explained that there remains a strong possibility for the diversion of feces and must be prepared for wearing a colostomy bag, if it is necessary.

CARE OF SEPTIC ABDOMEN AND PERFORATED DIVERTICULITIS

Technique for Transverse Loop Colostomy

Patient is placed in supine position on the operating table. The skin preparation and layout of the drapes have been described in other abdominal operations.

Initially, minilaparotomy is carried out through a midline incision made in the lower abdomen. If the source of the fecal peritonitis is in the sigmoid colon or in the cecum, the wound is extended up for a better exposure. The final operative procedure depends upon the finding of the lesion.

After establishing the source of fecal or purulent peritonitis, concentration is focused on the surgical toileting of the abdomen. In some cases, solid feces could be found in the pelvis and in other cases; subphrenic abscess and paracolic abscess could be found. These offending materials need to be evacuated and the peritoneal cavity needs to be thoroughly washed out and cleaned. The greater omentum and the small intestine are pushed aside or put inside a plastic bag. Then all feces are manually removed by scooping out with the right hand.

Once this has been removed, the peritoneal cavity is next mopped out with wet pack. At this stage, saline washout should not be used, because of the fact that this infected fluid would be absorbed rapidly.

In contrast, manual removal of feces reduces the risk of the fluid being absorbed into the circulatory system. Before saline washouts are given, the perforations of the sigmoid diverticula are closed.

The holes, through which the mucosa has protruded out more often, seem to be looking like a small umbilicus. These holes are closed with interrupted sutures. These are temporary measures that would stop discharging the feces into the abdomen. While the sutures are inserted, it is important to check that the colonic mucosa that has spouted through the holes has been pushed back into the hole.

The diseased segment of the colon would appear to be heavily inflamed, indurated and swollen that would appear to be fusiform in shape. In some cases, it could be found stuck to the parietal wall due to edematous mesocolon. Sometimes, it would be difficult to differentiate the inflammatory mass from the colonic carcinoma.

After this repair has been carried out, the saline washouts at room temperature are given in a systematic way, in that a small amount is poured at a time and it should be quickly aspirated back. Every corner of the abdomen has to be cleaned, until the peritoneum looks clean and healthy.

Surgical toileting entails cleaning of the small intestine with the wet pack and later with the saline wash outs. In this way, the upper abdomen, subdiaphragmatic space, all paracolic gutters and around the liver and spleen are washed out with saline. Pouring of large volume of warm saline into the peritoneal cavity should be avoided, because of the fact that a major portion of the fluid could be absorbed, before all of it is aspirated back from the abdomen.

After the surgical toileting being carried out, the next job is to deal with the diseased bowel.

For the perforated sigmoid colon, any one of the operative procedures, as outlined below could be performed. These are the operative procedures available for the perforated colon:

1. Construction of a transverse loop colostomy is carried out, after the repair of perforations being done, but the closure of the perforations may breakdown a few days later. Proximal third of the transverse colon is separated from the greater omentum.

For the construction of the transverse loop colostomy, a transverse skin crease incision is made 2 inches below the right subcostal margin and an inch lateral to the midline or away from the laparotomy incision. The rectus sheath incised transversely and the right rectus abdominis muscles are made split up between the parallel fibers. The opening should be adequate that can permit at least three fingers through the wound.

The parietal peritoneum under the muscles is opened but care is taken that other structures such as gallbladder or gut are not injured. A window is created through the mesocolon and it should be right side of the middle colic artery. A rubber tube or a long swab is passed through this window. The ends of the rubber tube or the swab are brought out through the colostomy wound.

The loop of the transverse colon is pushed slowly through the colostomy wound from inside and at the same time, it should be brought out by pulling the ends of the rubber tube or by the ends of the swab. Both pushing from inside the peritoneal cavity and pulling of the rubber catheter from outside the peritoneal cavity should be carried out concurrently.

Care is taken about the size of the colostomy wound to be constructed. It should not be too small that might cause strangulation of the colon. It would be difficult to get the loop of the colon negotiated through the small colostomy wound and colostomy may not start working, if the size of the wound is too small to pass flatus. A detailed description of the operative technique has been described in the previous chapter.

2. The second alternative procedure is a major operation. It requires technical experience and confidence in undertaking this major procedure in the middle of the night. It would be a combined procedure, in which the diseased colon is mobilized from the left parietal wall, with a view to carrying out the resection with end-to-end anastomosis. It would be similar to left sigmoid colectomy. After resection of the diseased segment of the colon, end-to-end anastomosis is carried out. This could be done either by the interrupted single layer sutures or by an old conventional method in two layers anastomosis. At the conclusion of this procedure, a transverse loop colostomy should be performed as described before.

3. The next alternative procedure is the Hartmann's operation. In this approach, the diseased segment of sigmoid colon is mobilized from the parietal wall, as described with other colonic operations, and the diseased part of the colon is resected between the two clamps. The proximal transected descending colon is brought out for the construction of the terminal colostomy. The distal transected sigmoid or rectosigmoid colon could be brought out through a separate wound to act as a mucocutaneous fistula.

Or it could be closed by hand suture either by interrupted stitches or by continuous suture in two layers. The primary closure of the distal transected end is buried with the invagination of seromuscular sutures. There remains a risk of blow-out of the closed stump of the distal end of the rectum. In this procedure, manual evacuation of feces from the proximal part of the descending or transverse colon would be unnecessary.

4. Alternatively, the distal transacted end is closed with the staple gun, using TA 55. It is left behind in the pelvis. Once the patient has recovered from these operative procedures, reversal of the Hartmann's procedure could be undertaken after a few months. With that procedure in mind, the distal stump is anchored with a loop of long nylon threads that would assist the surgeon to identify the distal stump from the depth of the pelvis and lots of adhesions, covering the stump, when the second operation for the reversal of Hartmann's procedure would be undertaken a few weeks later.

5. The modified Paul Mikulicz procedure is not a popular choice and it would be a relatively lengthy procedure that requires mobilization of the descending and the sigmoid colon along with the diseased bowel. The length of the double barrel colon up to the loop of the diseased colon should be three inches in length, before the loop is brought out through a separate wound made in the left lumbar region. The two parallel segments of the colon are sutured together by continuous stitches that go through the seromuscular layer, preferably through the taeniae coli.

After surgical toileting, the abdominal wound is closed in the usual way. This wound is covered with the dressing. This is necessary to protect the wound from contamination. The loop of the perforated segment is excised, leaving behind double barrel terminal colostomies. The transected ends of the double barrel colon are sutured with the surrounding skin wound. These two transected ends will act as colostomies independently, but a large colostomy bag would be necessary to cover all around the colostomies. At a suitable time interval, both stomas are anastomosed together—thus restoring the continuity of the colon. This second stage closure of stomas could be done without opening the abdomen.

The decision to pick up any one of those procedures depends upon the level of experience. At the conclusion of the definitive procedure being undertaken, as described in the respective section, metronidazole lavage with 1.5 gm in 300 ml, which is used for intravenous infusion, is performed. It must not be mixed with saline and must not be aspirated back straightaway. All the areas of the abdomen including the subdiaphragmatic spaces are squashed with this solution. Some solution is left in the 20 ml syringe to be added into the abdominal wound, before it is closed.[8,9]

Redivac drainage tubings are inserted through a separate stab wounds. One is put in the pelvis and one in upper abdomen. Abdomen is closed in the usual way. The drainage tubes are left clamped for 2 hours, before the vacuum in the bottles is put on.

Postoperative Care

Patient continues to receive all supporting therapy. Postoperative care would be no different from other septic abdomen. Poor renal function, pulmonary edema, chest infection, metabolic acidosis and anemia need to be looked at in perspective. Although the colon is affected in the operation, oral fluid must not be commenced until the patient has passed wind through the colostomy or through the back passage. Physiotherapy, oral mouthwash and hygiene and antithrombotic measures must be carried out, like any other postoperative cares.

Postoperative Complication

This includes wound infection, intraperitoneal abscess, chest infection or consolidation of the lung, pulmonary embolism, and other complications associated with colostomy.

ANGIODYSPLASIA

Angiodysplasia is an unusual clinical condition presented with massive rectal bleeding. It is due to bleeding from abnormal bleeding vessels developed in the colonic mucosa. It is regarded to be a paramount clinical emergency, because of painless profuse rectal bleeding. It is a rare pathology and puts the surgeons in a difficult situation on how this massive rectal bleeding could be managed, when the primary source of hemorrhage remains unknown, despite a lot of investigation being carried out. Uncertainty in the outcome of both investigations and the conventional treatment seems to be the major concern to the clinician. Author had experienced with the massive colonic bleeding in a limited number of cases.

Let me highlight the experience in dealing with these cases, in which the line of treatment is either total or subtotal colectomy, if the patient does not respond to blood transfusion along with other conservative regimen. In view of these uncertainties, total colectomy seems to be a blind procedure among the elderly patients, many of them may not be a fit person for such major operation. To overcome these risks, a new therapeutic approach was adopted in order to see any benefit among those patients. The outcome was encouraging.

Over a period of 7 years, only seven patients presented with massive colonic bleeding were included in the new therapeutic regimen. This was a new medical approach, which has never been reported in the literature. The therapeutic value of drug known as ethamsylate commercially known as dicynene has been established in various trials. Massive postoperative hematuria after open or TURP has been stopped by this drug, given by injection of 500 mg of ethamsylate intravenously every six hours for five days.

With this knowledge and experience, this new therapeutic drug was used in all those patients presented with massive colonic hemorrhage. None of the patients were on anticoagulant therapy nor was there any evidence of von Willebrand or cardiac disease apart from cardiac flatter present in one male patient. No other hemostatic agent was used to treat the massive colonic bleeding.

Massive bleeding from the lower digestive tract presents a diagnostic dilemma that delays the treatment at the moment of clinical urgency, and in the state of acute hemorrhagic shock.

Angiodysplasia is a rare benign pathology usually among the ageing population, but concomitant dual pathology, such as diverticulosis or malignant lesion is more frequently present in this age group.

Common types of investigation used in establishing the source and location of hemorrhage are simple sigmoidoscopy, upper and lower gastrointestinal tract endoscopy, selective angiogram, and red-cell radionucleotide scanning, better known as red cell tagging (RCT).

The criterion for confirming this rare disease either by selective angiogram or by RCT is the rate of bleeding per minute. It should be at least 0.5ml per minute. Otherwise, the result could be a false-negative. There are other pitfalls in this investigation that could also lead to a misleading report.

Therefore, reliability of all these investigations remains in question, in that the incidence of a false–positive was reported to be 9 percent in one study[13] and 42 percent in another study.[14]

The primary objective is to treat the shock first and then to contemplate how to stop bleeding. Uptill now, there has been no established noninvasive medical treatment available in the literature that could effectively be employed in order to stop the bleeding from the lower gut. But the diagnosis for acute bleeding should not be an immediate aim until the general state of health being improved and stabilized. Nevertheless, time is an essential factor in the management of this disease.

PATHOLOGY

Angiodysplasia comprises of ectatic blood vessels in the mucosa of the gut. Thinning of overlying colonic mucosa with or without ulceration seems to be the primary pathology for causing massive bleeding. The commonest site is on the right side of the colon. But the diverticula could be an alternative source of hemorrhage, but the true incidence of this condition is between 3 and 5 percent.[15,16]

Conservative Treatment

The conventional therapy for the angiodysplasia is a local application of monopolar electrocoagulation,[17] or injection of ethanolamine[18] or application of laser directly to the bleeding vessels.[19] It requires expertise in order to carry out this sort of local treatment through the colonoscope, but the outcome remains doubtful even in the hands of an expert. In some cases, technical difficulties may be encountered with the procedure, due to poor visibility, abnormal anatomical state of the colon and lack of expertise or those facilities.

Eventually, surgical intervention has to be contemplated, in those cases in which, the local treatment appears to be ineffective. In contrast, these modalities are inappropriate, if the source of bleeding is from the diverticula, in which cases bleeding stops spontaneously in 76 percent, but 99 percent of them may require up to 4 units of blood transfusion.[20]

Ethamsylate is not a new drug. It is known to be effective in reducing postoperative blood loss after transurethral resection of the benign prostate,[21] and for the treatment of menorrhagia,[22] but its potential therapeutic application to colonic hemorrhage has never been reported. In my past experience, this drug was found effective in reducing the postoperative blood loss from the denuded pelvic wall after abdominoperineal excision of the rectum. Although the results were not reported in my articles;[23,24] it compared favorably to my previous series.[25]

With this experience in my mind, this drug was used in the treatment of massive bleeding from the colon. The result in my first patient prompted me to extend this treatment to all cases of colonic bleeding. In this report, it is of paramount clinical importance to highlight the non-invasive treatment that provides a potential benefit to the sick patients, presented with massive colonic bleeding.

PHARMACOLOGICAL ACTION OF THE DRUG

Ethamsylate, known as dicynene is a nonhormonal agent that reduces capillary bleeding. And it acts as platelets plug in order to seal the leaking capillaries and induces capillary resistance. It has no effect on the coagulation, nor does it interfere with the platelet counts or function.[26]

A NEW THERAPEUTIC APPROACH

Between 1995 and 2002, seven patients aged between 38 and 89 years were included in this treatment, but one of them was an elderly woman. Among the men, one was only 38 years old. All other patients were between 58 and 89 years of age. No one was excluded from this treatment. None of the patients was on anti-coagulant therapy and none of them was associated with cardiac heart-valve dysfunction or von Willebrand disease.

Every patient was given injection of ethamsylate (dicynene) through the intravenous route for five days. The initial loading dose was 750 mg. It was followed by 500 mg given slowly every six hours. The treatment is to be discontinued, if there is any adverse reaction, encountered with this drug. None of these patients was treated with any other hemostatic agents, such as fresh frozen plasma, platelet infusion tranexamine acid or argon-plasma coagulation.

1. The first patient was a 38 years old man, presented with a massive colonic bleeding. On admission, he was very pale white and in a state of shock, lying in a large pool of his own blood in the stretcher, when he was brought to the hospital. Obviously, the primary diagnosis was not my initial concern, but the primary aim was to deal with the acute hemorrhagic shock. His past medical history suggested that, 4 years ago, he had another episode of mild rectal bleeding but all investigations were normal. In this emergency admission, acute peptic ulcer disease was the initial diagnosis, but gastroscopic examination undertaken within a few hours ruled out the diagnosis of the peptic ulcer disease.

The routine blood tests were normal apart from a high leukocytes count and low hemoglobin, which was around 5 gm/dl. The report of emergency selective angiogram suggested suspicious looking abnormal vessels in the right colon. This could not be confirmed on colonoscopy, done two days later. Barium enema was normal. During the supportive therapy for shock, the patient was commenced with intravenous injection of ethamsylate.

The initial dose was 750 mg, given straightaway after testing for allergic reaction. It was reduced to 500 mg, given at every six hours for five days. The patient had responded dramatically to the treatment, although 12 units of blood were transfused, in order to replace those units of blood being lost prior to admission. He remained well after leaving the hospital.

2. In 1996, a male schoolteacher, aged 58 years was having recurrent massive bleeding from the lower gut, while having investigations. For every episode of acute bleeding, he was transfused with 3-4 units of blood but on the night of my on-call duty, he was having further massive bleeding.

Upper gastrointestinal endoscopy was normal, so all other blood investigations, apart from low hemoglobin (8 gm/dl). Altogether, around 10 units of blood were transfused in less than one week. In view of the repeated episodes of massive bleeding, he was included in this new therapy, waiting for the investigation of a selective angiogram that was carried out on the following day.

The report suggested abnormal blood vessels in the area of ascending colon. Colonoscopy done 2 days later found a small area of inflammation in the proximal part of the transverse colon, but this finding was not consistent with the Crohn's disease. Nevertheless, both investigations had identified the same anatomical site. He remained well since then, but a few years later he developed Crohn's ileitis, which was far different from the previous colonoscopic finding. Massive bleeding from the Crohn's ileitis has never been reported to the literature.

3. In November 1999, angiodysplasia was diagnosed by red cell radionucleotide scanning done in a 70 years old man, presented with massive colonic bleeding. The location of the disease was in the cecum and the sigmoid colon. Apart from innocent diverticulosis in the sigmoid colon, no other pathology was found on a limited colonoscopy. He was initially treated with 12 units of blood, transfused over three days, but his hemoglobin persistently remained low at 8.6 gm/dl.

Therefore, emergency total colectomy was arranged, despite the fact that he was known to have a cardiac flutter. In view of his cardiac condition, he was treated with a new drug, in order to see any response to this treatment. In fact, he didn't need this major operation, and was discharged home a week later. In this case, the risk of postoperative morbidity or death had been averted.

Among the other four patients, ischemic colitis was diagnosed in one of them on a contrast CT scan. But the etiology of acute hemorrhage could not be established in other three patients on endoscopy. Perhaps, the diagnosis was missed due to the effect of the new drug therapy, poor bowel preparation and presence of blood mingled with soft feces in the proximal part of the colon.

Routine barium study did not suggest any colonic tumor. There was no conclusive evidence to suggest that the source of acute hemorrhage could be derived from the diverticula. Further specific investigations were considered inappropriate in the absence of further active bleeding. The total number of blood transfusion was between 5 and 7 units in two days.

RESULTS

Among the seven patients, ischemic colitis was found in one elderly man, and angiodysplasia was diagnosed in other six patients. This diagnosis was relied upon the combination of selective angiogram and colonoscopy in two and RCT and colonoscopy in one patient. Among the other three patients, concomitant diverticulosis was also found on emergency colonoscopy but there was no conclusive evidence to suggest that the source of massive bleeding was from the diverticula.

No adverse drug reaction was noticed in any patient, but the therapeutic response was unsatisfactory in one elderly man, who was later found to have ischemic colitis. Among the other six cases, emergency surgical intervention was considered imminent in three but it was averted because of the satisfactory response to the drug therapy. There was no further bleeding from these patients, since they were discharged from the hospital. None of these patients was on aspirin or anticoagulant therapy. And their platelets counts were within normal range.

BACKGROUND OF THE DISEASE

The average incidence of angiodysplasia is between 3 and 12 percent among the cases of colonic bleeding.[27-30] In this situation, a case control study presents a difficult task. The primary aim of the treatment is to stop the bleeding, while having supportive treatment for acute hemorrhagic shock. When the patient's general condition is stabilized, it is a paramount medical emergency to carry out both upper as well as lower endoscopy. But the benefit of emergency colonoscopy through the massive pool of hemorrhage remains in doubt.

And it is debatable, whether it is a safe procedure to carry out this invasive procedure, if they remain in a state of hemorrhagic shock. Despite this risk, the diagnosis of angiodysplasia may be missed due to large pool of blood, and poor bowel preparation.

The chances of missing the diagnosis would be greater if the colonoscope could not reach to the cecum due to some technical difficulty, in those cases in which, the favorite site for angiodysplasia remains in the area of cecum and the ascending colon.[31] In fact, 50 percent of the angiodysplasia lies in the cecum or in the right side of the colon.

In most cases, bleeding may stop spontaneously but it tends to recur more frequently. In these circumstances, emergency surgical intervention should be considered, when the patient general condition is not getting better, despite several units of blood being transfused. Surgical intervention is a clinical decision that is based on the arbitrary criteria, defined in the literature.[20,32,33] It states that surgical intervention is imminent if the blood transfusion exceeds the 4 units in less than 24 hours or more than 10 units in one week.

In those cases, in which preoperative or peroperative localization of the bleeding source could not be ascertained by the investigations, total colectomy remains the choice of operation. Alternative to this radical surgery is the blind segmental resection of the colon that may lead to a greater risk of morbidity with a higher incidence of recurrent bleeding.[34,35] Previous studies suggested that the risk of recurrent bleeding after segmental resection would be less, if the anatomical site of bleeding were known prior to resection. In this case, the incidence was reported to be 8.6 percent, but it could rise to 37 percent, if blind resection being undertaken.[35,36]

In my experience, noninvasive medical treatment is rational. In this report ethamsylate has proved to be effective in all six cases of this series, which is consistent with my previous unpublished studies[23-25] and it is in agreement with other studies.[21,22]

In my experience, the pharmacological effect of this drug has been targeted upon the bleeding vessels, irrespective of the pathological lesions. Hence, an accurate diagnosis is not a mandatory requirement for this drug to be used. Whether the source of massive colonic bleeding was from the diverticula or Crohn's colitis was not important to the clinician at that emergency situation.

Nevertheless, massive bleeding from the Crohn's colitis or Crohn's ileitis is very rare or unknown in the literature, but among those cases treated with this new drug therapy, Crohn's ileitis was diagnosed in one of them a few years later. And colonoscopic examination in other patients did not reveal that diverticula were the source of bleeding. The therapeutic value of this new approach has to be judged on balance whether this new therapeutic approach reduces the demand for blood transfusion and whether the major emergency colonic surgery has been averted, because of the fact that the drug starts working immediately on the bleeding capillaries.

It is debatable whether this new therapeutic approach should be delayed in order to reduce the risk of false-negative result with selective angiogram or RCT. The reason for false-negative diagnosis in those investigations was the therapeutic effect of ethamsylate that started working on the bleeding vessels straightaway. Although clinical diagnosis is necessary, this drug therapy that acts upon the bleeding vessels should be the priority for the safety and uneventful recovery of the patients.

My experience supports my strategy that our primary concern is to treat the shock along with noninvasive drug therapy. The response of the therapy has to be evaluated in perspective, whether the patients are benefited from conservative treatment alternative to emergency colonic surgery. In my view, there was no reason to delay the treatment, if this therapy will not interfere with other invasive investigation and concomitant local treatment.

On the contrary, I consider that delaying the treatment may attribute to a potential risk of other complication or may lead to a hasty decision in favor of emergency colectomy. Of the seven patients included in this prospective study, emergency colectomy was averted in three of them.

Although the therapeutic value of this drug in massive colonic bleeding remains a clinical importance, the prevalence of this rare disease may raise a problem in setting up a case control study. Nevertheless, it seems to be a beginning of a new therapeutic dawn that would encourage the clinician for setting up multi-center trials.

Efficacy, among other local treatments such as monopolar electrocoagulation,[17] ethalomine sclerosing injection[18] or laser coagulation,[19] remains in question, in certain circumstances, in which, the services of expertise are not always available in all hospitals, but it is not absolutely necessary for commencing this drug therapy. In conclusion, I recommend that this new therapy should be used routinely as a first line of treatment for all cases of massive colonic bleeding.

REFERENCES

1. Noer RJ, Hamilton JE, Williams DJ, Broughton DS. Rectal haemorrhage: Moderate and severe. Ann Surg 1962;155:794.
2. Noer RJ. Haemorrhage as a complication of diverticulitis. Ann Surg 1955;141:674.
3. Rushford AJ. The significance of bleeding as a symptom in diverticulitis. Proc Roy Soc 1956;49:577.

4. Dunning MWF. The clinical features of hemorrhage from diverticula of the colon. Gut 1963;4:273.
5. Salgado I, Wlodek GK, Mathews WH, Robertson HR. Massive haemorrhage due to diverticular disease of the colon: A case illustrating the bleeding point. Canad J Surg 1961;4:473.
6. Slack WW. The anatomy pathology and some clinical features of diverticulitis of the colon. Brit J Surg 1962;50:185.
7. Saha SK. Treatment of angiodysplasia: A new therapeutic approach, 2000.
8. Saha SK. Efficacy of metronidazole lavage in treatment of intraperitoneal sepsis: A prospective study. Digestive Diseases and Sciences 1996;41:1313.
9. Saha SK. Peritoneal lavage with metronidazole. Surg Gynecol Obstet 1985;160:335.
10. Uden P, Eskilsson P, Brunes L, Matzsch T. Clinical evaluation of postoperative peritoneal lavage in appendicitis. Br J Surg 1983;70:348.
11. Madden JL, Tan PY. Primary resection and anastomosis in the treatment of perforated lesions of the colon with abscess or diffusing peritonitis. Surg Gynecol Obstet 1961;113:646.
12. McKenna JP, Currie DJ, McDonald JA, et al. The use of continuous postoperative peritoneal lavage in the management of diffuse peritonitis. Surg Gynecol Obstet 1970;130:254.
13. Vellacott KD. Early endoscopy for acute lower gastrointestinal haemorrhage. Ann R Coll Surg Engl 1986;68:243.
14. Caos A, Benner KG, Manier J, McCarthy DM, Blessing LD. Acute rectal bleeding. J Clin Gastroenterol 1986;8:46.
15. McGuire HH, Hayness BW. Massive haemorrhage from diverticulosis of the colon: Guidelines for therapy based on bleeding patterns observed in fifty cases. Ann Surg 1972;175:847.
16. Judd ES. Massive bleeding of colonic origin. Surg Clin North Am 1969;49:977.
17. Rogerss BHG. Endoscopic diagnosis and therapy of mucosal vascular abnormalities of the gastrointestinal tract occurring in elderly patients and associated with cardiac, vascular, and pulmonary disease. Gastrointestinal Endosc 1980;26:134.
18. Bemvenuti GA, Julich MM. Ethanolamine injection for sclerotherapy of angiodysplasia of the colon. Endoscopy 1998;30:565.
19. Jensen DM, Machicado GA. Bleeding colonic angioma: Endoscopic coagulation and follow-up (abstract), Gastroenterology 1985;88:1433.
20. McGuire HH. Bleeding colonic diverticula: A reappraisal of natural history and management. Ann Surg 1994;220:653.
21. Symes DM, Offen DN, Lyttle JA, Blandy JP. The effect of dicynene on blood loss during and after transurethral resection of the prostate. British J Urol 1975;47(2):203.
22. Harrison RF, Cambell S. A double blind trial of ethamsylate in the treatment of primary and intrauterine-device menorrhagia. The Lancet 1976;2(7980):283.
23. Saha SK, Robinson AF. A study of perineal wound healing after abdominoperineal resection. British J Surg 1976;15:287.
24. Saha SK. Care of perineal wound in abdominoperineal resection. J of the Royal College of Surgeons of Edinburgh. 1983;28:324.
25. Saha SK. A critical evaluation of dissection of the perineum in synchronous combined abdominoperineal excision of the rectum. Surg Gyne & Obst 1984;158:33.
26. Ethamsylate (Dicynene) injection, manufactured and marketed by Lorex Synthelabo UK and Ireland Ltd. Edited in Data Pharm Publication Ltd, 12 Whitehall, London. 1999-2000:777.
27. Richter JM, Christensen MR, Kaplan LM, Nishioka NS. Effectiveness of current technology in the diagnosis and management of lower gastrointestinal haemorrhage. Gastrointestinal Endoscopy. 1995;41:93.
28. Colacchio TA, Forde KA, Patsos TJ, Nunez D. Impact of modern diagnostic methods on the management of active rectal bleeding –ten year experience. Am J Surg 1982;143:607.
29. Bramley PN, Masson JW, McKnight G, Herd K, Fraser A, Park K, et al. The role of an open-access bleeding unit in the management of colonic haemorrhage: A 2-year prospective study. Scand J Gastroenterol 1996;31:764.
30. Farrands PA, Taylor I. Management of acute lower gastrointestinal haemorrhage in a surgical unit over a 4-year period. J R Soc Med 1987;80:79.
31. Foutch PG, Rex DK, Leiberman DA. Prevalence and natural history of colonic angiodysplasia among healthy asymptomatic adults. Am J Gastroenterol 1995;90:564.
32. Newhall SC, Lucus CE, Ledger wood AM. Diagnostic and therapeutic approach to colonic bleeding. Am Surg 1981;47:136.
33. Field RJ, et al. Total abdominal colectomy for control of massive lower gastrointestinal bleeding. J Miss State Med Assoc 1994;35:29.
34. Hunter JM, Pezim ME. Limited value of technetium 99m-labeled red cell scintigraphy in localization of lower gastrointestinal bleeding. Am J Surg 1990;159:504.
35. Drapanas T, Pennington G, Kappelman M, Lindsay E. Emergency subtotal colectomy: Preferred approach to management of massive bleeding diverticular disease. Ann Surg 1973;177:519.
36. Browder W, Cerise EJ, Litwin MS. Impact of emergency angiography in massive lower gastrointestinal bleeding. Ann Surg 1986;204:530.

17 The Vermiform Appendix

SURGICAL ANATOMY AND CLINICAL PATHOLOGY

The appendix is a tubular worm-like structure, derived from the base of the cecum. Its length varies from 1 to 10 cm. The appendix has a narrow lumen; its diameter is around 2 mm, similar to that of a matchstick. And it is lined by a mucous membrane, which has a single layer of columnar epithelium. On cross section, the lumen of the appendix is lined by the mucous membrane, then by mucosa, submucosa, and by circular muscle, finally covered by the longitudinal muscle. The whole length of the appendix is invested by the peritoneum, apart from the line of attachment of the mesoappendix.

The mucous membrane is resistant to bacterial invasion. Unlike the colon, appendix has abundant lymphoid follicles in the mucosa that provide immunity to the body against the bacterial invasion and they are known as abdominal tonsil, and this protective power seems to be very important to the young babies and in adolescent life. But its function ceases after they are atrophied, usually after 30 years. Then how our gut is protected later in life remains unknown in medicine?

The main arterial supply is the branch of the right ileocolic artery. It passes behind the terminal ileum and enters into the mesoappendix near the base of the appendix. It continues distally along the free edge of the mesoappendix—thus supplying the tributaries to the body and apex. These vessels could be visualized through the mesoappendix, when the appendix is lifted up by the two pairs of Babcock forceps, one holding at the distal and other one at the proximal end of the appendix. Identification of these vessels is very important in order to divide either each branch separately or en-mass during appendicectomy. This will be highlighted later.

The osteum of the lumen has mucosal valves but they remain open among the younger person, but with the age, the opening gets smaller and its lumen gets obliterated. Because of these reasons, appendicitis is rare in children and also in older age group. It contains bacteria, parasites and foreign bodies.

The anatomical position of the appendix varies, depending upon the descent of the cecum. Due to incomplete descent, the cecum may settle in the subhepatic position. Appendicitis in this position may turn out to be a difficult diagnosis. And appendicectomy may be a difficult task technically, because of inaccessible position of the inflamed appendix, if the incision has been made in the true McBurney's point over the right iliac fossa. As a result, a lot of operative morbidity may be encountered with this operation. Nevertheless, even in the normal position of the cecum, the appendix may lie in different position with relation to the cecum. They are retrocecal, retroileal, pelvic and paracecal position.

Among these variations, the incidence of the retrocecal position is very high compared to the pelvic type or any other positions. In rare cases, appendix may be found missing at operation. This could be due to congenital phenomenon, or autoappendicectomy resulting from the spontaneous resolution of previous acute appendicitis.

Among other congenital conditions, appendix could be of duplex variety or it could be found located in the left iliac fossa. This is due to transposition of the heart, known as dextrocardiac. In this developmental condition, liver, gallbladder, and spleen will change their positions.

DISEASES OF THE APPENDIX

a. Acute appendicitis.
b. Carcinoid tumor.
c. Adenocarcinoma.
d. Diverticulosis.

Acute Appendicitis

Acute inflammation of appendix may occur in any age group, but its frequency is rare below the age of 4 and among the older age group of patients.

EPIDEMIOLOGY OF THE APPENDICITIS

It is the disease of the western people and among the upper social communities. It is rare in Asian and African countries and also rare among the people who are brought up primarily with vegetarian diet and less among the nonvegetarians who hardly consume meat in their regimen of diet. In fact, appendicitis tends to develop among the people whose diet contains a high proportion of meat protein and less of vegetables. In fact, the prevalence of this condition remains with the habit of diet and bowel movements.

ETIOLOGY

In the midst of body's protective power, the children and young subjects are often confronted with a life-threatening disease, and its outcome would have been uncertain, if surgical services are not available at hand. Because of this reason, a lot of interests have been generated in understanding the pathogenesis of this disease.

Epidemiological studies suggest that individual diet habit may contribute to one-third of the total number of appendicitis, but all others are believed to be affected by other factors. All the evidences suggest that obstruction to the lumen is the incriminating pathological condition for the development of acute appendicitis. This is caused by the fecolith or any other foreign materials.

The lumen may be occluded by secondary factors. They are blood-borne infection arising from the tonsillitis, or sore throat. This is referred to as catarrhal inflammation in which the lymphoid follicles are inflicted with bacterial invasion, thus causing inflammation, leading to edematous mucosa. This eventually leads to acute appendicitis. Hence, it could be divided into two main groups. One is obstructive and other one is nonobstructive type of appendicitis.

OBSTRUCTIVE APPENDICITIS

Of all the foreign materials, fecolith is frequently present in the lumen and it causes intraluminal obstruction. The incidence of acute appendicitis by the fecolith is 80 percent.[1] There are other foreign materials, which may also cause obstruction. They are roundworms, threadworms, and intestinal parasites.

The lumen may also be occluded secondary to other pathological conditions. They are cecal carcinoma, carcinoid, kinking, or inflammation of the lymphoid follicles or mucosa.

PATHOLOGICAL CHANGES

When the osteum of the appendix is occluded, the lumen of the appendix would appear to be a blind tube. At the site of impaction with the fecolith, the mucosa undergoes pressure necrosis. Bacterial floras, present inside the lumen of appendix, start proliferating and invade the mucosa through the damaged mucosa. This sets in acute inflammation in the mucosal layer, producing secretion from the goblet cells. And this secretion is pent up, causing the intraluminal pressure leading to ulceration or breakdown of the mucosal barrier or hemorrhage.

At the same time, lymphoid follicles present in the mucosa are enlarged, due to inflammation because of bacterial assault, thus causing further obstruction to the lumen of the appendix.

Eventually, within 12-18 hours, the appendix gets gangrene, distal to the obstruction and it is due to thrombosis of the appendicular arteries, being an end artery running through the intramural part of the terminal appendix.

In some cases, perforation of the appendix may occur through the site of impaction of fecolith. This is due to pressure necrosis. It may also cause perforation through the site of gangrene which could be at the distal end. As a result, the pent up purulent fluid escapes into the peritoneal cavity, before the appendix gets wrapped up by the greater omentum, which is regarded to be policeman of the abdomen. The infective fluid spreads up rapidly into the peritoneal cavity.

The speed of the pathological changes depends upon the virulence of the pathogens present in the lumen of the appendix.

COMPOSITION OF FECOLITH

It is a pea-sized round or oval-shaped dry and hard feces, developed from inspissated feces, containing calcium, magnesium, carbonates, phosphates and bacteria. It is radiopaque. In the plain X-ray of the abdomen, it would appear to be whitish calcified round opacity in the right side of the pelvis. It would be much brighter on contrast CT scan, if taken for resolving the debate on the question of appendicitis.

APPENDICITIS DUE TO PARASITES

Roundworm, known as *Ascaris lumbricoides* may be isolated from the lumen of the appendix. It may cause appendicular colic and may produce appendicitis. It is very common in the developing countries.

Threadworms, known as *Oxyuris vermicularis,* are not directly causative factor for developing acute appendicitis, but they attribute to recurrent attack of mild type of pain in abdomen, and in particular, children are often affected with these worms in the developing countries. The commonest site is near the opening of the appendix and the female worms use the appendix as a breeding ground for laying down ova near the base of the appendix.

Serial histological section would confirm that the worms have invaded the mucosa, and they could be seen deep in the mucosa and closer to muscular coat. And also it would show minute ulceration and hemorrhage within the wall of the appendix. These are probably the predisposing factors for causing infection of the appendix and generalized colicky abdominal pain, without any evidence of tenderness. Empirical treatment on the intestinal parasites may improve the symptoms.

NONOBSTRUCTIVE APPENDICITIS

The pathogenesis of the initial inflammation in the mucous membrane is not fully understood and debatable. Nevertheless, unlike the obstructive variety, it is a slow process. It may resolve spontaneously or continue having recurrence of mild attack of pain, often referred to as grumbling appendicitis or chronic appendicitis.

One school of thought suggests that the lymphoid follicles present in the mucosa are inflicted by the blood-borne infection remote from the appendix, and this could be associated with catarrhal infection. The mucous membrane becomes inflamed, congested and swollen due to edematous condition. This may cause ulceration or hemorrhage.

The appendix appears to be swollen and inflamed. In this situation, the infection may spread to serosal surface where fibrinous flakes are formed around the appendix. It may cause exudation and serous collection in the peritoneal cavity and the mesoappendix will turn out to be turgid and edematous.

In these cases, mesenteric lymph glands are found enlarged and appear to be fleshy in the mesentery, which are often referred to as mesenteric adenitis, but in many cases, the appendix has been found normal at the operation. It is often associated with sore throat and tonsillitis.

Although patient may complain of pain in abdomen, there will be a history of sore throat, cough, or a high rise of temperature, despite having normal appendix. More often, the symptoms settle down.

But in some cases, the enlarged lymphoid follicles present in the mucosa of the appendix may cause obstruction to the lumen. Some of these cases may resolve and in other instances, it may turn out to be acute appendicitis.

Another school of thought suggests contrary to the former view that lymphoid follicles are less likely to be first affected, but the acute inflammation sets in the mucosal layer. This is referred to as catarrhal appendicitis. In this case, the obstruction to the lumen is due to inflammation and edematous state of the mucosa. It is a slow process and it may resolve spontaneously or with conservative treatment.

In rare cases, collection of serous fluid continues in the obstructed lumen of the appendix. This is due to the secretion of the goblet cells present in the mucous membrane. In the absence of infection, it may lead to formation of mucocele of the appendix.

If it does not settle, then the inflammation and infection spreads up. The final state of the pathology could be resolution, fibrosis, or it may turn into suppuration and gangrene. The latter is attributable to the occlusion or thrombosis of the intramural part of the terminal artery that is an end artery to the terminal part of the appendix. Because of a slow progression, the greater omentum protects the inflamed appendix, by wrapping around the cecum and appendix.

Clinically, appendicular mass is palpable in the right iliac fossa. This implies that the infection and the inflamed appendix have been wrapped up by the greater omentum, thus preventing the spread of infective fluid from the right iliac fossa. This takes 2-3 days to be clinically palpable. This is referred to as appendicular mass. It comprises of collection of inflammatory and purulent fluid, wrapped up by the greater omentum around the inflamed or gangrenous or perforated appendix and around the cecum, and dilated terminal ileum.

In summary, there are not many differences in the pathogenesis of the acute appendicitis, whether or not the primary causative factor is either obstructive or nonobstructive appendicitis.

These would be the eventual outcomes of the acute appendicitis:
a. Acute inflammation of the appendix.
b. It may resolve, or it may recur with similar attack of inflammation.
c. Mucocele of the appendix.
d. Ulceration or pressure necrosis of the mucosa.
e. Gangrene.
f. Perforation.
g. Localized peritonitis.
h. Appendicular abscess, pelvic abscess.
i. Generalized peritonitis.

Bacteria present in the lumen of the appendix are normal bacterial floras. They are *E. coli,* enterococci, streptococci, *Cl.welchii* and anaerobic bacteria such as bacteroides, and anaerobic streptococci.

SYMPTOMS OF ACUTE APPENDICITIS

In most cases, the symptoms of acute appendicitis remain consistent, irrespective of the anatomical position of the appendix and types of appendicitis. There could be a marginal difference in severity of presentation between the obstructive and nonobstructive appendicitis. This will be highlighted later.

In most instances, patients experience first with discomfort around the umbilicus and then they start complaining of spasmodic type or constant pain around the umbilicus. It develops more often in the early morning. After few minutes, they feel nauseated and start vomiting.

They feel anorexia, and later the pain shifts to the right iliac fossa that takes around 6 hours. They prefer to lie on the right side with the knees bringing towards the belly. This relieves the psoas spasm and makes the abdominal muscles relaxed—thus relieving the pain. If the symptoms continue over 12 hours, they start vomiting violently and complain of pain all over the abdomen. Patients are often constipated but a few of them may open soft or loose motion a few times.

It is important to obtain any other history that would be suggestive of food poisoning, gastroenteritis, or dull aching or sharp pain in the loin or in the right lumbar region. Patient should be asked with a specific question whether the sharp pain radiates down to the right testis, or to the front part of the thigh or whether he is having watery motion, not associated with the vomiting, frequency of micturition and nocturia. Further history should be obtained about the color and smell of the urine, rigors, any hematuria, any pain referred to the tip of the shoulder, or radiating to the right shoulder blade.

Patient should be asked about past history of biliary dyspepsia, peptic ulcer disease, whether he or she is on regular medications such as aspirin, nonsteroidal antiinflammatory tablets. Many of these symptoms are usually related to a particular age group that could be above 20 years of age.

In case of female patients, particular history should be secured, related to contraceptive pills, white and foul vaginal discharge, last menstrual date, morning sickness, or having any intrauterine devices. All these history and those symptoms would be required in order to differentiate the acute appendicitis from other diseases, such as acute cholecystitis, pyelonephritis, renal or ureteric stone, peptic ulcer perforation, ectopic pregnancy, ovulation pain, salpingitis, ovarian cyst, cystitis, and so on. These will be highlighted separately later.

Murphy states: "If vomiting or distinct nausea precedes pain, the case is not acute appendicitis."

Clinical Assessment

On admission, nurse takes the oral temperature, but for the children, axillary temperature is safe. For, there remains a risk of breaking of the thermometer, if the child gives a bite to it. These days, electronic thermometer is used to record the temperature of the middle ear.

However, the temperature would be either normal, if the temperature is taken immediately, after being admitted to the ward. This would be a misleading temperature, because of the fact that the body temperature has been lost in air while walking through the cold atmosphere.

Therefore, patient's body should be allowed to pick up the room temperature. And temperature should be taken 2 hours later. More often, it would reflect the true body temperature. In acute appendicitis, the initial temperature is not very high. More often, it is around 37.2°C. And this is an early signal of acute appendicitis that should not be ignored.

Again, if the initial temperature, recorded on admission is around 39°C without any evidence of peritonitis, it is more likely not to be associated with gangrenous or perforated appendicitis. In this situation, one should look for tonsillitis, urinary tract infection, chest infection (pneumonia).

If the temperature is around 38.5°C, and there is no evidence of tonsillitis, this pattern of elevated temperature is suggestive of advanced acute appendicitis which could be perforated or gangrenous appendix. However, the pulse rate in acute appendicitis is also goes up with the rise of temperature and it is usually between 80 and 90 per minute.

GENERAL INSPECTION AND EXAMINATION

When the patient has settled and is in a comfortable position in his bed, he should be examined thoroughly. First a general inspection is carried out. It begins with the color of the skin, sclera of the eyes, and inspection of the mouth. Inside the mouth, particular attention is focused on the under surface of the tongue, whether there is a tinge yellow color in the mucosa.

To examine the color of the sclera and the conjunctiva of both eyes, the lower eyelid is gently retracted down by the tip of the index finger, placed just below the edge of the eyelashes of the lower eyelid. Jaundice patient will reveal yellowish color in the sclera and anemic patient will show pale color in the conjunctiva, when the lower eyelid is pulled down.

Patient is next asked to open the mouth. He will be asked to stick the tongue out. It will show coated and dry tongue. A fetor smell will be noticed in his breath. Then his oral cavity, sides and dorsum of the tongue, gum and buccal mucosa, and tonsillar fossa are examined methodically. This is done by using a tongue spatula under a bright light.

The disposable wooden tongue spatula is used to elevate or to push the sides of the tongue away from the gum. This will reveal the sides of the gum and buccal mucosa. During this examination, a good illumination is necessary and a pencil torch held by one hand should be used, while the wooden tongue spatula, held by other hand is tempted, pushing the buccal mucosa and angle of the mouth away from the tongue.

The back of the tongue and oral feces are examined by a tongue depressor under a pencil torch. The tongue depressor held by the left hand keeps the dorsum and back of the tongue down, while inspecting the back of the oral cavity and tonsillar fossa with the pencil torch held by the right hand.

Patient may be coughing from time-to-time and may be uncomfortable while undertaking this inspection. Sometimes, patient may not allow the clinician or may turn the mouth away or may push the clinician's hands away from the mouth. In these situations, gentleness and reassurance are both necessary. Patient must be explained about the purpose of this examination and repeated approach may be required to see inside and around the oral cavity.

In the palpation of the neck, examination is continued around the mandibular gland, angle of the jaw, and along the sternomastoid muscles. Any evidence of enlarged lymph glands in the neck is suggestive of glandular fever (mononucleosis). And if they are tender to touch, or appear to be inflamed, then look for infection in the mouth or aural fauces.

The possible source of primary infection could be tonsillitis, ulcer of the tongue, tooth abscess or stone in the submandibular salivary gland. Tuberculous lymph-adenitis should be suspected, if there is a history of long-standing painless discharge from the cervical lymph nodes in the neck.

There are many other conditions that may give rise to palpable cervical lymph nodes, which should be looked for a differential diagnosis, if suspicion arises. One should not forget to examine the axilla. Axillary lymph glands should be examined, whether they are tender to touch, or rubbery in consistency. A detailed account of the palpation should be recorded for any differential diagnosis.

ABDOMINAL EXAMINATION

Patient is asked to lie flat on the back in supine position with both knees lying flat on the couch. His head is rested on a single pillow, if he feels uncomfortable and both hands are kept along the side of the body. Reassurance to the patient is important. He will be asked to show the site of pain in the abdomen should be advised to locate the pain by his right index finger.

More often, patient puts his palm vaguely around the lower abdomen, but once they are advised to pin-point the exact site of pain by using the index finger, they, then, put the tip of the index finger onto the correct place.

After a few talks, patient is asked to breathe slowly and deeply. The purpose is to look for the free movement of the abdominal wall. It is important to be sure that the patient is not keeping the abdomen rigid voluntarily. In normal circumstances, the abdominal wall moves in pari passu with the movement of the chest during inspiration and expiration, but in acute peritonitis, the abdominal wall remain rigid, during inspiration.

If there is generalized peritonitis, patient will be unable to carry out a deep breathing and there will be evidence of some restriction of the movement of the abdominal wall.

After this test, patient is next advised to turn his face to other side and then asked to give a cough. And he will be asked whether he has experienced any pain in abdomen, if so, ask him to put his hand on the particular site.

If the site of pain is in the upper abdomen, both hypochondrium or on a particular site, then this pain could be due to pleurisy or pneumonia or it could be due to lesions in the upper abdomen, which could be acute cholecystitis, pyelonephritis, pancreatitis or peptic ulcer disease.

If the pain is not in the upper abdomen, more often, he will put his palm over the right iliac fossa.

Before palpating the abdomen, it is important to make sure that your hand is warm. If the patient is a young child, it is a good practice to palpate his abdomen through his palm, placed over his belly and press down his palm passively on his abdomen, by your hand placed on the dorsum of the patient's hand. This reassures the child that he is not going to be hurt.

Palpation should be done over the left iliac fossa first, then over the left hypochondrium and then right hypochondrium. This will give him confidence that you are not going to hurt him. And he will enjoy examining his own abdomen by his own palm.

This passive palpation is carried out methodically, as outlined just before. This will divert the attention of the patient, but he will resist pressing his palm further down, when his hand will be brought down over to the right iliac fossa, where you would experience the resistance through his hand. And you would be unable to carry out a deep palpation through his palm over the site of peritonitis.

After this round of examination is finished, further palpation could be repeated without the assistance of the patient's hand. It would reveal that right iliac fossa is tender to touch and appears to be guarding and there could be rebound tenderness, when the hand or fingers are gently lifted off suddenly.

Apart from these evidences, a vague palpable mass or fullness in the right iliac fossa could be identified. Outside the margin of the guarding, there would be a palpation of softness without tenderness, and guarding. This would be the vague margin of the appendicular lump when you would palpate it by the tip of your fingers. If this is possible to map it out, it should be marked out with a skin pencil.

If the palpation reveals that the whole abdomen is diffusely tender, guarding or rigid, and rebound tenderness has been elicited, then the clinical diagnosis would be generalized peritonitis. In some cases, the generalized rigidity may not be clinically evident, if the duration of peritonitis has exceeded over 12 hours.

■ Other Test

Rovsing's sign is another test. In this case, the left iliac fossa is pressed down in order to find out whether the patient experiences a pain in the right iliac fossa. In this case, loops of the small intestine have pushed to the right iliac fossa, thus interfering with the position of the inflamed appendix.

McBurney's sign: McBurney's point is the landmark at the junction between the lateral one and medial two-third of an oblique line drawn between the anterior superior iliac spine and the umbilicus. This landmark is used for making a grid iron incision for appendicectomy. In clinical examination,

McBurney's sign is referred to as positive in acute appendicitis, if tenderness is elicited on the said landmark point on a deep palpation.

■ Psoas Test

There are two clinical tests to elicit psoas spasm and obturator internus spasm. The first condition is attributable to retrocecal appendicitis and pelvic appendicitis, and the latter is due to only pelvic type appendicitis.

In retrocecal appendicitis, patient tends to keep the right hip joint in flexion position. Extension of the hip joint will lead to abdominal pain. If this pain seems to be equivocal, the patient is turned to lie on the left lateral position and the right hip joint is made hyperextended by pulling the right thigh backwards. Patient will notice abdominal pain because of pulling of the psoas muscle.

For pelvic type appendicitis, the spasm of the obturator internus is elicited on internal rotation of the hip joint. To demonstrate this test, the right hip joint is first flexed. It is then first rotated externally and then internally. Psoas spasm may also be elicited on hyperextension of the hip joint. All these maneuvers suggest that the inflamed appendicitis is in the pelvic position, causing irritation of psoas muscle and obturator internus muscle.

Psoas spasm may also be elicited in other surgical conditions. They are psoas abscess, ureteric stone, salpingitis, ovulation pain, and pyelonephritis.

After palpation, percussion is carried out gently on all parts of the abdomen and particularly over the appendicular mass and both sides of the pelvis. This may reveal a note of dullness on percussion in the pelvis which could be pelvic abscess, ovarian mass or ovarian cyst.

The inguinal regions are also palpated in order to exclude the inguinal hernia and any evidence of tenderness on either side of the bladder in female patient. In male patient, both testes are palpated to exclude torsion of the testis. And finally, bowel sounds should be heard with the stethoscope. Absent bowel sounds suggest paralytic ileus. But it has very little clinical importance, if the patient admits that he has passed wind per rectum.

At the completion of abdominal examination, both loins are palpated simultaneously. This is done by placing four fingers of the right hand behind the left loin and left fingers on the right loin of the patient. The purpose is to find out whether the loin is tender and whether the quadratus lumborum muscle appears to be rigid, which would suggest whether it is due to retrocecal appendicitis or pyelonephritis or perinephric abscess.

Patient is asked to be relaxed and to lie back on both hands of the clinician placed over the loins, instead of raising the back away from the hands or the bed. This would cause stiffness of the muscles of the back. As a result, the finding may be misleading.

Once you find that the patient's back is resting gently on your hands, then press gently the loins simultaneously by fingers of both hands and keep on watching on the face whether there is any facial expression of discomfort, if not, then ask the patient whether you are hurting the loins; if so, which one of the loins is getting hurt on palpation.

Rectal digital examination should be done at the end, if patient agrees for this internal examination. Vaginal examination requires permission of the patient and this examination must be done in the presence of a nurse or a relative. In most cases, tenderness in the rectovesical pouch or pouch of Douglas may be elicited. It would be marked, when the index finger is directed towards the right side.

Fullness or bulging of the pelvic floor associated with tenderness is suggestive of pelvic abscess or ovarian mass in woman, if clinically indicated. Tenderness may not be elicited for retrocecal appendicitis.

■ Investigations

Blood Tests

FBC, Hb, LFT, serum electrolytes, urea, creatinine, ESR, C Reactive protein.

USS of the abdomen – This includes liver, GB, pancreas, kidneys, and pelvis (ovary and uterus).

X-ray of the chest and abdomen, (in younger women, pregnancy test must be done before X-ray of the abdomen is taken).

MSU (Midstream urine) is sent for microscopical examination and for culture and sensitivity test.

SURGICAL PHYSIOLOGY OF PAIN AND VOMITING IN ACUTE APPENDICITIS

■ Significance of Shifting Pain and Vomiting

Before the symptoms of acute appendicitis become apparent to the patient, the cecum tends to remain quite from its peristaltic activity, thus protecting the inflamed appendix from any disturbance. This is only possible if the ileocecal valves remains shut, thus causing dilatation of the terminal ileum.

And this local dilatation is a unique feature that becomes apparent at the operation. Of course, this dilatation of the terminal ileum could be attributable to paralytic ileus because of local infection.

The pathogenesis of this condition is less important in this case, whether or not the dilatation is attributable to local paralytic ileus. This may result from local peritonitis. Regional dilatation of the terminal ileum may also be attributable to defunctioning of the ileocecal valve.

The distention of the terminal or midgut, whatever may be the attributing factors, may cause irritation of the parietal peritoneum in the central abdomen, affecting initially around the umbilicus. This raises the first alarm of uneasiness and awareness of something expecting to happen. Patient experiences discomfort initially and later spasmodic or continuous type of pain. The latter could be the result of acute peritonitis.

This distention leads to a reverse peristalsis, but the stomach needs to be emptied first in order to accommodate the back pressure of the gut. As a result, further protective measure begins with the pylorospasm. This leads to a feeling of nausea first and then it is followed by vomiting, thus making the stomach empty. This whole process allows the proximal gut contents to be refluxed into the empty stomach by reverse peristalsis. Further vomiting continues, thus helping the gut to be less distended.

The sequence of events continues, until the inflamed appendix is wrapped up by the greater omentum in the right iliac fossa. As a result, peritonitis develops that remains localized in the right iliac fossa. By the time, local parietal peritoneum is inflicted with infective and inflammatory materials; acute pain is triggered off in the right iliac fossa. It takes a few hours before the central abdominal pain is shifted to right iliac fossa. Eventually, the inflamed and edematous appendix is wrapped up by the greater omentum in most cases.

The whole process probably takes around 6 hours. Therefore, accurate history and duration of pain is very important. This will assist the surgeon, whether the severity of the symptoms is attributable to nonobstructive or obstructive type of appendicitis. But in clinical practice, such fine analysis is not practical.

All studies suggest that obstructive appendicitis produces symptoms rapidly, mimicking acute intestinal obstruction. The greater omentum fails to limit the spread of infection within a short spell of time because of the fact that obstructive appendicitis gets swollen up rapidly, causing a spread of cellulites, collection of infective exudates and perforation or gangrene of the appendix.

In sharp contrast, nonobstructive appendicitis, the symptoms develop slowly, inflammation gets out of the appendix slowly and sometimes it may resolve or it continues progressing slowly. As a result, perforation or gangrene of the appendix is a late sequel that is sealed off by the greater omentum. This sets up the appendicular lump.

Significance of Age in Acute Appendicitis

Appendicitis is very rare in extreme age groups. It is uncommon under the age of 3-4 years old, and rare above the age of 70. But age is no bar in developing acute appendicitis.

If younger children are presented with symptoms of appendicitis, the condition becomes a great concern to both parents and the clinician. The clinical diagnosis becomes much more complicated if there is a concomitant tonsillitis, chest infection and diffuse tenderness without guarding or peritonitis. In some cases, the infant may develop generalized peritonitis very rapidly. This rapid presentation could be explained by the fact that the greater omentum is not fully developed, it would look like a thin paper and not long enough to reach to the inflamed appendix.

In this critical situation, surgeons are often in dilemma and arrive at judgement, not often consistent with true diagnosis. One of the factors is the dual pathology and other factor is the age. It would be a dilemma to the surgeon whether or not to operate upon the infant. Its mortality is very high and could be as high as 80 percent.

Among the young children, vague pain in abdomen associated with tonsillitis, sore throat or cough and high temperature may also present a difficult problem in arriving at a correct diagnosis. If there is no clinical evidence of guarding on palpation of the abdomen and patient remains free of symptom in between the attack of pain, but cervical lymph nodes are palpable, mesenteric adenitis is more likely to be the clinical diagnosis in these age groups. The diagnosis of glandular fever (mononuleosis) should be suspected.

In this case, the duration of symptoms is crucial. The initial approach is to treat the tonsillitis and chest infection with appropriate combined antibiotics and to keep observing the temperature and pulse rate for 3-6 hours. If no change, then operative decision should be taken.

If the clinical examination reveals generalized peritonitis and the child has a very high temperature and tachycardia, then sooner the operation is done is better.

The incidence of acute appendicitis is very high among the adolescent and younger people between 20 and 30 years of age.

Among the elderly patients, appendicitis does present classical clinical features, in that the abdomen does not show classical features of guarding or peritonitis within a permissible duration of symptoms, although acute appendicitis has already developed. In this age group, temperature is not elevated for some-time and white cell counts remain within a normal range in most cases.

All these findings delay the surgical intervention and if the clinical diagnosis is regarded to be acute appendicitis, at operation it may turn out more often to be cecal carcinoma. Therefore, it is important to bear in mind the possibility of cecal carcinoma and patient must be warned with this possibility.

CLINICAL FEATURES ASSOCIATED WITH UNUSUAL TYPE OF APPENDICITIS

Tenderness in the loin may indicate retrocecal appendicitis, pyelonephritis, pyonephrosis; but tenderness over the cecum is much less in retrocecal and retroileal appendicitis.

Pyelonephritis is associated with a frequency of micturition, rigors and high temperature which could be 39°C. The color of urine should be cloudy and concentrated. Urine examination will reveal pus cells and evidence of infection, In young female patient, presented with ascending bilateral pyelonephritis, vesicoureteric reflux should be suspected. In some cases, acute appendicitis is diagnosed and a normal appendix is removed at emergency operation. In these cases, micturating cystogram should be done after a few months. This would assist in resolving the true diagnosis.

MSU may also reveal microscopical RBC. This could be attributable to stone in the kidney, renal pelvis, ureter or bladder, or inflamed appendix lying across the ureter. Plain X-ray of the kidney, ureter and bladder will resolve the confusion. If there is any opacity along the line of ureter, or in the renal parenchyma, IVP should be done to exclude the renal tumor, stone and obstructive uropathy.

In other cases, simple tenderness of the cecum without guarding or palpable lump may present a difficult clinical problem. In this case, analysis of the symptoms is very crucial and it is important to find out whether there is a history of painless watery or loose motions, with or without any symptoms of vomiting. *Salmonella enteritis* is often associated with watery diarrhea without any symptom of pain in abdomen.

In this clinical condition, the cecum may be tender on deep palpation. This is due to excessive purgation. Patient may be dehydrated and may have a rise of temperature. Rectal digital examination would be negative in most cases. Stool culture should be done straightaway. Contrast CT scan may assist in the management of this case. If the duration of symptoms is over 3-4 days and there is no evidence of localized peritonitis, conservative line of management should be continued with nil by mouth. Daily pulse and temperature chart should be observed carefully.

If the symptoms persist, despite conservative treatment being continued, appendicectomy should be carried out but the specimen of stool from the appendix should be sent for further stool culture in order to exclude salmonella organism.

The reason for recommending appendicectomy is the possibility of retroileal appendicitis, or pelvic abscess. In the position of pelvic or retroileal appendicitis, abdominal examination may not reveal classical features of tenderness and guarding.

DIFFERENTIAL DIAGNOSIS WITH OTHER ABDOMINAL CONDITION

Acute appendicitis seems to be straightforward surgical admission, but it may present a difficult task in differentiating it from other acute surgical and medical admissions. These are as follows:

- Tonsillitis
- Sore throat
- Chest infection — Basal pneumonia, pleuritic pain
- Peptic ulcer perforation
- Acute cholecystitis, empyema of the gallbladder
- Right-sided pyelonephritis, right-sided pyonephrosis
- Right-sided perinephric abscess
- Right renal or ureteric stone
- Nonspecific mesenteric adenitis
- Meckel's diverticulum
- Carcinoma of the cecum
- Crohn's ileitis
- Nonspecific enterocolitis (Salmonella)
- Tuberculous enteritis
- Carcinoid tumor of the appendix
- Salpingitis, right-sided pyosalpinx, hydro-salpinx
- Right tubal pregnancy, ruptured ectopic pregnancy
- Ruptured corpus luteal cyst
- Right twisted ovarian cyst
- Cystitis
- Intestinal obstruction
- Diverticulitis.

IMPORTANT DIFFERENTIAL DIAGNOSTIC FEATURES

Differential Diagnostic Features in Peptic Ulcer Perforation, Acute Cholecystitis

Problem may arise; when the abdomen appears to be markedly rigid or guarding and tenderness is elicited all along the right paracolic gutter from the right hypo- chondrium right down to the pelvis.

History of previous peptic ulcer disease may not resolve the difficult diagnosis. But a few important past clinical history or symptoms may unravel the mystery of the abdomen.

The first question needs to be put to the patient whether he takes aspirin or nonsteroidal antiinflammatory drugs for arthritis and whether the pain in abdomen has also been referred to the tip of the right shoulder.

If the answer is yes, then perforated duodenal or gastric ulcer should be suspected. In this case, temperature remains normal despite having high leukocytes count, the abdomen will not move with the inspiration and expiration and it would appear to be diffusely tender associated with a cardboard rigidity and dull on percussion, if the duration of pain is around 6 hours, but the rigidity would be much less after 6-12 hours.

An X-ray of the chest in erect position may reveal a gas shadow under the diaphragm in most cases. Sometimes, it could be seen under the diaphragm on both sides, which is a suggestive of perforation of the gastric ulcer. Clinician should be trained how to read the plain X-ray of the chest and abdomen, when the consultant radiologist is not available. In this case, it is also important to know the difference between the gas shadow present within the fundus of the stomach and that remains outside the fundus.

In the former case, the size of the gas shadow would appear to be wider compared to that lying outside the fundus and under the left half of the diaphragm. In the latter case, it would appear to be a narrow strip, usually above the shadow of the fundus. Furthermore, chest X-ray will exclude basal pneumonia, pleural effusion and collapsed lung or spontaneous pneumothorax.

The second question is whether he had noticed sickly feeling, after fatty food, or biscuit and whether the pain radiates around the right chest towards the right shoulder blade. If the answer is yes, finding of tenderness and guarding in the right hypochondrium or further down to the right lumbar region would suggest acute cholecystitis, or empyema of the gallbladder. This will be associated with a high rise of temperature. This needs to be confirmed by the USS of the abdomen.

A plain X-ray of the abdomen may reveal a typical faceted multiple stones or a round concentric type of a single gallstone.

RIGHT RENAL AND URETERIC STONE

Acute pain arising from the renal or ureteric stone has characteristic and classical features, quite different from any other pain. Patient will experience with pin pointed pain, similar to that of a needling into the skin surface or a sharp pain like a toothache or stabbing type of pain. It radiates down to the groin, testis or over the front part of the right thigh. This distribution of pain is unique and distinct from any other type of pain. It originates due to irritation of the genito-femoral nerve (L_1 and L_2), by the stone in the ureter overlying the nerve.

The pain referred to the testis in males or to the vagina in females is due to irritation of the genital branch, and that radiating down to the thigh is due to irritation of the femoral branch of the genitofemoral nerve. Patient will not experience pain in the right iliac fossa on coughing, which is in contrast to the acute appendicitis. MSU may reveal trace of RBC and pus cells, in both conditions, due to the fact that the appendix may lie across the ureter.

Plain X-ray of the abdomen may reveal tiny opacity along the line of ureter or in the shadow of renal parenchyma. To identify its clinical and radiological significance, two plain X-rays are taken; one on inspiration and other one on expiration. This will distinguish the renal stone from the calcified lymph nodes.

In the case of a renal stone, its position with relation to the distance between the cortical border of the kidney and the opacity present in the cortex or in the renal calyx will remain constant in both X-ray films, despite the fact that soft tissue shadow of the kidney has moved up with expiration and down with inspiration. But these X-ray films will not confirm the ureteric stone. In this case, IVP should be done.

CLINICAL FEATURES OF PYELONEPHRITIS

In the case of pyelonephritis, there should be a dull aching pain in the loin and lumbar region. Other clinical symptoms are a frequency of micturition, smelly cloudy urine, rigor and high temperature, which could be around 39°C. On palpation, the tenderness may be elicited in the loin. These are suggestive of urinary tract infection. MSU may reveal pus cells greater than 5 per field, and bacterial growth may be found on culture. If it is sterile pyorrhea, the suspicion of tuberculous nephritis should be raised.

CROHN'S ILEITIS

In rare cases, Crohn's ileitis may mimic appendicitis. If there is a past history of loose motion several times per day, a soft tender lump is palpable in the right iliac fossa and blood test showed a very high ESR, and an X-ray of the abdomen may reveal dilatation of small intestine, Crohn's ileitis should be suspected.

BILATERAL ACUTE SALPINGITIS

Pain in both groins, associated with a vaginal discharge, which could be foul smelling whitish or brown in color are suggestive of acute salpingitis. In most cases, the ascending infection from the vagina causes acute inflammation in both fallopian tubes. A marked tenderness is elicited around the inguinal region on both sides. The cervix will be tender to touch on vaginal examination or through the rectal digital examination. The latter is done by touching the cervix, indirectly through the wall of the rectum.

TWISTED OVARIAN MASS

Clinically, it would appear to be an appendicular mass in the right iliac fossa. If the tender mass is palpable in the right iliac fossa and appears to be large in size, a bimanual examination should be carried out through the vagina or through the rectum with the permission of the patient and in the presence of a nurse. This will reveal an irregular solid mass in the pelvis.

If it seems to be solid in consistency and dull on percussion, it could be any one of the following pathological lesions. They are follicular cyst, corpus luteal cyst or dermoid cyst or papillary carcinoma of the ovary.

A dermoid cyst is a form of teratoma, and may occur at any age group. It is a slow growing tumor and its size is no greater than a fist of the hand, but a malignant change may be possible. It is a rare variety and represents an incidence of 10 percent of all cases of ovarian tumor. The incidence of bilateral tumor is around 10 percent. It has a pedicle that may undergo into torsion.

The X-ray of the pelvis may show soft tissue shadow. USS will confirm the diagnosis of an ovarian mass. Malignant tumor is most likely to be the case if the patient is above 35 years old, and if there is no rise of temperature, appendicular mass or abscess is very unlikely.

After pregnancy test, CT scan should be done. This may reveal many abnormal embryonic tissues within the ovarian mass. The commonest varieties are skin, hair, bone, and less common varieties are teeth, cartilage, brain and striated muscles. If clinically, the tender palpable mass is evident in the right side of pelvis, an urgent exploration should be done.

RUPTURE OF THE RIGHT CORPUS LUTEAL CYST

Among the benign cysts, follicular cyst is a commonest variety, and it may undergo torsion and infarction. In an early childbearing age, woman often experiences mild type of pain in the right iliac fossa that occurs in the midcycle of the menstruation. This is commonly referred to as an ovulation pain. In these cases, the corpus luteal cyst in midcycle of menstruation may rupture, causing hemorrhage in the peritoneal cavity. This may cause a peritoneal irritation.

The pain in the lower part of the right iliac fossa is mild with a slight tenderness and without much guarding. The symptom would be similar to a tubal pregnancy, but there would be no history of missed period and no sign of soft cervix.

The hemorrhage in the center of the mature corpus luteum cyst may increase in size or may undergo a resorption and replaced by a clear fluid or jelly-like fibrin within the cyst. It is larger than a follicular cyst and it is usually single in number but multiple cysts may be present. In extreme clinical condition, operation is necessary.

RUPTURED ECTOPIC PREGNANCY

The tubal pregnancy may rupture into the pelvis. In most cases, the right-sided tubal pregnancy seems to be more common. Patient is admitted to the surgical ward because of acute pain in the right iliac fossa, consistent with that of an acute appendicitis.

Patient may be in a state of shock. There could be some pain referred to the shoulder, if the foot end of the bed is kept elevated for a few minutes. There will be history of missed period and pregnancy test will be positive.

Hemoperitoneum causes peritoneal irritation and may present with diffuse tenderness and some degree of guarding and rebound tenderness on palpation in the lower abdomen.

Rectal digital examination will be tender and the cervix will appear to be soft and very tender on vaginal examination.

NONSPECIFIC ACUTE MESENTERIC ADENITIS

Children are more often affected, and it is rare after adolescence. In most instances, appendix is not involved, but the ratio between the acute appendicitis and acute mesenteric lymphadenitis is reported to be 10:1.

Etiology is not known, but it follows the respiratory tract infection in 25 percent of the cases.

Symptoms: The central abdominal pain that comes and goes in every 20- 30 minutes remains remission in between the attack of a pain. And it is relieved on lying on to the left lateral position. These are distinct features, quite different from the acute appendicitis. Vomiting is common but bowel movement is not associated with the diarrhea.

Examination may reveal diffuse tenderness and mostly around the umbilicus and shifting tenderness could be demonstrated when the patient turns to the left lateral position. No guarding is elicited, but rectal digital examination reveals tenderness anteriorly. Oral fauces, tonsil and chest are examined. Acute inflammation in the oral fauces or respiratory infection may be found in this condition. Neck glands must be examined.

Other findings are a high temperature (38.5°C) and a high leukocytes count (> 10000 per cmm).

Despite all these clinical differences, it is not always possible to be certain in the diagnosis of acute nonspecific mesenteric adenitis.

Treatment is conservative. If no difference in symptoms is evident, appendicectomy should be done. Although it does not help for further attack of abdominal pain, it resolves diagnostic dilemma at least that the recurrence of abdominal pain is unlikely to be acute appendicitis, but it could cause many other problems. They are pain in the appendicular scar, incisional hernia, numbness in the groin or neuralgia, recurrent mild abdominal pain which could be due to subacute intestinal obstruction, or acute intestinal obstruction resulting from adhesion of the gut with the appendicular scar or intraperitoneal adhesions.

At the operation, mesenteric lymph glands remain with the peritoneal coverings, and it could be enucleated easily by making an incision over the peritoneal covering. Its sizes are variable, but the largest one could be around a size of walnut.

It should be sent for histological examination in order to exclude tuberculous adenitis.

TUBERCULOSIS OF THE MESENTERIC LYMPH NODES

It is very rare disease because of dramatic public health improvement. Nevertheless, in the absence of pulmonary tuberculosis, milk containing the bovine type of tuberculous bacilli is the primary source for the transmission of infection to the mesenteric lymph nodes. It is still prevalent in the developing countries, where cows remain the primary source of carrying with this type of tuberculous bacilli. Once these bacilli are swallowed with the milk, the mesenteric lymph nodes are affected through the Peyer's patches.

Age is no bar despite the fact that children are more vulnerable to this debilitating disease. A loss of appetite, loss of body weight, pale color, evening rise of temperature and a vague central abdominal pain are the general clinical features. Sometimes, abdominal pain may be acute, associated with vomiting. Abdomen may appear to be protuberant centrally. It may contain some degree of ascitic fluid due to tuberculous peritonitis. It would be difficult to differentiate the tuberculous lymphadenitis from nonspecific lymphadenitis or appendicitis.

Among all routine investigations, the following specific investigations should be done: These are chest X-ray, sputum test for acid fast bacilli, blood test for FBC, Hb, ESR, and Mantoux test and stool test for parasites.

In addition, USS, plain X-ray of the abdomen and CT scan should be done, if there is such suspicion of TB intestine. In this case, calcified mesenteric lymph nodes may be present in the plain X-ray of the abdomen, but their positions will appear to be inconsistent with the X-ray of the abdomen, taken on expiration or inspiration. This does not suggest that these features could be associated with TB lymphadenitis. For tissue diagnosis, needle biopsy from those enlarged lymph nodes could be done under the guidance of CT scan.

Small bowel enema should be done to exclude stricture in the terminal ileum or filling defect in the colon.

PATHOLOGY OF THE APPENDICULAR MASS OR ABSCESS

Despite the symptoms being known to the patient, admission to the surgical ward is delayed over 6–12 hours. And it could be a few days, if the patients are from the villages. By the time, the patient is examined in the ward; the total duration of symptoms has probably passed at least 12 hours. If the palpation reveals a well-defined tender mass in the right iliac fossa, it is more likely that the total duration of the symptoms has exceeded over 2 days.

In this case, either perforation or gangrene of the appendix has taken place. To conceal the perforated or gangrenous appendix, the greater omentum has wrapped up the appendix and the cecum.

The common site for perforation is usually at the distal end, where the appendix may appear to be gangrenous state. This is due to thrombosis of the terminal artery. Perforation may also occur at the site of impaction of the fecolith. This is due to pressure necrosis, caused by the fecolith.

Initially, there would be a diffuse tenderness associated with a guarding in the right iliac fossa. This is due to the infective and inflammatory collection of fluid accumulated around the cecum, inflamed or gangrenous or perforated appendix. In some cases, the appendix will appear swollen and edematous. Within 2 days, the area is sealed off by the small intestine and greater omentum. This forms a well-defined mass because, the rigidity surrounding this mass is less marked or worn off. It takes around three days to be localized.

The boundary of the lump could easily be marked out by a gentle palpation with the tip of the fingers. This boundary of the palpable mass is marked with a skin pencil between the soft non-tender and the tender edge of the palpable mass. Rest of the abdomen will appear to be soft and non-tender.

Temperature will continue to swing up and down for a few days, but its pattern will start falling downwards after 2 days since the conservative treatment has been commenced with intravenous infusion of fluids and appropriate antibiotics.

This implies that the patient is responding to the conservative treatment. Furthermore, the size of the tender mass should be evaluated everyday and its boundary should be marked out everyday with a skin pencil. This will show whether or not the size is getting smaller. Patient will admit that he has passed wind per rectum and feels hungry. Patient may start having bowel movement and the motion could be soft or loose in consistency.

COMPOSITION OF THE APPENDICULAR MASS

The appendix could be inflamed, edematous, swollen and perforated or gangrenous.

In addition cecum may be edematous, fecolith may be lying outside the appendix, surrounded by the collection of purulent fluid, fibrinous flakes, dilated loops of the terminal ileum and greater omentum.

In elderly patients, the cecal carcinoma should be suspected within the appendicular mass. During taking the history, patient should be asked for any change in bowel habit over the last few weeks, loss of body weight, poor appetite and tired or sickly feeling or fullness in the lower abdomen. In the blood tests, the striking finding would be low hemoglobin. In this case, USS, and Plain X-ray should be done.

SURGICAL PROCEDURE FOR ACUTE APPENDICITIS

Emergency appendicectomy is the bread and butter for the trainee surgeons. This provides the opportunity to be a self-trained surgeon and more often the opportunity comes at night or in the weekend, where the senior surgeons are not available to teach or to supervise the trainee surgeons.

Despite the opportunity being available, safety and well-being of the patients have to be the prime concern to all surgeons. Emergency appendicectomy could provide a cutting experience, but one should not take the advantage of the trust and poor clinical judgement.

The criteria for emergency appendicectomy are the duration of the symptoms, evidence of raised temperature, (around 37.2°C or above), raised pulse rate, tenderness in the right iliac fossa (RIF), associated with the guarding. A high temperature, rigors, and tenderness in the loins are more likely to be related to a urinary tract infection or pyelonephritis. Decision to operate upon the patient may be influenced by additional findings, which are rebound tenderness in the RIF, and tenderness on rectal digital examination.

THE CRITERIA FOR DEFERRING THE OPERATION

a. Duration of symptoms over 48 hours.
b. Well-defined tender lump in the RIF without generalized peritonitis.

A high white cell count, guarding and rebound tenderness around the lump, swinging temperature are the evidences of appendicular mass or abscess. In these cases, patient may have diarrhea.

For a benefit of doubt, these cases should be treated with conservative regimens. These are nil by mouth, hourly aspiration by the NG tube, intravenous antibiotics covering for both aerobic and anaerobic bacteria, intravenous fluids, hourly recording of temperature, pulse rate and urine output. In most cases, they begin to feel better within 48 hours.

If the operation is deferred for the next 24-48 hours, the palpable lump in the RIF should be marked with a skin pencil. This will guide the surgeon whether it is getting smaller and softer.

The reason for deferring the operation or to adopt a policy of wait and watch is to avoid the risk of spread of pus from the localized area to all over the peritoneal cavity, leading to a generalized peritonitis. This may cause a serious intraperitoneal sepsis such as subphrenic abscess, paracolic abscess or pelvic abscess.

It would be unwise to interfere with the body's defence in which the omentum has provided the protection of the peritoneal cavity from the risk of generalized purulent peritonitis, by wrapping up the inflamed or gangrenous appendix, thus forming an appendicular mass or abscess in the RIF.

EVIDENCES OF RESPONDING TO CONSERVATIVE TREATMENT

1. Swinging temperature is falling everyday.
2. Pulse rate is returning towards a normal range.
3. Palpable lump is getting softer and smaller in size.
4. No evidence of a generalized peritonitis.
5. Has passed wind per rectum.
6. Tolerating oral fluid and appetite is getting better.
7. WCC count is back to a near normal.
8. CRP will be coming down.

If the patient develops a generalized peritonitis, operation must be carried out.

INITIAL THERAPEUTIC MEASURE

There is no detrimental effect, for commencing an intravenous infusion with dextrose saline, before a full investigation is carried out. On the contrary, it would assist in the correction of preexisting dehydration. Patient should be advised not to drink, until further review is carried out. Due to dehydration and starvation, patient may suffer from ketoacidosis, and acetone will be detected in the ward urine test. Nurses are advised to keep recording hourly intake and output chart, hourly pulse rate and temperature chart, and to keep the patient nil by mouth until a final decision is made.

Antibiotic therapy should be commenced based upon the clinical diagnosis, and if the blood test shows the leukocytosis counts above the normal range and elevated C reactive protein.

PREOPERATIVE PREPARATION

Patient must receive supportive treatment for tissue hydration, and to combat systemic infection. It is also equally important that patient is having a good urine output before the operation being done.

TECHNIQUE FOR APPENDICECTOMY

A wider skin preparation with antiseptic solution should be done; in case a laparotomy needs to be done through a separate incision or the existing wound needs to be extended in either direction.

A grid iron oblique incision is made at the McBurney's point in the right iliac fossa.

The line of incision should be made at the junction of a lateral one-third and a medial two-third of the line drawn between the anterior superior iliac spine and umbilicus. And two-third of the incision should be towards the medial side and one-third towards the lateral side from the said point (Fig. 17.1).

One needs to know the surgical importance of the landmark for the proposed incision to be made. If the incision is made more medially, it would be over the anterior rectus sheath. If the incision is made more laterally, extension of the wound would be limited and delivery of the cecum would be struggling and the scar will be close to the iliac bone. In most cases, the appendix remains sitting over the iliac fossa.

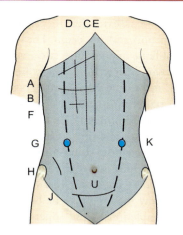

Fig. 17.1: The site of grid iron oblique incision is shown at H

The length of the incision should be around 2 inches for children and 3 inches for the adults but it could be extended medially or laterally that could be done by splitting up the longitudinal muscle fibers of the external oblique aponeurosis, if the position of the appendix is not easily accessible through the existing wound.

After the incision is made, the subcutaneous fatty tissues are cut by the knife along the line of the same skin incision. The bleeding vessels are picked up by a small curved artery forceps. These vessels could be ligated with a fine thread or coagulated but the skin edges must be protected from the thermal heat.

The fatty layer is separated by the scissors and they are held apart by the self- retaining retractor or by the Langerbeck retractors. The shining aponeurotic fibers could be seen running obliquely up and down. They are the external oblique aponeurotic fibers. It is incised for 2 cm with a knife, an inch medial to the anterior superior iliac spine.

The cut edges, picked up by the two artery forceps are lifted up, thus permitting the surgeon to pass the scissors under the aponeurotic fascia. The window is next extended in both directions by scissors. Each aponeurotic flap is mobilized medially and laterally from the underneath muscles. They are held apart by the retractors.

The transversus abdominis muscle fibers could be seen running transversely away from the anterior superior iliac spine. Underneath these muscles lie the internal oblique muscles. Both are split up by putting a straight scissors between the parallel muscle fibers.

Cleavage is created between the parallel muscle fibers, when the scissors is opened up. This maneuver is repeated until all the muscle fibers are separated from each other. The scissors is next inserted into the same cleavage, but it is opened up in an opposite direction between the muscle fibers, thus opening the cleavage wider so that these muscle fibers could be retracted further by the index fingers or by the Langerbeck retractors, inserted inside the cleavage.

Once both right and left index fingers have been put in the cleavage, the fibers are pulled apart and are held apart by the retractors. And this separation should be closer to the edge of the rectus sheath. Because, the ilioinguinal and iliohypogastric nerves pass between the transversus abdominis and internal oblique muscles, and they are situated by the side of the anterior superior iliac spine. These nerves should not be damaged or caught in the stitches.

The transversalis fascia and the peritoneum are picked up and lifted up by the two artery forceps. The tent of the peritoneum is examined by a palpation to be sure that intestinal wall has not been caught up by the two artery forceps. A small nick is made between the two artery forceps, peritoneal fluid will start emerging through the tiny window. The suction tube is inserted through the hole.

Under the peritoneum, edematous greater omentum could be seen floating. This is pushed inside either by the suction tube or by the nontooth forceps. The window is extended under protection of the nontooth forceps that is put under the peritoneum, thus guarding the gut or omentum from being caught up by the tip of the scissors. If these structures are protruding through the peritoneal wound, they should be pushed back, by inserting the wet swab, which is held in position by the retractors, inserted inside the peritoneal cavity, thus keeping the greater omentum and the small intestine away from the wound.

It is common to see the dilated terminal ileum around the RIF, obscuring the finding of the cecum and appendix. This dilatation is the localized paralytic ileus that resulted from the infection. The cecum is picked up by the Babcock forceps and it is delivered out of the peritoneal cavity. This will bring the base of the appendix with it. Pus swab is sent for culture.

The cecum is held by the wet warm swab outside the peritoneal cavity. The appendix is next held by the Babcock forceps in order to define the boundary of the mesentery.

Some surgeons advocate for a single mass ligature of the mesoappendix. This is done by making a small window in the mesentery at the angle between the cecum and the base of the appendix. Through this hole, the ligature is passed to be ligated around the free edge of the mesoappendix. Having done this ligature, the mesentery is cut along its attachment to the appendix. But there remains a risk of bleeding from the vessels, if the vessels slipped out from the mass ligature, applied around the free edge of the mesoappendix.

Alternatively, individual appendicular vessels could be divided between the artery forceps, passed transversely below the appendix. They are ligated separately.

Now, only the appendix needs to be amputated from its base. For this purpose, a pair of small artery forceps is applied across the proposed level of amputation of the appendix, a little above the base of the appendix. Then, a ligature is put around the base 2 cm below the clamps applied to the appendix. A purse string suture is next applied around the base of the cecum and away from the junction of the appendix, and it should be 2 cm proximal to the ligature.

The appendix is transected by a knife, but it should be 1 cm distal to the ligature. The appendix is sent for histology. The knife and swab that is used to wipe out the appendicular stump are put in the separate tray. They are contaminated. The stump is next buried into the cecal wall by the purse string suture. For a safety reason, a piece of omental graft or remnant of the mesoappendix could be used to cover the said burial site of the cecum by a few stitches.

The cecum is put back into the peritoneal cavity but the terminal ileum is pulled back instead. The purpose is to look for Meckel's diverticulum, which is expected to be present 2 ft away from the ileocecal junction and its incidence is about 2 percent among the population. It is important to examine the small intestine in all cases of appendectomy. Once this has been done, the intestine is put back in the same order, as they were brought out.

Finally, the suction tube is put inside into the bottom of the pelvis to be sure that there is no collection of pus. Saline wash out should be given if there was collection of pus around the cecum. Like other cases, wound lavage with metronidazole 500 mg should be done. A drainage tube should be left into the peritoneal cavity, if there were gangrenous appendix or puss found in the area.

The peritoneal edges are picked up by the artery forceps. It is closed with a continuous suture. The internal oblique and transversus abdominis muscles are closed together with two interrupted sutures. The corners and the edges of the external oblique aponeurotic fascia are picked up by the artery forceps and they are closed with continuous sutures. Fatty layer may need to be sutured, if necessary. The skin wound is closed in the usual way. If the drain has been brought out through a separate wound, it is anchored with a silk suture. Finally, wound dressing is applied.

DEALING WITH THE PROBLEMS

The cecum is not in the normal anatomical position, and the appendix is not visible at the initial examination. In these cases, the right index finger is inserted in order to find out the position of the cecum and the appendix and the left index finger is used to examine the pelvis. In female patient, sometimes ovarian cysts may be palpable but it should not be excised.

In many cases, an inflamed and swollen appendix remains behind the cecum or in the pelvis or higher up in the RIF. If the cecum could not be pulled out due to adhesion, or it is located higher up, the wound needs to be extended in either direction in line with the skin incision.

The skin incision is extended in accordance with the position of the appendix and the cecum. The longitudinal fibers of the external oblique aponeurotic fascia are also cut along its fibers in the same direction. Swabs are put inside the peritoneal cavity, to protect the intestine, before the internal oblique and the transversus abdominis muscles are divided.

The transversus abdominis muscle fibers and the internal oblique muscle fibers are identified. Only the upper or lower part of the muscle fibers need to be cut with the scissors that depend upon the exact position of the appendix or the cecum. The peritoneum is next incised in that direction. This wide exploration will allow the cecum to be brought out into the wound for the completion of the appendicectomy.

Despite all these procedures being followed up, the base of the appendix may not be accessible for appendicectomy. In this case, the taeniae coli of the cecum are followed up that may lead to the base of the appendix. In elderly patient, either sigmoid colon or the transverse colon may be pulled out by mistake. Surgeon must be aware of the abnormal position of the colon.

And if the base of the appendix is not easily visible, the dissection of the mesoappendix is commenced from the tip of the appendix, by dividing and ligating the vessels and the mesentery, one by one individually. This retrograde dissection is continued towards the base of the appendix. At last, the appendicectomy is completed as described before.

At the completion of the appendicectomy, the corners of the peritoneum are picked up from where the continuous suture begins. After this closure, the transected muscles are sutured together in line with its fibers and then the split section of the internal oblique and transversus abdominis muscle are sutured with 2-3 interrupted sutures, thus obliterating the cleavage that was initially created with scissors. The rest of the wound closure is straightforward.

In certain cases, appendicectomy must not be done, in those cases in which, the terminal ileum reveals the features of Crohn's ileitis. If by mistake, it has been done, there remains a risk of blow-out of the appendicular stump. In other cases, Meckel's diverticulum could be resected if it is present on initial examination, but there remains a risk of intestinal obstruction, if anastomosis is not carried out with due care; the anastomosis may breakdown, resulting in fecal peritonitis in the postoperative period. These complications must be kept in mind, while dealing with those pathological conditions.

If the appendicular abscess resolves with the conservative treatment, an interval appendicectomy is recommended. If an elderly or middle-aged person is admitted with acute appendicitis or with a tender palpable lump in the RIF, this case should be investigated to exclude carcinoma of the cecum or regional ileitis. Eventually, a laparotomy should be undertaken, despite the fact that all investigations turned out to be normal.

POSTOPERATIVE CARE

Routine observation is carried out.

Oral fluid is commenced after 24 hours and feeding is commenced, if the patient has passed wind per rectum and patient is discharged home after he opens the bowel, and the temperature remains normal over 48 hours. He should stay in the hospital, until the drainage tube or corrugated sheet has been removed or the wound appears to be inflamed.

Further investigation may be necessary if the histology report suggests that there was carcinoid in the appendix. Right hemicolectomy should be considered at some stage.

POSTOPERATIVE COMPLICATIONS

a. Internal bleeding from the mesenteric vessels due to slip ligature.
b. Wound infection.
c. Pelvis abscess.
d. Appendicular stump blow-out and fecal peritonitis.
e. Chest infection or collapsed lung.
f. Intestinal obstruction.
g. Deep vein thrombosis and/or pulmonary embolism.
h. Incisional hernia.
i. Pain in the scar or in the groin due to entrapment of nerves in the wound.
j. Risk of damage to the wall of the intestine by the suction drainage tube, if the suction pressure is kept very high and if the size of the holes on the wall of the drainage tube are greater than 2 mm.

Patient may develop a wound infection or pelvic abscess after a few days or weeks. In these cases, patient may need to be readmitted. In some cases, the early sign for pelvic collection is the rise of temperature that could be swinging up and down. Or there could be a feeling of nausea or vomiting associated with or without a soft or loose motion. In some cases, patient may show features of septicemia, which could be paleness in skin color, rapid pulse rate, hypotension, severing along with a rise of temperature and vomiting.

These patients require an immediate resuscitation with intravenous infusion and antibiotics. Abdominal examination will reveal either a localized or generalized peritonitis, dull on percussion over or around the pelvic abscess or around the appendicular scar.

Investigations include a plain X-ray of the chest, X-ray of the abdomen and abdominal USS. Routine blood tests are FBC, Hb, CRP, electrolytes and urea.

The plain X-ray of the abdomen may show features of dilated small and large intestine right down into the rectum. These are referred to as a paralytic ileus, provided, the bowel sounds are found absent on auscultation.

The X-ray of the chest may also reveal a basal consolidation or collapsed lung. These findings may give rise to elevated temperature and tachypnea. And the chest infection may refer to abdominal symptoms and paralytic ileus. It is equally possible that all these findings in the X-ray of the chest may be attributable to subphrenic abscess.

After reviewing the results and further examination, decision is taken whether an emergency laparotomy is necessary. Conservative approach may be considered, if the abscess remains localized and the temperature is coming down.

TUMORS OF THE APPENDIX

They are adenoma, adenocarcinoma and carcinoid. Among these rare varieties of the tumors, carcinoid is common and its incidence is 0.4 percent among the pathological lesions developed in the appendix. It affects the women more than the men and its incidence could be as high as 80 percent. And the age group is between 20 and 30 years, but some literature refers to between 10 and 60 years. Outside the appendix, carcinoid may be found in the small intestine and it is rare in the colon and rectum.

PATHOLOGY

It is present in the distal part of the appendix and lies in the space between the mucosa and the serosal layer of the appendix. It appears to be a circumscribed nodule that could be recognized by its golden color on naked eye, because of presence of lipoid contents within the tissue. When it increases its size, it causes obstruction to the lumen of the appendix, thus causing acute appendicitis.

In most cases, it does not metastasis unless it invades the mesoappendix. In all instances, appendicectomy is carried out; further surgical intervention depends upon the histology report and other 24 hour urine test for 5- hydroxyl indole acetic acid. This test would suggest whether or not the metastasis has already occurred in the liver.

If the tumor has invaded the mesoappendix found at the operation, right hemicolectomy should be carried out. This is an academic advice, but it would not cause any adverse effect by delaying this major operation. In this case, one should wait for the histology report and on the merit of this report, further consultation should be carried out with the patients with a view to considering a right hemicolectomy.

BIOCHEMICAL EFFECT OF THE TUMOR

This tumor arises from the cells known as Kulchitsyk present in the crypts of Lieberkühn. It is related to autonomic nervous system and it has a characteristic affinity for silver stains. Because of this observation, it is also known as argentaffin tumors. It liberates a chemical known as 5-hydroxy tryptamine, also known as serotonin. It has a profound effect upon the gut motility resulting in an increased peristalsis. It may cause constriction of the bronchus and pulmonary hypertension. The latter is due to vasoconstriction of pulmonary arteriole.

When it is injected into the tissue, it may produce local congestion and it may cause flushing on the face and hands like a brilliant brick red color. If the tumor causes metastasis in the liver, this chemical is then changed to 5-hydroxyl indole acetic acid which is excreted in the urine.

Carcinoid tumor is a slow growing and low grade tumor. In the small intestine, the terminal ileum seems to be the common site for developing this tumor. It may give rise to abdominal pain, diarrhea, and loss of body weight. And in advanced condition, it may lead to intestinal obstruction. It may metastasis to the mesenteric lymph nodes and then to the liver, where, much of its chemical products are metabolized. In these cases, prognosis is poor.

REFERENCE

1. Wangensteen OH, Bowers WF. Arch Surg 1937;34:490.

18 Reversal of Transverse Loop Colostomy

The closure of loop colostomy is a simple procedure that could be employed either with extraperitoneal or intraperitoneal approach; but the decision is taken after the result of barium enema being known to the surgeon. This particular investigation is done a few weeks after the resection of the diseased segment of the left colon or the rectum has been done.

PREOPERATIVE ASSESSMENT

Complete evacuation of the hard feces and inspissated barium from the colon and rectum has to be carried out. This requires laxatives to be inserted into the colostomy for the clearance of hard feces present in the distal colon. In addition, phosphate enema, followed by soap and water enemas is given from the rectum. After this procedure being done, rectal examination and sigmoidoscopy are carried out. Postoperative anastomotic leakage may occur if the distal bowel clearance remains unsatisfactory.

Patient is kept on oral fluid after oral laxative is given for the clearance of the proximal colon. The risk of wound infection, fistula formation and incisional hernia has to be highlighted to the patient before consent is obtained from the patient.

Patient remains nil by mouth for 12 hours prior to surgery and should have nasogastric tube before going to the theater table. All other prophylactic measures as described before with other major operations must be adopted in this operation.

Patient needs a final rectal digital examination and sigmoidoscopy, when lying on the Lloyd Davis Table. The rectal digital examination may reveal a degree of anal stenosis. This could be the result of disuse action of the anal orifice, and is also due to maintaining of a high sphincteric muscle tone. This may result from the diversion of the feces that is drained through the loop colostomy.

In physiological terms, this is referred to as disuse anal stenosis. If this is the apparent clinical features around the circular muscle of the sphincters, there could be a similar condition around the site of anastomosis and all along the left colon and the rectum. The latter may provide some degree of intraluminal resistance to the propagative peristalsis after the colostomy is closed.

In the literature, anastomotic dehiscence after closure of the colostomy has been reported. The possible explanation for this postoperative complication in those reported cases could be attributable to disuse anal stenosis. This dysfunctional state of the distal colon, the rectum and the anal sphincters could be overcome by the following measures and treatment.

Apart from the mechanical evacuation of the hard feces, the anal orifice is dilated by three fingers and rigid sigmoidoscopy is carried out. This procedure assists in overcoming the temporary disuse activity of the circular muscles of the rectum and the sigmoid colon by the mechanical dilatation and by the inflated air. Since these therapeutic measures have been implemented in all cases, there was not a single case of anastomotic leakage occurring in those postoperative patients.

TECHNIQUE FOR INTRAPERITONEAL CLOSURE

Skin preparation and draping around the operative area remain the same. The mucocutaneous edges of the colostomy are lifted up by the Allis Tissue Forceps. This would make the skin edge taught—thus assisting the surgeon to make elliptical incisions around the mucocutaneous edge of the colostomy. The line incision should be 0.3 cm away from the edge (Fig. 18.1).

After cutting the edge all around by a small knife, the subcutaneous tissues are dissected out by the fine scissors and a cleavage is created under the cut edge of the skin, while the edge of the colostomy is held up and away from the skin edge (Fig. 18.2).

The skin cut edge is retracted by a small Langerbeck retractor. This would assist the surgeon to identify the serosal wall of the colostomy from the surrounding parietal wound.

Eventually, the colostomy edge is lifted further up from the depth of the wound and the peritoneal cavity as shown

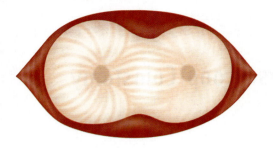

Fig. 18.1: Showing a transverse elliptical incision made around the edge of the colostomy

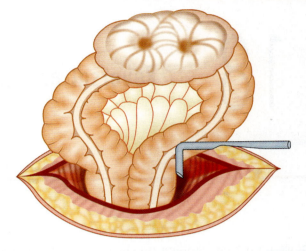

Fig. 18.3: Showing the two limbs of the transverse colostomy separated from each other, thus displaying the transverse mesocolon. Rectus abdominis muscle is kept holding retracted by the Langerbeck retractor

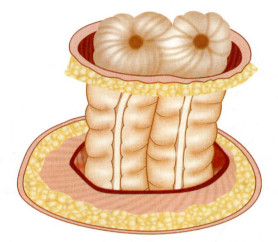

Fig. 18.2: The loop colostomy has been dissected out from the surrounding area of the skin edges

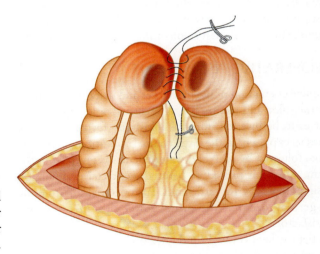

Fig. 18.4: Showing how end-to-end anastomosis is commenced by interrupted sutures

in the Figure 18.2. By doing so, the peritoneal cavity is opened at one side that would assist the surgeon for further mobilization of the colon. This is done by the index finger that is inserted around the colon into the peritoneal cavity.

The colostomy will be eventually separated from the surrounding fibrinous or omental adhesions by inserting the index finger into the intraperitoneal cavity. The taeniae coli of the colon will guide the surgeon in order to identify the proximal and distal limbs of the transverse colon. By a gentle clearance of all those fibrinous adhesions or omental bands, both limbs are separated from each other (Fig.18.3). Once complete separation has been done, the fibrosed mucocutaneous ring around the colostomy is excised with the scissors.

Normal mucosal edge will appear, and the blood vessel starts spurting from the cut edges of the mucosa. There is no need to excise the posterior colonic wall that would be the only continuity left between the two limbs of the colon.

Now, intraperitoneal anastomosis between the two stomas is commenced either by interrupted hand sutures or by autosutures. For the purpose of hand sutures, stay suture is inserted at each corner (Fig. 18.4).

The end-to-end anastomosis begins with interrupted sutures, the technique of which has been described in previous section. The anastomosis could be done safely by single layer interrupted stitches (Fig. 18.5) or by two layers that depend upon the practice of the operator.

At the end, each interrupted suture is ligatured. The threads are cut. The proximal colon is next milky out towards the distal colon. This is done between the index and middle finger towards the distal colon. The purpose is to see any evidence of leakage of air bubbles and liquid feces, coming out through the spaces in between the sutures, holding the cut edges of the anastomosis.

Once this has been satisfied, the anastomosis should be concealed with the omental graft. The colon is next put back into the peritoneal cavity. Local wash out with saline is first

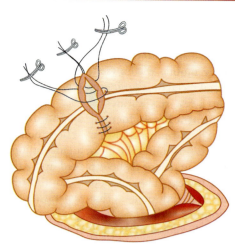

Fig. 18.5: Showing the technique how anastomosis is carried out by a single layer interrupted sutures, inserted between the two cut edges of the stomas

given. It is next followed by metronidazole (500 mg) lavage, as described before.

It is important to put a drain into the peritoneal cavity, but what sort of drainage system is to be used depends upon the experience and confidence of the surgeon.

In uncomplicated cases, a redivac drain is left in the right side of the abdomen and it is brought out through a stab wound. The suction should not be commenced until 2 hours have passed.

In other cases, where there remains a risk of leakage of feces, a corrugated or a tube drain could be used. This sort of drainage may assist in the discharge of pus or feces, if anastomotic dehiscence occurs later. And a fistula track may develop between the colon and the parietal wound after the drainage is removed. This fistula will heal slowly if there is no distal colonic obstruction. Hence, surgeon needs to decide about the type of drainage to be inserted into the peritoneal cavity, before the abdominal wound is closed in layers.

TECHNIQUE FOR EXTRAPERITONEAL CLOSURE

In this approach, the mucocutaneous edge of the colostomy is dissected out from the skin as described before. The loop of the colostomy is mobilized from the parietal walls of the abdomen without entering into the peritoneal cavity. After adequate mobilization of each side of the stomas, the mucocutaneous rim of fibrous tissue is excised all around. Index finger is passed into the lumen of both proximal and distal colon. The aim is to see any obstruction inside the lumen.

For end-to-end anastomosis, stay suture is inserted through each corner of the stomas for defining the boundary of the stoma that needs to be sutured with interrupted stitches, as described before. This anastomosis could be done in two layers or it could be carried out with autosuture. The colon is put back inside the abdomen. As before, wound lavage with metronidazole should be done. A drainage tube is left nearby before the parietal wound is closed in the usual way.

POSTOPERATIVE CARE

The postoperative care would be no different from any other colonic surgery. Hence, prophylactic antibiotics are continued. For the first few days, regular aspiration through the NG tube is carried out and the oral fluid is restricted until the patient has passed wind per rectum. It takes more than 4 days after operation is done. If there is no rise of temperature, and the patient has tolerated the oral fluid day-by-day, light diet could be commenced initially.

If the patient feels hungry and has opened soft feces per rectum, solid diet could be given. Drainage tube is removed after defecation and no collection of purulent fluid is evident in the bottle. Skin sutures are removed on the 10th postoperative day.

POSTOPERATIVE COMPLICATIONS

Patient may complain of discomfort and distention of the abdomen, associated with or without vomiting in the postoperative period. If there is no evidence of peritonitis, conservative regimen should be adopted. This includes hourly NG tube aspiration, nil by mouth and intravenous infusion. Plain X-ray of the abdomen is arranged and blood investigations are carried out.

If there is swelling and inflammation around the wound, this could be abscess that may start discharging spontaneously through the scar. Pus swab is sent for culture and sensitivity test.

If the underlying abscess is related to anastomotic dehiscence, either fecal peritonitis or colocutaneous fistula may develop. In the absence of peritonitis, colostomy bag is put around the fistula. If there is no distal obstruction, it will close slowly over three months. Local wound dressing would be necessary. If the fistula does not close, reexploration would be necessary. For cases with peritonitis, reexploration is to be done as an emergency procedure. In this case, the anastomosis needs to be re-done.

REVERSAL OF THE HARTMANN'S PROCEDURE

Preoperative Preparation and Consultation

Patient is given oral laxatives in order to keep the colon empty and through the anal orifice, evacuation of feces would be necessary. These could be done with a phosphate enema, followed by a soap and water enema. Patient should be on oral fluids for 24 hours prior to the operation. Intravenous infusion with normal saline could be commenced if necessary. The rectum must be examined with the sigmoidoscope after rectal wash out has been given.

Patient must be warned that anastomosis may breakdown or reversal may not be feasible technically, despite exploration of the abdomen being carried out. There could be fistula, pelvic abscess, wound dehiscence or intestinal obstruction.

Operative Procedure

Patient is placed on the Trendelenburg lithotomy position on the Lloyd-Davis Table. Foley's catheter is inserted into the bladder and its residual volume is recorded. Preoperative prophylactic antibiotics, covering for both aerobic and anaerobic bacilli are given and should be continued for 5-7 days.

Rectal digital examination and sigmoidoscopy should be done before the operation is commenced. If there is evidence of tightness around the anal orifice, it should be dilated with three fingers.

Skin preparation and the layout of the draping are carried out like APR. Through the old scar, the abdomen is opened and the wounds are retracted with the self-retaining retractors. There could be lots of fibrinous adhesions among the loops of the small intestine and under the abdominal scar. These adhesions are carefully separated from the scar, from the pelvis, from the area around the left lumbar region and around the segment of the terminal colostomy. All these guts are pushed to the upper abdomen and tucked under the packs.

Concentration is focused on the identification of the distal stump. If the nylon thread could be traced out from the scar tissue, this will guide the surgeon to dissect out the distal rectal stump. Despite this approach being adopted, the rectal stump may not be possible to be located in the pelvis. In this situation, either the assistant or the surgeon could pass the sigmoidoscope through the anal orifice and it has to be passed under a direct vision, until the blind end of the rectum is in sight. From the abdomen, the tip of the instrument could be felt and this will assist the surgeon to dissect the stump out from the surrounding adhesions.

The blind end of the rectum is picked up by two pair of Babcock forceps before the sigmoidoscope is removed from the rectum. The distal stump is mobilized from the pelvic wall, until it is fully mobile with attached mesentery. The blind end of the distal rectal or colonic stump is excised and its edge is held up by a few stay sutures.

Now, concentration is focused on the dissection and detachment of the terminal colostomy. This is done by putting an elliptical incision around the mucocutaneous junction. The rim of the mucocutaneous tissue is picked up by the Babcock or other tissue forceps. The dissection is continued all around from outside the abdomen— thus separating it from the parietal abdominal wall.

The terminal colostomy is pushed inside the peritoneal cavity or alternatively it could be dissected out from inside the abdomen. If the length of the terminal colostomy appears to be short or inadequate, it may require to be mobilized from the parietal wall, until a reasonable length of the descending colon is mobilized with a view to carrying out end-to-end anastomosis without tension.

Once this has been done, the rim of mucocutaneous tissue is excised all around to be sure that the capillary vessels are spurting from the cut edge of the mucosa. The continuity of the gut is restored by end-to-end anastomosis with interrupted stitches or by Stapling Gun (EEA), as described before.

At the completion of the anastomosis, a tube drain is left in the pelvis. Wound lavage is carried out as described before. The colostomy wound is closed from inside the abdomen and the dead space should be obliterated by interrupted strong Vicryl No.1 sutures. At the end, the skin wound is closed from outside. Abdominal wound is closed in the usual way.

POSTOPERATIVE CARE AND COMPLICATIONS

Routine procedure is followed in this case, like any other colonic surgery. The drainage tube should not be removed until the bowels open.

Among the complications, anastomotic leakage, fecal fistula, pelvic abscess, wound infection and chest infection are possible.

19 The Anus

It comprises of anal canal, anal sphincter, and anal orifice. It seems to be of less clinical importance but treatment of many complicated diseases developed in this anatomical site could be a difficult task to the clinician. As a result, these may lead to chronic conditions.

Common diseases are:
- Hemorrhoids, known as piles
- Perianal abscess
- Perianal fistula
- Fissure-in-ano
- Pruritus ani
- Papilloma known as anal warts.

Other rare varieties related to other primary diseases. These are:
- Proctitis
- Crohn's disease
- Tuberculous lesion
- Anal stricture

Malignant tumor
- Squamous cell carcinoma
- Basal cell carcinoma
- Adenocarcinoma
- Malignant melanoma.

All these diseases will be described in that order.

HEMORRHOIDS

Background of the Hemorrhoids

Hemorrhoids are also referred to as piles. They are in fact dilated venous plexus like tortuous varicose veins in the lower limb. They are also located in the anal canal that is the dependent part of the portal system as well as the dependent part of the left colon and rectum and these veins do not have valves, but these venous plexus are formed by the radicals of the superior, middle and inferior rectal veins. Although, hemorrhoids are attributable to local factors, men are more frequently affected than women. The reason for this difference is not known.

ETIOLOGY

1. Idiopathic varieties are those cases where no cause for developing the piles could be identified. The majority cases belong to this category.
2. Obstruction of the venous return to the portal vein could be due to the local attributing factors. These are rectal carcinoma at the rectosigmoid region, pregnant uterus, constipation, and bladder outlet obstruction due to enlarged prostate or urethral stricture. Surprisingly, no association has been found between the cirrhosis and the piles.
3. Heredity seems to be prevailing among the family members like varicose veins. In fact, piles and varicose veins are found frequently in the same person concurrently. There could be congenital defect in the venous wall of the piles.
4. Chronic obstructive airway disease may contribute to delayed venous return to the portal veins.

PATHOLOGY

Piles are of two types, one is known as internal piles while the other one is known as external piles. The anatomical sites for the internal piles are consistent with the anatomical distribution of the superior hemorrhoidal or rectal artery. The latter is first divided into right and left branches and the right branch is again divided into anterior and posterior branches, which follow down along 7 and 11 o'clock positions on the right side, but the left branch descends and lies at the 3 o'clock position on the left side of the anal canal. The venous return from the anal canal follows along the superior rectal arterial trees.

Hence, the sites of the piles or hemorrhoids lie at 3 o'clock, 7 o'clock and 11 o'clock positions within the wall of the anal canal. Internal hemorrhoids are covered by the anal mucosa and by contrast, the external hemorrhoids, although they are the propagation of the internal hemorrhoids, are covered by the skin below the level of dentate line.

The external piles could be seen around the anal orifice and their anatomical sites remain consistent with that of the internal hemorrhoids. But additional smaller piles could be seen in between the primary piles. Within the tuff of the dilated varicose venous plexus lie tributaries of the superior rectal arteries.

In sharp contrast, bleeding from the piles is bright red blood, seen in the commode or toilet wiping papers. This raises a question in the pathogenesis of piles as to why venous blood is rarely seen in the commode at defecation and as to why the piles are not found among the patient developing cirrhosis of liver.

A new research is necessary to establish the etiological factors, whether the composition of piles is primarily of dilated superior hemorrhoidal arteries that enhance to tortuous and dilated veins.

Apart from the anatomical distribution, piles could be classified into three categories, on their behavior. If the piles protrude into the lumen of the anal canal and lie above the dentate line, it is called first degree internal piles.

If they descend further and protrude down through the anal orifice on straining at defecation, but they return to its original position spontaneously at the end of defecation, they are called second degree piles.

If the piles descend through the anal orifice and remain outside all the time or are needed to be pushed back into the anal canal by the finger, they are called third degree piles.

At times, these third degree piles may drop out of the anal canal on coughing or sneezing. In these situations, they need to be pushed back digitally. This is an embarrassing situation.

The third degree piles may be strangulated, once they are hanging outside the anal orifice and they may be strangulated by the external anal sphincter that may lead to thrombosis and later ulceration. Also they may discharge mucoid materials, causing pruritus ani.

■ Symptoms

In majority of cases, first degree piles remain silent. If they bleed, the bleeding is painless and it splashes in the pan or they are often recognized seeing the bright red blood soaked in the toilet paper used in wiping the bottom.

If the rectal bleeding is associated with acute and sharp pain in the anus and the pain persists for a few days after being to the toilet, acute fissure-in-ano is likely to be the cause for the rectal bleeding. Alternative diagnosis would be thrombosed external piles, or strangulated internal piles. Patient may complain of only irritation around the anal orifice or may notice some foul smelling and mucus discharge or staining of the underpant.

Although the main symptom is related to painless rectal bleeding, other enquiries, related to bowel actions, appetite, body weight, consistency of the feces are made and all these evidences should be recorded in the case notes. Until internal examination is made, diagnosis should be kept open in mind. Age, family history, pregnancy, cirrhosis of liver and urinary symptoms are all taken into consideration in the differential diagnosis.

■ Clinical Examination

In the general examination as described before, patient may appear to be pale and anemic. Although the symptom may be related to painless bleeding per rectum at defecation, examination should be carried out methodically, as highlighted in other chapters. Palpation of the abdomen should be carried out methodically. Patient is asked to lie flat on the back. Particular attention should be focused on pulsatile mass (aortic aneurysm), enlarged liver, spleen and any palpable mass in the pelvis or along the left colon, like any other abdominal examination.

Patient is next asked to turn on the left side and lie on the left lateral position, bringing both knees towards the left groin.

With the permission of the patient, the anal orifice is first inspected under bright light. This may reveal any evidence of external piles, anal skin tags or prolapsed or thrombosed piles. If nothing is apparent on inspection, then it is possible that internal hemorrhoids, which could be of second or third degree piles, have been pushed back spontaneously or by the patient, before coming to the clinic.

To confirm whether or not there are second or third degree internal piles, patient is requested to give a few coughs. As a result, internal piles will emerge through the anal orifice. If they return inside the anal orifice after a few minutes, then the diagnosis of second degree internal piles is confirmed.

If they remain hanging outside the anal orifice and are needed to be pushed back inside, then third degree piles are diagnosed. Apart from this confirmation, there could be features of inflammation ulceration on the surface of the prolapsed piles. This could be the result of rubbing of a pile with the contralateral piles or with the clothes, while sitting on the chair. In long-standing condition, the lining epithelium may undergo metaplastic changes to squamous type. In advanced cases, pruritus ani could be seen around the perianal skin.

If there is no evidence of external piles, the next approach is to exclude fissure-in-ano. Anal verge on both sides is retracted away from the anal opening by placing left and right fingers over the edge of the anal verge. This may reveal posterior or anterior acute or chronic anal fissure. All cases of painless bleeding should be investigated in order to exclude the carcinoma. These include rectal digital examination, proctoscopic, and sigmoidoscopic examination.

In the absence of anal fissure, rectal digital examination with right index finger is carried out as described before. During this examination, external piles or prolapsed third degree piles are evident on the surface without internal examination. Nevertheless, all routine procedure must be completed as described before.

After this examination, proctoscopy is inserted into the anal canal. And its obturator is withdrawn. The proctoscope is slowly withdrawn or moved around inside the anal canal, the internal piles could be seen bulging into the lumen of the proctoscope or in the anal canal.

After this procedure, sigmoidoscopy is carried out.

In the routine investigations, blood profile should be done. And barium enema and colonoscopy must be arranged in order to exclude any other lesion developed in the colon.

Once the hemorrhoids have been confirmed, the treatment is contemplated that depends upon the degree of hemorrhoids, found on examination.

■ Complications

1. Anemia – This is due to repeated rectal bleeding.
2. Pruritus ani.
3. Prolapse of the internal hemorrhoids, if they are left untreated.
4. Strangulation of the prolapsed internal piles associated with pain.
5. Thrombosis and ulceration of the prolapsed piles, if left untreated.
6. Fibrosis in 2-3 weeks time, if left untreated.
7. Thrombosed external piles associated with acute pain. After a few days, it may discharge old blood clots and later healed spontaneously. The end result would be fibrosis and anal skin tags.

INDICATION FOR HEMORRHOIDECTOMY

Excision of the piles should be carried out for those piles that need to be pushed back. These sort of prolapsed piles are referred to as third degree internal piles.

Unlike the internal piles, external piles in most cases are skin tags. They do not bleed but may cause irritation around the anus. In some rare cases, bulky external piles may develop. Excision of both prolapsed piles and those large external piles is recommended.

All other varieties of internal piles, which are either first or second degree, could be treated with a high-fiber diet. In this line of management, patient is encouraged drinking plenty of plain of fluid and to cut down the daily consumption of tea and coffee. If they do not make any difference, the piles could be treated with the injection of phenol 5 percent in almond oil or with rubber band ligation. These procedures are done at the outpatient clinic.

In both treatments, patient should be explained that there could be some degree of discomfort felt in the anus after treatment.

The injection therapy may need to be repeated in every three to six weeks, but after three course of treatment, further injection needs to be assessed, whether the treatment is effective to the piles. If there is acute fissure-in-ano, proctoscopy should be avoided. In this case, anal dilatation remains the choice of treatment that may resolve both the conditions.

TREATMENT OF PILES WITH INJECTION OF PHENOL IN OIL

Under direct vision, the piles are identified through the proctoscope, phenol, 5 percent in almond oil is injected to the site of the piles but the amount of solution to be injected should not exceed 5 ml in one pile and more than two piles should not be injected in one seating.

In rare cases, the site of injection may be ulcerated or may develop submucosal abscess.

TREATMENT OF PILES WITH RUBBER BAND LIGATION

Rubber band ligations are effective for the second degree piles and no more than two piles should be treated with rubber band ligatures at one seating. They could be repeated six weeks later. In some occasion, bleeding may occur from the sites of rubber band ligation later. This is due to mucosal necrosis.

OPERATIVE TREATMENT FOR LARGER PILES

■ Preoperative Consultation and Preparation

Patient needs to be explained that reactionary or secondary hemorrhage may occur after operation. Patient may need to be taken back to the theater for dealing with the bleeding. Constipation and retention of urine is not uncommon after operation. Anal stenosis, recurrence of piles or anal fissure may develop in some cases.

Preoperative bowel preparation is done with phosphate enema followed by soap and water enema. This procedure is done a few hours before the operation. Overnight bowel preparation is no longer advocated.

TECHNIQUE FOR HEMORRHOIDECTOMY

Patient is placed in lithotomy position on the Lloyd Davis Table. The buttock is rested on the sand bag or on a transverse rubber cushion. The anal orifice should be a few inches away from the said cushion. It is examined with index finger, then with proctoscope and finally with sigmoidoscope in that order. If the rectum remains empty, hemorrhoidectomy should be undertaken.

Before cleaning the bottom, anal dilatation is carried out. The perineal region and the anal canal are cleaned with Savlon solution. Both legs are covered with trousers type drapes. A separate towel is placed under the buttock. Small dry swab is put inside the anal canal and it is pulled back to be left in the anal orifice. This brings the piles from inside the anal canal.

Each pile is picked up by two pairs of the curved artery forceps; one will be holding the outer skin margin that will be hanging from the anal verge and the other one to the anal mucosa covering the pile. They are held by the left hand, but the tip of the left index finger will keep supporting the pile from inside.

By the gentle pull of the forceps that brings the pile downwards and medially, the left index finger of the surgeon keeps supporting, and pressing firmly on the pile from inside the anal orifice. The tongue-shaped prolapsed pile and anal skin is excised commencing from its edge with a curved Mayo's scissors, and this cut would be from both edges of the piles, thus producing a V-shaped skin margin over the anal verge, the apex of which lies just over the subcutaneous external sphincter (Fig. 19.1).

This dissection is done by the tip of the curved Mayo's scissors and is continued towards the anal orifice, by following the direction and distribution of the longitudinal fibers of the anal canal. Some of these longitudinal fibers pass across the subcutaneous external anal sphincter, and others descend to be attached to the mucocutaneous junction, but the venous plexus remain medial to the longitudinal fibers.

The blunt mobilization is carried out by a combination of a swab soaked in savlon and fine dissection. It is continued medially, thus revealing circular fibers of the subcutaneous external anal sphincter. The wedged-shaped anal skin along with the bunch of anal vessels and mucosa is separated from the internal sphincter.

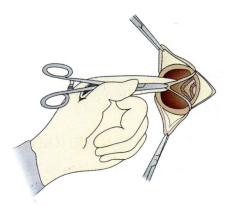

Fig. 19.1: Method of excision of the piles

The pedicle of this pile is transfixed with sutures and the distal stump is excised 2 cm distal to the ligature and the threads are cut 2 inches longer from the knot. Any remaining bleeding point is stopped with diathermy.

In this way, each pile is dissected out from the anal verge and excised after transfixation suture is inserted, but a change of hand would be necessary for the dissection. There should be a strip of skin bridging between the two pear-shaped wounds. Each wound is covered with jelly nets.

A tube drain either alone or wrapped up with jelly net is inserted inside the rectum; but care should be taken that the stump of the piles is not pushed inside with the tube or they are not torn.

A safety-pin is inserted through the tube. Its purpose is to prevent the tube from being slipped into the rectum. Furthermore, jelly net is put around the tube under the safety-pin. This will protect the perineal skin from being injured by the pin. It acts as a pressure dressing in order to stop bleeding from the wounds. Other benefit is to let the flatus pass through the tube, thus relieving wind pain but the tube itself would be uncomfortable to the patient. Dressing pads are put over the perineal wound. These are held over the buttock by the T bandage that is applied across the pelvis.

POSTOPERATIVE CARE

Postoperative analgesic must be given regularly. It is important to see the dressing pads whether it is soaked with blood. It is also important to check whether the bladder is distended or the patient has passed urine within the last 12 hours. On the following day, the tube drain should come off while having a warm sitz bath or it could wait for another day. Oral laxative such as liquid paraffin should be prescribed on the first postoperative day. Once the patient has opened motion, he could be discharged home. Daily sitz bath should be encouraged.

POSTOPERATIVE COMPLICATIONS

1. Pain is the most important postoperative complaint from the patients. The severity of the complaint varies from person-to-person. And it is inevitable due to the insertion of the tube drain wrapped around with jelly net. In my experience, pain seems to be less in those cases in which the anal orifice has been dilated by three fingers before the resection of the respective pile is carried out. This simple maneuver takes away the tension and spasm of the anal sphincters.

Nevertheless, patients tend to lie on the lateral position with the knee bringing towards the belly, believing that this would relieve the pain. Some patients have described the nature of pain by referring to bites of broken glass.

During my postoperative ward round, a male patient was found lying on the lateral side, holding both knees together by his both hands, but he never complained of pain from the site of operation. His respiration rate went up to 28 per minute, which should have been below 20 per minute.

For measuring his pain threshold level, Omnopon 10 mg (Morphine mixed with papaveretum) in 10 ml saline was given slowly through the intravenous route. By the time 5 mg was infused, he started extending his both legs downwards and a few minutes later, he changed from lateral position to supine position with both legs lying flat on the bed. His respiration rate came down to 18 per minute.

He seemed to be relaxed and started smiling, telling me his experience with excruciating pain and the difference between before and after the injection of narcotics given through the vein. The pain threshold level in his case was 7 mg.[1]

In most cases, patient had also experienced with similar pain on the defecation on the following day. Tube drain and all jelly net dressing are expelled out, while having defecation. It is a routine practice that all patients are asked to have a warm bath immediately after defecation on the first postoperative day. This warm bath provides a soothing effect to the wound.

2. Bleeding may occur from the slip of the ligature or from the vessels that were overlooked at the operation. This is referred to as reactionary hemorrhage that may occur a few hours after the patient is transferred to the ward or postoperative recovery room. Patient is taken back to the theater for stopping the bleeding from the stumps.

3. Retention of urine: This could be related to postoperative pain, enlarged prostate or impacted feces in the rectum in the postoperative period. Acute pain in the perineum interferes with the relaxation of the urethral sphincters; while voiding urine, even in women.

Sometimes, too much morphine injection given for pain may remove the urgeness to void and also inhibits the sphincteric function. If palpation of the lower abdomen suggests that bladder has been distended right up to the umbilicus, this should be relieved by the insertion of an indwelling catheterization. And catheter should be left *in situ* for 2-3 days, until the muscle tone of the bladder has returned.

4. Constipation: If the patient has not opened motion after 3-4 days, internal examination should be done under local anesthesia.

This procedure could be done in the side room but lignocaine jelly 1 percent, soaked in gauze should be left over the anus or it could be instilled directly around the anal orifice 1 hour before the rectal digital examination being contemplated. In most cases, the rectum could be found impacted with hard lumpy feces. In these cases, olive oil enema should be given. If the result seems to be unsatisfactory, manual evacuation under general anesthesia should be done in the theater.

5. Secondary hemorrhage: This is the most serious postoperative complication. It remains unnoticed due to the fact that slow bleeding continues and blood clots are accumulated inside of the anal canal for some days. It occurs between seventh and tenth postoperative days.

Etiology of this secondary hemorrhage is the infection developed at the pedicles that cause softening of the arterial pedicle within the ligature. Defecation or straining may lead to bleeding from these pedicles. Patient ignores small streak of blood at defecation not realizing the seriousness of the problems, when the bleeding has been continuing inside the rectum.

Clinically, patient will look pallor, pulse rate will be running higher and blood pressure will drop. In this situation, urgent investigation should be carried out and infusion therapy with saline should be commenced straightaway waiting for the result of blood hemoglobin. If it turns out to be very low, blood transfusion should be given; and patient should be taken to the theater for internal examination with proctoscope under general anesthesia.

In the theater, patient is put on lithotomy position. Rectal digital examination will reveal soft clots in the rectum. To identify the source of bleeding requires rectal wash out with saline at room temperature. Warm saline may increase capillary dilatation leading to further oozing from the denuded surface and from the fine capillaries present in the hemorrhoidectomy bed.

Treatment of the Bleeding Points

It depends upon the degree of hemorrhage. Conservative approach should be adopted for a small oozing. Patient needs a bed rest, sedation and oral fluids.

Diathermy to the active spurting vessels may be attempted but it is not a reliable procedure. Alternative to this procedure is the transfixation sutures with Vicryl, under direct vision. In this case, the anal orifice is kept retracted with self-retaining bivalve speculum in order to display the sites of hemorrhages. With a long needle holder, the bleeding sites or bleeding points could be controlled with a few transfixation sutures.

Other schools of thought suggest packing the anal canal with tube wrapped up with paraffin gauze, thus exerting pressure upon the vessels. In this case, it is recommended to pass the said tube through the proctoscope, and the latter is slowly withdrawn when the tube wrapped up with paraffin gauze is pushed inside the rectum.[2] A large-sized safety-pin is inserted through the tube and gauze that are left outside the anal orifice.

The anal sphincters contract, thus exerting pressure around the tube, which itself act as a pressure upon the denuded vessels. Both flatus and blood stained fluid may pass through the tube. This will reveal the progress whether or not bleeding stopped.

In the postoperative period, hourly observation on the pulse rate, blood pressure and the perineal wound dressing should be continued for the first day. Blood transfusion may be required, if the hemoglobin is less than 10 gm/dl. Otherwise, patient could be advised to take oral iron tablets, if it is around 10 gm/dl. The tube drain and jelly net dressings are removed on the third postoperative day after giving injection morphine sulphate 10 mg.

6. Anal Fissure: This is very rare and resulted from poor healing of the wound, present in the original site of the piles, located at 7 O'clock or 11 O'clock position. For some reasons, the location of this fissure seems to be associated with the anterior or posterior branch of the right superior hemorrhoidal artery. This poor healing could be due to poor blood supply to the affected site.

The fact needs to be recapitulated about the distribution of the superior hemorrhoidal artery. The right branch divides into the anterior and posterior branches.

This suggests that each branch that supplies to the sites of 7 O'clock and 11 O'clock position of the anal orifice carries a half of the blood to those sites. Hence, poor healing at 7 O'clock and 11 O'clock positions seems to be directly attributable to the reduced blood flow in those two branches of right superior hemorrhoidal artery.

This rare complication is treated with anal dilatation done under general anesthesia, if it persists for several weeks.

7. Stricture of the anal orifice: This is also rare, but its etiology is not fully understood. In my judgment it is believed to be associated with the faulty operative technique. I have witnessed the faulty operative technique in which a part of the circular fibers of the internal sphincter has been implicated in the transfixation suture inserted through the pedicle of the respective pile, thus reducing the size of the anal orifice at the outset, by this faulty technique.

It is the consensus that lack of skin-bridge between the piles is attributable to postoperative anal stenosis.

The treatment is regular anal dilatation to be carried out by the patient. For this application, St. Marks' dilator has been designed. If it does not resolve the problem, anal dilatation should be done under general anesthesia.

Later, it could be done at the outpatient clinic with anal dilator. High fiber diet and plenty of drinks of plain water are encouraged.

TREATMENT FOR THROMBOSED PILES

It is often referred to as perianal hematoma. It develops in the external piles. In fact, it develops at the defecation when the patient tends to strain at the hard bolus of stool. As a result, one of the veins breaks down, which results in bleeding in the subcutaneous tissue. That is the reason that it remains confined to a small area, forming a black cherry on the anal verge.

It is a very painful condition. Patient finds difficulty in sitting on the buttock. To avoid the distress, patient tends to sit on the healthy side of the buttock.

EXPECTED OUTCOME OF THE ACUTE THROMBOSED PILES

Over a few days, it may resolve spontaneously but it may burst out spontaneously, in which case, the extrusion of a small solid clot may stick to the edge of the skin or it could be infected resulting in abscess and fistula formation.

If the pain seems to be persisting over a few days, interfering with the day-to-day work, the patient should be taken to the theater for the evacuation of solid clots. And this is done by a radial incision made over the black skin. Overlying thrombosed skin should be excised. Jelly net dressing is applied over the wound, supported by T bandage. Patient is encouraged to have warm sitz bath twice daily.

STRANGULATED PROLAPSED PILES

This is a very difficult surgical problem. It occurs in the prolapsing piles. For the first few days, conservative approach is adopted, in that, rest in bed with the foot end of the bed being elevated and application of ice packs in surgical gloves is placed over the piles, alternatively, warm saline packs could be placed, if the cold packs appear to be uncomfortable.

Under the application of 2 percent lignocaine jelly, manual reduction of the prolapsed piles could be tried, but more often it does not sustain inside the anal canal very long. It slips back within a few hours. In minor cases, resolution may take place after a week.

There remains a risk of ulceration due to strangulation. In this potential risk of infection, hemorrhoidectomy should be undertaken, as soon as the local edema and inflammation have subsided. This will relieve the discomfort sooner.

REFERENCES

1. Saha SK. Continuous infusion of papaveretum for relief of postoperative pain. Postgraduate Medical Journal 1981;57:686.
2. Lockhart-Mummery JP. Diseases of the Rectum and Colon, Second Edition London: Bailliere 1934.

20 Anorectal Abscess

Anorectal abscess may present in various ways. It could be referred to as perianal abscess, ischiorectal abscess, submucous abscess and pelvirectal abscess. These classifications are based upon the anatomical locations. Many of these abscesses may turn into a fistula-in-ano. Anorectal abscess develop more among the men than among the women. The reason for this difference is not known.

The basic principle involved in the pathogenesis of abscess in any part of the body requires a thorough understanding of surgical pathology. The pathogenesis of perianal abscess would be no different from that of other abscess developed in other parts of the body. Obviously, a bacterial invasion is necessary to develop abscess in the tissue planes, but how this invasion takes place in the tissue planes in the anorectal region remains enigmatic to the clinicians.

In all instances, bacterial invasion is the single etiological factor for the pathogenesis of an abscess, whether it develops in the lymph glands, sweat glands, sebaceous glands, hair follicles, hematoma or in the inflammatory fluid, collected in the cavity such as, joint spaces, peritoneal cavity or in the anatomical spaces.

Clinical presentation would vary that depends upon how the particular site being inflicted with the pyogenic pathogens. At the outset, a painful swelling would appear, but it is later invaded by the bacteria leading to acute inflammation and cellulites. Finally it would turn up into a fluctuating inflamed swelling, what is known as abscess.

The same mechanism is involved in the intraperitoneal or perianal abscess, but in the case of perianal abscess, pathogenesis remains obscured. This seems to be related to difficult access. The fact findings reported in the surgical books are mainly based upon the retrospective studies, carried out in 1920s and 1930s. In those years, a full surgical finding was not possible at operation because of the fact that anesthesia was primitive. Hence, the findings of retrospective study compiled in the Textbook of surgery may not be comprehensive.

Despite the advancement in Surgical practice, a very little difference in the description of the surgical pathology of the perineal abscess or perianal fistula has been noticed in the present surgical books. Hence, the merits of those findings and the pathological features need to be highlighted in the light of present clinical experience.

Background of the Diseases

In those years, public was probably less concerned of their personal health care, and were not fully aware of the consequent effect for delay in seeking the treatment. These could be related to lack of facilities, pressure at work, economy, social environment and standard of living. Those who were aware of the symptoms but they probably delayed seeking any treatment with the hope that it would resolve spontaneously.

They were only forced to seek a medical advice, when problems were unmanageable. Among all these problems, access to the site of abscess was probably another reason for the patient to be less concerned. And it was also possible that it was not easy for the surgeon to deal with the abscess promptly and efficiently, because of poor primitive anesthetic service.

According to the retrospective study, men were found affected more frequently and its ratio between man and woman was 3:1; and it is very rare among the children, but male babies, who are under a year old, are invariably affected.

Etiology

Even today, the etiology is not known. But it is surrounded by divergent and controversial concepts in the pathogenesis of the anorectal or perianal abscess.

In one school of thought, it has been claimed that the infection develops in the intersphincteric anal glands that led to suppuration locally. This raises two important issues, one of the factors is whether there is any conclusive anatomical evidence that anal glands do exist in the space between the internal anal sphincter and the longitudinal muscles of the anal canal, if so, how the infection reaches to these glands. These issues have not been clarified in the literature. The issue of anal glands in the etiology of perianal abscess had been

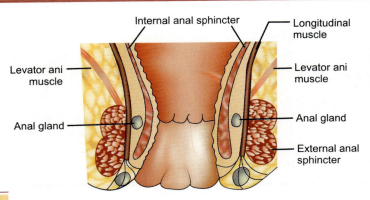

Fig. 20.1: Showing the anal gland in the space between the longitudinal muscles and the circular muscles of the internal sphincter. It was reproduced by courtesy from the Surgery of Anus, Rectum and Colon, 1967

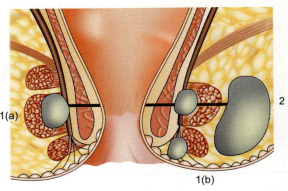

Fig. 20.2: Perianal abscess, defined by Sir Alan Parks in 1961. 1a= Suppuration of anal glands, 1b= Perianal abscess, 2= Ischiorectal abscess

highlighted in the literature by many surgeons;[2-4] but there are many unanswered questions in the merits of their fact findings.

Sir Alan Parks has reported in the literature that anal glands were found to be present in the space between the circular muscles (internal sphincter) and longitudinal muscles of the anal canal (Fig. 20.1). As a rule, 4-8 of the glands were found located in the wall of the normal anal canal. These were referred to as intersphincteric anal glands. Each one drains into the apex of an anal crypt and it has also been emphasized that rarely two glands open into the same crypt.

But 50 percent of the crypts in any anal canal do not have any communication with those glands,[4] whether these anal glands are regarded to be lymph glands or mucous secreting glands have not been clarified in the literature. If they are lymph glands, its location seems to be in conflict with the distribution of other intestinal lymph glands, which are present over the serosal surface of the rectum and colon and they are known as epicolic glands.

If they are mucous secreting glands, they are not present within the muscular layer in other parts of the gut, apart from the Peyer's patches which are the lymphoid follicles, present in the submucosal space of the terminal ileum. In contrast, these findings were found inconsistent with the Textbook of Anatomy.[5]

To resolve the controversy, dissection of the anal canal was carried out on seven cadaveric specimens in the Department of Anatomy at the NRS Medical College in December 2007. And none of the dissected anal canals revealed any evidence of glands within the muscular layers of the anal canal and within the muscular layers of the anal sphincter.[6]

This finding is in conflict with the previous claim reported in the literature and is in conflict with the claim made in the Surgery of the Anus Rectum and Colon, second edition 1967.[7]

According to the literature,[4] the purulent fluid, resulting from the suppuration of the anal glands may pass downwards because of gravitational force along the intermuscular space, until it forms an inflamed swelling over the anal verge—thus forming a perianal abscess. In other cases, it may traverse laterally through the longitudinal muscles of the anal canal and through the deep external sphincters into the ischiorectal fossa, forming the ischiorectal abscess (Fig. 20.2). In some cases, the infection may traverse upwards through the same space between the internal sphincter and longitudinal fibers of the anal canal in order to develop a high intermuscular abscess.[8]

It is debatable, whether the purulent fluid can get through the muscular wall or through the thick external sphincters into the ischiorectal fossa seems to be contrary to the principle of surgical pathology of abscess developed in different anatomical sites. It is more likely that the purulent fluid takes the least resistance pathways and in most instances, it follows the anatomical cleavage or path present between the layers of muscles, through the pre-existing drainage track, or operative scar, before it is clinically evident.

Another school of thought has postulated that mucosal abrasion or tear in the wall of the anal canal may be inflicted by the fish bone. But this seems to be erroneous hypothesis to implicate the fish or meat bone in the abrasion of the lining of the anal canal. It seems to be rational that the mucosal tear could be the primary etiological factor for developing infection in the perianal region. The actual mechanism how this tear may occur is not known.

It seems to be more likely that perianal abscess has resulted from the thrombosed or prolapsed piles or perianal subcutaneous hematoma, if they are not surgically evacuated. Abrasion of the overlying skin or in the anal wall may be the portal of bacterial entry into the hematoma or into the submucosal plane. Eventually, this may turn into a perianal abscess.

Although the mucosal tear may not be evident, by the time the patient is taken to the operating room or it is possible that it was overlooked during proctoscopy and sigmoidoscopy before the perianal abscess or ischiorectal abscess was surgically drained. Despite a meticulous examination, it may not be possible to identify the tear of the anal mucosa through the pool of feces. This sort of investigations at the emergency operation is practically not possible, because of the fact that these minor operations are performed by the most inexperienced junior doctors.

In most instances, the likelihood explanation could be postulated that tear of the lining of the anal canal is a well-known surgical condition and it is regarded to be anal fissure, in the absence of perianal hematoma or thrombosed piles. In both circumstances, patient could experience with acute pain in the anal region that initiates the spasm and contraction of the circular muscles of the anal sphincters, thus keeping the anal orifice closed for a while. As a result, it could be presumed that anal pressure has been built up for sometimes.

In this situation, it could be a possible explanation that the flatus or feculent fluid is held up for a while inside the anal canal. At the same time, the denuded mucosal lining that may act as a portal of bacterial entry may give way for these infected flatus or fluid to get into the least resistance cleavage present in the wall of the anal canal.

Tension builds up within its limited submucosal space. It eventually is released through the least resistance pathways into the different anatomical cleavages. A few bacteria are necessary to cause inflammation and to develop abscess in the loculated inflammatory fluid. In these circumstances, the flatus may act as vehicle for the bacteria to traverse through any one of the following pathways.

The anatomical routes that could provide a least resistance to the pressure of the flatus or feculent fluid are anal crypts, mucocutaneous junction around the dentate line or abrasion of the anal lining.

Once the infection sets through any one of these routes, it may then pass around the lower end of the internal anal sphincter or between the latter and the longitudinal muscles of the anal canal or it may leak through between the superficial and deep external anal sphincter or between the latter and the levator ani muscles. These are possible routes through which the infected flatus or purulent or feculent discharge can traverse, before a full blown abscess is produced, known as perianal or ischiorectal abscess.

In some instances, infected flatus or feculent fluid could stay in the space between the submucosa and internal sphincter, thus forming submucous abscess. In other instances, all these pathogens could pass through any one of those anatomical cleavages, but they may not be possible to pass directly through the posterior wall of the anal canal because of anococcygeal raphe. Therefore, Goodsall's rule that has been defined in relation to anal fistula supports the concept of the fissure-in-ano in the pathogenesis of a perianal abscess and ischiorectal abscess (Fig. 20.3).[9]

In this case, it is more likely that the flatus and/or the inflammatory fluid may traverse through those routes. For instance, it may run downwards, because of gravitational force. It may then take the course either medial to or lateral to the subcutaneous external sphincter— thus presenting as perianal abscess (Fig. 20.4-1a and 1b).

Or it may travel upwards along the same plane and the infection may leak into the ischiorectal fossa either through the cleavage between the superficial and deep external sphincter or between the latter and the levator ani muscles (Fig. 20.4-2).

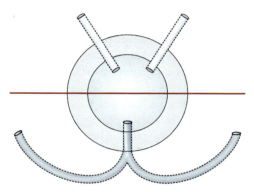

Fig. 20.3: Goodsall's rules states that if the external opening of the anal fistula is anterior to the horizontal line that divides the anal orifice, the tract would be straight and the internal opening of the respective anal fistula would be in the anterior wall of the corresponding side of the anal canal. On the other hand, if the external openings are found located posterior to the said horizontal line, the tracks of these external openings would be curved that would be directed away from the midline of the anus but their tracks would be arising from a single internal opening that would be in the posterior wall of the anal canal

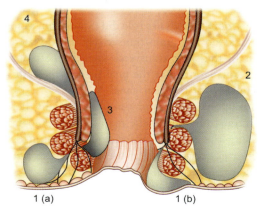

Fig. 20.4: Locations of varieties of anal-rectal abscess. 1a= Perianal abscess; 1b= Another variety of perianal abscess; 2= Ischiorectal abscess, 3= Submucous abscess,; 4= Anorectal abscess

But the ischiorectal fossa is filled up with fatty tissue along with a poor vascularity. Hence, purulent fluid is built up within the fossa at the sacrifice of fat-necrosis, thus developing the ischiorectal abscess.

There may be further debate between the two schools of thoughts that could be resolved by the Goodsall's rule.[9] The position of the external openings of the fistula tracks would indicate, whether the fistula tracks would appear to be straight or curved like horseshoe-shaped tracks (Fig. 20.3).

In early stage, the track arising from the posterior opening will tend to turn curved away from the midline. This deviation is presumably due to anococcygeal raphe present along the posterior wall of the anal canal. But it would tend to open one of the ischiorectal fossa, thus causing an ischiorectal abscess.

If this abscess is not promptly surgically drained, the same track that had turned to one direction may also turn to the opposite direction in order to open in the contralateral ischiorectal fossa, forming another ischiorectal abscess. The two curved tracks would appear to be like a horseshoe-shaped tracks, under the skin surface, but these two curved tracks would have a single internal opening that is located in the posterior wall of the anal canal. These tracks will eventually open externally, forming perianal fistulae, if they are not surgically drained.

This implied that the location of the internal opening is more likely to be arising from an anal fissure in the posterior wall and that was the primary source for the abscess developed in the ischiorectal abscess, whether or not it is located either in the anterior or posterior wall of the anal canal, but unlike the anterior fistula track, the posterior fistula track, arising from the posterior anal fissure cannot drain directly posteriorly behind the anus. The reason for this difference is due to anococcygeal raphe present in the posterior anal canal that prevents the fistula track to open directly behind the posterior anal orifice.

Furthermore, Goodsall's rule did not explain as to why the fistula tracks do not drain transversely on the lateral side of the anus in the same transverse line. This strengthens the possible explanation that the anal fissure does not occur in the lateral wall of the anal canal.

This supports the second school of thought that the anal fissure seems to be one of the many other etiological factors for causing the perianal abscess. It is presumed that the intersphincteric anal glands, if present at all, are irrelevant in the etiology of the perianal abscess. If they are regarded to be the source of primary suppuration, then the abscess could have drained through the same route into the anal canal.[7]

Apart from these concepts, perianal abscess may result from the infection developed in the hair follicle, sebaceous or sweat glands present in the perineal regent. It may result from Crohn's or ulcerative proctitis, tuberculous proctitis.

Classification of Perianal Abscess

According to the anatomical sites, perianal abscess could be classified into several names. These have been delineated in Figures 20.2 and 20.4. These are as follows:

(i) Perianal abscess— It may lie deep to the subcutaneous external anal sphincter (Fig. 20.4-1a).

Or

It may be found superficial to the subcutaneous external anal sphincter (Fig. 20.4-1b, Fig. 20.2-1b).

(ii) Ischiorectal abscess— It occupies the huge fatty space lateral to the external sphincters (Fig. 20.2-2, Fig. 20.4-2).

(iii) Submucous abscess— It may be in the space between the internal anal sphincter and anal mucosa (Fig. 20.4-3).

(iv) Pelvirectal abscess— It remains in the pelvis above the levator ani muscles and under the pelvic peritoneum (Fig. 20.4-4).

PERIANAL ABSCESS

Clinical Features

It has been suggested that perianal abscess commences in the anal glands,[4] but such claim requires a conclusive anatomical evidence. The commonest pathogens found in the culture of the pus are *E. coli* (60%), *Staphylococcus aureus, Bacteroides, Streptococcus* and *Bacillus proteus* in 23 percent. And the sources are from the infected hematoma, anal mucosal tear, infection of the anal gland or blood-borne infection. There may be other sources of infection. These are Crohn's proctitis, ulcerative colitis or proctitis, tuberculosis and malignant tumor.

Pathogenesis of Perianal Abscess

The exact mechanism how the abscess developed in different sites around the anal canal is not known. It has been postulated that the anal glands are infected and it tends to suppurate, discharging purulent fluid in the space outside the anal canal. From this focus, infection spreads into different direction. The sites of abscess are perianal abscess (60%), ischiorectal abscess (30%), submucous (5%), intermuscular and pelvirectal abscess.

It is also possible that patient develops painful hematoma after defecation and it is more likely the primary etiological factor for perianal abscess. It is more often associated with constipation, in which case, hard bulky motion tends to stretch the sphincters and overlying skin during defecation that may cause hemorrhage over the anal verge, forming a round hematoma about a size of a cherry. It may also result from acute fissure-in-ano. If the hematoma is not evacuated surgically, infection may supervene into this subcutaneous hematoma that may turn into a superficial perianal abscess, over the lateral side of the anal orifice. It is less painful than ischiorectal abscess.

Periurethral abscess may also develop anterior to the anal orifice and by the side of the bulbar urethra. It is more often related to the infection, extended from the anus or related to urethritis or urethral stricture.

All these cases are admitted as an emergency condition. In the clinical examination, concentration is focused around the perineal region and groins. On palpation, an inflamed and localized lump is visible on the site of the anal verge. Internal examination must not be done, because of very painful condition around the anal orifice and it would not be possible to insert the index finger through the tight anal orifice. The localized swelling may appear to be firm, or fluctuating on a gentle palpation by the palmar surface of the index finger.

If the buttock lateral to the anal orifice appears to be indurated and bulging, ischiorectal abscess should be suspected. It would appear to be an ill-defined swelling or induration and tender to touch. Apart from these findings there should have constitutional symptoms, associated with a high rise of temperature.

All these cases require examination under general anesthesia.

Treatment

The inflamed lump, whether it is a perianal hematoma, abscess, or ischiorectal abscess needs to be surgically evacuated. And sooner it is done is better. It would relieve the pain, and it would stop spreading the infection or communicating with other sites, forming a fistula. Systemic antibiotic should be prescribed, despite the fact that it may not reach to an optimum therapeutic level in the abscess cavity, because of a dead space and a poor vascularity in the ischiorectal fossa or in the inflamed swelling. A combination of two types of antibiotics covering for aerobic and anaerobic bacteria should be commenced, before the patient is taken to the theater.

OPERATIVE PROCEDURE FOR DRAINAGE OF ABSCESS

In the theater, patient is placed on the lithotomy position. Anal orifice and the canal are digitally examined. This is followed by proctoscopy and sigmoidoscopy. The purpose is to look for any local inflammation such as Crohn's or ulcerative proctitis, anal fistula, piles, perianal hematoma and chronic or acute fissure-in-ano or tumor.

The perineum is cleaned with a savlon solution. A separate sheet is put underneath the buttock. The surgical treatment entails the deroofing of the abscess. Therefore, cruciate incisions are made across the roof of the abscess and the corners of the skin edges are excised. The pockets of the abscess are broken down by inserting the finger. A pus swab is taken for culture and sensitivity test for the bacteriological study and for antibiotics.

The cavity is examined with the index finger. In rare cases, feces may be found emerging. In this case, the etiology of the abscess would be the perianal fistula. At this stage, no attempt should be made to find out the fistula track. If such an attempt is made, it is more likely that a false passage has been made inadvertently which could be alleged that a surgeon-made fistula has resulted from such procedure.

The abscess cavity should be wiped out with gauze before it is packed with small ribbon gauze, soaked in proflabin solution. This is left *in situ* for 48 hours. If it is removed sooner, the wound will close sooner, leaving behind the infection and a dead space under the healed scar.

Wound packing is very important and it should be continued until the healing by a granulation tissue starts filling up the cavity from the depth of the wound. Superficial dressing and sitz bath is recommended until the cavity is filled up with the granulation tissue.

Therefore, an acute infection and inflammation around the abscess cavity should be treated by a regular wound packing. No further surgical intervention should be done until the acute condition has settled down with the local wound dressing and salt-bath.

After a few weeks, further investigation is undertaken to establish the cause for delayed healing or persistent wound discharge, whether or not it was attributable to anorectal fistula. Wound dressing is continued as in all other case.

If the wound discharge continued over several months, this could be attributable to persisting infection or sinus track. After a necessary investigation being completed, patient should be taken to the theater in order to deal with the discharging sinus or perianal fistula.

Ischiorectal Abscess

The etiology is unknown. The possible source of infection could be from the old perianal hematoma, pelvic abscess, posterior fissure-in-ano. In rare cases, the sources of infection could be attributable to Crohn's proctitis, ulcerative proctitis or carcinoma in the anus or the rectum. Tuberculous infection should be suspected in the absence of other lesions.

It is presented with a large area of induration and cellulites by the side of the anal orifice. Patient may complain of throbbing pain in that region. Fluctuation would be elicited at last when the condition has been worse. In this situation, it may burst into the rectum. Infection may spread to the contralateral side of the ischiorectal fossa via the postsphincteric space, if the abscess is not drained urgently.

Surgical intervention should be urgent. This requires rectal digital examination, followed by proctoscopy and sigmoidoscopy.

Operative Treatment

In the theater, the patient is placed on the lithotomy position. Proper draping is carried out around the perineum and the buttock. On the site of induration and inflammation a large cruciate incision is made. The wound is made large by excising the skin corners and deeper by breaking the septum, present within the ischiorectal abscess. This is done with the index finger. The size of the cavity would appear to be much larger than what appears to be on the skin surface. Pus swab is sent for bacteriological study and culture.

Moderate-sized ribbon gauze soaked in proflabin solution is used to pack the abscess cavity, starting from the depth. A large dressing pad is left over to cover the wound packs. Postoperative wound dressing remains the same, consistent with the principle of wound packing. The packing is continued over a few weeks, until it heals completely.

Submucous abscess occurs above the dentate line and results from the injection of piles. It settles down spontaneously and surgical intervention is unnecessary.

Pelvirectal abscess is literally pelvic abscess that develops from other primary sources of infection. They are appendicitis, salpingitis, diverticulitis and parametritis. It lies in the space formed between the pelvic peritoneum forming a roof and the levator ani muscles acting as a floor of the abscess.

Clinically, it presents with swinging temperature and not very well. There may be symptoms of loose motions. Patients do not complain of pain in the rectum or anal canal.

Abdominal examination may reveal some degree of fullness or resistance in the lower part either on the right or on the left iliac fossa, clinical impression would be salpingitis in female patient and diverticulitis or chronic appendicitis in either sex.

Rectal digital examination may reveal bulging higher up associated with the tenderness or some mucus discharge may be seen on the finger stall. It is possible that the pus may drain rectally spontaneously or it may extend downwards involving the ischiorectal fossa.

If the ischiorectal fossa has been involved by the pelvic infection, the rectal wall will appear to be tender and bulging on rectal digital examination. If one ischiorectal fossa seemed to be affected, it is important to palpate the contralateral wall of the rectum and the corresponding ischiorectal fossa.

In female patient, tenderness in the cervix uteri may be elicited through the rectal digital examination. Above all, vaginal examination should be done with prior permission and in the presence of a lady nurse. And bimanual examination should be carried out in order to feel any palpable mass in the fornix.

Clinical diagnosis is established by the ultrasound scan, CT scan, and by the blood tests. The latter may reveal raised leukocytes count, and by the high elevation of C reactive protein.

Eventually, pelvic abscess may require to be drained either through the laparoscope or through laparotomy that depends upon the primary source of the infection. In the theater, the same examination should be repeated under anesthesia. And proctoscopy and sigmoidoscopy should be carried out before operative procedure is undertaken. If abscess has developed in the ischiorectal fossa, then it should be drained separately.

In this procedure, curetting of the abscess cavity is carried out, but a cautious approach should be adopted in order to assess the upper limit of the perianal abscess or fistula tract by the probe or sinus forceps. It is unlikely that these instrumentations may cause accidental injury to the levator ani muscles from below —thus spreading the infection into this space from below. The technique for surgical drainage for perianal or ischiorectal abscess remains the same.

Tuberculous abscess may manifest as perianal or ischiorectal abscess, but clinically it would appear to be less tender and may burst before the surgical intervention is undertaken. Unlike the pyogenic abscess, the discharge is watery. Suspicion should arise in this case.

Pus and granulation tissue are sent for both histology and TB culture. Diagnosis is made on the culture report confirming the evidence of tuberculosis.

If Crohn's disease is excluded by the histology report, other investigation should be done in order to exclude TB. These investigations are X-ray of the chest, sputum for AFB, and blood test for ESR. A Mantoux skin test, ultrasound scan of the abdomen, and guinea-pig inoculation test for TB should be arranged. Tuberculous intestine must be excluded with a small bowel enema, barium enema and colonoscopy. If mesenteric lymph glands are found to be enlarged, lymph node needle biopsy should be done through the CT scan.

Etiology for Recurrent Infection or Recurrence of Abscess

Despite the surgical intervention and regular wound dressing, wound discharge may continue. This could be attributable to persisting infection. There are many etiological factors that may cause persisting infection or recurrent abscess.

If the infection keeps recurring and recurrence of abscess becomes a problem, this may lead to a chronic granulomatous

tract which could be a sinus or fistula tract. The local causative factors for the persisting discharge are as follows:
(a) Repeated contamination by the discharge of flatus, feces, or both in combination. These inhibit the healing of the abscess or fistula track.
(b) Repeated trauma by the sphincteric activity during and after defecation. This interferes with the healing of the fistula track.
(c) Persistent anal pain produces spasm of the external anal sphincter and particularly the subcutaneous external anal sphincter that tends to keep the anal orifice closed because of contraction of the circular muscles of the subcutaneous external anal sphincter. This may raise the pressure high within the anal canal. Because of this resistance around the anal orifice, flatus and/or feculent discharge may be redirected through least resistance pathways and this may cause delay in wound healing both by recurrence contamination and by disturbances at defecation.

PERIANAL FISTULA

Definition of Fistula

Fistula is a track that forms a communication between the two viscuses or between a cavity and a viscus and it is lined by a chronic granulomatous tissue. Both openings could be internal or it could be a combination of internal and external openings. It is referred to by the names of two organs or viscera such as colovesical, rectovaginal, colocutaneous, ileocolic or gastrocolic fistula or fistula-in-ano.

Its etiology varies but primarily it may result from an injury, drainage of an abscess, chronic inflammatory disease, and invasion of the tumor or pressure necrosis. The track between the two cavities or walls develops slowly in chronic debilitating diseases, and its communication remains unknown for several weeks until it is clinically evident by the discharge of its contents or pus.

By and large, its basic principle for draining the contents follows the least resistance path, or it may follow from a high pressure to a low pressure zone or from a higher level to a lower or dependent level because of gravitational force.

Etiology

Etiology of perianal fistula could be associated with a benign perianal abscess or with the chronic debilitating or malignant disease. They are:
(i) Pulmonary tuberculosis, only 2-3 percent of the fistula could be tuberculous.
(ii) Crohn's disease.
(iii) Ulcerative proctitis.
(iv) Colloid carcinoma or anal carcinoma.
(v) Bilharziasis.
(vi) Lymphogranuloma inguinale.
(vii) Chronic recurrent perianal abscess.
(viii) Actinomycosis.

Its pathogenesis remains obscured, for various reasons. The most important factor for developing in chronic state is the delay in seeking medical advice. As a result, the primary etiology of the infection and the true sites of suppuration remain unknown for a long time, until unbearable problems force the patient seeking for the treatment.

Therefore, the pathology of the fistula-in-ano remains enigmatic to the surgeons. The results compiled in the Textbook of Surgery were obtained from the retrospective studies in those years when the anesthesia was primitive and our knowledge was limited. Therefore, it may not reflect the true prevalence of the disease among the public at large and the incidence of an individual type of anal fistula may not represent a true statistical prevalence among those cases, treated in the district hospital.

For some reasons, men are affected more frequently and its ratio between men and women is 3:1 and it is very rare among the children, but male sex is invariably affected among the babies under a year old.

Classification of the Perianal Fistula

It is a granulomatous track that has resulted from the abscess at the outset whether or not it is connected to the anal canal or the rectum. It has been classified into two groups, based upon the position of the internal opening. It would be referred to as a high perianal fistula, if the fistula track opens in the canal above the dentate line and a low fistula, if the said opening remains below the dentate line.

Milligan and Morgan have produced a detailed classification of anorectal fistula.[10] These are: (1) Subcutaneous fistula, (2) Submucous fistula, (3) Low anal fistula, (4) High anal fistula, (5) Anorectal fistula (Fig. 20.5).

In practical point of view, the surgical treatment entails excision and laying open the track that should be the basic principle, involved in the surgical care of the chronic infective process.

Clinical Feature

It is related to a high or low anal fistula.

Low Anal Fistula

There will be a past history of spontaneous discharge of pus or previous operation for the perianal abscess, but patient may not recollect the previous episodes, until he was questioned for such symptoms of discharge or perianal abscess. During consultation, patient should be asked about bowel habits,

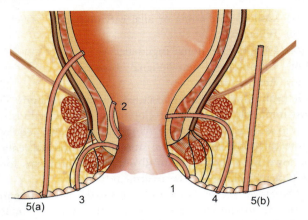

Fig. 20.5: Perianal and anorectal fistula. 1= Subcutaneous fistula, 2= Submucous fistula, 3= Low anal fistula (below the dentate line), 4= High anal fistula (above the dentate line), 5a= Anorectal fistula, 5b= Another type of anorectal fistula (Supralevator ani fistula, described by Sir Alan Parks)

appetite, body weight and past history of pulmonary tuberculosis, and whether he had any contact or lived with any patient suffering from pulmonary tuberculosis. Nevertheless, these are the classical presentations, when they are attending to the hospital.

(a) Persisting purulent or feculent discharge that may cause irritation around the external opening. This discharge may produce a foul or feculent smell.
(b) It remains painless, but patient experiences a pain or discomfort around the fistula opening, when it stops discharging. If the external opening closes, there would be a building up of pus inside the track that may cause a pain and throbbing. This is attributable to a recurrence of abscess. In most instances, it discharges either through the same opening or through a new opening.
(c) The location of the external opening is within 4 cm from the anal verge and a single opening is present but it could be multiple, and surrounded by induration, skin discoloration and they remain close together. Granulation tissue could be seen pouting from inside the opening.
(d) The opening could be in the anterior or in the posterior part of the anus.
   - If ischiorectal fossa on both sides is implicated with the infection, there would be two external openings— one on each side of the anal orifice, but there would be a communication between these two openings under the anal skin and behind the anal orifice. This subcutaneous track would be a horseshoe-shaped, connected to a single internal opening draining into the posterior anal canal.
   - If the external opening is present anterior to the anal orifice, the fistula track would be straight arising from a single internal opening located in the anterior wall of the anal canal (Fig. 20.3).

HIGH ANAL FISTULA

This is referred to as a high fistula if the internal opening is above the dentate line and below the anorectal ring. According to Park classification, there are:
(a) High intersphincteric fistula.
(b) Trans-sphincteric fistula.
(c) Supralevator ani fistula.

The symptoms from these fistula tracks will be no different from the low anal fistula in most cases. In the course of investigation, these types of fistula are usually recognized.

Clinical Examination

After recording a detailed history, patient is asked to lie on the left lateral position and to take off the clothes from the vest and the patient is asked to bring both knees towards the pelvis. Under a bright illumination, initial examination is carried out in order to see the number of external opening, sentinel piles, anal skin tags, external piles and skin color around the fistula tract.

Then the external fistula opening or openings are palpated by the right index finger in order to feel any induration around the fistula opening and the fistula tracks. If induration is suspected, the area is palpated by two fingers.

If there is any external discharge coming from the sinus, swab is taken for a bacterial culture and the discharge is put on the slide for staining in order to exclude tuberculous lesion.

After external palpation, the anal canal and the rectum is palpated by inserting the index finger. This digital examination may reveal any induration, stricture, tumor and mucopurulent discharge. On withdrawing the finger from the anal canal, inspection of the finger-stall may reveal any blood stained discharge around the finger stall.

Like all other cases, the anal canal and the rectum are examined with proctoscope and sigmoidoscope. These instrumental examinations may reveal internal opening, papilloma, discharge of pus, or inflammation of the mucosa, contact bleeding, or malignant tumor.

A tubular type proctoscope should be used and its full length with obturator should be inserted. After the obturator is removed, the proctoscope is moved around in order to look for internal opening that is recognized by the discharge of fluid, when a gentle massage is given by other hand and an area of inflamed induration may be evident in the wall of the anal canal. This finding may be more evident, when the proctoscope is slowly withdrawn from inside the anal canal.

If there are evidences of contact bleeding or patchy mucosal or granular mucosal appearance, biopsy should be taken to exclude Crohn's or ulcerative proctitis.

Investigations

Routine investigation includes X-ray of the chest, blood tests and ESR. If there is any doubt, all other tests should be done to exclude pulmonary tuberculosis.

If the clinical and local examination indicates for ulcerative colitis or Crohn's disease, then, small bowel enema, barium enema should be done. Colonoscopy will be considered, if necessary.

Radiopaque contrast would not be able to demonstrate the internal opening of the fistula track because of the fact that the track has a long-standing fibrous tissue along its wall and it contains thick granulation tissue in its tunnel that would not permit the contrast to get through and through into the anal canal or the rectum, unless it is injected with force. And on the operating table, demonstration of the internal opening would be much more difficult. In fact, it may cause more damage than any benefit being achieved from its identification. Therefore, it would be a theoretical and academic issue whether or not it is a true fistula or sinus or whether it is a low or high fistula.

The demonstration of the internal opening of the fistula is not an easy task. Particularly it would be technically impossible to confirm whether the fistula has a low or a high track above the dentate line, until they are examined on the operating table. Having known these difficulties, every investigation should be carried out, whether or not the outcome would be of any benefit to the line of treatment.

Operative Procedure

A good bowel preparation is necessary, before patient is put on the operating table in lithotomy position.

Local digital examination around the fistula opening is very important. This may reveal, whether there is any induration or watery discharge or whether the discharge is thick passé or mucoid in character. In rectal examination, it is possible to palpate the induration or papillomatous or raised mucosa on the side wall of the anal canal or rectum and whether some induration could be felt by bidigital examination between the two index fingers, one is inside the anal canal and the other one is placed on the side of the discharging wound.

During digital examination, a sinus probe should be passed through the external opening slowly, while this is advancing slowly without any force, the index finger that has already been inside the anal canal should feel any abnormal sensation or could feel a pin-pointed probe touching the finger from outside the mucosal wall of the anal canal. This does not indicate that the internal opening of the fistula is very close to the anal canal. Pus swab should be taken for microscopical examination and for culture.

After the digital examination, proctoscopic examination should be done in order to identify any abnormal area or papilla seen on the wall of the anal canal or any discharge is emerging on external massage, applied by the finger around the affected side of perineal region.

To look for the internal opening, bivalve anal speculum should be used that could be moved around, when a sinus probe is advanced slowly through the external opening. More often, a false passage is created by this maneuver.

Finally, sigmoidoscopy should be carried out in order to exclude Crohn's disease, ulcerative proctitis, ulcerative colitis or malignant growth present in the rectum.

If the internal opening has been identified by the sinus probe, this track is excised for the purpose of tissue diagnosis. Apart from the diagnostic point of view, this exploration of the fistula would be necessary for the purpose of therapeutic wound dressing.

The sinus probe with its groove facing the skin surface is left within the track (Fig. 20.6). The roof of the fistula track is incised with a fine knife, facing upwards that goes through the groove of the sinus probe all along up to the margin of the anal verge. The sinus probe is removed temporarily with a view to examining the floor of the fistula track.

If it confirms that its wall has scar tissue and its cavity contains the granulation tissue, swab is taken from the area for culture. Further examination is carried out in order to find out any side track, connected to this fistula. During this examination, the wound is palpated, whether there is any extension of the induration.

At the completion of the examination, the fistula track is next curated with the sinus scraping spoon. After this has been done, the remaining part of the track needs to be examined whether it has the features of fistula track or it is a false passage made by the sinus probe.

If it contains infected or scar tissue within its track, then the sinus probe is put back into the fistula track with a view

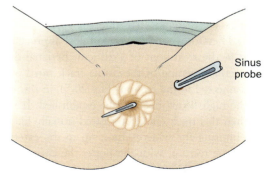

Fig. 20.6: Shows the sinus probe inside low anal fistula

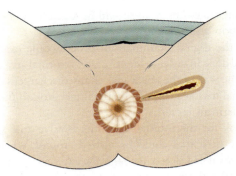

Fig. 20.7: It shows that the fistula track has been excised and left open, to be healed by the granulation tissue

to excising it and keeping it wide open. It may be necessary to divide the subcutaneous external anal-sphincter. This will not cause incontinence.

At the end, the whole fistula track is excised with the scissors, thus making the wound much wider, and it would appear pear-shaped, the broader base of which would be directed around the external opening and the narrower end would be going through the wall of the internal sphincter. The fistula track is sent for histology and the wound cavity is packed with the proflabin or any other suitable antiseptic dressing available in the theater (Fig. 20.7).

If there is no such internal opening into the anal canal, in that case, the infected track is excised in order to laying it open and a similar line of treatment should be continued until the wound cavity is filled up with a healthy granulation tissue.

If a wider area needs to be excised for the multiple fistula tracks, then the skin graft is recommended, but its merit is debatable. The reasons are recurrent wound contamination and trauma. This would interfere with the implantation of the skin graft or it may cause a disruption of the new growth of granulation tissue or epithelialization.

Apart from wound contamination, trauma to the wound is another detrimental factor for wound healing. This trauma could be of various natures. This could be due to cleaning of the perineum, rubbing with the clothes or sitting on the buttocks.

In many cases, a repeated exploration of the same track may be necessary that may frustrate the surgeon as well as the patient. Therefore, conservative surgical approach should be adopted in the treatment of a difficult perianal discharge.

If the internal opening of the fistula track turns out to be high and connected to the rectum (Fig. 20.5), in this case, the cause for the high fistula needs to be established. If no cause is found, then this track could be treated initially like a sinus tract, thus limiting the wide excision up to the external anal sphincter or the rectum, with the hope, the cavity would be filled up by the granulation tissue from deep to the skin surface and the internal opening may heal on its own.

If no improvement is in sight, and there is a conclusive evidence of discharge of feces coming through this fistula track, then diversion of the feces is to be carried out, instead of putting the patient at a risk of developing fecal incontinence that may result from excising the internal opening of the fistula.

In this case, the fistula would heal, if the feces could be diverted by the construction of a pelvic loop colostomy. This would be a major operation and further consultation is necessary for this procedure. To avoid major laparotomy, telescopic pelvic loop colostomy could be constructed in the first attempt, if the surgeon is trained to do this job. In this procedure, two teams are necessary; one team will carry out the endoscopic work using a flexible sigmoidoscope that would assist the second team, where a circular incision is to be made in the left iliac fossa. In the dark theater room, illumination will be seen coming through the left pelvic wall. Construction of loop colostomy will be carried out, as described in the previous section.

After a few weeks, gastrograffin enema should be done in order to be sure that the internal opening of the high anal fistula has healed. On the basis of this result, the loop colostomy is closed.

Complications

Despite a meticulous wound dressing, complete healing may not be possible. Recurrence may occur. In addition, a partial mucosal prolapse of the rectum would be an added morbidity. And if it does occur, there could be a mucous discharge, ulceration of prolapsed mucosa, bleeding, and incontinence. Therefore, surgeon should be cautious in dealing with the perianal fistula.

Sequel of Untreated Anal Fistula

In most cases, patients do not take any notice about the recurrent minor discharge from the external wound. They do hope it would stop discharging eventually. There is a common observation that all internal openings of the colocutaneous fistula would heal spontaneously, if there is no distal obstruction. This implied that regular defecation is very important in the management of colocutaneous fistula. I believe the treatment of perianal fistula obeys the same basic principle.

However, pain, repeated spasm or sphincteric dysfunction may be the causative factor for the recurrent transmission of infection from the anal canal.

Nevertheless, the management of the anal fistula is unpredictable. Although, the discharge from the fistula track remains insignificant in most of the time, it does not cause a great deal of disadvantage to the individual's day-to-day work. In some cases, it stops spontaneously for a temporary period, until a further collection is accumulated inside the track, and then it would burst again, and starts discharging spontaneously. This is one type of sequel.

In other cases, the tiny track may be filled up with a chronic granulation tissue. This may be organized into a scar tissue—thus assisting the internal opening to be closed by the epithelialization. The track turns into a fibrous scar, which does not get re-infected. It is very rare.

Among other rare varieties, the squamous epithelium, arising either from the external or internal opening of the track may cover the lining of those tracks, which are either low anal fistula or subcutaneous fistula. These two varieties of cases are self-limiting conditions that do not require surgical intervention.

Therefore, a careful review is necessary over many months in order to assess the sequence in the pattern of discharge and patients' disability. In the meantime, wound dressing and salt bath is continued. After a full evaluation, a balanced decision should be taken on how to improve the healing of the track. Treatment of anal fistula is very complicated and a slow process that may bring unhappiness among the patients and the family members, if a prolonged procrastination continues over many months. It is a no win position in some cases, despite an honest attempt is made to treat the chronic fistula track.

In all instances, it is important to exclude evidence of Crohn's or ulcerative proctitis, TB intestine. The fistula will not heal until all the primary debilitating diseases are treated. In most cases, no active intervention is necessary for the anal fistula, once those diseases are treated satisfactorily.

REFERENCES

1. Gabriel WB. The Principle and Practice of Rectal Surgery, Third Edition, HK Lewis & Co. 1945.
2. Lockhart-Mummery JP. Discussion on fistula-in-ano. Proc Roy Soc Med 1929;22:1331.
3. Gordon-Watson C, Dodd H. Observation on fistula-in-ano in relation to intramuscular perianal glands. Brit J Surg 1935;22:303.
4. Parks AG. Pathogenesis and treatment of fistula-in-ano. Brit Med J 1961;1:463.
5. Last RJ. Anatomy Regional and Applied, Fourth Edition, J & A Churchill Ltd, London, 1966.
6. Chatterjee S, Gupta I, Dasgupta (Mrs) H, Saha SK. Dissection of the anal canal in seven cadaveric specimens, Department of Anatomy NRS Medical College, Kolkata, December 2007 (Unpublished report).
7. Goligher JC. Surgery of the Anus, Rectum, and Colon, Second Edition. Bailliere, Tindall & Cassell Ltd. London 1967.
8. Eisenhammer S. The internal anal sphincter and anorectal abscess. Surg Gyne Obst 1956;103:501.
9. Goodsall DH. In Goodsall DH, Miles WE. Disease of the Anus and Rectum. Pt. I. Longmans:London. 1900.
10. Milligan ETC, Morgan CN. Surgical anatomy of the anal canal with special reference to anorectal fistulae. Lancet, 1934;2. 1150;1213.

21
Fissure-in-Ano

A sharp pain at defecation associated with a bright red bleeding is the classical symptoms for acute fissure-in-ano. Pruritus ani is often complained off by the patient. Constipation and soft motions are often the predisposing factors—thus contributing to this condition.

PATHOLOGY

Anal fissure is a linear longitudinal tear at the mucocutaneous junction. It lies between the anal verge and the dentate (pectinate) line. The commonest location is in the posterior wall and it is less frequently located in the anterior wall of the anal canal. The women of childbearing age group seem to be more vulnerable than any other age group or in men. But surprisingly, it does not occur on the lateral wall of the anal canal of either sex. Its reason is not known.

The prevalence of this benign condition is more among the young and middle-aged persons than any other age groups, but it is not uncommon among the young children. The etiology for the anal fissure seems to be attributable to constipation. The reason for this association is probably related to reduce muscular activity of the anal sphincters in between the action of defecation. This leads to hypertonicity of the striated circular muscles of the anal sphincter.

Fissure-in-ano may be found among other diseases. These are ulcerative colitis, Crohn's disease, tuberculous ulcer, pruritus ani and anal carcinoma.

Acute fissure-in-ano is a very painful condition. Sharp pain is experienced, as if the skin has been cut by a knife or glass. Bleeding associated with a sharp pain is the classical presentation of acute anal fissure. Painless bleeding at defecation is considered to be piles or is associated with malignant lesion.

There are two types of fissure-in-ano. One is the acute fissure-in-ano and other one is chronic fissure-in-ano. Recurrent episodes of tear or delayed healing may lead to a chronic fissure-in-ano, resulting in fibrosis around the scar and developing anal skin tag, known as sentinel pile that keeps hanging from the lower end of the fissure. Anal stenosis could be the end sequel of untreated fissure-in-ano, but it is rarely seen.

Divergent Opinion about the Disease

Although, the anal fissure seems to be simple and self-limiting disease, a lot of divergent theory has been postulated surrounding its surgical anatomy, pathogenesis and treatment. In the past it was the view of many surgeons that anal fissure lies over the subcutaneous part of the external sphincter.[1-4] It was disputed by others.[5] A few years later, it was claimed in the literature that anal fissure lies over the lower edge of the internal sphincter.[6,7] In the illustration of the anal sphincter, the lower level of the internal sphincter has been depicted to be below the dentate line of the anal canal.[8]

It is also debatable whether the initial tear is at the mucocutaneous junction or below the above junction. If the former finding is believed to be correct, then patient does not need sitting on the one buttock and changing its position now and then. The question would be whether the evidence reported in the literature[6,7] was based upon the clinical examination conducted at the outpatient clinics or upon the anatomical dissection of the anal fissure made on the cadaveric specimens.

The striking presentation is the sharp acute pain in the perineum. It has been the accepted postulation that spasm of the internal sphincter is believed to be the causative factor for the acute anal pain. Because of spasm, the anal orifice tends to remain closed. This spasm drags the anal orifice inwards between the two buttocks. The purpose is to protect the tear from the repeated rubbing against the clothes or from sitting on a chair.

For avoiding the discomfort, patient tends to sit on the one buttock by tilting the body to the other side and a few minutes later the position is changed by sitting on the contralateral buttock. The purpose of sitting on one buttock and then changing its position is to keep the anal fissure away from the direct contact or pressure. This is a classical experience described by the patients. In this way, direct contact of the fissure is avoided while sitting on the chair. This was my personal experience and I found a similar experience with other patients.

In most instances, the anal orifice remains retracted inwards between the two buttocks as if it looks like a funnel, when the patient lies on the lateral side of the buttock. This position becomes apparent in some cases, if the patient is examined a few months later, but in other cases where the duration of the anal fissure is very short, the anal orifice does not appear to be retracted and it remains at the same level with the buttocks.

It could be postulated that the former shape could be attributable to the long-standing contraction of the longitudinal muscle of the anal canal—thus pulling the subcutaneous external anal sphincter inwards. This mechanism could be explained by the anatomical distribution of the longitudinal muscle fibers of the anal canal and rectum. Some of these fibers pass laterally over the circular muscles of the subcutaneous anal sphincter. This explains how the anal verge is pulled inwards. Its purpose is to protect the anal fissure from a direct contact with the seat or clothes, thus keeping it within the anal orifice.

In these cases, it is not easy to see the anal fissure. And demonstration of anal fissure may not be easy, unless the lateral part of the anal verge and perianal skin is retracted sideways. This is done by the fingers of both hands. For this display, the left hand is placed over the right side and the right one placed over the left side of the perineum – a little away from the anal orifice.

Both sides of the anal verge are then gently retracted away from the anal orifice, in order to see the anal fissure. Of course, spasm of the sphincters that keep the anal orifice closed would resist against this maneuver for the inspection of the acute fissure-in-ano. But the issue is whether it is the subcutaneous external sphincter or internal sphincter or both in combination induce spasm, needs to be highlighted in perspective.

Etiology of Anal Pain

In the literature, spasm of the internal sphincter or poor blood supply has been incriminated in the pathogenesis of the anal pain and slow healing of anal fissure.[9-11] The answer to the contentious issue on the etiology of the acute anal pain lies probably in the surgical anatomy of the anal orifice.

Before proceeding further, it is important to highlight inconsistency with the anatomical description of the internal anal sphincter in different surgical and anatomical books.[8,12] Therefore, these differences need to be highlighted in order to understand the true anatomy and true pathology of the benign condition.

The illustration of the internal sphincter as defined in Figure 21.1 seems to be inconsistent with other Textbook of Anatomy and Surgery. In those literatures, the internal sphincter has been shown to have ended at the level of the dentate line (Fig. 21.2).

Although all this literature did not produce any photographic evidence from the cadaveric specimen, nevertheless, to resolve the confusion, dissection of the anal canal retrieved from a cadaveric male body was carried out at the department of Anatomy of NRS Medical College and hospital in February 2009. The colored photograph (Fig. 21.3) would confirm that the internal sphincter was found absent below the level of the dentate line.

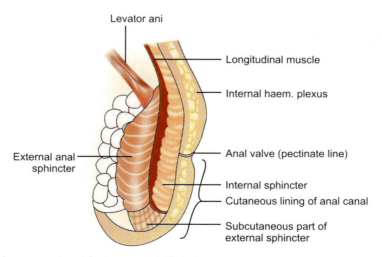

Fig. 21.1: This illustration has been reproduced by courtesy of JC Goligher from the Textbook of Surgery of the Anus, Rectum and Colon, Second Edition published by Bailliere, Tindall and Cassell, London in 1967 and it was also reported by JC Goligher in Disease of the Colon and Anorectum, ed. R. Turrel, Philadelphia: Saunders in 1959[8]

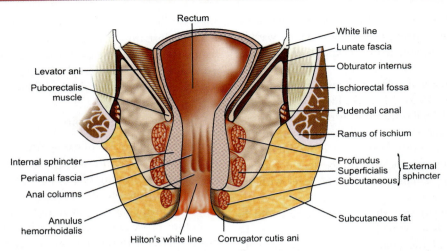

Fig. 21.2: Shows the internal anal sphincter at the level of dentate and above the attachment of the longitudinal muscles of the anal canal By Courtesy of Prof RJ Last from his book "Anatomy—Regional and Applied, Seventh Edition, published by English Language Book Society and Churchill Livingstone Longman Group Ltd 1986.[12]

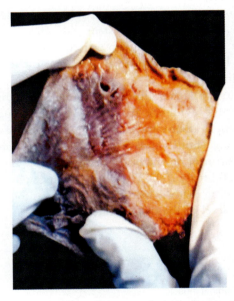

Fig. 21.3: Dissection of the anal mucosa, displaying the circular muscles of the anal canal. The lower edge of the specimen held by the right thumb and index finger is the site of the anal orifice, now opened. The bluish color shown on the left side of the dissected specimen and held under the two thumbs is the anal mucosa that has been turned over on the left side, after it has been dissected out from the circular muscles of the anal canal. Below the level of the transverse fibers which are circular muscles of the anal sphincter, no such muscles fibers are present in this specimen. It was covered by yellowish fatty like tissue (By courtesy of SK Saha and SK Chatterjee)[17]

In the dissection, the anterior wall of the anal canal was opened by a longitudinal incision, thus displaying the mucosal wall of the anal canal. The anal mucosa was gently dissected out from one cut edge of the specimen and ended at the other cut edge of the anal canal. The dissected mucosa was then turned over towards the other edge. It came out easily from the circular muscle, like a peeling of the skin from the orange. It seems to be loosely attached with the circular muscles of the internal sphincter.

When the mucosa was turned over on the left side as held by the left thumb and index finger, the circular muscles became clear with a distinct muscular fibers lying transversely across the wall of the anal canal, but it was found absent in the lower part of the anal canal, below the dentate line. In fact, the lower part of the anal canal seemed to be covered by a layer of yellowish fatty tissue.

Furthermore, the inner surface of the anal mucosa has been turned inside out, after it is dissected out from the circular muscles. It revealed clearly the features of corrugations which seem to be an imprint of each fiber of the said circular muscle over the mucosa, and it was like a fingerprint of the transverse muscular fibers of the circular muscles; but it is absent in the lower part of the same mucosa, thus confirming the fact that the circular muscles do not exist below the dentate line of the anal canal.

It was evident in the colored illustration that the horizontal grooves, like corrugation printed over the anal mucosa are present along its attachment with the circular fibers of the anal canal, but these indentations in the mucosal wall are absent in the lower part of the same mucosa This is another evidence to support the finding that the circular muscles of the anal canal does not exist in the lower part of the anal canal. This evidence is consistent with all other textbooks of anatomy and operative surgery.

THE ANATOMY OF THE ANAL CANAL

The anal canal commences from the lower end of the rectum, at the level of the puborectalis muscles and it extends down to the anal orifice. It is around 4 cm long; but upper two-third of it is covered by the mucous membrane, composed of columnar epithelium and it is loosely attached, but it has a number of longitudinal folds known as anal columns. These anal columns are joined together at its lower ends by crescentic folds known as anal valves. It lies a little above the level of Hilton's white line or known as pectinate line.

The part below this line which is lower one-third is covered by the modified stratified hairless skin. The stratified skin covering this part has a limited elasticity, compared to the anal mucosa. This anatomical difference in the lining of the anal canal is related to embryology. The upper two-thirds of the anal canal are derived from the endoderm and the lower one-third from the ectoderm. The reason for a limited elasticity of the stratified skin is partly due to characteristic feature of the skin itself, but its main reason is in contact with the anococcygeal raphe that may inhibit its maximum stretching limit at defecation.

The junction between the endoderm and the ectoderm is the Hilton's white line, which is also known as pectinate line in the anatomical book (Fig. 21.2). In this figure, the fascia, derived from the longitudinal muscles of the rectum is attached to the pectinate line and the circular muscles of the anal canal, anatomically known as internal sphincter ends just above the attachment of the longitudinal muscles that lies at the level of the Hilton's white line.

This anatomical description seems to be consistent with the embryology, but some surgical book has described it differently (Fig. 21.1), not consistent with other textbook of anatomy (Fig. 21.2). In this respect Figure 21.2 seems to be consistent with that of Figure 21.4, included in another textbook of operative surgery. All those illustrations referred to in those books are consistent with the recent dissection of the cadaveric specimen of the anal canal (Fig. 21.3).

According to the textbook of anatomy, the subcutaneous external sphincter has been delineated below the Hilton's white line. Furthermore, the subcutaneous anal sphincter that encircles around the anal orifice constitutes the anal verge. It is a striated circular muscle and are voluntary muscle, separated from the internal sphincter and other external sphincters by a fascia derived from the longitudinal muscle of the rectum. It is around 1 cm in diameter. Furthermore, it has no bony attachment, but it is free from the anococcygeal raphe or the coccyx. It acts independently and as a wiper of the bottom at defecation (Fig. 21.5).

By contrast, the internal anal sphincter that ends at the level of the Hilton's white line or pectinate line is composed of circular muscles, which are continuation of the circular muscles of the rectum and colon. They are smooth and involuntary muscle. Its thickness is around 3 mm.[6] Hence, it is unlikely to induce pain due to acute anal fissure, but the discomfort or acute sharp pain arising from the acute fissure-in-ano, experienced by

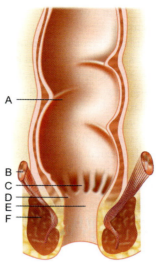

Fig. 21.4: In this figure, the lower end of the internal anal sphincter (D) is above the attachment of the longitudinal muscles of the anal canal (B) and it lies at the level of pectinate line /Dentate (E).[13] (By courtesy of the publishers and authors, this figure has been reproduced from the "Farquharson's Textbook of Operative Surgery, Sixth Edition 1978)[13]

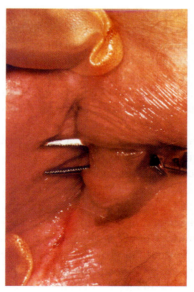

Fig. 21.5: Displaying the thick circular muscles of the subcutaneous external anal sphincter

the patient is a somatic pain. Furthermore, the force of contraction exerted by the circular muscles of the anal canal would be much weaker than that of the subcutaneous external anal sphincter (Figs 21.2 and 21.4).

Long-standing Controversy of the Internal Sphincter

In late 1930s, eminent surgeons like Morgan, Milligan and others described the surgical anatomy of the internal sphincter of the anal canal,[1,3,11,14] but a decade later, this was questioned by other eminent surgeons.[6,7,15]

It seems as if what had been taught to us yesterday turned out to be different a few years later and who knows what would be taught tomorrow could be quite different from today.

Despite this conflicting anatomical description, the anal canal and in particular to the internal sphincter, described in one textbook of anatomy[12] seems to be in conflict with other teachers.[6,7,15] In this anatomy book,[12] the internal anal sphincter has been delineated to be at the level of Hilton's white line, known as pectinate line.

I always believe that human anatomy remains undisputed, once printed in the textbooks of anatomy, but it is apparent that the surgical literature seems to have been evolving, whether or not the facts reflect a true feature of medical science.

To resolve the conflicting report, dissection of the rectum and anal canal was carried out on a cadaveric specimen, preserved in formalin. And it was carried out at the anatomy department of RG Kar Medical College, Kolkata.[16]

Although the cadaveric specimen of the rectum and anal canal was found shrunken, due to use of preservative of formalin, the thickness of the circular muscle of the internal sphincter was found to be no more than 2 mm.

Its separation or dissection was found to be tedious either from the longitudinal muscles or from the anal mucosa, despite using a sharp knife or scissors and there were a clear evidence of longitudinal mucosal folds in the lower part of the anal canal and they were joined together at the bottom known as anal valves. The latter were present a few mm above the Hilton's white line.

In brief, this study confirmed that the anatomical position of the internal sphincter was found consistent with what has been described in the textbook of anatomy.

Further study was carried out on the male cadaveric specimen at NRS Medical College and Hospital in Kolkata and a different approach was adopted in order to find out the exact level of the circular muscles of the anal canal.[16] And this dissection confirms the previous one that was carried out a year earlier.

In this respect, it is worth highlighting the sphincteric function of the anal sphincter. As I understand the morphology of all other sphincters, the behavior of the anal sphincter would be the same. And in fact, they keep the anal orifice closed at rest. It has no power to operate independently in opening the anal orifice, but it can keep the anal orifice closed voluntarily.

Furthermore, the internal sphincter has no independent function in closing and opening of the anal orifice, when it cannot stop passage of wind per anus, but the discharge of flatus per rectum is held back by the anal columns and anal valves present in the lower part of the anal canal. Their physiological function has never been described in the literature, to my knowledge. In fact, the flatus is discharged at times, when the rectal air pressure exceeds the tone of those anal columns and anal valves.

Suspicion arose during the dissection of the internal sphincter, as to how the internal sphincter, which is less than 3 mm in thickness, can contract or can act as a sphincter independently, when it was found inseparable from the longitudinal muscle of the anal canal and when it is encircled by the powerful striated muscles of the external anal sphincter. I wonder whether it can act as internal anal sphincter independently alone or at all.

In fact, the thickness of the circular muscles around the anal canal was no thicker than those around the rectum. Therefore, it seems to be a misnomer referring to the circular muscles of the anal canal to be the internal sphincter, when it would not be able to contract voluntarily or it can induce spasm independently, in those circumstances in which, these circular muscles are surrounded by other surrounding muscles and it is embraced by the thick striated muscles constituting the external anal sphincter.

The striated muscles encircling the lower part of the anal canal would prevent the circular muscles of the anal canal to work independently as an internal sphincter. In the operation of the abdomen, the small intestine has been found contracting circumferentially that implies that both longitudinal and circular muscles of the intestine work together. Hence, it was wrong to assume differently in the function of the same muscles in the anal canal. Hence, the circular muscles of the anal sphincter cannot work independently without the longitudinal fibers of the anal canal being involved.

Furthermore, the physiological function of the anal columns and the anal valves has not been clearly defined in the literature, but it is reasonable to assume that they act as a cushion, filling the lumen of the anal canal in order to make the anal canal, air-tight at rest, thus preventing the leakage of flatus through the anus all the time. They can only lose their feature of longitudinal mucosal folds passively either at the time of discharging the flatus or at the defecation of feces. Its main physiological function is to keep holding back the flatus within the ampulla of the rectum and anal canal.

It is postulated that the anal columns and anal valves supported by the circular muscles of the anal canal act as a cushion within the anal canal, thus maintaining the continence of the flatus. In this respect, they all act as an internal anal sphincter for the purpose of maintaining the continence of the flatus. The discharge of the flatus is permitted at times, when the tuft of venous flexus that lies within the anal columns and anal bulbs are squashed. This is only possible when the rectal air pressure exceeds the resting pressure of these anal columns and the anal valves.

We all know that discharge of flatus makes an embarrasing noise, which is not possible to stop and its mechanism of producing such noise is no different from playing the clarinet or a similar musical instrument.

It suggests that the anal columns and anal valves gives way to the rectal air pressure in the similar way of blowing the flute. The circular muscles of the anal canal play no part in regulating the discharge of the flatus. It is a passive action. The flatus could only be withheld voluntarily by the sphincteric function of the external anal sphincters and not by the so-called internal sphincter or by those anal columns. Incontinence of flatus can occur when these anal columns cannot maintain the airtight cushion within the anal canal.

The evidence that internal sphincterotomy causes anal incontinence in certain number of cases does not imply that the circular muscles of the internal sphincter have lost its sphincteric function. This concept could have been accepted, if the flatus can be withheld voluntarily by the contraction of the internal sphincter alone.

Therefore, the true mechanism for the incontinence of flatus or feces that may be encountered with the internal sphincterotomy in certain cases seems to be quite different from what has been universally accepted.

The fact that division of the circular muscles of the anal canal makes a longitudinal groove under the anal mucosa has never been questioned in the clinical practice. The reason is that the smooth muscle of the intestine has an elastic property like rubber. Once it is incised, it would retract. In the dissection of the cadaveric specimen, anal mucosa was found loosely attached to the circular muscles of the internal sphincter.

Hence, the transected circular fibers would remain retracted from each other, thus making a groove under the anal mucosa. This would increase the girth of the anal canal and at the same time, the overlying anal mucosa would be pushed to fill up the said groove. The consequent effect would be loosing the depth of corrugation of the anal columns and its anal valves—thus resulting in loss of depth of cushion.

This change in surgical anatomy has resulted from the change in diameter of the anal canal. Because of this new situation, the anal columns and anal valves become loose, failing to maintain the air-tight cushion within the canal. As a result, they cannot maintain the continence of flatus and motion in certain cases after the operation is done. It seems these anal columns and valves behave like washer of the tap water within the anal canal.

To support this evidence, another example could be cited in this context that anal incontinence has also been encountered with the anal dilatation, in certain cases in which, the anal orifice has been dilated beyond the tensile strength of the muscle tone of the circular muscles of the anal sphincters. The mechanism in these cases is no different from the internal sphincterotomy.

Although the internal sphincterotomy has been accepted to be a gold standard in the treatment of acute anal fissure, the rationality of this approach has to be questioned in perspective, after the revelation of controversy of the true surgical anatomy of the internal sphincter in those dissections of the cadaveric rectum. Time will tell us which way the future generation will lead the operative approach to the anal fissure.

BACKGROUND OF THE ETIOLOGY OF ANAL FISSURE

Elasticity of the smooth muscle of the internal sphincter and its overlying mucosa is no different from other circular smooth muscles of the gut. But it has to be recognized that it has much greater power of elasticity than that of the modified stratified skin and the striated muscle of the subcutaneous external anal sphincter.

Hence, the modified stratified anal skin will tend to split up in response to any pull of force that may be encountered with the defecation, causing anal dilatation. Although the modified stratified anal skin is present all around the anal orifice below the Hilton's white line, acute anal fissure does not occur in the lateral wall of the anal canal but in most instances, the linear tear of the anal skin or mucosa occurs in the posterior wall of the anal orifice.

The etiology for the tear in the posterior wall is related to the anococcygeal raphe that restricts the elasticity of the overlying stratified anal skin. It is possible that the overlying stratified skin cannot get stretched bilaterally away from the posterior wall in pari passu with the dilatation of other area of the anal canal during defecation. As a result, it splits up longitudinally, in the posterior wall along the longitudinal fibrous strands of the anococcygeal raphe.

To limit the discomfort, and to keep the torn skin edges protected from the potential injury, the circular muscles of the subcutaneous anal sphincter tend to remain contracted, thus keeping the anal fissure within the anal canal. As a result, the torn skin edges of the anal fissure are protected from any injury, while sitting on the chair. This preventive measure would reduce the tension upon the torn skin edges thus relieving the pain.

Hence, it is rational to believe that the spasm of the subcutaneous anal sphincter relieves the acute pain of the anal fissure. How the internal sphincter which lies above the dentate line could lead to spasm on its own, when the dissection confirms that it remains inseparable from the longitudinal muscle fibers and the surrounding sphincteric muscle. It is presumed that the spasm of the anal canal is probably accompanied by the contraction of the surrounding muscles, such as external anal sphincters.

Although the internal sphincter is anatomically separated from other anal external sphincters, they all constitute one composite structure. The question remains to be resolved is whether the internal sphincter, which is entirely composed of involuntary muscle of the gut can induce spasm physiologically, and if so it seems to be physiologically incomprehensible without longitudinal muscle fibers and other anal sphincters being involved in such contraction. In fact, contraction of involuntary circular muscles of the internal sphincter would be resisted by the external anal sphincters that keep encircling around the internal sphincter.

Hence, it is debatable whether the internal anal sphincter alone goes into spasm at all or whether it works in combination with the subcutaneous external anal sphincter. It is also arguable whether the resting high anorectal pressure associated with the anal fissure is attributable to spasm of the internal sphincter or subcutaneous external sphincter or both in combinations has never been questioned, despite the fact that a high resting anorectal pressure has been reported in the literature.[10,18-20]

PATHOGENESIS OF ANAL FISSURE

The rectum and the anal canal is one tubular structure, lying upon the sacral curvature but why the anal fissure occurs in the lower part of posterior wall of the anal canal in most cases remains unknown. During defecation, sky-bolus of hard feces descends through the rectum and anal canal. It eventually strikes behind the anal verge.

Although the anal canal is stretched all around by the descent of the round feces, the stratified anal skin gets splitted on the posterior wall, not on the lateral wall of the anal canal and rarely, it occurs anteriorly. Obviously, there must be reason for the fissure occurring in the posterior wall.

It is presumed that the modified stratified anal skin, covering the lower third of the anal canal is subjected to undue stretch by the passage of hard bulky motion, but its power of elasticity seems to be restricted by the fibrous strands of the anococcygeal raphe supporting this particular site.

During defecation, the distention of the side walls of the anal canal keeps on pulling the anal skin in all direction, but the strip of the modified stratified anal skin covering the narrow strip of anococcygeal raphe cannot expand concurrently in pari passu with the expansion of the side wall of the anal canal. It seems such action is like a tug of war. In this case, this bilateral pull leads to a linear tear of the skin in the posterior wall of the anal canal. This occurs when it exceeds its limit of elasticity or its elasticity is restricted by the fibrous strands supporting the back of the anal skin.

In contrast, the subcutaneous anal sphincter formed by the thick circular muscles is also dilated in all direction without its fibers being torn, before the hard feces is delivered, but unlike the stratified anal skin, the thick circular muscle fibers are free from such restriction.

There must also be some reason for not having a similar tear in the lateral wall of the anal canal. The reason is that anococcygeal raphe is absent in the side and anterior walls of the anal canal. Because of this variation, anal fissure does not occur in the lateral wall and it may occur rarely in the anterior wall among the childbearing age group of women.

As a result, patient would experience an acute pain straightaway and it is associated with a fresh red bleeding, spurting in the commode, and a burning sensation may be felt. Such a pain may be experienced around the anus, while washing the anal orifice with water.

The position of the tough fibrous strands on the posterior wall seems to be the reasonable etiological factor for having the tearing of the anal skin posteriorly and over the anal verge (Fig. 21.6).

The etiology for the slow healing is very unlikely to be related to poor blood supply. In fact, perineum has a rich blood supply.[21, 22] Hence, the reasons for slow healing are due to repeated injuries and recurrent infection from the feces. In fact, the delay or slow healing could be attributable to the fibrous strands of the anococcygeal raphe interfering with the healing of the wound.

■ Examination

Inspection is the most important part of examination in the diagnosis of the acute fissure-in-ano. In this procedure, patient is requested to lie on the left lateral position with both knees bringing together towards the belly. Patient is also reassured to be relaxed. Under a bright light, the anal verge of both sides is retracted away from the anal orifice gently. This retraction

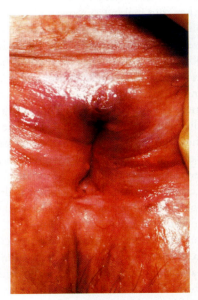

Fig. 21.6: Shows a triangular-shaped skin tear in the posterior wall of the anal verge

is done by pulling the skin of anal verge with the fingers of both hands, placed over the sides of the anal orifice.

If difficulty is experienced because of noncooperation of the patient or because of anal spasm, lignocaine jelly 2 percent soaked in swab could be applied locally over the anal orifice for 5-10 minutes. This may relieve the pain and spasm. This would help the surgeon to re-examine the fissure. In view of this painful condition, internal examination should be abandoned.

Patient may need to be examined under general anesthesia in order to establish any other pathological lesions present in the anal canal and rectum, if patient does not respond to conservative treatment, or patient may need minor operation at some stage.

Eventually, a full inspection is possible, acute fissure will appear like a slit in the midline of the posterior anal orifice. Minimum inflammation is evident.

In chronic cases, fissure-in-ano will appear like a pear-shaped ulcer. It may be associated with a sentinel skin tag, hanging from the lower edge of the fissure (Fig. 21.6). It may be oval-shaped and edematous. This may result from recurrent trauma and infection. It provides protection of the fissure. Infection and abscess may develop around the fissure and in some cases, superficial fistula may develop. It may be covered with a chronic granulomatous scar tissue.

At the operation, the sentinel pile and surrounding overhanging skin edges should be excised and sent for biopsy. This will exclude Crohn's or any other lesion. The lateral edges of the fissure could be found retracted from each other, thus keeping the floor of the fissure covered with the granulation or fibrous tissue.

Differential Diagnosis

1. Pruritus ani is associated with multiple fissures, and there are many other local conditions producing pruritus ani. These are piles, fistula, vaginal discharge, and poor hygiene. In most idiopathic condition, multiple superficial cracks lie radially from the anal orifice. But sharp pain and anal spasm are often absent in those conditions.
2. Anal fissure may be associated with the classical clinical features of ulcerative colitis or proctitis. Sigmoidoscopy and other radiological investigations will confirm the diagnosis. In these cases, the fissure is painful, broad, deep and septic. It may develop fistula.
3. In Crohn's disease, there may be more than one anal fissure, but it is confirmed by the histology. In addition, there will be evidence of other sites inflicted with Crohn's disease. It is usually confirmed by other investigations and histology.
4. Tuberculous ulcer may present as a form of anal fissure, and it is rare, but it is indistinguishable from true anal fissure apart from the undermined skin edge present around the fissure. It requires confirmation by biopsy of the ulcer and guinea-pig inoculation test.
5. Malignant growth in the anus could be differentiated from the anal fissure by the digital palpation which will reveal a deep and wide induration around the carcinoma. Patient will experience severe pain on defecation and enlarged lymph glands are palpable in the inguinal region.
6. Anal chancre presents as a painful ulcer. Spirochetes could be identified from the serous discharge. It is collected by a glass pipette and is placed on a slide to be examined under a dark ground illumination.

Treatment

Conservative Treatment

In the treatment, conservative approach should be the primary aim, due to the fact that it tends to recur. Hence, patients are encouraged to stay on high-fiber diet and to drink plenty of plain water and are discouraged in having too many cups of tea and coffee (< 4 cups/day).

For the relief of pain, lignocaine jelly (1%) in a swab should be applied locally several times per day, after being to the toilet. In addition, Glycerine trinitrate ointment (0.2%) could be applied locally. This enhances increased vascularity, thus promoting quick healing, but it may cause headache.

If patients are not benefited, the first line of intervention would be anal dilatation under general anesthesia. Ulcerative colitis, proctitis, Crohn's disease and malignant condition should be excluded from this procedure.

Technique for Anal Dilatation

In this case, the patient is placed on the lithotomy position and buttock remains on the soft cushion. Anesthetist must be warned before anal dilatation being undertaken.

First, internal examination of the anal orifice is done with both hands. The main objective is to establish the diagnosis of the anal fissure. This is done by retracting the anal verge by placing two fingers (index and middle) on each side of the anal verge. While the anal verge is held apart, tear of the anal skin could be seen. It may extend further inside the anal canal up to the dentate line.

After this examination, the anal canal is inspected using proctoscope and the rectum is examined by rigid sigmoidoscope. This investigation will exclude ulcerative colitis, Crohn's disease and carcinoma of the rectum and anal canal.

At the completion of all these procedures, the anal canal is dilated, using first two index fingers. Right index finger is placed at 3 o'clock and left one at 9 o'clock positions. These two fingers are slowly stretched away from the center and are held in position for a minute. These two fingers are replaced by index and middle fingers on each side of the anal canal.

Clinical Practice and Surgery of the Colon, Rectum and Anus

It is again dilated in the same way. Finally, the dilatation is completed by three fingers, using index, middle and ring fingers. The same principle is followed. Too much dilatation should be avoided. This may lead to fecal incontinence.

If the patient is having recurrence of acute fissure-in-ano, lateral subcutaneous internal sphincterotomy should be done. Patients must be explained about the technique to be used. Postoperative complications must be discussed with them. There remains a risk of incontinence of feces, and flatus. There could be hemorrhage within the anal orifice that may lead to formation of hematoma and infection in the postoperative period. Recurrence of fissure is also possible in some cases.

Operative Technique for Lateral Subcutaneous Internal Sphincterotomy

Patient is placed on the lithotomy position. Anal canal and the rectum are examined as described before, and in addition, the clinical state of the anal fissure is evaluated by a palpation and by an inspection.

Alan Park's anal speculum is inserted into the anal canal with two curved blades, facing each other, in that one blade is held at 6 o'clock and other one at 12 o'clock position. It is opened slowly, thus keeping the anal orifice and canal wide apart. This procedure acts as a dilator and at the same time it assists the surgeon in the identification of the groove present between the internal and external sphincters.

The left index finger is inserted into the anal canal in order to palpate the dentate line and it is kept inside the anal canal; until the sphincterotomy is completed. The next procedure is to feel the groove at 3 o'clock position of the anal verge by the tip of the right index finger. A pen knife is inserted through this groove and its sharp edge is either directed downwards or upwards while it is slowly advanced between the external and internal anal sphincters, until its tip has reached to the level just below the dentate line. The left index finger could feel the knife, passing through the wall of the canal.

The sharp edge of the knife is next turned inwards, facing its sharp edge at the pulp of the left index finger kept inside the anal canal. Bear in mind that the thickness of the internal sphincter is around 2-3 mm; and they are smooth circular muscles that lie between the mucosa and the longitudinal fibers of the rectum.

Hence, it is important to be careful in this blind procedure that the knife does not make a hole in the mucosa and injure the finger. The knife is next slowly withdrawn from inside out—thus cutting the circular fibers of the internal sphincter, when the left index finger is also withdrawn concurrently.

The left index finger is inserted again in order to palpate the same side of the anal wall. A groove under the anal mucosa is felt by the palmar surface of the index finger, confirming the division and retraction of the circular muscles. No suture is necessary. A soft dressing is left over the anal orifice.

Although this procedure has been universally accepted, its rationality and reliability requires further highlight, in perspective of the conflicting evidences of the surgical anatomy of the internal sphincter. This is a blind procedure; complete cut of the circular fibers by this blind procedure is also to be questioned.

It is debatable whether the benefit from this blind procedure is attributable to this technique or due to anal dilatation that is done by the Anal Park's retractor, inserted into the anal canal prior to undertaking the procedure of subcutaneous internal anal sphincterotomy.

Complication

The risk of incontinence of feces and flatus is possible if the dentate line is divided inadvertently. The incidence could be as high as 35 percent.[23,24] Wound infection or abscess formation is possible.

Treatment for Chronic Fissure-in-ano and Anal Stenosis

The treatment of anal stenosis is a difficult problem. In this case, the anal orifice may admit only index finger, on rectal digital examination. This is attributable to contracted subcutaneous external sphincter muscles. This may result from the disuse functional state of the sphincters. The common clinical presentation is the constipation and anal skin tags that keeps hanging from the inferior edge of the fissure. These are known as sentinel piles. In some cases, skin edges from the side of the fissure creep over the fissure, thus inhibiting the healing of the chronic anal fissure.

Repeated anal dilatation may not resolve the problem. Following the internal examination, and anal dilatation, the skin tags along with the chronic fissure should be excised. The wound is left open to be healed slowly. The excision should be undertaken like the excision of a pile and the circular muscle under the floor of the fissure should be incised concurrently. This procedure should be avoided if the fissure-in-ano is associated with Crohn's disease or malignant condition.

If anal stenosis is evident on rectal digital examination, lateral subcutaneous external anal sphincterotomy is recommended. This operation used to be a popular choice in 1930s for acute fissure-in-ano.

The subcutaneous external anal sphincter is a round circular muscle. It is over 1 cm in diameter, much thicker and stronger than the internal sphincter. It is not attached to the anococcygeal raphe and is separated from the deep external sphincter by the septum, formed by the longitudinal fibers of the rectum. It acts like a wiper of the anus and it is a striated muscle. It constitutes the anal verge. Division of this muscle does not cause incontinence of flatus or feces.

PREOPERATIVE PREPARATION

Bowel preparation is very important, before the operation being undertaken. Oral laxative should be prescribed 3-4 days prior to the operation and enema should be given on the day of operation.

Operative Procedure

Patient is placed on the lithotomy position. Anal canal and rectum are examined with proctoscope and sigmoidoscope. This has to be done to exclude other pathological disease, such as Crohn's disease, ulcerative colitis, carcinoma or nonspecific proctitis. With the permission of the anaesthetic colleague, anal sphincter is dilated. Manual evacuation of feces may be required.

The perineum is next cleaned with Savlon. Alcohol-based antiseptic solution must not be used for the skin preparation. Gloves are changed. Sterile drapes are applied around the perineum. The technique for subcutaneous anal sphincterotomy has been depicted in Figures 21.7A and B.

A radial incision is made at 3 o'clock or 9 o'clock position (Figs 21.7A and B). It should be just outside the anal verge. The length of the incision should be around 2 cm. The skin edges are separated from the muscles by blunt mobilization. Longitudinal fibers coming from the rectum could be seen across the circular muscles. These are subcutaneous external anal sphincter. The outer edge of this muscle is identified by blunt dissection, using the tip of the curved artery forceps. Once its outer edge is defined, artery forceps are passed slowly under the circular muscle, until its tips have emerged from other end of the muscle.

The artery forceps lying under the muscle act as a platform, upon which the fibers are divided. Once the collar of circular muscle is fully defined and isolated, it is divided by a cutting diathermy needle or by a knife. Once fibers are divided completely, each cut end will retract away from the artery forceps.

There should not be any residual fibers under the handles of the artery forceps. A septum between the subcutaneous external sphincter and deep external sphincter becomes apparent. Bleeding points are controlled. The skin wound is closed with interrupted mattress sutures, using 2/0 prolene. Jelly-net dressing is applied, before a T bandage is put across the perineum.

Postoperative Care

For a few days, patient should be on restricted oral feeding. When bowels open, the area needs to be cleaned with a salt

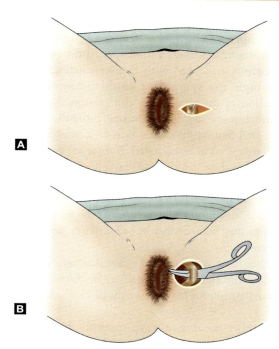

Figs 21.7A and B: Operative technique for subcutaneous external sphincterotomy

or sitz bath. Sutures are removed after two weeks. Results in 25 consecutive cases were excellent, with no evidence of incontinence of feces. The result of this operation is consistent with the surgical anatomy and pathology.

PRURITUS ANI

Pruritus is a medical condition but it may be present, secondary to other surgical pathology, in that discharge of mucoid fluid may cause irritation or itching at the anus and around the perineal region. Multiple skin cracks are encountered in the area. There are many reasons to cause itching around the anus. Men are frequently affected and it is rare among the children, unless they suffer from the threadworms.

Etiology

(a) Idiopathic.
(b) Secondary pathological conditions:
  (i) Poor local hygiene.
  (ii) Parasites infestations.
  (iii) Fungal infection.
  (iv) Allergy to the fibers of the clothes.
  (v) Excessive sweating.

Clinical presentation: Although the itching begins in the anal skin folds, it may extend beyond the perianal region. In male patient, back of the scrotum, and in female, vulva is also affected.

Local finding is variable, in some cases; the perianal skin folds may appear to be thickened and exaggerated around the anus. In other cases, there would appear to be excoriation of the epidermis associated with many scratches.

Although the symptoms could be minor, internal examination of the anal canal, and rectum should be done with a proctoscope and sigmoidoscope. From the surgical point of view, anal fissure, piles, anal skin tags, anal fistula, polyps or papilloma need to be excluded. If these are present, surgical treatment for these conditions may alleviate the symptoms. In some cases, the symptoms may be attributable to the first degree of internal piles. In these cases, injection therapy with phenol (5%) in almond oil may improve the symptoms. Several procedures may be necessary in order to get any benefit from this treatment.

In other cases, excision of the anal skin tag, fibrous polyps protruding through the anal orifice, or electrocauterization for perianal papilloma may reduce the discharge to the perianal region.

In all other nonsurgical cases, patients should be advised to seek further advice from other specialty.

MALIGNANT TUMORS OF THE ANUS

Although malignant tumor is rare finding in the anal canal or anal orifice, the common varieties are:
  (a) Squamous cell carcinoma.
  (b) Basal cell carcinoma.
  (c) Malignant melanoma.

Apart from these tumors, adenocarcinoma may be found within the anal canal. In advanced stage; the tumor protrudes through the anal orifice. But in fact, it arises from the rectal mucosa. Exact mechanism is not clearly understood that how does it arrive at the anal canal or protrude through the anal orifice, it is possible that during defecation, the tumor tends to be dragged downwards through the anal orifice.

The squamous cell carcinoma may also grow upwards, involving the rectum. It can arise at the pectinate line, chronic anal fistula or in the anal orifice. Again, it can move upwards in contrast to the adenocarcinoma. However, there is a distinct difference in consistency when the two malignant tumors are palpated in that the adenocarcinoma would appear to be soft in consistency and it tends to be friable. And it may discharge colloid material, but in contrast, the squamous cell carcinoma would be firm or very hard in consistency.

Prevalence and Sex Distribution

Among the cases of adenocarcinoma found in the rectum, anal canal, and anus at the St. Mark's Hospital, the prevalence of the squamous cell carcinoma was 3.5 percent[25] but it was 4.7 percent reported from the Massachusetts hospital.[26] It is evident that it is a very rare variety of all malignant tumors grown in the rectal and anal canal regions.

Furthermore, it was reported from the St. Mark's hospital that the distribution of the squamous cell carcinoma was found equal both sexes;[25,27,28] but adenocarcinoma was found more among the men compared to women.

The report also states that men are affected more than women if the squamous cell carcinoma arises from the anal orifice, but in contrast, the incidence would be greater among the women; if the same variety of tumor arises from the anal canal.[25] The study also suggested that pruritus ani was found associated with the carcinoma developed in the anal orifice. Its significance has not been highlighted but it is presumed that the discharge from the tumor may cause irritation to the local skin.

Apart from the sex distribution with relation to the site of the tumor, it has been reported that those squamous cell carcinoma found among the men are frequently a low grade malignancy and those among the women are by contrast a high grade malignancy.[29] Furthermore, the tumors arising from the region of the anal canal are poorly differentiated and those from outside the anal canal are well-differentiated.

Pathology

In early stage, a wart-like growth or an ulcerated lesion with an irregular margin develops usually in the anterior aspect of the anus. It gradually progresses all around, thus forming an annular type hard tumor mass within the anus and its surface could be ulcerated and fixed to the tissue underneath the base of the tumor. An area of indurated edge over the intact skin could be felt outside the true edge of the tumor.

Clinical Presentation

In most instances, patients complain of various types of symptoms arising from the growth developed in the anal canal or anal orifice. These are pain at defecation, bleeding, some feeling of lumpiness around the anus, discharge, irritation, or foul smelling, because of soggy stained in the underpant, or incontinence of feces. In female patient, there may be discharge of feces through the vagina. Sometimes, perianal warts are present without knowing the serious nature of the disease. One of my female patients had presented with acute ischeorectal abscess. It was due to invasion of the tumor into the ischeorectal fossa.

All these insignificant symptoms require a thorough clinical examination and local examination. In the groin examination, superficial inguinal glands could be palpable either in one or both groins. In this palpation, concentration is focused whether the glands are soft or hard and whether they are fixed and matted together. Some of the enlarged lymph glands may be affected by the transmission of infection from the ulcerated tumor of the anus. In these cases, glands would appear to be soft on palpation and it could be tender to touch. By contrast, the metastatic lymph glands would be found hard in consistency and matted together on palpation.

In these cases, glans penis in male and vaginal canal in female patients must be examined to exclude any malignant growth. In addition, lower limbs are examined to exclude lymphedema or pitting edema and whether there is any evidence of deep vein thrombosis in the calf of each leg.

At the end of all clinical examination, rectal digital examination should be done, but it may not be possible to get into the anal canal due to ulcerated growth present inside the anus. In other cases, ulcerated tumor mass could be seen peeping through.

In these cases, diagnosis would be obvious. Proctoscopy would be impossible. In other cases, when the digital examination would be possible, the rectal digital examination would reveal the classical presentation of a hard indurated and raised ulcerated growth and it could be fixed to the wall of the anus.

These classical findings would suggest a tentative clinical diagnosis of malignant tumor. After digital examination, proctoscopy, if admissible through the anal orifice, should be done, but biopsy should be taken under general anesthesia.

After proctoscopic examination being done, sigmoidoscopy should be done to exclude any other lesion in the rectum and the sigmoid colon; but it may mislead the surgeon by failing to recognize the tumor in the anal orifice or in the anal canal, when it would pass through the tumor. For the examination of the anal canal or for taking tissue from the anal canal, sigmoidoscope should not be used at all.

The tumor tissue should be obtained under general anesthesia either through the proctoscope or by the guidance of the left index finger inserted through the anus. Once the left index finger has been inserted into the anal canal and the tumor is palpated, the biopsy forceps is next passed along the side of the index finger. The tip of the forceps is then directed by the tip of the finger towards the lesion in order to take a tissue from the ulcerated growth.

A few such biopsies should be taken for a better histology report. Sometimes, it has been experienced that tissue sent for histology may not contain the tumor tissue or the forceps could not bite the tissue in the first attempt because of hardness of the tumor mass and what was sent in the preservative was a few necrotic tissue. A negative report does not exclude malignancy of the ulcerated growth.

Differential Diagnosis

In the early clinical presentation, diagnosis may not be straightforward in certain cases, in which the lesion could be of various presentations. They are:

- Papilloma or anal warts.
- Prolapse thrombosed pile.
- Ulcerated lesion which could be due to Crohn's disease.
- Chronic anal fissure.
- Condylomas.
- Primary chancre.

Of course, a careful examination and tissue diagnosis must be done before contemplating any kind of surgical treatment. One of my female patients was having a repeated electrical cauterization of anal papilloma over a few years but no histology was done prior to the treatment.

In fact, it turned out to be squamous cell carcinoma. Another male patient had presented with a small nodule in the midthigh and histology report suggested that it was squamous cell carcinoma, but the patient had very little bowel symptoms and he was not aware of any ulcerated lesion in the anus. Eventually, the primary tumor was squamous cell carcinoma found on rectal digital examination. Hence, it is important to establish the tissue diagnosis first before undertaking any operation, however a small lesion it could be.

TREATMENT OF THE CARCINOMA OF THE ANUS

The treatment of the anal carcinoma is much more complicated and controversial than that of the rectal carcinoma. This is probably related to many factors involved. These are related to:

(a) The site of the tumor whether it is above or below the pectinate line of the anal canal.
(b) Mode of therapeutic approach related to the evidence of palpable or non palpable inguinal lymph glands.
(c) Local radiotherapy with or without colostomy.
(d) Surgical treatment with or without preoperative radiotherapy.
(e) Surgical therapy with or without bilateral block dissection of the inguinal lymph nodes.
(f) Surgical treatment for local excision or radical abdominoperineal excision.

Furthermore, one cannot acquire expertise in surgical practice, if the prevalence of the anal tumor is less than 4 percent among all patients presented with malignant tumors in the rectum and anal canal.

However, for a better understanding of the management, the cases with squamous cell carcinoma could be divided into three groups. These are:

(a) Group one includes those tumors arising from the area above the pectinate line.
(b) Group two includes those tumors arising from below the pectinate line.

(c) Group three include those tumors, which could not be differentiated between the two sites.

These findings are important in order to decide the methods of treatments suitable to each type of case. Eventually, a final decision should be in consultation with the oncologist, whether the tumor of the first group should be treated with abdominoperineal excision and the second group with radiotherapy or with local excision or combination of radiotherapy followed by surgical ablation.

The third group could be treated by any one of the three modalities that depends upon the stage of the tumor, general health of the patients and skill of the surgeon.

Apart from the treatment modality used, prognosis of survival rate is related to the metastasis either into the inguinal lymph glands or into the mesenteric or pelvic lymph glands. In this respect, it is important to understand the lymphatic drainage from the anal canal.

It states that the lymphatic plexuses drain from the area below the pectinate line into the inguinal lymph glands and those above the pectinate line follow the superior hemorrhoidal and middle rectal vessels. Those lymphatic channels follow the superior rectal arteries drain eventually to the mesenteric lymph glands, lying along the inferior mesenteric vessels and those follow the middle rectal vessels drain to the lymph nodes lying along the internal iliac vessels.

If the inguinal lymph glands are found to be enlarged, hard and matted together, it is presumed that the primary site of the tumor could be below the pectinate line. This is an apparent clinical assessment. And the prognosis in these cases is poor, despite undertaking a bilateral block dissection.

On the other hand, absence of palpable inguinal lymph glands does not imply that the primary site of the tumor is above the pectinate line. Hence, decision for operative treatment for the inguinal lymph glands is to be judged on the merit of clinical assessment.

It is a universal agreement that the squamous cell carcinoma responds well to the deep X-ray therapy, whether or not the primary site of the tumor is above the pectinate line. All patients presented with squamous cell carcinoma could be treated with deep X-ray therapy and this should be the first line of treatment modality. Contrary to this policy, all statistics suggest that five year survival rate was reported consistently better with abdominoperineal excision, compared to local excision and/or radiotherapy.

If the tumor is treated with deep X-ray therapy, temporary diversion of feces may be required, if there is evidence of difficulty in defecation. Temporary colostomy would provide a comfort and improve the general health and quality of life, after radiotherapy is given. This consideration has to be taken in conjunction with the oncologist, dealing with the radiotherapy. In some advanced stage of the tumor, pelvic loop colostomy should be done prior to radiotherapy.

The next consideration is to evaluate the merit of surgical ablation of the tumor. Here lies the disagreement between the two schools of approach. This will be highlighted with reference to the survival rate.

Apart from the local adjuvant radiotherapy, there are two types of surgical treatment available with or without the block dissection. In the absence of palpable inguinal nodes, the anal tumor could be excised locally or it could be treated by radical abdominoperineal resection of the rectum and anus, whether or not the squamous cell carcinoma had originated from the area above the pectinate line of the anal canal.

It is the consensus that surgical excision of the tumor is unnecessary in those cases, in which, the tumor arises from the area below the pectinate line. These patients should be treated with deep radiotherapy.

The next treatment policy is to be determined whether a prophylactic bilateral block dissection of the inguinal lymph glands should be carried out routinely, whether or not the primary tumor has been treated either with radiotherapy or abdominoperineal excision. There is no consensus on this modality.

Some school of thought suggests wait and watch, in those cases, in which, the inguinal lymph glands are not clinically palpable. But these patients require reviewing in the follow-up clinic every month for six months and then every two months for the next two years. Goligher does not recommend for lymph gland biopsy for histological evidence prior to undertaking the block dissection. I agree that one or two lymph nodes biopsy may not provide conclusive evidence whether or not other inguinal lymph nodes are infiltrated by the metastasis.

If bilateral block dissection is necessary, then it is advisable that it should be done six weeks after the primary treatment being carried out. But patient must be explained that there remains a risk of developing wound infection, slow postoperative recovery, and persistent drainage of lymphatic fluid in the suction bottle over a month. The permanent morbidity would be a permanent bilateral lymphedema in both lower limbs and around the genital area. Patient is advised using a tight stocking (TED) in both lower limbs during the day time.

Surgical Treatment

These are the options available to the patients:
1. (a) Abdominoperineal excision of the rectum and anus could be carried out, and a detailed technique for this procedure has been described in the chapter of the rectum.
   (b) Alternatively, local excision of the squamous cell carcinoma is undertaken by using a cutting diathermy needle. The technique is similar to the resection of the villous papilloma in the rectum. It requires excision of

the tumor with a wide skin margin of about 1 inch, away from the edge of the tumor all around, but this local excision should be abandoned, if such clearance is not possible between the upper edge of the tumor and the pectinate line. In this case, abdominoperineal resection should be employed.

2. If the deep X-ray therapy has resolved the tumor completely, it is debatable whether or not further ablation surgery is indicated. One has to evaluate the merits between the radical surgical operation and local radiotherapy. If the inguinal lymph glands are clinically palpable, the tumor should be treated with radiotherapy alone.

3. Bilateral block dissection of the inguinal lymph glands— It should be done six weeks later after the primary treatment is completed.

■ Operative Technique for Block Dissection of the Inguinal Lymph Glands

Apart from the anal carcinoma, lymph glands could be invaded by other malignant carcinoma developed in the penis, the prostate gland, pigmented skin lesion (melanoma), fatty lump (liposarcoma), and in the female genitalia.

As pointed out before, patient must be explained about the permanent morbidity associated with this operation, if the metastatic tumors in these glands could not be treated with local radiotherapy. Unilateral block dissection is done if the source of the primary tumor is in the lower limb, but bilateral block dissection of the inguinal lymph glands are carried out in all other cases of malignant tumor developed in the penis, prostate, anal orifice and female genitalia.

An indwelling Foley catheter either No. 16FG or 18FG is passed into the bladder before operation. A wide skin preparation is done, covering the lower abdomen, genital area, upper part of the thigh, lateral part of the pelvis and thigh. Sterile drapes are applied all around the field of operation.

Block dissection could be done either by making a curved incision, two inches below the inguinal ligament or by "T" shaped incision, where the longitudinal incision is commenced from the middle of the transverse skin crease incision, made below the inguinal ligament in the upper part of the femoral triangle and it is continued down along the line of femoral vessels.

There are some advantages and disadvantages in all approaches. Wound healing is better with a skin crease transverse incision, but the exploration of the glands along the femoral vessels may be limited in some instances. If T incision is employed, good exploration is achieved but there remains a small risk of poor skin wound healing over the "T" junction.

If a transverse incision is made over the femoral triangle, it should be between the anterior superior iliac spine and pubic tubercle. The upper skin flap is dissected out from the fascia of Camphor and fascia of Scarpa. Dissection is continued upwards beyond the inguinal ligament. All the fatty layers and the glandular tissues are stripped off from the aponeurotic layer of the anterior rectus sheath right down to the inguinal ligament. All blood vessels are ligatured. Dissection is continued further down below the inguinal ligament.

The lower skin flap is next dissected and retracted down by the Langerbeck retractors. The long saphenous vein is next divided between the two ligatures at the level of 3-4 inches below the inguinal ligament. All the fatty layers along the cluster of enlarged glands are slowly dissected out, using a fine scissors. Dissection is continued upwards, carrying with the proximal segment of the long saphenous vein, until the saphenofemoral junction is reached, where it is divided between the two ligatures.

The whole fatty tissue along with the long saphenous vein and chains of lymph nodes are slowly stripped off, around the femoral vessels and from the femoral canal. A good hemostasis is achieved. Redivac drainage tubing is left into the wound, before the skin wound is closed with interrupted prolene sutures. The specimen is sent for histology.

Alternative to the transverse curved incision, block dissection could be carried out through a "T" type skin incision, in that the transverse skin crease incision is made across the upper part of the groin. It should be between the anterior superior iliac spine and pubic tubercle and an inch below the inguinal ligament.

In addition, a longitudinal incision is made, commencing from the center of the transverse incision, and it is continued down until it reaches the lower end of the femoral triangle. The upper skin flaps is lifted upwards across the inguinal canal. All the fatty layers along with the vessels are stripped off from the aponeurotic layer of the abdomen right down to the groin.

The vertical skin flap is next dissected, commencing from the center and the dissection of each skin flap begins from the vertical incision. They are retracted away from the center. The long saphenous vein is next identified and is divided between the two ligatures. This division is done at the level with the apex of the femoral triangle.

All fatty layers and the chains of lymph nodes are meticulously dissected out from the floor of the femoral triangle and around the femoral vessels by the scissors. This specimen along with the proximal segment of the long saphenous vein are dissected out and removed in en bloc. All tributaries draining to the long saphenous vein are excised with the specimen.

In this dissection, lymph glands from the femoral canal are also cleared off. A good hemostasis is achieved. Redivac drainage tubing is left inside the wound before the skin flaps are closed with interrupted prolene sutures.

Postoperative Care

The drainage tubing should be kept *in situ* even after the patient is discharged home. Because the collection of lymph will continue in the bottle for many weeks after the operation, but arrangement should be made to change the bottle as and when necessary, until it stops discharging. Sutures are usually removed in 2 weeks, if there was no infection and good healing has been achieved. But in most cases, healing is slow due to lymphedema in the skin edges. The lower limb should be worn with crape bandage, tube-grip, or long thromboembolic deterrent (TED) stocking from the toes to midthigh all the time.

Merits of the Operative Techniques and Survival Rate

The survival rate is worse in the treatment of squamous cell carcinoma of the anus compared to carcinoma of the rectum, but the results with abdominoperineal resection of the rectum and anus for the squamous cell carcinoma compares favorably from the local excision of the tumor.

This is a bird eye review of the literature. The five year survival rate is influenced by many factors related to the clinical stage of the tumor, site of the tumor and treatment modalities.

In one study, the incidence was found to be 17.3 percent, among those patients treated with a combination of radiotherapy and surgery, but the same author claimed in his study that the five year survival rate was much better with radical operation than with radiotherapy alone, in that the incidence was 30 percent among the cases included in abdominoperineal resection. In sharp contrast, it was 5 percent among the 19 patients treated with radiotherapy alone.[26]

In other study, the incidence of five year survival rate was 63 percent, among the squamous cell carcinoma included in the surgical treatment.[30] The author stated that the reason for this result was attributable to early stage of the growth included in the operation. In Mayo clinic, the five year survival rate was 53.4 percent but in other series in which the cases were included in abdominoperineal excision, the overall five year survival rate was 62 percent.[31] It was another contrast results between the cases operated upon by abdominoperineal excision and those by local excision, reported in 1957. The incidence was 58 percent compared to 28 percent respectively.[32]

All these data are encouraging and provide a good reference to other surgeons whether or not the patients would be benefited from a local or abdominoperineal excision, but these results did not disclose a detailed analysis of the tumor sites and metastasis into the inguinal lymph glands.

In that respect, much clinical information was included in the results of five year survival rate, reported by the St. Mark's hospital. For instance, survival rate was 59 percent among those cases of squamous cell carcinoma, developed at the anal margin or around the perianal region treated by local excision, but it was 51 percent among the cases of squamous cell carcinoma in the anal canal, operated upon by abdominoperineal excision.[33]

In Mayo Clinic, the five year survival rate was found much worse among those cases of metastasis in the inguinal lymph glands arising from the squamous cell carcinoma, located either in the anal canal or in the anus, and none of those patients survived for five years.[34]

All these statistics convey one message that the prognosis is very poor among the cases with the inguinal lymph gland metastasis and the survival rate over 5 years would be better with abdominoperineal resection than with local excision of the tumor or with radiotherapy.

It requires more study in order to develop a conclusion whether the radiotherapy to the squamous cell tumor provides a better survival rate compared to radical excision of the tumor.

Management of Another Rare Malignant Ulcer in the Anal Region

It is a basal cell carcinoma like a rodent ulcer developed in the face. It is extremely rare in the anal region. It is often referred to the clinic as piles, but unlike the piles, it has an indurated ulcer with a raised irregular margin. It is usually located over the anal margin or anal verge. Average size is 1 × 2 cm in diameter. It does not metastasize like rodent ulcer on the face. Suspicion should arise because of nature of ulcer in the anal region among the older age group.

Although biopsy should be taken, prior to excision of the ulcer, but there would be no harm in total excision of the lesion from the region prior to histology report, but it could be established later by sending the entire specimen to the pathology. The local wound is treated with wound dressing. Primary wound closure may not last due to infective site and recurrent trauma.

Alternative to excision is the radiotherapy. In that case, a small surgery is necessary for tissue diagnosis before referring to radiotherapy. It would be too much hassle when the outcome is no different from the primary excision.

Another Rare Variety of Malignant Skin Lesion

It is a malignant melanoma that is presented as piles or a thrombosed piles in the anal orifice. In some cases, a small polypoidal skin lesion is presented over the anal margin or in the anal canal. Its surface may be ulcerated.

Clinical symptoms could be of many forms, such as pain, discharge of pus or hemorrhage from the ulcerated site or patient may complain of change in bowel habit and discharge of slime. All these symptoms are typical nature of malignant growth in the anal orifice. But a mistaken diagnosis is made as thrombosed piles because of bluish skin color.

In advanced condition, inguinal lymph glands may be found enlarged and hard. Such finding is a poor prognosis.

Treatment

A wide excision remains the only option for all malignant melanoma, and prophylactic block dissection provides an added benefit but in most cases, the prognosis is uncertain or poor. In early stage of the tumor, abdominoperineal resection of the rectum and anus is a widely acceptable method of treatment, but an urgent tissue diagnosis must be made before proceeding with this radical surgery. Bilateral block dissection of the inguinal glands could be done after the patient has fully recovered from the previous operation. There is no role for radiotherapy and chemotherapy in the treatment of malignant melanoma.

REFERENCES

1. Milligan ETC, Morgan CN. Surgical anatomy of the anal canal with special reference to anorectal fistula. Lancet 1934;1213.
2. Blaisdell PC. Pathogenesis of anal fissure and implications as to treatment. Surg Gynec Obstet 1937;65:672.
3. Milligan ETC. Section of Proctology: The surgical anatomy and disorders of the perianal space. Proce Roy Med 1943;36:365.
4. Gabriel WB. Principal and Practice of Rectal Surgery. 4th ed. London: Lewis.
5. Miles WE. Observations upon internal piles. Surg Gynec Obstet 1919;29:497.
6. Eisenhammer S. The internal anal sphincter: Its surgical importance. S Afr Med J 1953;27:266.
7. Goligher JC, Leacock AG, Brossy JJ. Surgical anatomy of the anal canal. Brit J Surg 1955;43:51.
8. Goligher JC, Duthie HL, Nixon HH. Surgery of the anus, rectum and colon. Second Edition, Bailliere, Tindall & Cassell, London, 1967.
9. Schouten WR, Briel JW, Auwerds JJA. Relationship between anal pressure and anodermal blood flow: The vascular pathogenesis of anal fissure. Dis Colon Rectum 1994;37:664.
10. Schouten WR, Briel JW, Auwerds JJA, De-Graaf EJR. Ischaemic nature of anal fissure. Br J Surg 1996;83:63.
11. Klostererhalfen B, Vogel P, et. al. Topography of the inferior rectal artery: A possible cause of chronic primary anal fissure. Dis Colon Rectum 1989;32:43.
12. Last RJ. Anatomy, Regional and Applied, Fourth Edition, published by J & A Churchill Ltd 1966.
13. Rintoul RF. Farquharson's Textbook of Operative Surgery, Sixth Edition, published by The English Language Book Society and Churchill Livingstone.
14. Morgan CN. The surgical anatomy of the anal canal and the rectum. Postgrad Med J 1936;12:287.
15. Parks AG. The surgical treatment of haemorrhoids. Br J Surg 1955;43:337.
16. Saha SK, Seth T, De (Mrs) A, Sengupta (Mrs) RB. Dissection of the anal canal about the anatomical position of the internal sphincter. RG Kar Medical College and Hospital, Kolkata, February 2008 (unpublished).
17. Saha SK, Chatterjee SK. Dissection of the internal anal sphincter of a cadaveric male body, NRS Medical College and Hospital, February 2009 (unpublished).
18. Hancock BD. The internal sphincter and anal fissure. Br J Surg 1977;64:92.
19. Chowcat NL, Araujo JG, Boulos PB. Internal Sphincterotomy for chronic anal fissure: Long-term effects on anal pressure. Br J Surg 1986;73:915.
20. Farouk R, Duthie GS, et al. Sustained internal sphincter hypertonic in patients with chronic anal fissure. Dis Colon Rectum 1994;37:424.
21. Saha SK. Care of perineal wound in abdominoperineal resection. J Royal College of surgeons of Edinburgh, 1983;324.
22. Saha SK. A critical evaluation of dissection of the perineum in synchronous combined abdominoperineal excision of the rectum. Surg Gynec and Obstet 1984;158:33.
23. Khubechandani IT, Reed JF. Sequalae of internal sphincterotomy for chronic fissure-in-ano. Br J Surg 1989;76:431.
24. Sharp FR. Patient selection and treatment modalities for chronic fissure-in-ano. The American. J Surg 1996;171:512.
25. Morson BC. The pathology and results of treatment of cancer of the anal region. Proc Roy Soc Med 1959;52(Suppl.):117.
26. Sweet RH. Results of treatment of epidermoid carcinoma of the anus and rectum. Surg Gynec Obstet 1953;84:967.
27. Gabriel WB. Squamous cell carcinoma of the anus and anal canal. Proc Roy Soc Med 1941;34:139.
28. McQuarrie HB, Buie LA. Epithelioma of anus. Post grad Med 1950;7:402.
29. Broders AC. The grading of carcinoma. Minn Med 1925;8:726.
30. Grinnell RS. An analysis of forty-nine cases of squamous cell carcinoma of the Anus. Surg Gynec Obstet 1954;98:29.
31. Richards JC, Beahrs OH, Woolner LB. Squamous cell carcinoma of the anus, anal canal and rectum in 109 patients. Surg Gynec Obstet 1962;114:475.
32. Dillard BM, Spratt JS Jr, Ackerman LV, Butcher HR Jr. Epidermoid Cancer of the anal margin and canal. Arch Surg 1963;86:772.
33. Gabriel WB. Principles and Practice of Rectal Surgery, 5th Ed. London: Lewis, 1963.
34. Judd ES, Jr, De Tar BE. Squamous cell carcinoma of the anus: Results of Treatment. Surgery 1955;37:220.

22. Volvulus of the Colon and Intussusception of the Intestine

VOLVULUS OF THE COLON

Definition of Volvulus

Rotation of the gut or viscus around its axis, causing obstruction is known as volvulus. It may occur in the stomach, gallbladder, small intestine, cecum and sigmoid colon. It may occur in neonates and middle-aged and elderly patients.

The main causative factor for the volvulus of the small intestine is the congenital defect, failing to rotate the small intestine. The most common site is the lower ileum and it occurs around a band connected between the antimesenteric border of a loop of intestine and the umbilicus. In some cases, a remnant of Meckel's diverticulum may act as a string between the gut and the umbilicus.

Volvulus of the Colon

Volvulus of the cecum and ascending colon occurs due to a loose peritoneal attachment to the parietal wall. It is also a congenital defect, failing to keep the cecum and ascending colon adherent to the parietal wall. It tends to rotate in a clockwise direction involving the ascending colon in the first instance and then it brings a part of the terminal ileum in the rotation, causing small bowel obstruction.

Females are frequently affected and the common symptom is the abdominal pain in most instances (90%), less frequently is the nausea and vomiting (70%) and other symptom is constipation that could be around 60 percent.

Clinical Examination

On examination, a mobile and well-defined mass could be felt initially in the right side of the umbilicus. But later the mass in most cases tends to occupy around the center of the abdomen or in the left side of the abdomen. If it is tympanitic on percussion, volvulus of the cecum should be suspected. Rectal digital examination and sigmoidoscopy would be unhelpful in establishing the diagnosis.

A plain X-ray of the abdomen will show a grossly dilated cecum full of air far away from the original site, and more often it would occupy in the left side of the abdomen. Plain X-ray will also show distended loops of small intestine but no colonic gas shadow will be evident in the X-ray.

Barium enema should be done but CT scan and MRI scan would provide a definitive diagnosis. If laparotomy is necessary, barium enema should be avoided because, clearance of barium from the distal colon would pose a difficult task in undertaking the resection of the gut, if it appears to have developed ischemic change in the antimesenteric border of the cecum or colon.

Treatment

Patient needs parenteral infusion for correction of dehydration and NG gastric tube in the stomach for hourly aspiration. Catheter is inserted into the bladder for measuring hourly urine output. Prophylactic appropriate antibiotics are commenced. After resuscitation, laparotomy should be carried out, sooner the better, if gangrene of the gut is to be prevented.

Patient is next prepared for emergency laparotomy that is done through a midline incision. Some surgeons may prefer to open the abdomen through the right paramedian incision.

At the operation, there are a few options available. It depends upon the condition of the cecum. First, it is untwisted through anticlockwise rotation and then to assess the viability of the cecal wall. If it appears to be in a satisfactory condition, the choice of operation is either fixation of the parietal cecal wall and ascending colon to the posterior wall of the abdomen, but there remains a further risk of recurrence.

To avoid this risk, cecostomy should be done. This will serve the purpose of decompression of the cecum and the terminal ileum. At the same time, it would encourage adhesion of the cecum to the parietal wall.

If the cecum appears to be near gangrenous or if it is perforated, then right hemicolectomy remains the choice of operation. After resection of the terminal ileum, cecum and ascending colon, end-to-end anastomosis between the ileum and the distal ascending or proximal transverse colon should be carried out in the usual way as described before. Rest of the operative procedure remains the same.

VOLVULUS OF THE SIGMOID COLON

Sigmoid volvulus occurs around its axis in the root of the narrow mesentery. It is prevalent among the elderly people and in those cases, in which the colon is distended with loaded feces due to habitual constipation. It is common in Russia, Scandinavia, Asia, and particularly in India, Central Africa, and Eastern Europe and very rare in Western Europe and North America. This epidemiological difference is not known.

Etiology is not known but the contributing factors are a long and narrow pedicle present at the root of the mesentery, but it has a broader mesentery like a fan-shaped along the long loop of distended sigmoid colon, loaded with feces. In some cases, a loose string or band may be found attached between the loop of the antimesenteric border of the colon and the parietal wall.

Pathology

Unlike the cecal volvulus, sigmoid volvulus rotates in anticlockwise direction around the narrow pedicle (Fig. 22.1). The broad loop of the sigmoid colon loaded with feces may induce rotation, when the patient starts straining at defecation. Venous obstruction tends to occur with one and a half turns.

In this situation, the colonic wall will initially appear to be congested and edematous, but it would turn into gangrene if the duration of the obstruction exceeds six hours. In other cases, total vascular obstruction occurs, if the pedicle rotates more than one and a half turn and the colon will turn into gangrene.

The whole episode occurs very quickly, by a sudden acute colicky pain. No other colonic obstruction gives rise to this sort of abnormal clinical presentation. The incidence is much greater among the men and it could be four times more in men than in women. Again, reason for this sex difference is not known. Furthermore, volvulus occurs more in the sigmoid colon than in the cecum and ascending colon.

Clinical Features

Classical symptoms are sudden onset of colicky pain in the left side of the abdomen. It may recur from time-to-time with a spontaneous resolution, but it is often associated with the passage of large volume of flatus and bowel action. It recurs with a half turn and returns to normal position spontaneously. When it resolves on its own; patient passes a lot of flatus and loose motion.

Initially, the large colonic swelling is palpable in the left side of the abdomen, but very soon, it would occupy the whole abdomen, thus pushing the diaphragm higher up.

The symptoms of sigmoid colon volvulus would be closely similar to that of acute colonic obstruction due to carcinoma. The only difference is the presentation of acute cramp-like abdominal pain in the left side of the abdomen and a gross distention of the central abdomen associated with absolute constipation. Nausea and vomiting will be a late presentation. Again the evidence of the tympanic mass in the center of the abdomen would suggest strongly in favor of sigmoid volvulus. Such evidence is unknown in any other large bowel obstruction.

In clinical examination, a soft palpable mass could be palpable in the central part of the abdomen. And percussion will reveal a tympanitic note over the palpable lump. If the clinical features appear to have developed for a longer duration, there may be tenderness and guarding with or without rebound tenderness that depends upon whether the colon is strangulated by more than one and a half turn of the twist around the root of the pedicle of the sigmoid colon.

Investigations

At the end of clinical examination, parenteral infusion therapy should be commenced as soon as possible. Blood is sent for routine biochemical tests and other blood tests.

Indwelling catheter is passed per urethra for decompression of the bladder and for assessing the hourly urine output.

Plain X-ray of the chest may show a gas under the diaphragm which will be elevated. It may also reveal other abnormalities such as pleural effusion, basal congestion and enlarged heart.

Plain X-ray of the abdomen will show an enormous sized gaseous distention within the thick colonic outline in the central part or on the right side of the abdomen. USS of the

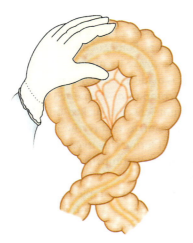

Fig. 22.1: Volvulus of the sigmoid colon twisted in anticlockwise direction

abdomen would confirm the radiological diagnosis. Other complementary investigations are CT scan or MRI scan that will assist the diagnosis.

If there are no features of peritonitis or no evidence of localized rebound tenderness, sigmoidoscopy or colonoscopy should be done with a view to untwisting the volvulus.

Treatment

Patient is asked to lie on the left lateral position. The sigmoidoscope is passed, it should reach up to the level of angulation of the colon and then a long soft rubber tube, well-lubricated with KY jelly, is passed through the sigmoidoscope until it reaches the other end, from where the soft rectal tube is gently advanced through the narrow or angulated lumen of the colon by a half-twisting clockwise and anticlockwise direction. This may allow advancing the tip of the rubber tube into the lumen of the sigmoid colon. This will deflate the colon straightaway by the passage of wind and watery motion. Blood stained watery motion would be a confirmatory evidence of sigmoid volvulus.

The sigmoidoscope is slowly removed leaving behind the rectal tube *in situ* and fixed to the left thigh for 48 hours, or until the colon is fully deflated and there would be no residual lump palpable in the abdomen. Postreduction plain X-ray of the abdomen is again taken in order to be sure that there is no residual collection of gas in the colon. If deflection is unsuccessful, laparotomy must be carried out.

It needs a definitive decision on the merits of age, general health and past history. In most cases, patients are grossly dehydrated and pale with depletion of electrolytes. Volvulus tends to recur; but surgical correction is a major operation. A balance has to be achieved between the symptoms of recurrence of volvulus and a poor health condition.

It is advisable to carry out a definitive surgery, if there is a history of recurrent symptoms and patient is reasonably fit for the major operation. Furthermore, the volvulus of the sigmoid colon, which would appear to be a size of a rugby ball, will lose its muscle tone because of gross dilatation. In this situation, its physiological function of the atony gut remains in doubt. Hence, the conservative management by untwisting the colon and by decompression of the dilated atony colon may not work.

Therefore, the volvulus part of the colon should be resected, if general condition of the patient remains reasonably fit. This will remove the uncertainty and further morbidity, if everything goes well in the operation.

Before the surgery is undertaken, patient needs resuscitation and correction of dehydration, and depletion of electrolyte and to establish the good renal function. The site of left pelvic colostomy should be marked with a skin pencil, before the patient is taken to the theater.

■ Operation

Before proceeding with a laparotomy, a long lubricated rectal tube is passed into the rectum through the sigmoidoscope, if it has not been done before. The sigmoidoscope is withdrawn, leaving behind the rubber tube inside the rectum. The size of the tube should be of an index finger. Foley catheter should not be used. It would not serve the purpose, due to the fact that eyes of the catheter will be blocked by the feces and the size of the lumen would be too narrow to drain the loose motion.

However, the outer end of the rubber catheter should be connected to an air-tight suction chamber or jar. This will prevent leakage of foul gas in the operating room and spilling of the feces on the operating table and theater floor.

Before the laparotomy is undertaken, the assistant is explained about his role in dealing with the rectal tube. During operation, he will be advised to advance the tube from outside and the surgeon will advance it from inside in order to push it further up into the dilated segment of sigmoid colon.

OPERATIVE PROCEDURE

Abdomen is prepared with antiseptic solution. Sterile drapes are laid around the operative field. The peritoneal cavity is opened through a midline incision. The volvulus is first untwisted in clockwise direction. It may require several times until, both limbs of the pedicle are found separated or untwisted and lie parallel to each other.

The assistant could advance the said rectal tube by pushing it from outside the perineum and the surgeon could get hold of the tube from outside the colon and it could be advanced further through the lumen of the colon, using both hands—in that one hand keeps holding the tube and other hand is sliding the colon over the shaft of the tube. The distended colon will be found collapsed. Rectal tube is next pulled out, if its purpose has been served.

Alternatively, the sigmoid colon could be decompressed by the Savage's decompressor. First a purse string suture is inserted over the antimesenteric border of the colon. Rest of the abdomen and the wound is covered with large warm packs.

A small nick is made in the center of the purse string suture. The Savage's decompressor is inserted through the nick and the gas and liquid feces are sucked out through the suction tube. It is important to empty the proximal colon beyond the level of twist. During this manual evacuation, anesthetist should infuse saline to compensate the loss of fluid that has been sucked out.

Once the procedure is completed, the redundant loop of the sigmoid colon is resected with a view to undertaking an end-to-end primary anastomosis, provided that both transected limbs to be anastomosed appear to be healthy and not edematous. There are three options available to the surgeon.

These are:
1. Paul-Mikulicz procedure: In this case, the diseased dilated segment of the colon is excised, using TIA 90 or using Demartel clamps or Zachary Cope clamps. Both terminal ends of the transected colon are held together by a continuous seromuscular sutures.

   The side wall of the respective terminal transected colon is sutured together at least for three inches in length and the sutures should go through the taenia coli of the respective segment of the colon. Eventually, it would be looking like a barrel-shaped two colostomies; similar to that of Paul-Mikulicz procedure, but it is a modified technique. These two barrel-shaped colonic tubes, which remained closed either by the autosutures or by the clamps are brought out through a separate wound made in the left iliac fossa.

   Both transected colonic ends are converted into terminal colostomies and the transected ends are sutured to the skin edge of the new stoma's sites. This final procedure is done after the main abdominal wound is thoroughly cleaned and washed with saline and then with metronidazole lavage (1 gm IV solution).

   It is necessary to leave a drainage tubing inside before the abdominal wound is closed in layers, as described before.
2. Alternative approach is to do terminal colostomy like a Hartmann's procedure. The distal rectal stump is closed, as described before and it left behind in the pelvic. There remains a risk of blow-out of the blind rectal stump.
3. Alternative to the above procedure, the proximal transected end of the descending colon is brought out through a separate wound made in the left iliac fossa with a view to constructing a terminal colostomy, as described before and the distal rectal stump is brought out in order to construct a rectal fistula. This is done through a separate wound. This is regarded to be a safe procedure that would avoid any risk of blow-out of the distal rectal stump. In all these procedures, reversal of colostomies could be carried out three months later.
4. If both limbs of the colon seem to be healthy, then primary end-to-end anastomosis could be undertaken either with a single layer interrupted hand sutures or with stapling autosutures gun. For any fear of anastomotic dehiscence, transverse loop colostomy should be constructed, as described in an other section.
5. In long-standing cases of the volvulus, the dilated loop of the colon may appear to be gangrene at the operation. In this case, the narrow pedicle formed by the long mesocolon that lies between the proximal and distal limbs of the pelvic colon may be found twisted which could be of several turns, like cork-screw appearance. The mesenteric vessels supplying to the distended loop of the colon would be strangulated, because of multiple rotation of the colon around its mesenteric pedicle of the colon (Fig. 22.2).

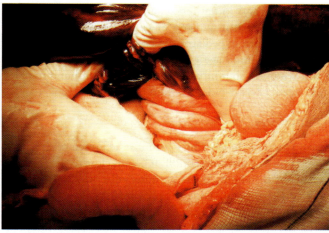

Fig. 22.2: This illustration shows the rotation of the colon and black segment of the Colon (By Courtesy of Mr C Peach and Medical library of doctors.net.uk)

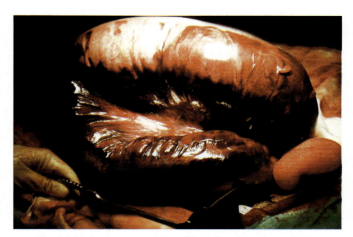

Fig. 22.3: Gangrenous state of the sigmoid colon volvulus

The loop of the volvulus needs to be untwisted very quickly. The viability of the gut requires to be assessed by covering its wall with warm wet packs. In most instances, it may not recover and require resection of the pelvic colon (Fig. 22.3).

This figure shows the pathological changes of the sigmoid volvulus. Final decision is taken on the operating table, whether or not primary end-to-end anastomosis is possible, as outlined before.

Postoperative care is carried in the usual way, until oral feeding is commenced.

INTUSSUSCEPTION OF THE INTESTINE

Epidemiology

Babies with intussusception are frequently admitted under the care of the pediatric consultant physician. After a full investigation and initial resuscitation, child is then handed over to the pediatric surgeon or general surgeon who has a particular interest in pediatric surgery for emergency operation. The most common age group among the babies is between 4 and 9 months, but intussusception has been found in older child aged 12-year-old. It is rare in adults.

Pathology

Invagination of the proximal gut into the lumen of the distal gut is known as intussusception. It begins close to the adjacent side of the distal gut. It has an outer tube which is the part of the distal gut embracing the proximal gut. The outer tube is known as intussuscipiens and the proximal gut that gets inside the intussuscipiens is known as intussusceptum. The distal invaginating end is called apex and the proximal junction between the outer wall and the inner wall of the distal gut is called the neck of the intussusception (Fig. 22.4).

Etiology

The etiological factor for presenting with intussusception is quite different between the two groups.

Among the babies below the age of 9 months, inflammation of the Peyer's patches in the terminal ileum is the trigger factor for causing intussusception.

Among the teenage or adolescent people, inverted Meckel's diverticulum may lead to develop intussusception but among the middle-aged group of patients, papilliferous carcinoma, or submucosal lipoma is the causative factor for developing intussusception. The barium enema shows a classical feature of spiral coils in the apex of colocolic intussusception (Fig. 22.5).

Among all varieties of intussusception, ileocolic intussusception has been reported to be around 77 percent and all other varieties such as ileoileal, ileoileal colic and colocolic are very small. It ranges from 2 to 12 percent.

Clinical Presentation

The classical symptoms are sudden onset of colicky abdominal pain associated with screams. Baby tends to bring both the knees together to the belly. Child continues having recurrence of similar symptoms every few minutes. In between the attack of spasmodic pain, child remains lethargic and looks tired, pale. With the passage of time, vomiting becomes a prominent feature and later baby may pass red-currant jelly-like soft motion.

On examination, warm palm must be used to palpate the abdomen and it is advisable to palpate the belly under the blanket or bedsheet. Palpation should be carried out in between the spasmodic pain. Initially, abdomen remains flat and no cecal lump is palpable in the right iliac fossa or the latter will appear to be empty, but palpation along the anatomical site

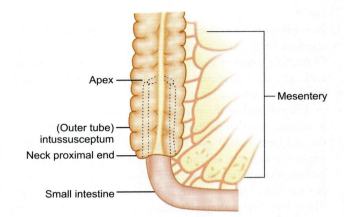

Fig. 22.4: Intussusception of the terminal ileus has invaginated through the ileocecal valve into the ascending colon

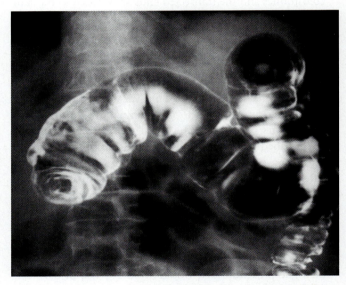

Fig. 22.5: Barium enema showing colocolic intussusception. It shows a classical feature of spring-coil at its apex (By courtesy of Dr AK Dutta-Munshi)

of the colon may reveal a sausage-shaped lump either in the right hypochondrium or in the upper abdomen.

Distention or guarding of the abdomen may be noticed if the duration of the symptom is longer than 12 hours. Rectal digital examination may reveal blood stained mucus and nothing else could be felt. In the literature, it has been reported that intussusceptum mass could be felt rectally, if the patient has a long mesentery.

Investigation

The plain X-ray of the abdomen will show no gas in the colon, but small intestine will appear to be dilated. Urgent barium enema should be done for diagnosis which may show a claw feature because of barium entering into the intussusception. This sort of evidence is only present if the intussusception is of ileocolic type. It would be absent in other types.

In this case, apart from the diagnostic value, barium enema also has a therapeutic value, in that it would act as a hydrostatic pressure pushing the apex of the intussusceptum back. But the result of this approach depends upon the duration of the intussusception.

Treatment

At the outset, infusion therapy with dextrose and saline must be commenced to compensate the fluid and electrolyte depletion. Nasogastric tube of a suitable size is inserted for hourly aspiration and a catheter is also passed per urethra into the bladder for recording hourly urine output.

Surgical intervention is imminent if resection of the gut is to be avoided. Prior to laparotomy, attempt should be made for the reduction of the intussusception under hydrostatic pressure, while the child remains under general anesthesia.

To accomplish this procedure, a Foley catheter (18FG) without lubrication is passed into rectum and the balloon is inflated with 10 ml water. The other end of the catheter is connected to the saline reservoir held in a stand at a height of 1 meter from the operating table.

Saline solution is allowed to run into the rectum for four minutes, and both buttocks are held together in order to stop leaking of solution. The catheter is then removed. The fluid is allowed to escape into the proximal part of the colon. After a few minutes, the fluid is allowed to drain out per rectum. Blood stained fluid will return. Procedure is repeated. At the end, the successful outcome would be recognized by the passage of flatus and motion. If the outcome is doubtful, laparotomy should be made.

Although this conservative approach seems rational, it is not without a problem, in that over-loading of saline absorption from the colon is possible and a risk of perforation through the gangrenous wall of the intussusception could not be ruled out.

The alternative approach is to do manual reduction. This is done through a midline incision. At the operation, the segment of the intussusception is examined about its color and vascularity.

Index or little finger is first passed through the neck into the space between the outer wall and inner wall of the intestines. It is then moving around the inner tube—thus breaking down any soft fibrinous adhesion developed within the space and it would assist to expel some feces from the lumen of the intestine. Reduction would be much easier by this maneuver.

Then the outer wall of the intussusceptum is squeezed just distal to the apex of the intussusceptum between the thumb and index finger of both hands. This squeeze is done slowly and progressively in order to push the apex of the intussusceptum proximally, thus expelling a part of the intussusceptum from inside out. The procedure is repeated in order to expel a little by little until the final part is fully out.

Some surgeons recommend to anchor the cecum and the terminal ileum to the parietal peritoneum, but the outcome has been questioned. The cecal adhesion will prevent from recurrence.

If the intussusception seems to be gangrene, then right hemicolectomy remains the choice of operation. This procedure does not require further operative description. Peritoneal cavity is washed with saline and then with metronidazole lavage (200 mg) and a tube or suction drainage tube is left in the right paracolic gutter, before the abdominal wound is closed.

Postoperative Care

Routine regimen for postoperative care is followed in the usual way. Patient must be given prophylactic infusion of antibiotics and analgesic drugs in the usual way as outlined before. Postoperative fluid infusion must be guided by the pediatrician, if the child is less than 2-year-old.

23 A Bird's Eye View of the Surgical Practice

It is an imperative to be fully aware of the potential problems that may occur in the course of surgical treatment. Because of these reasons, a bird's eye view of all those problems has been compiled in this section for every surgeon intended to be specialized in a particular field of surgical practice, so that they should have an overall vision in the surgical care of his or her patient, whether or not his team or a subspecialty team being involved in undertaking a particular treatment modality. The surgeon remains the captain of the ship. Because of this clinical responsibility, a short review of potential risks of clinical and operative problems is highlighted in this section.

POTENTIAL RISK OF PROBLEMS AT INDUCTION

We must appreciate that an uneventful postoperative recovery is the result of a careful care, dedication and innovative general anesthesia. Nevertheless, unexpected adverse event may occur in the induction room, in the theater or in the recovery room. The overall responsibility remains to the surgeon or clinician in charge of the patients for a month after the patient being discharged from the hospital. Hence, the surgeon needs to be fully aware of any potential complication that may occur with the intubation of general anesthesia or it could occur at any time during or after the operation being successfully performed. These are summarized below:

a. Difficulty in intubation: This could be a lack of experience of the anesthetist, or it could be due to a short neck of the patients or inappropriate size of the endotracheal tube used. In some cases, patient may go into a laryngeal spasm that may result from asphyxiation of gastric contents. To stop having aspiration of stomach content, patients are kept on nil by mouth overnight or the stomach contents are aspirated by the NG tube before general anesthesia is given in emergency operation.

b. In other circumstance, there could be a sudden fall of blood pressure, during general anesthesia. This could be due to cardiac arrest, allergic reaction to anesthetic drugs, empty oxygen cylinder or unilateral ventilation of the lung. The latter is due to an error in intubation, in which the endotracheal tube has been inserted into the right bronchial tube because of its relatively vertical position. As a result, the left bronchial tree becomes obliterated—resulting in collapse of that lung. This may momentarily lead to hypoxia and retention of carbon dioxide that may lead to peripheral capillary vasodilatation. Other possible cause could be the compression of the inflated right lung upon the right atrium, thus interfering with the venous return. Further knowledge should be sought in the Textbook of Anesthesia.

In this situation, the operation should be cancelled. Necessary investigations should be carried out. These include blood gas analysis, cardiac enzymes, blood sugar, and a portable plain X-ray of the chest. The chest X-ray may reveal that the endotracheal tube is in the right bronchus and that the left side of the chest would appear to be featureless opacity. Patient may expire, as a result of faulty intubation, but it is very rare. Postmortem examination would reveal a gross disparity between the two sizes of the lungs.

These unexpected events are very rare. Anesthetist plays an important part in assisting the surgeons in many respect, one of the art is to control the capillary bleeding in the wound. This is done by just expelling the excess amount of CO_2 from the circulation. This enhances capillaries vasoconstriction due to increased oxygen saturation. It is important to know the physiology that retention of carbon dioxide causes capillary vasodilatation and a high concentration of oxygen in the blood induces capillary vasoconstriction.

PROBLEMS DEVELOPED IN THE OPERATING ROOM

a. In the theater, there could be accidental injury to major vessels. These are pedicle of the splenic vessels or renal vessels. In some cases, inferior vena cava or common iliac vein may be injured. Other accidental damages are common bile duct, or ureter. There have been many incidents of litigation that at the completion of operation, instrument, needle or swabs have been left behind into the abdominal cavity before the parietal wound has been closed. It is important to count all instruments and swabs before the wound is closed. If such incident of carelessness occurs, patients' life would be at risk of untold sufferings and surgeon's confidence and integrity would be lost forever.

b. During the operative procedure, patient may have a cardiac arrest or kidneys stop producing urine. The possible causes are gross perioperative hypotension, endotoxin shock or transfusion of incompatible blood.

c. Despite a lot of improvement in the apparatus of electrocoagulation, electrocution has been reported in the past, and it may result from the faulty electrical connection, forming a short circuit. In other occasions, we have noticed that patient had suffered from skin burn. This could be attributable to a pool of ether or alcohol-based antiseptic agents, collected in the umbilicus, groin, or under the buttocks or due to faulty application of the coagulation forceps to the bleeding vessels, just under the subcutaneous tissue. Diathermy does not interfere with the modern types of pacemaker inserted into the heart, but it should be used with a prior knowledge and cautious approach in those cases in which prosthesis has been implanted to the heart or in the joints.

d. In some cases, operation could be performed on the wrong site, if preoperative skin mark on the site of the operation has not been done, before the patient has been transferred to the theater. The common error is on the breast lump, epigastric or inguinal hernia, testis, kidney or ureteric stone, varicose veins. There have been many cases of litigation for removing a healthy kidney instead of removing a nonfunctioning kidney. It is very important to examine the IVP film before the patient is placed on the operating table and turn the body to the appropriate site. In some cases, it has been the case that femoral artery has been stripped off or femoral vein has been ligated and divided by mistake. These sorts of irreparable damages had occurred during the varicose veins operation.

e. It is very important job of the resident doctor to record the amount of blood lost in the swabs or any other fluid collected in the suction bottle. For the purpose of assessing the fluid deficit, wet swabs should be measured in weight. These measurements would reveal the amount of blood or fluid lost in those swabs, in which, one gram in weight is equivalent to one ml of blood lost. These data must be recorded in the fluid balance chart and it would be necessary to adjust the infusion at the end of the operation or in the circumstances in which the patient is in a state of hypovolemic shock or hourly urine output has dropped.

PROBLEMS IN THE RECOVERY ROOM

In most instances, recovery from the general anesthesia is expected to be an uneventful occurring, but unexpected complication may be encountered with the withdrawal of endotracheal tube. Patient may expire due to asphyxia, resulting from falling back of the tongue into the back of the mouth causing airway obstruction. This sort of oversight does occurs by not putting the airway tube into the mouth after the endotracheal tube being removed and when the patient has not fully awakened from the general anesthesia.

In all instances, patient will push the airway out, as soon as he has regained a full conscious. In other rare cases, patient may need assisted ventilation for sometime after the operation is completed. It has been noticed that patient went into acute bronchospasm immediately, as soon as the endotracheal tube was withdrawn. There could be several factors, but aspiration of gastric contents is a mortal postoperative complication. In these cases, patient may appear to be cyanosed and needs assisted ventilation. Chest X-ray should be taken.

If this has occurred, patient is transferred to the intensive care unit. Again in rare circumstances, tracheostomy may be necessary if ventilation is necessary for more than a week. This would spare the vocal cords from being damaged by the pressure of the endotracheal tube, but the ventilation may continue through the tracheostomy tube for a longer period. And in other emergency conditions, tracheostomy may be needed. These are Ludwig angina, diphtheria, thyroidectomy.

The ventilation is not without problem. Its consequent effect could be multiple. These are bilateral pulmonary edema, chest infection, gross peripheral tissue edema, bed sores, catheter cystitis and bacteremia. Many of these conditions could be attributable to overtransfusion, hypoalbuminea, and peripheral venous stasis. Again the peripheral tissue edema could be the result of positive pulmonary pressure inhibiting the venous return from the lower limb. Again, this venous return may be affected by muscular inactivity of the limbs because of the fact that the patient is kept on sedation during the period of ventilation.

In short, the peripheral tissue edema may be attributable to venous stasis, over transfusion and hypoalbuminea. Infusion of parenteral TPN, containing 50 percent glucose may contribute to retention of water in the body tissue, what is commonly referred to as water-logged. Plain chest X-ray will show multiple cotton balls appearance in both lungs or consolidation in the base of the lung. If the patient does not recover, the cause of death is often referred to as multiorgan failure or adult respiratory distressed syndrome, in short it is known as ARDS.

PROBLEMS IN THE RECOVERY WARD

Hemorrhage

There are three types of hemorrhage. They are known as:
a. Primary hemorrhage that occurs from the operative procedure, undertaken in the theater.
b. Reactionary hemorrhage that occurs within a few hours in the recovery ward.
c. Secondary hemorrhage that occurs between one and two weeks after the operation being performed.

Reactionary Hemorrhage

In the recovery or in the postoperative ward, there could be evidence of excessive discharge of blood through the drainage tubing, or in the wound.

It may result from slip ligature of the artery, or bleeding from the capillaries due to massive blood transfusion. The latter may cause low platelet count, low serum calcium, and it could be due to cumulative effect of anticoagulants agents added in the storage of blood that depends upon number of units of blood transfused at a time.

There could be oozing from the wound or from the denuded surfaces of the operative area. This may be encountered among those patients, operated upon by those surgeons who are known to be popular among the nurses and junior doctors, because of their fast operative technique. The only way to finish the operation very quickly is to omit the steps of procedure, not paying due care to the tissues or not dealing with the bleeding from the capillary vessels.

These capillaries that remain shutting due to postoperative shock may start bleeding after recovery of postoperative shock. In the latter condition, transfusion of blood or colloids may improve the blood pressure—thus filling up the collapsed veins, which were overlooked during operation. In some cases, venous bleeding could be excessive in the circumstances of repeated cough or chronic obstructive airway disease—thus inhibiting the venous return and raising the venous pressure or capillary dilatation due to retention of CO_2.

In some cases, patient may present with tachycardia, perspiration, hypotension and pale looking face. The possible causes are internal bleeding, cardiac arrest, or fluid deficit or low hemoglobin due to loss of blood at operation that has not been replaced in the theater.

Secondary Hemorrhage

It may occur between one and two weeks after operation. It may result from the erosion of the major vessels by the drainage tubing. In rare cases, melena could be noticed in colonic surgery or postoperative gastric surgery. This may result from the bleeding from the mucosa. In some cases, persisting slow oozing from the sites of the operation may be due to the effect of aspirin, low platelets count or on anticoagulant therapy.

Blood Transfusion

If the patient has received many units of blood during and after operations, there could be many complications resulting from blood transfusion. These are:

Cardiac failure due to overtransfusion.

Acute hypotension due to transfusion of incompatible blood.

Rigors and rise of temperature due to transfusion of old stored blood, or due to pyrogens present in the blood.

A fall of fibrinogens and low platelets counts (thrombocytopenia)—It may be due to intravascular hemolysis, known as disseminated intravascular coagulation (DIC).

A lot of hemorrhage or oozing is possible due to low platelets counts and low serum calcium or abnormal coagulopathy.

Oliguria or anuria—It may result from gross dehydration, hypotension, irreversible shock, endotoxin shock, or acute renal tubular necrosis.

Cardiac arrest—It may result from the preexisting medical conditions. Because of this reason, preoperative cardiac function, blood pressure and ECG are routinely done.

POSTOPERATIVE CHEST PROBLEMS

Chest Infection

Predisposing Factors

a. Smoking.
b. Chronic lung disease.
c. Sore throat.

A detailed clinical features and management has been described in the chapter of postoperative care. In this section, a broad outline is highlighted.

From the second postoperative day, a rise of temperature is an early sign for the hidden chest infection. In addition, there could be shortness of breath, difficulty in breathing or bronchitis.

If these initial features are not dealt with immediately, these symptoms may lead to collapsed lung, basal consolidation and lung abscess.

Among the predisposing factors, operation should be deferred for a month until the smoking being stopped. No one, with a sore throat should be allowed working in the theater, or operation should be stopped if the patient, anesthetist, nurse or the surgeon suffers from a sore throat.

In my experience, one of my patients developed a serious postoperative septicemia due to transmission of β-hemolytic

Streptococcus bacteria, during intubation of general anesthesia. The investigation revealed that the source of transmission of organism was from the anesthetist who had a sore throat, before coming to the theater.

Apart from the pre-existing risk factors, chest infection may develop due to:
1. *Pain:* It inhibits the deep breathing and cough reflex —thus retaining the mucus secretion in the bronchial tree.
2. Anesthetic agents reduce the ciliary's action resulting in accumulation of bronchial secretion. The effect of atropine, given along with other premedication, for general anesthesia may produce viscid secretion in the bronchus in the postoperative period.
3. Analgesic narcotics cause deep sedation, thus inhibiting the cough reflex. As a result, the viscid mucus materials tend to trickle down at a deep sleep and eventually, it may occlude the bronchial tree or bronchiole. As a result, the air present in the lung distal to the blockage is absorbed leading to atelectasis. Secondary infection gets into the collapsed lung from the upper respiratory tract—thus producing lung abscess.
4. Distention of the abdomen due to paralytic ileus, or pain in the abdominal wound will cause a similar chest infection.

DISTENTION OF THE ABDOMEN

After a few days, usually after 48 hours, distention of the abdomen becomes apparent all around the abdomen. This could be attributable to many conditions. They are:
- Swallowing of air.
- Retention of gastric secretion.
- Chest infection.
- Paralytic ileus and sequestration of a lot of intestinal fluid.
- Analgesic drugs such as morphine sulphate.
- Effect of epidural analgesia.
- Low serum potassium.
- Low serum albumin.
- Uremic state.
- Anticholinergic drugs.
- Constipation.

Despite of all these clinical conditions, in most cases, patient recovers uneventful and is discharged home in less than 12 days, but some of those symptoms may persist. Among these cases are rise of temperature, vomiting, loss of appetite and colicky abdominal pain.

In most cases, the differential diagnosis would be between postoperative paralytic ileus, septic abdomen or mechanical obstruction or something else outside the primary operation.

Again apparent mechanical obstruction of the small intestine could be attributable to paralytic ileus or twisting or strangulation of the intestine or fibrinous adhesions between the loops of the intestine. Bear in mind, these clinical conditions may be encountered after a few weeks. This will be discussed later.

One needs to understand the mechanism and physiology of intestinal obstruction due to paralytic ileus. Although it stops discharging the flatus per rectum because of lack of peristaltic movements of the gut, it may cause kinking of the small intestine at the sites of bend, like a kink of garden hosepipe. Because of the kinking, there would be excessive secretion from the congested mucosa, and diffusion of gas from the loops of dilated gut. These are the result of venous stasis that usually occurs at the site of mesentery attachment with the intestine and also along the antimesenteric border of the gut, where the thin-walled veins are subjected to be collapsed by the pressure, exerted from inside the distended intestine. As a result, venous return from mucosa would be delayed resulting in mucosal congestion.

Untreated cases may cause gangrene or perforation and the usual site for the ischemic change is the antimesenteric border of the distended gut. A detailed account of this condition has been described in the section of postoperative care.

Again, the etiology of paralytic ileus is related to clinical and gastrointestinal surgery. It may also occur in other traumatic conditions. They are:
a. Pleuritic pain, chest infection.
b. Subphrenic, paracolic, pelvic abscess.
c. Fracture spine.
d. Hip surgery.

Again, postoperative sepsis develops usually after a week. It could be attributable to anastomotic dehiscence, infected hematoma, and secondary infection to the pool of inflammatory fluid, accumulated in the anatomical pockets, in the space within the loops of intestine, paracolic gutter, or pelvic cavity. The intraperitoneal sepsis may interfere with the gut motility due to peritonitis.

It has been my personal experience among those noninfective postoperative cases in which patient experiences distention of abdomen in some cases where the serum albumin remains below the level of 25 gm/l. And they have responded dramatically to infusion of human albumin given to those cases. It is postulated that serum albumin improves the cardiac output and blood pressure because of increased absorption of tissue fluid. As a result, it improves the oxygen saturation that leads to increased neural response and gut motility.

Intestinal Obstruction

It may result from paralytic ileus as described before. In untreated cases, fibrinous adhesions develop between the loops of the small intestine resulting in subacute intestinal adhesion.

Acute intestinal obstruction may occur due to twisting of the gut or faulty layout of the small intestine at the completion of operation or by omental bands going around the root of the mesentery. It has been found that the loops of the small intestine, which were brought out of the peritoneal cavity or pushed higher up in the upper abdomen during primary operative procedures, are dumped back or put back into the abdomen in haphazard way, before the peritoneum is closed. In these reckless works that seem to be hurrying in closing the abdomen, the loop of the intestine is left in half-twisted fashion into the peritoneal cavity. As a result, strands of the greater omentum may lie around the loops of the intestine without recognizing the potential risk of complication. These sorts of cases may present later with intestinal obstruction.

To avoid all these potential complication, the jejunum should be put back first in the left upper abdomen, then midgut in the central abdomen and in the pelvis and finally the terminal ileum and the cecum in the right iliac fossa. The greater omentum should be spread out covering the site of operation and all those loops of intestine. It acts like a policeman of the abdomen.

ATTENTION TO THE ACUTE ABDOMEN

In the midst of these clinical conditions, clinical examination of the abdomen, blood tests and the plain X-ray of the chest and abdomen would assist the surgeon to unravel the differential diagnosis, as outlined before in other chapters. At least, paralytic ileus could be differentiated from mechanical intestinal obstruction by a simple plain X-ray of the abdomen, which would show gas shadows present in the sigmoid colon and rectum.

WOUND HEMATOMA AND INFECTION

Another complication is the bruise around the wound margin or hematoma that may develop in the parietal wound. It is often encountered with a poor surgical technique, or a very quick operative procedure. To save time, some surgeons intend to omit certain steps of the procedure, as a result, capillary bleeding vessels are overlooked with the belief that they would stop spontaneously in due course.

But in fact, these vessels continue bleeding into the tissues, resulting in a big hematoma. A few of these cases need evacuation of the clots under general anesthesia. And in other cases, it may resolve spontaneously, but it would take two to three months' time before it resolves completely or it may start discharging blood stained fluid through the wound or it could be infected resulting in formation of an abscess. Hence, curtailing the operative steps and the theater time does not improve the postoperative recovery.

If the wound hematoma remains dry with no evidence of inflammation or discharge, it should be treated conservatively. No surgical evacuation is necessary, provided it is no more than an inch in size, but perianal hematoma should be evacuated, before it gets infected.

If there are clinical features of wound infection, it takes several days to develop infection and the usual time is between 5 and 10 days. In some cases, it develops after the patient being discharged home. The usual period for delayed wound infection is between 2 and 4 weeks.

In the initial stage, while staying in the ward, wound infection becomes evident in the parietal wound by inflammation, induration, diffuse swelling and a slow discharge soaked through the wound dressing.

In some cases, staining of the wound dressing provides an alarming sign for primary wound infection. The dependent and lower part of the wound is commonly affected. If there is any evidence of fluctuation around the wound, a few stitches should be removed. This will allow discharge of infected or inflammatory fluid—thus relieving the local tension and pain.

There could be anastomotic dehiscence of the gut on the fourth or fifth postoperative day. It is presented with a rise of temperature, bile or feculent discharge through the drainage or through the main wound. There could be localized abscess, pelvic abscess, paracolic abscess or subphrenic abscess. Eventually, a fistula track may develop.

After 10 days, there could be an early sign of burst abdomen. Discharge of serous fluid, commonly known as pink fluid, noticed in the wound dressing is an early sign of burst abdomen. Eventually, omentum and loops of small intestine protrude through the peritoneal gap and may stay in the extraperitoneal pocket under the skin wound. A full fledged burst abdomen becomes evident after the sutures are removed and after a violent cough is given. A detailed account of management has been described in the chapter on postoperative care.

DEEP VEIN THROMBOSIS AND PULMONARY EMBOLISM

It may present initially with an aching in the calf a few days after the operation is done. Suspicion should arise if there is a swelling of one leg, accompanied by dilated superficial veins and unexplained rise of temperature at the end of first week. In most cases, deep vein thrombosis develops on the operating table but it takes 2 weeks to develop the clinical presentation, after the operation is done, and its incidence could be as high as 30 percent among the postoperative patients over the age of 30 years.

It commonly develops in the tributaries of the leg veins or in the pelvic veins. Because of this reason, the prophylactic antithrombotic measure is applied around the lower limbs, using a graded stocking (TED) in both lower limbs, before the operation begins. This stocking will obliterate those tributaries, thus stopping the platelets to be accumulated within these veins.

The primary causative factor is the platelets adhesiveness that increases after the operation is done. Study shows that the risk of developing DVT is greater among the smokers or if a second operation is undertaken within a month. In postoperative period, platelets count increases and it tends to be sticky or adhesiveness is present in the damaged wall of the vein. There would be an increased amount of fibrinogen that is deposited over the platelets—thus producing thrombosis in the vein. This continues propagating proximally, until it blocks the lumen of a larger vein completely or partially. This causes delay in venous return, thus developing swelling of the distal limb and particularly in the calf muscles.

A few days later, patient experiences aching and notices swollen calf. On examination, the overlying skin would appear to be shining and there would be pitting edema over the dorsum of the foot and increase in girth around the midcalf of the leg compared to the other leg. Further examination will reveal tenderness on deep palpation of the calf muscle and Homan's sign would be positive. This clinical diagnosis could be confirmed by Doppler ultrasound sonic aid, placed over the femoral vein. The Doppler sound may be absent or partially reduced that depends upon the degree of patency of the femoral vein.

Other investigation is venogram or isotope scan using Iodine 125 fibrinogen.

Detailed clinical features and treatment has been described in the previous chapter.

PULMONARY EMBOLISM

It results from the dislodgement of a thrombus or multiple thrombi from the pelvic veins or from the veins of the leg. It may remain silent and in other extreme cases, patient found dead in bed. The latter condition is attributable to the blockage of the right heart with a massive embolus. In some cases, patient asks for a bedpan, but by the time the nurse brings the bedpan, patient is found dead in bed. This sort of experience is not unknown to the resident doctors and nurses.

In between these extreme presentations, patient may complain of pleuritic pain, retrosternal pain, hemoptysis, shortness of breath and sweating, low blood pressure. Clinical examination may reveal dilated jugular veins, pleural rub, and cyanosis, rapid pulse rate and a rise of temperature. There may not be any evidence of DVT in the calf muscles in some cases.

In these presentations of symptoms, initial investigation is ECG, blood test for fibrogen degradation product (FDP) and coagulation screen and X-ray of the chest. But on the basis of ECG report, which may reveal right heart strain, anticoagulant therapy, as described in the treatment of DVT, should be commenced without any delay on the basis of clinical diagnosis, provided the platelets counts and coagulation test are within a normal range. If the patient's condition seems to be satisfactory, ventilation perfusion scan could be arranged. This specific investigation would guide the clinician whether or not a long-term anticoagulant therapy should be continued.

These are the clinical problems that may be encountered at any time since the patient is operated upon. The management for respective problems has been described in the appropriate chapter.

OTHER CHRONIC DEBILITY CONDITIONS

Chronic necrotic slough at the wound edges, wound discharge, sacral bed sores, malnutrition, breathing problems, urinary problems or catheter cystitis may be encountered in some cases for some reasons beyond one's imagination. These problems require continuous clinical care with a different line of investigations and supportive treatment, and finally this patient may require rehabilitation in the community or at home. Resources, manpower and patients are important factors in dealing with these problems.

Although many of these postoperative complications are treated by appropriate clinician, the overall care remains initially under the leadership of the surgeon. Hence, the surgeons should have a good experience in dealing with all these problems at the initial stage, before referring to the appropriate team. In other words, you need to be a good physician to be a good surgeon.

DELAYED COMPLICATIONS

Among other postoperative patients who have been discharged home, a few of them may be readmitted a few weeks later with an acute abdomen. The most likely complications could be projectile vomiting, associated with a colicky abdominal pain, or a rise of temperature, peritonitis, or discharge of purulent fluid or feces through the drainage site or through the abdominal wound, or with a deep vein thrombosis.

It would be the responsibility of the surgical team to investigate and to treat the conditions that had contributed to the unexpected postoperative complications. These unexpected complications may cause distress to the patient and his family. These emergency admissions should be investigated as outlined in the management of postoperative complications. The treatment for the respective clinical pathology should be carried out in accordance with the clinical diagnosis and the results of investigations.

All these postoperative morbidities should be dealt with by the surgeons who had a full knowledge of the previous operative care of his or her patients. I hope these compilations would assist the trainee surgeons to be cautious and alert against any risk of unwanted encounter in the management of his patients.

Index

A

Abdominal
    examination 229
    pain 21, 22, 54
    rectopexy 168
Abdominoperineal resection 142, 144
Acetone smell in breath 73
Actinomycosis 257
Acute
    abdomen 288
    appendicitis 225, 227, 231, 235
    colonic obstruction 179
    dilatation of colon 54
    diverticulitis 54
    ulcerative colitis 53, 54
Adenocarcinoma 225, 245
Amebic
    colitis 6, 206, 207
    dysentery 207
Ampulla of rectum 64
Amputation
    and reconstruction of ileostomy 203
    of ileostomy spout 203
Anal
    carcinoma 257
    dilatation 269
    fissure 268
    fistula 260
    pain 263
    sphincteric dysfunction 138
    stricture 245
Anastomotic
    clamps 82
    leakage 114, 136
    stricture 139
Anatomy of anal canal 264
Angiodysplasia 220
Anorectal abscess 251
Anterior resection 116
Antibiotic therapy 88
Antidiuretic hormone 38, 83
Anus 1, 245
Appendicectomy 236
Appendicular mass 48, 235
Ascending colon 15
Ascites 53
Assessment of delayed morbidity 138
Autosutures using clips 78

B

Bacillary dysentery 207
Background of
    diseases 222, 251
    etiology of anal fissure 267
    hemorrhoids 245
Barium enema 37
    study 41
Basal cell carcinoma 245
Benign
    colonic lesions 6
    epithelial tumor 6
    lesions 6
    lymphoma 6
    tumors 6
Bilateral acute salpingitis 233
Bird's eye view of surgical practice 284
Bisacodyl suppositories 42
Bladder dysfunction 155
Blood
    tests 230
    transfusion 73, 286
Bowel preparation 54
Buscopan 54

C

Carcinoid
    syndrome 6
    tumor 225
        of appendix 232
Carcinoma of gallbladder 48
Cardiac
    attack 66
    disease 37
Care of
    colostomy 152
    septic abdomen 171
    urethral catheter 152
    wound 201
Causes
    for leakage of ileostomy 202
    of ulceration of ileostomy 202
Central venous pressure 72, 175
Centrally bulging abdomen 29
Certain pharmacological restrictions 87
Change in bowel habit 21
Chest infection 93

Choices of treatment modalities 10
Chronic
    anal fissure 273
    bronchitis 94
    debility conditions 289
    lung disease 286
    pulmonary disease 37
    recurrent perianal abscess 257
Classification of perianal
    abscess 254
    fistula 257
Clinical application of nasogastric tube 85
Closed drainage system 96
Clostridium difficile 87
Closure of burst abdomen 79
Colloid carcinoma 257
Colon 99
Colonic
    carcinoma 15
    diseases 6
    hemorrhage 218
Colonography 37, 48
Colonoscopy 43, 53, 55
Colorectal carcinoma 19
Colovesical fistula 216
Complication of
    colonoscopy 66
    ileostomy 201
    pelvic loop colostomy 125
    postoperative pain relief 93
    procedure 8
    rectal stump 201
    telescopic colostomy 125
    appendicular mass 235
Composition of Fecolith 226
Computerized tomography scan 37
Condylomas 273
Conservative treatment 221, 269
Constipation 21, 97
Construction of
    loop ileostomy 131
    pelvic loop colostomy 124
    telescopic colostomy 125
    terminal ileostomy 133
    transverse loop colostomy 122
Continuous
    blanket suture 78
    mattress suture 78
    perineal wound irrigation 157

subcutaneous suture 78
suture 78
Crohn's
colitis 6, 205
disease 205, 208, 245, 257, 269
proctitis 207
CT scan 48
Curative and palliative resection 158

D

Daily
fluid requirement 69
wound discharge 95
Deep vein thrombosis 97
and pulmonary embolism 288
Definition of volvulus 278
Dehiscence of
abdominal wound. 93
anastomosis 93
Dehydration 54
Delayed
complication of ileostomy 202
venous filling rate 73
Delorme's operation 166, 167
Descending colon 15
Description of
proctoscope 31
sigmoidoscope 32
specific complications 202
Devadhar operation 166, 168
Dextran 68
Dextrose 68
Diabetes 94
Diazepam 54
Dilated biliary ducts 48
Diseases of
appendix 225
colon 6
Distention of abdomen 287
Distribution of carcinoma 15
Divergent opinion about disease 262
Diverticula of colon 209
Diverticulosis 210, 212, 225
Dukes classification of rectal carcinoma 157
Dukes stage of colorectal tumor 19
Dysfunction of ileostomy 204

E

Elective
operative treatment 214
surgery 67
Emergency
laparotomy 183
operative procedure 173
surgery 175

Endoscopy 37
Epidemiology of
appendicitis 226
prolapse rectum 164
Evidences of
colonic obstruction 42
dehydration 72
overhydration 73
rehydration 73
Examination of
abdomen 26
ascending colon and cecum 66
Expected outcome of acute thrombosed piles 250
Extraperitoneal closure 243

F

Feeling of thirst 72
Fibroid of uterus 48
Fissure-in-ano 245, 262
Fluid thrill 29
Full blood count 37
Function of colon 3

G

Gallbladder 86
Gallstones 48
Gastric aspiration 86
Glycerine suppositories 42
Gonorrheal proctitis 207

H

Habitual constipation 42
Hamartomas 6
Hartmann's procedure 120
Hemangioma 6
Hematological blood profile 180
Hemorrhage 286
Hemorrhagic shock 53
Hemorrhoidectomy 247
Hemorrhoids 245
Hepatic flexure 15
Hepatitis 53
High anal fistula 258
Hirschsprung's disease 53, 54
Hydronephrosis 48
Hydrosalpinx 232
Hydroureter 48
Hypertrophied anal polyp 6
Hypokalemia 54
Hyponatremia 54
Hypotension 66
Hypovolemic shock 54, 68

I

Ileitis 204
Ileocolic fistula 216
Immediate complication of ileostomy. 201
Incidence of anastomotic leakage 137
Inflammatory diseases 6
Initial therapeutic measure 236
Inspection 26
Internal
fistula 216
herniation of small intestine. 204
Interrupted
mattress suture 78
suture 78
Intestinal obstruction 54, 232, 287
Intraperitoneal
abscess 3
closure 241
Intravenous pyelogram 47
Intussusception of intestine 281
Ischemic colitis 53, 54, 206
Ischiorectal abscess 255

J

Juvenile polyp 6

K

Ketone in urine 73
Klean preparation 42

L

Laparoscopy 43
Laparotomy 37, 43
Left hemicolectomy 109, 110
Lipoma 11
Liver 48
function test 37
Low
anal fistula 257
anterior resection 134
serum
albumin 287
potassium 287
Lymphatic spread 16
Lymphogranuloma inguinale 207, 257
Lymphoma 11

M

Macroscopical
appearance of tumors 13
changes in colon 14
Magnesium sulfate 54

Index

Magnetic resonance
   cholangiopancreatic scan 37
   image scan 37
Malignant
   growth in anal canal 24
   melanoma 245
   skin lesion 277
   tumor 6
      of anus 272
      of colon, rectum and anus 13
Management of
   constipation 97
   deep vein thrombosis 97
   diverticulosis 213
   ileostomy 201
   obstruction 204
   ulcerative colitis 198
   wound drain 95
Mantoux
   skin test 47
   test 235
Massive colonic hemorrhage 54
Meckel's diverticulum 232
Megacolon 42, 53, 54
Method of
   perineal dissection of rectum 147
   proctoscopy 33
   small bowel enema 46
Midazolam 54
MRI scan 48

N

Nausea 42, 54
Neurofibroma 6
Nonmalignant disease 43
Nonobstructive appendicitis 227
Nonspecific
   acute mesenteric adenitis 234
   enterocolitis 232

O

Occult blood test 43
Open drainage system 95
Operating room 284
Oral
   lavage regimens 42
   laxatives 42
Ovarian cyst 48

P

Pain 94
   relief 92
Palpation of abdomen 180
Pancreas 86
Pancreatic mass 48

Papillae 6
Papilloma 245
   of anus 11
   or anal warts 273
Paralytic ileus 42, 54
Parastomal hernia 204
Parenteral infusion 68
Partial prolapse 164
Pelvic floor reconstruction 157
Perianal
   abscess 245, 254
   fistula 245, 257
Perineal wound closure 156
Peritoneal collection 48
Peritonitis 42, 53, 54
Persistent wound infection 90
PET scan 37, 48, 51
Pethidine 54
Phosphate enema 42
Plain X-ray of
   abdomen 181
   chest and abdomen 180
Plasma 68
Pneumatosis cystoids intestinalis 6
Policy for
   antibiotic therapy 87
   oral
      bowel preparation 54
      feeding to postoperative patients 86
   parenteral fluid infusion 67
   postoperative parenteral infusion 84
Polycystic kidney 48
Polyp in gallbladder 48
Polypectomy 7
Polyps 212
   Peutz-Jeghers syndrome 6
Postradiation proctitis 207
Primary
   chancre 273
   wound healing 89
Principle and policy for postoperative care 83
Principle of
   anastomosis 81
   bowel preparations 42
Proctitis 207, 245
Proctoscopy 33
Prolapse
   of rectum 164
   thrombosed pile 273
Protuberance of umbilicus 29
Pruritus ani 245, 271
Pseudopancreatic cyst 48
Psoas test 230
Pulmonary
   embolism 289
   tuberculosis 257
Pyelonephritis 233

R

Reactionary hemorrhage 286
Recent heart attack 53
Recovery
   room 285
   ward 286
Rectal
   carcinoma 31
   digital examination 29
   enemas 42
Rectosigmoidectomy operation 166
Rectum 15, 115
Refashioning of
   ileostomy. 203
   terminal ileostomy 203
Relocation of ileostomy 203
Renal
   cyst 48
   stones 48
   tumor 37, 48
Respiratory distress 66
Review of barium enema study 42
Right
   corpus luteal cyst 234
   hemicolectomy 102
   renal and ureteric stone 233
   sided pyosalpinx 232
   twisted ovarian cyst 232
Ringer's lactate solution 68
Ruptured
   corpus luteal cyst 232
   ectopic pregnancy 234

S

Saha retrograde dissection of rectum 148
Saliva 86
Salmonella typhoid 3
Salpingitis 232
Selection of colonoscope 55
Septic shock 54
Serum
   creatinine 72
   electrolytes 37
   potassium 70
   sodium and chloride 69
Sigmoid myotomy 215
Sigmoidoscopy 34, 35
Size of spleen 48
Skin preparation 75, 145
Small
   bowel enema 37, 43
   intestine 86
Soap and water enema 42
Spleen 48
Splenic flexure 15

Spread of
    cancer by transplantation 19
    colonic and rectal carcinoma 15
Squamous cell carcinoma 245
Stapling gun 82
Stenosis of skin stoma 204
Stomach 86
Stone in bile duct 48
Strangulated prolapsed piles 250
Study of septic abdomen 173
Sunken eyes and face 72
Suture materials 80

T

Techniques for palpation 26
Telescopic pelvic loop 125
Terminal colostomy 125
Thiersch operation 166
Thromboembolic deterrent 276
Total
    loss of water 69
    proctocolectomy 198
    water lost for humidifying 69
Transcelomic spread 19
Transverse
    colon 15, 107

loop colostomy 218, 241
Treatment of
    bleeding points 249
    carcinoma of anus 273
    hyperkalemia 71
    hypokalemia 70
    piles with rubber band ligation 247
Tuberculosis of mesenteric lymph nodes 234
Tuberculous
    enteritis 232
    intestine 53
    proctitis 207
Tumors of appendix 240
Twisted ovarian mass 233
Types of
    anastomosis 100
    bowel preparations 42
    colitis 205, 206
    drainage systems 95
    immediate complication of ileostomy 202
    skin sutures 78

U

Ulcerative proctitis 257
Ultrasound scan of abdomen or pelvis 37
Urinary tract infection 93

V

Venous
    invasion 140
    spread 18
Vermiform appendix 225
Villous papilloma 6
Volvulus 42, 54
    of colon 278
    of sigmoid colon 279
Vomiting 42, 54

W

Well's operation 166, 169
Wound
    healing 156
    hematoma and infection 288
    infection 93, 206

X

X-ray of chest 47